2nd Edition of Innovation in Chemical Plant Design

2nd Edition of Innovation in Chemical Plant Design

Guest Editors

Roberta Campardelli
Paolo Trucillo

MDPI

Basel • Beijing • Wuhan • Barcelona • Belgrade • Novi Sad • Cluj • Manchester

Guest Editors

Roberta Campardelli
Department of Civil,
Chemical and Environmental
Engineering
University of Genoa
Genoa
Italy

Paolo Trucillo
Department of Chemical,
Material and Industrial
Production Engineering
University of Naples Federico II
Napoli
Italy

Editorial Office
MDPI AG
Grosspeteranlage 5
4052 Basel, Switzerland

This is a reprint of the Special Issue, published open access by the journal *Processes* (ISSN 2227-9717), freely accessible at: https://www.mdpi.com/journal/processes/special_issues/V67XVDS9IM.

For citation purposes, cite each article independently as indicated on the article page online and as indicated below:

Lastname, A.A.; Lastname, B.B. Article Title. *Journal Name* **Year**, *Volume Number*, Page Range.

ISBN 978-3-7258-6111-8 (Hbk)
ISBN 978-3-7258-6112-5 (PDF)
https://doi.org/10.3390/books978-3-7258-6112-5

Contents

About the Editors

Paolo Trucillo

Paolo Trucillo is currently an assistant professor at the Department of Chemical, Materials, and Industrial Production Engineering of the University of Naples Federico II, Italy. His scientific activity focuses on the design of sustainable materials, drug delivery systems, and the mechanical behavior of polymer-based structures. He belongs to the Foamlab research group, where he is involved in the design of advanced polymeric carriers for controlled drug release, particularly through the use of bio-based materials and physical foaming processes. His recent work has been focused on the modeling of release kinetics of active compounds within biodegradable matrices, with applications in pharmacology and tissue engineering. He has also coordinated interdisciplinary studies on the environmental impact of polymer production and the substitution of fossil-based plastics with renewable alternatives. He is the author of several peer-reviewed articles and a guest editor of many Special Issues for Processes. His work is driven by a strong interest in combining material science with biomedical applications to develop efficient and eco-sustainable solutions for the healthcare industry.

Roberta Campardelli

Roberta Campardelli, since 2022, is an Associate Professor in the scientific field of chemical plants in the Department of Civil, Chemical, and Environmental Engineering (DICCA) at the Polytechnic School at the University of Genoa. She is a professor for the course on Unit Operations, Bachelor's Degree in Chemical Engineering, for the course Chemical Plant Design, Master's Degree in Chemical Engineering, and for the course on Innovation in Unit Operations, for the PhD course at DICCA. She is a member of the Research Center of Biologically Inspired Engineering in Vascular Medicine and Longevity (BELONG) at the University of Genoa, a joint center with the School of Medicine, where innovative and functionalized biomaterials are investigated to develop new biodegradable vascular prosthesis and hydrogel-based wound dressing. She is co-founder of an academic spin-off, BEST SRL, for innovation in the agricultural field that uses novel biostimulants.

Roberta Campardelli's research activity has been continually focused on chemical engineering, food engineering, and biomaterials, with a constant focus on process and product innovation through the design, development, and implementation of new plant solutions. In particular, her research activity is focused on the field of nanotechnology that is used for the controlled and targeted release of drugs, using polymeric nanoparticles or nanoemulsions, and the development of innovative food packaging materials derived from natural sources.

Preface

The design of chemical plants is undergoing a profound transformation, driven by the urgent need for sustainability, flexibility, and digital integration. This Special Issue, the *2nd Edition of Innovation in Chemical Plant Design*, emerges as a platform for showing novel ideas and multidisciplinary approaches that can redefine the future of process engineering. By merging classical design principles with advances in artificial intelligence, process intensification, circular economy strategies, and renewable resources, the issue seeks to connect academic research with practical industrial implementation. Contributions explore how smart control, modular construction, and eco-efficient materials can reduce environmental impact while enhancing productivity and safety. The editors hope that this collection will inspire researchers, engineers, and practitioners to envision chemical plants not only as production systems, but as dynamic, adaptive entities capable of responding to global challenges, toward a truly sustainable and resilient process industry.

Roberta Campardelli and Paolo Trucillo
Guest Editors

processes

MDPI

Editorial

Editorial Overview of the Special Issue "Second Edition of Innovation in Chemical Plant Design"

Paolo Trucillo [1,*] and Roberta Campardelli [2]

1 Department of Chemical, Materials and Industrial Production Engineering, University of Naples Federico II, Piazzale Vincenzo Tecchio 80, 80125 Naples, Italy
2 Department of Civil, Chemical and Environmental Engineering, University of Genoa, Via Opera Pia 15, 16145 Genoa, Italy
* Correspondence: paolo.trucillo@unina.it

Plant innovation extends beyond equipment and process layout to the smart integration of materials science, reaction engineering, and system design [1]. Several studies address this coupling by developing intensified and integrated processes that reduce energy consumption and waste [2,3]. For example, new conceptual and pilot-scale schemes for the production of cosmetic emulsions from Amazonian oils demonstrate how process intensification can translate natural feedstocks into high-value products with lower environmental impact than traditional methods [Contribution 1]. Through careful analysis of hydrodynamics, emulsification kinetics, and economic parameters, these studies show that combination of extraction and formulation in a single modular unit can minimize water and energy intensity [Contribution 2]. Other contributions focus on the integration of renewable energy within conventional systems. The thermal coupling of solar fields to combined cycles exemplifies how hybrid energy integration can reduce carbon emissions without sacrificing power output, thus merging process engineering with sustainable energy management [Contribution 3].

This Special Issue also includes research that expands the concept of process intensification beyond energy and mass transfer, addressing instead the challenge of waste valorization and resource recovery. The design of a biorefinery based on non-marketable edible mushroom waste illustrates how circular-economy principles can be applied to convert residues into chitin, citric acid, and organic fertilizer [Contribution 4]. By combining process simulation, economic assessment, and environmental analysis, the authors highlight the feasibility of such biorefineries as viable routes to close material loops and diversify the bioeconomy. Likewise, the coupling of energy integration and inherent safety evaluation in suspension-polyvinyl-chloride production underscores that process optimization must always be balanced by safety considerations, prompting the need for new design strategies that simultaneously optimize efficiency and safety [Contribution 5].

Innovation in chemical plant design is increasingly linked to the development of novel materials. The synthesis of porous zinc nano-wafer aerogels, for instance, introduces an advanced nanostructured electrode for high-performance supercapacitors, combining lightweight architecture with superior electrical properties and durability [Contribution 6]. In parallel, biologically derived stabilizers and biosurfactants are explored as eco-friendly tools for nanoparticle production and hydrocarbon remediation. The use of fungal biosurfactants as stabilizers for polymeric nanoparticles demonstrates the potential of biologically sourced amphiphiles to replace synthetic surfactants in colloidal processing [Contribution 7]. Similarly, sophorolipid biosurfactants show excellent emulsification performance in oil recovery and marine clean-up, bridging biotechnology and environmental engineering [Contribution 8]. Multifunctional hydrogels and composite exhibit dual capabilities for dye adsorption and antibacterial activity, highlighting how multifunctional materials can support sustainable remediation and water-treatment operations [Contribution 9].

Some works of this issue address reaction kinetics and separation processes under complex conditions, providing insights that are essential for the rational design of large-scale units. The kinetic study of barium sulfate precipitation in the presence of organic additives elucidates the interplay between solvent composition, supersaturation, and crystal morphology, offering strategies to control fouling and particle formation in industrial crystallizers [Contribution 10]. Similarly, the selective extraction of nitrogen-containing heterocycles from crude methylnaphthalene oil through formamide demonstrates how tailored solvent systems can enhance the purification of aromatic streams and improve downstream product quality [Contribution 11]. Other contributions analyze adsorption–desorption cycles for dye removal from tanning wastewaters and critically review biological and hybrid systems for the treatment of tannery effluents, with a particular focus on nitrogen and sulfur species removal [Contribution 12, Contribution 13]. These works emphasize the importance of coupling experimental studies with modeling and process evaluation to ensure scalability and robustness in real-world applications.

Complementing these investigations, comparative studies on photocatalysis, sonophotolysis, and sonophotocatalysis offer a systematic understanding of advanced oxidation processes for wastewater treatment [Contribution 14]. The kinetic and energetic analyses performed highlight both the potential and the limitations of these emerging technologies when applied to complex organic mixtures. The integration of such oxidation systems into existing treatment chains could represent a decisive step toward achieving near-zero discharge targets in industrial water management.

Beyond these core themes, several unconventional but thought-provoking contributions broaden the traditional boundaries of chemical plant design. Numerical simulations of methane combustion in industrial gas turbine injectors provide a detailed analysis of flame stabilization, vortex formation, and pollutant formation, guiding more sustainable combustion strategies [Contribution 15]. The exploration of smart card-based vehicle ignition systems, incorporating materials science, sensor technology, and regulatory compliance, reflects the growing convergence between process engineering, electronics, and safety systems, integrating multidisciplinary knowledge to design safer, more efficient, and more sustainable systems [Contribution 16].

Studies included in this Special Issue capture the dynamism and breadth of contemporary research in chemical plant design. They demonstrate that innovation today lies not only in technological advancement but also in methodological integration. The interplay between intensified operations, advanced materials, kinetic understanding, and environmental responsibility is reshaping the landscape of process engineering. As digitalization, artificial intelligence, and process simulation tools continue to evolve, future plant designs will increasingly rely on real-time optimization, modular architectures, and closed-loop sustainability assessment.

The final message of this Special Issue is clear: the future of chemical plant design will depend on our ability to merge creativity with rigor, sustainability with profitability, and micro-scale innovation with macro-scale implementation, as affirmed by many researchers and colleagues [4]. Therefore, we extend our sincere gratitude to all authors for their contributions, to the reviewers for their invaluable insights, and to the editorial staff of *Processes* for their continued support. We hope that the ideas presented here will inspire further research, fostering innovation in chemical plant design toward a cleaner, safer, and more resilient future.

Funding: This research received no external funding.

Acknowledgments: The co-guest editors thank the authors for providing their excellent papers and sharing their knowledge and experience.

Conflicts of Interest: The authors declare no conflicts of interest.

List of Contributions

1. Scalvenzi, L.; Guardado Yordi, E.; Santamaría Caño, E.W.; Avilez Tolagasi, I.N.; Radice, M.; Abreu-Naranjo, R.; León Guardado, L.; Bravo Sánchez, L.R.; Pérez Martínez, A. The Design of an Intensified Process and Production Plant for Cosmetic Emulsions Using Amazonian Oils. *Processes* **2025**, *13*, 1923. https://doi.org/10.3390/pr13061923.
2. Guardado Yordi, E.; Guambuguete Guaman, I.S.; Freire Fuentes, M.E.; Radice, M.; Scalvenzi, L.; Abreu-Naranjo, R.; Bravo Sánchez, L.R.; Pérez Martínez, A. Conceptual Design of the Process for Making Cosmetic Emulsion Using Amazonian Oils. *Processes* **2025**, *13*, 1770. https://doi.org/10.3390/pr13061770.
3. Abdelhalim, A.M.; Meana-Fernández, A.; Suarez-Ramon, I. Integration of Thermal Solar Power in an Existing Combined Cycle for a Reduction in Carbon Emissions and the Maximization of Cycle Efficiency. *Processes* **2024**, *12*, 2557. https://doi.dor/10.3390/pr12112557.
4. Lazaro-Molina, B.; Lopez-Arenas, T. Design and Technical-Economic-Environmental Evaluation of a Biorefinery Using Non-Marketable Edible Mushroom Waste. *Processes* **2024**, *12*, 2450. https://doi.org/10.3390/pr12112450.
5. Mendivil-Arrieta, A.; Diaz-Pérez, J.M.; González-Delgado, Á.D. Effect of Energy Integration on Safety Indexes of Suspension PVC Production Process. *Processes* **2025**, *13*, 2926. https://doi.org/10.3390/pr13092926.
6. Ramkumar, R.; Koyyada, G.; Al Rabbi Abir, M.R.; Gurugubelli, T.R.; Kim, W.K.; Kim, J.H. Porous Zn Nano-Wafer Aerogels for Asymmetric Supercapacitors: Synthesis, Structural Engineering, and Performance. *Processes* **2025**, *13*, 1461. https://doi.org/10.3390/pr13051461.
7. Soares, A.R.; de Andrade, J.C.; Lacerda, C.D.; Azevedo, S.G.; Pérez, M.T.M.; Manzato, L.; Duvoisin Junior, S.; Albuquerque, P.M. Synthesis of Polymeric Nanoparticles Using Fungal Biosurfactant as Stabilizer. *Processes* **2024**, *12*, 2739. https://doi.org/10.3390/pr12122739.
8. Silva, I.A.; Alcântara Fortunato, J.G.L.; Gomes Almeida, F.C.; Nepomuceno Alves, R.; Costa Cunha, M.C.; Rufino, R.D.; Banja Fernandes, M.L.; Sarubbo, L.A. Production and Application of a New Biosurfactant for Solubilisation and Mobilisation of Residual Oil from Sand and Seawater. *Processes* **2024**, *12*, 1605. https://doi.org/10.3390/pr12081605.
9. Xie, L.; Zhang, Z.; He, Y.; Jiang, Y. Preparation of Polyvinyl Alcohol–Chitosan Nanocellulose–Biochar Nanosilver Composite Hydrogel and Its Antibacterial Property and Dye Removal Capacity. *Processes* **2024**, *12*, 2277. https://doi.org/10.3390/pr12102277.
10. Mechi, L.; Alshammri, K.S.K.; Alsukaibi, A.K.D., Azaza, H.; Alimi, F.; Hedhili, F.; Moussaoui, Y. A Study of the Kinetics, Structure, and Morphology of the Effect of Organic Additives on Barium Sulfate Precipitation Reactions in Propan-1-ol–Water and Ethanol–Water Mixture Solutions. *Processes* **2025**, *13*, 1471. https://doi.org/10.3390/pr13051471.

11. Kim, S.J. Study on Removal of Nitrogen-Containing Heterocyclic Compounds Contained in Crude Methylnaphthalene Oil by Formamide Extraction. *Processes* **2024**, *12*, 1550. https://doi.org/10.3390/pr12081550.
12. Trucillo, P.; Lancia, A.; Di Natale, F. Adsorption–Desorption Process to Separate Dyes from Tanning Wastewaters. *Processes* **2023**, *11*, 3006. https://doi.org/10.3390/pr11103006.
13. Ngobeni, P.V.; Mpofu, A.B.; Ranjan, A.; Welz, P.J. A Critical Review of Systems for Bioremediation of Tannery Effluent with a Focus on Nitrogenous and Sulfurous Species Removal and Resource Recovery. *Processes* **2024**, *12*, 1527. https://doi.org/10.3390/pr12071527.
14. Bognár, S.; Jovanović, D.; Despotović, V.; Finčur, N.; Putnik, P.; Šojić Merkulov, D. Advancing Wastewater Treatment: A Comparative Study of Photocatalysis, Sonophotolysis, and Sonophotocatalysis for Organics Removal. *Processes* **2024**, *12*, 1527. https://doi.org/10.3390/pr12061256.
15. Sehole, H.A.H.; Mehdi, G.; Riaz, R.; Maqsood, A. Investigation of Sustainable Combustion Processes of the Industrial Gas Turbine Injector. *Processes* **2025**, *13*, 960. https://doi.org/10.3390/pr13040960.
16. Vitiello, V.; Benazzi, A.; Trucillo, P. Smart Card-Based Vehicle Ignition Systems: Security, Regulatory Compliance, Drug and Impairment Detection, Through Advanced Materials and Authentication Technologies. *Processes* **2025**, *13*, 911. https://doi.org/10.3390/pr13030911.

References

1. Agnolin, S.; Di Felice, L.; Pacheco Tanaka, A.; Llosa Tanco, M.; Ververs, W.J.R.; Gallucci, F. Intensification of Hydrogen Production: Pd–Ag Membrane on Metallic Supports for Methane Steam Reforming. *Processes* **2024**, *12*, 40. [CrossRef]
2. Ramírez-Márquez, C.; Ponce-Ortega, J.M.; Segovia-Hernández, J.G.; Hernández, S. Process Intensification Control: Advancing Efficiency and Sustainability—A Review. *Chem. Eng. Process. Process Intensif.* **2025**, *216*, 110388. [CrossRef]
3. Srivastava, S.; Pandey, V.K.; Fatima, A.; Pandey, S.; Singh, R.; Dar, A.H.; Dhillon, B. A Literature Review on Process Intensification: An Innovative and Sustainable Food Processing Method. *Appl. Food Res.* **2024**, *4*, 100363. [CrossRef]
4. Mitchell, S.; Martín, A.J.; Guillén-Gosálbez, G.; Pérez-Ramírez, J. The Future of Chemical Sciences Is Sustainable. *Angew. Chem. Int. Ed.* **2024**, *63*, e202409953. [CrossRef]

processes

MDPI

Article

Effect of Energy Integration on Safety Indexes of Suspension PVC Production Process

Antonio Mendivil-Arrieta, Juan Manuel Diaz-Pérez and Ángel Darío González-Delgado *

Chemical Engineering Department, Nanomaterials and Computer Aided Process Engineering Research Group (NIPAC), Universidad de Cartagena, Cartagena 130015, Bolivar, Colombia; amendivila@unicartagena.edu.co (A.M.-A.); jdiazp3@unicartagena.edu.co (J.M.D.-P.)
* Correspondence: agonzalezd1@unicartagena.edu.co

Abstract: Polyvinyl chloride (PVC) is the third most widely produced plastic on an industrial scale, due to its diverse applications and physicochemical properties. Its production through suspension polymerization presents significant safety challenges due to the handling of hazardous substances. To assess the impact of energy integration on process risks, the inherent safety analysis was implemented to determine the characteristic hazards of PVC suspension production. The methodology's indicators were quantified by reviewing databases, literature, and safety data sheets, considering process steps such as vinyl chloride monomer recovery, PVC purification, and drying. The results revealed that the PVC production process under energy integration conditions is intrinsically unsafe, with a total inherent safety index (ISI) of 34. The chemical component would contribute 19 points, with VCM being the main chemical risk given its flammable and carcinogenic nature, contributing a value of 15, along with the heat released by the reactions. Process safety would contribute 15 points, associated with hazardous equipment such as furnaces, burners, and dryers, as well as risks related to inventories and similar plant accidents. To improve process safety, it is recommended to reduce VCM inventories, optimize operating conditions, and implement advanced control systems for possible accidental releases.

Keywords: plastics; PVC; VCM; polymerization; inherent safety analysis; energy integration

1. Introduction

Industrial process safety has acquired an increasingly important role in decision making within the petrochemical industry since its systematic incorporation more than 45 years ago [1]. This trend responds to the need to evaluate and optimize the intrinsic characteristics of the processes, which has a positive impact both in economic and environmental terms [2]. In this context, the large-scale production of polyvinyl chloride (PVC) represents one of the most critical operations, not only because of the production volume, but also because of the inherent risks associated with the handling of hazardous chlorinated compounds and the operation with high-intensity energy sources [3].

The main raw material in PVC production, vinyl chloride monomer (VCM), is a highly explosive, carcinogenic, and mutagenic compound, which requires extremely accurate leak detection systems as well as robust preventive measures to safeguard both personnel and the environment [4]. Against this backdrop, inherent safety is established as a fundamental strategy, as it allows for intervention from the initial design stages by replacing, minimizing, or simplifying hazardous operating conditions, thus reducing reliance on external protective barriers [2,5]. Suspension processing (s-PVC), widely used in industry, involves thermodynamically demanding conditions that require rigorous risk assessment using quantitative inherent safety analysis methodologies such as Computer-Aided Process Engineering (CAPE) indices and simulation tools integrated into platforms such as Aspen Plus V14 [6]. The application of such tools allows for the assignment of risk scores to the different stages of the process, identifying critical points for improvement, and facilitating decisions aimed at reducing operational risk [7].

Energy integration in large-scale chemical plants has proven to be a synergistic strategy that not only reduces specific energy consumption but also improves operational stability by reducing thermal gradients [8]. This type of integration also becomes a key element in the inherent safety analysis, since it allows for identifying operational strengths and areas with potential for improvement, where mitigation measures can be applied from the design stage [9]. This allows for reducing the costs associated with external control systems and significantly improving the overall sustainability of the plant. This is evidenced in the study carried out by Irene Chan et al., where they required the design and selection of the best heat exchange network, through the methodology of energy integration under considerations of inherent safety indicators, concluding that the most appropriate heat exchange network was the one that had inherent safety considerations, thus allowing for the extra reduction in capital costs going from 149,079 to 133,538 USD, reflecting a reduction percentage of approximately 10.42% [10]. This perspective becomes particularly relevant within contemporary frameworks of circularity and sustainable design, which seek to minimize environmental and social impacts [7].

In addition to approaches based on inherent safety principles, there are complementary methodologies widely adopted in the industry for systematic risk analysis, such as the HAZOP (Hazard and Operability Analysis) method, which is based on the identification of deviations in process behavior under normal operating conditions. While inherent safety acts at early stages and proposes root-cause solutions, HAZOP allows for the detection of possible failures at later stages, functioning as a corrective and diagnostic tool. This comparison highlights how both approaches, although different in nature, are complementary: one acts on prevention from design, and the other reinforces operational reliability during process implementation and operation [11]. The integration of HAZOP with inherent safety indicators strengthens the preventive approach, allowing for a better prioritization of corrective actions from conceptual design to operation. Likewise, the need to integrate inherent safety indices in dynamic simulation and multivariate analysis environments has been raised, thus consolidating a holistic approach for PVC process engineering [12]. Sano et al. evaluated an acrylonitrile production plant by applying Dow's Fire and Explosion Index (F&EI) together with Fault Tree Analysis (FTA), identifying critical accident scenarios such as reactor fires and explosions, and proposing investment prioritization strategies to reduce risks and ensure operational continuity [13]. This type of study demonstrates the relevance of inherent safety assessments and complementary methodologies to prevent human, economic, and environmental losses in the chemical industry. However, an aspect of increasing importance that has been less explored is the risk evaluation of processes that integrate energy efficiency strategies. Energy integration, while providing environmental and economic benefits, also increases operational complexity, thereby generating new risk scenarios [14]. In this context, our research introduces a novel contribution by incorporating inherent safety assessment into systems with energy integration, strengthening the link between sustainability and industrial safety and offering a more comprehensive framework for process design and operation. However, the growing use of Artificial Intelligence (AI) in engineering and industrial fields has had an extraordinary boom [15], and it is not surprising that the design of sustainable processes is influenced by the objective of optimizing processes and aiming to meet the sustainable development goals (SDGs) under the concept of Industry 4.0 [16]. Therefore, this type of research, where inherent safety methodologies are applied to biofuel production processes, allows for the generation of sufficient structured and concise documentation that functions as Big Data, so that AI can analyze different bibliographic sources and generate conclusions in the shortest possible time, facilitating the prevention of accidents in the biofuel industries [17].

2. Materials and Methods

2.1. Process Description

Figure 1 illustrates the industrial-scale suspension polymerization process for PVC production, as previously developed by the authors using operational data from industrial plants and literature sources. For more information on energy-integrated process simulation, please refer to the research conducted by Mendivil et al. [8]. A feed stream comprising fresh and recovered vinyl chloride monomer (VCM) enters the polymerization reactor (R-101), where it is dispersed in an aqueous suspension containing a stabilizing agent (polyvinyl alcohol, PVA) and a free-radical initiator (typically a peroxide). The polymerization reaction occurs at 70 °C and 9.8 bar. Polymer particles form within monomer droplets as the initiator decomposes, triggering an exothermic reaction with a typical conversion efficiency of approximately 85%. Upon completion of the reaction, the system yields a heterogeneous mixture (slurry) composed of suspended PVC, unreacted VCM, water, residual initiator, and stabilizer. The slurry remains at 70 °C and 3.4 bar. Due to the high toxicity of residual VCM, its concentration in the polymer must be reduced to below 1 ppm, in compliance with international safety regulations [18].

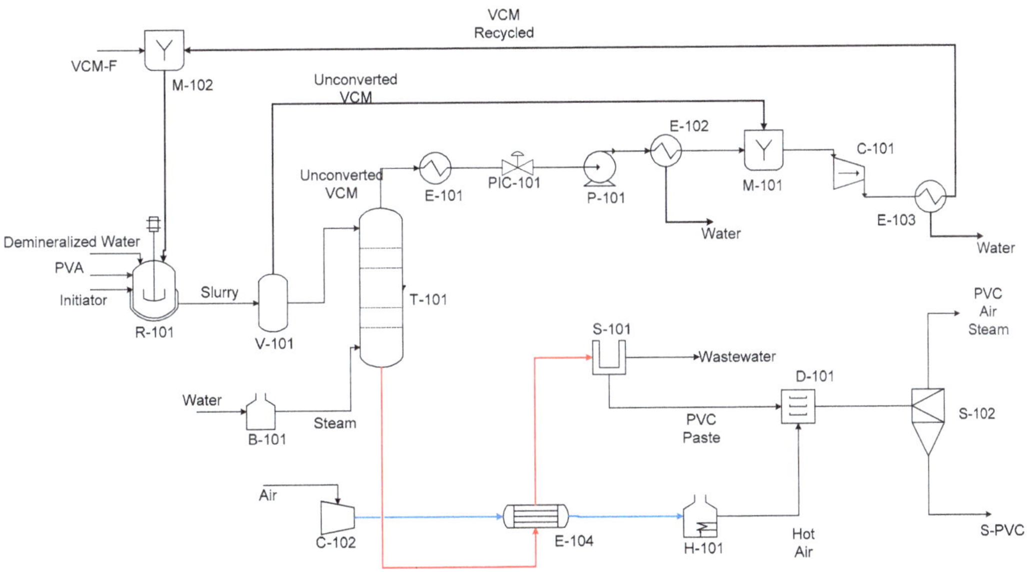

Figure 1. Process flow diagram (PFD) of energy-integrated PVC production.

VCM removal is accomplished through successive degassing and stripping stages. Initially, the system pressure is lowered to 1.7 bar, allowing for the release of approximately 95% of the unreacted VCM. The remaining 5% is removed in a stripping column (T-101), which consists of a tray tower into which superheated steam (13.7 bar, 225 °C) is introduced from the bottom. This step produces two streams: an overhead stream rich in VCM and a bottom stream containing the PVC slurry with less than 1 ppm of residual monomer.

The overhead stream from the stripping tower proceeds to a recovery unit, where unreacted VCM is separated from accompanying phases (e.g., water) and reconditioned for reuse via condensation. This recovery process involves a series of cooling and compression steps. The stream is first cooled to 50 °C, then subjected to vacuum compression below the water saturation pressure, enabling condensation and phase separation. Subsequently, gas-phase components are further purified. Stripped gases from the degassing stage are compressed to 3.4 bar—near the VCM saturation pressure—and efficiently condensed in a heat exchanger for reintegration into the polymerization cycle.

The stripped PVC slurry, now essentially free of monomer, undergoes mechanical dewatering via centrifugal separation (S-101) at 1800× g rpm, removing approximately 75% of the water content (initially ~70%). The expelled water contains minor fractions of PVC, PVA, and initiator. The resulting wet PVC paste is further dried in a rotary dryer, using a hot air stream at 250 °C. Following air mixing, the system stabilizes at 70 °C. The final moisture content of the dried PVC falls below 0.01% by weight, in accordance with product quality specifications.

The dryer's outlet consists of a gas mixture of air and water vapor entraining a small amount of polymer particles. These particles are recovered in a cyclone operating at standard atmospheric pressure. The cyclone's top stream, which contains approximately 0.2% of the total PVC produced, exits as air and vapor, while the solid polymer is discharged through the bottom with a final moisture content of 0.01%.

2.2. Energy Integration Using Aspen Energy Analyzer™ V14

Energy integration serves as a strategic approach to comprehensively analyze and optimize energy consumption within industrial systems. By establishing energy targets and maximizing heat recovery, it enables more efficient thermal energy management. This methodology requires detailed data on process stream properties, including inlet and outlet temperatures, specific heat capacities, and thermal loads associated with both process and utility streams. Energy integration through pinch analysis and the process data required to apply this methodology were presented in previous research conducted by the authors [8].

These results were subsequently utilized as inputs for Aspen Energy Analyzer™ V14, a specialized tool developed by AspenTech to enhance energy efficiency across various industrial sectors. Widely applied in energy-intensive industries, this tool functions as a decision-support system for the design and optimization of Heat Exchanger Networks (HENs). Software applies a systematic framework to generate near-optimal heat exchanger network configurations. It extracts thermodynamic data from simulations and employs graphical techniques—such as composite and grand composite curves—to minimize thermal utility consumption. The software also facilitates automatic targeting and screening of network alternatives, accounting for economic parameters such as capital investment and energy operating costs [19].

2.3. Process Safety Evaluation

At a global level, the concept of built-in safety was first introduced in 1976 by chemical engineer Trevor A. Kletz, when he described the nitroglycerin production process and discussed the inherent constraints of the process itself in achieving a safe design [20]. This concept was born from the need to avoid or reduce potential risks in industrial plants by implementing new process designs. Furthermore, Trevor recommends replacing hazardous substances in processes with others that represent a lower risk and, in turn, reducing their inventories. This took place due to the increase in safety concerns from political, social, and economic perspectives, which were represented by certain accidents in industrial plants between the 1960s and 1970s, such as Beek in the Netherlands, Seveso in Italy, Flixborough in the United Kingdom, and even the major Bhopal incident [21].

However, it was not until 1999 that Anna-Mari Heikkilä introduced the inherent safety index (ISI), which seeks to prevent process hazards instead of controlling them as other safety systems do, by seeking to reduce the presence of hazardous material and the number of stages or equipment that are a potential hazard for the plant, from the chemical and process safety point of view (variables, operating conditions and related characteristics), which are estimated under the selection of the worst possible case [22]. The total inherent safety indicator (I_{SI}) is estimated using the following equation:

$$I_{SI} = I_{CI} + I_{PI} \tag{1}$$

where I_{CI} corresponds to the inherent safety chemical index, and I_{PI} represents the inherent safety index of the process, and if the sum of both indicators yields a value greater than or equal to 24, the process is considered intrinsically unsafe.

2.4. Chemical Index of Inherent Safety (I_{CI})

Equation number 2 represents the chemical index of inherent safety of the process, which is estimated by taking into account the characteristics and physicochemical properties of the substances and reactions that take place in the industrial process. These include reactivity, flammability, flammability, and corrosiveness.

$$I_{CI} = I_{RM} + I_{RS} + I_{INT} + (I_{FL} + I_{EX} + I_{TOX})_{max} + I_{COR} \tag{2}$$

Figure 2 describes the types of reactions that can be classified based on the heat released or enthalpy of reaction, ranging from a score of 0, known as thermally neutral, to a score of 4 or extremely exothermic; said heats are quantified by Hess's law (measured in J/g), and the same figure applies to the main reaction subscript (I_{RM}) and the secondary reaction subscript (I_{RS}).

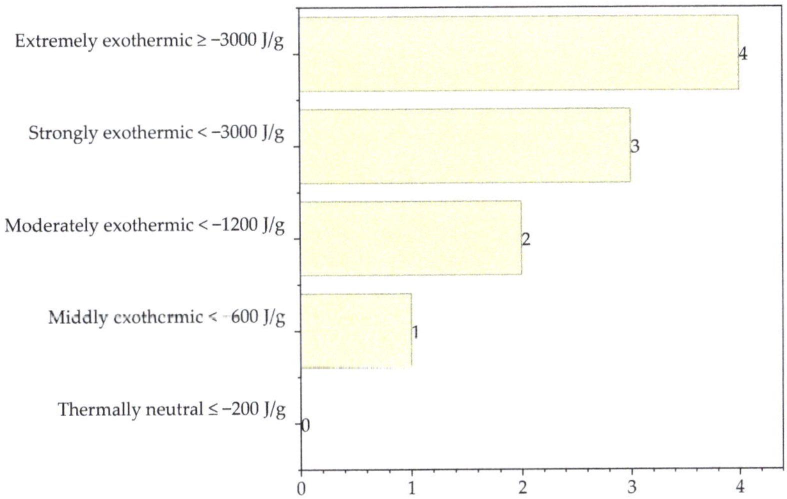

Figure 2. Subscripts by main chemical reaction (I_{RM}) and secondary (I_{RS}).

The subscript of chemical interactions (I_{INT}) that can occur in an industrial process generate a possible extra risk in production, given the possible interactions between the substances in the process and the environment itself (construction materials of the equipment or the air in the atmosphere). Figure 3 represents the types of interactions and the score that would be given to each one, ranging from the formation of heat (scores from 1 to 3 depending on the amount of heat released) to the production of soluble toxic chemicals (score of 1).

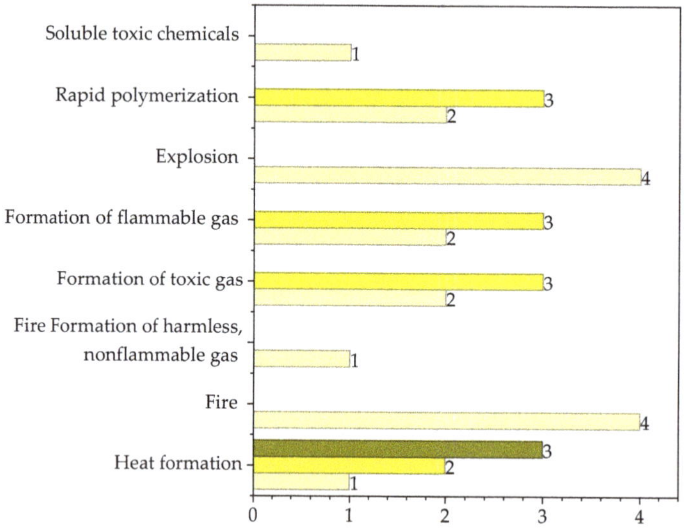

Figure 3. Subscript for chemical interactions (I_{INT}).

Figure 4 lists the flammability subindex (I_{FL}) from the concept of flash point, which ranges from a non-flammable category with a score of 0 to a highly flammable category with a flash point below 0 °C or a boiling point ≤ 35 °C, giving a value of 4.

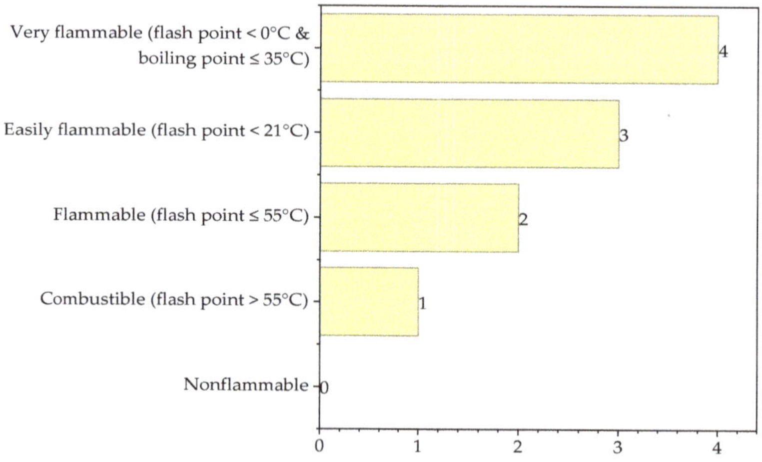

Figure 4. Flammability subindex (I_{FL}).

Given the existence of possible leaks of explosive substances in industrial processes, the explosiveness subindex, or I_{EX}, needs to be classified (Figure 5) according to the difference between its maximum (UEL%) and minimum (LEL%) concentration limits to generate a trend according to the formation of an explosive mixture between a substance and air.

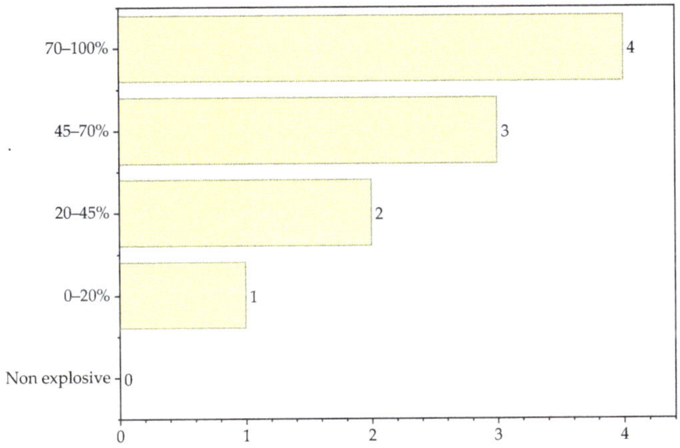

Figure 5. Explosiveness subindex (I_{EX}).

The Figure 6 shows the different classifications and scores according to the toxicological risks that different substances have in any process, and their mere presence can directly affect the inherent safety of the process, when there are compounds capable of generating physical effects on the workers of a plant, therefore, this indicator is broken down into 6 possible points according to their respective score, going from a TLV (toxicological threshold limit) greater than 10,000 ppm (substance with little toxicological risk and score of 0) to a TLV ≤ 0.1 ppm, classifying the substance or compound as an imminent risk to the worker or operator.

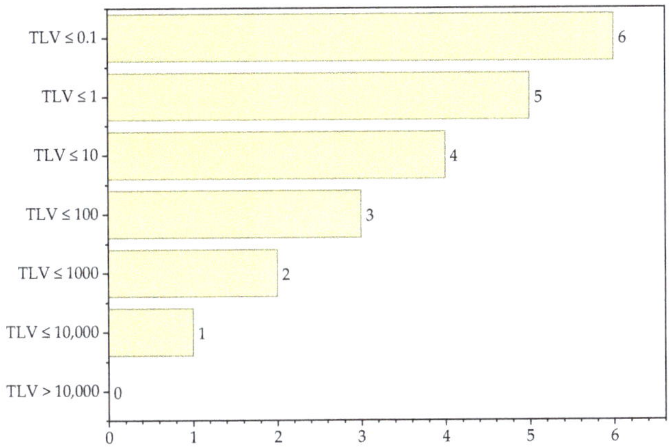

Figure 6. Toxicity subindex (I_{TOX}).

Now, after calculating the three previous subindices, it is necessary to select the substance with the highest risks, that is, select the substance or compound that can contribute the worst risk scenario to the process by adding the subindices of flammability, explosiveness, and toxicity. Finally, there is the corrosivity subindex, which is measured based on both the most hazardous substance and the process conditions. For proper selection, the author of the methodology recommends taking into account temperature and pressure to determine the conditions under which the mechanical stresses will occur, to which the equipment will be constantly subjected [22]. To this end, Figure 7 presents a range of values that depend on the type of material (some type of metal being the preferred option), going from carbon steel with a score of 0, then stainless steel (score of 1), and then, if the process requires a material much more suitable for the process, either due to chemical or process reactivity conditions, a score of 2 would be given.

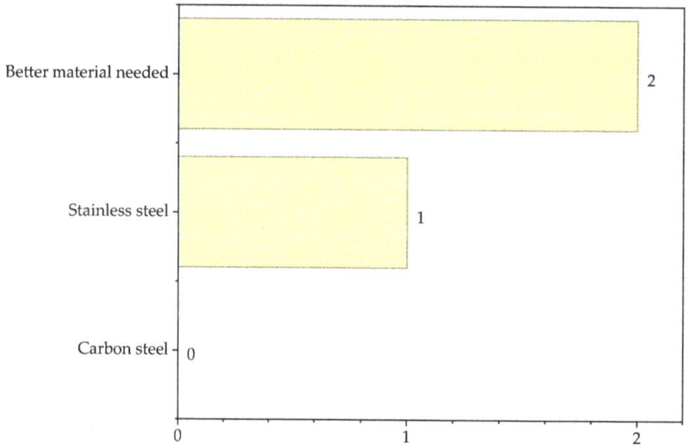

Figure 7. Corrosivity subindex (I_{COR}).

2.5. Inherent Process Safety Index (I_{PI})

The inherent process safety index is represented by equation 3, whose primary focus is on evaluating the safety of the process based on its operating conditions and structural design. The process safety index is also broken down into a series of subindexes that make it much more interesting from an engineering perspective. These are inventory; maximum operating temperature and pressure; the equipment safety index, which denotes the presence of equipment based on its location and proximity to the heart of the plant; and finally, the level of safe structure.

$$I_{PI} = I_I + I_T + I_P + I_{EQ} + I_{ST} \tag{3}$$

Figure 8 describes the different scores that can be assigned to the inventory indicator based on the total tons of raw materials and products handled during a one-hour residence time in the different process vessels (reactors, distillation columns, etc.). However, one of the main challenges is that the inherent safety index methodology is applied from the design stages, which makes it difficult to clearly identify all the equipment that will be involved in the final plant design. To this end, the author of the methodology recommends distributing the design equipment according to the internal battery boundaries (ISBL) and external battery boundaries (OSBL). This allows for the classification of the main equipment of interest to the production process, which would be located closest to the plant core (ISBL), while the rest is located outside the plant boundaries (OSBL).

Figure 8a shows that the ISBL inventory can range from 0 to 5 points, with a range of 0 to 1000 tons. Figure 8b shows the OSBL inventory with the same range of points, but with a higher capacity in tons, going from 0 to 10,000 tons.

In the design of industrial chemical plants, the maximum temperature must be reviewed to take precautions, given that the higher the temperature, the greater the amount of circulating thermal energy, which becomes a problem for the equipment's construction materials. The temperature subscript (I_T) is represented in Figure 9, which takes into account temperatures below 0 °C with a score of 1, 0 °C with 0 points, and up to 4 points for temperatures above 600 °C.

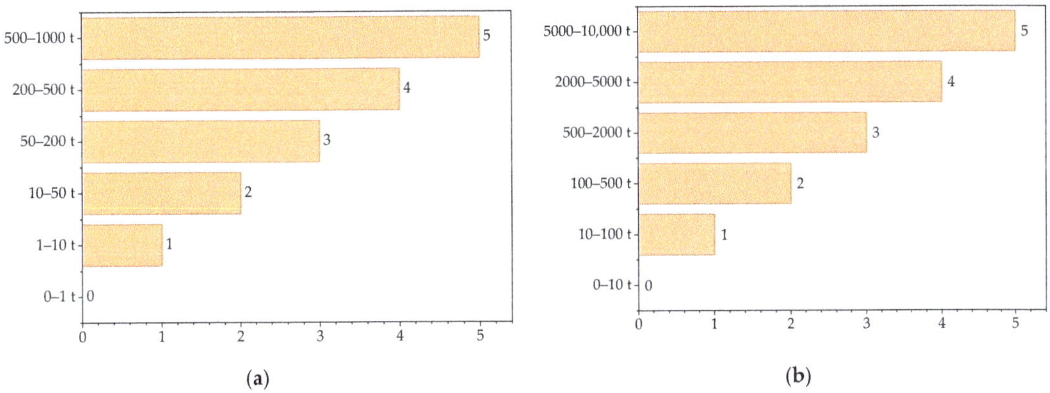

Figure 8. (**a**) Inventory subindex from internal battery limit (ISBL); (**b**) inventory subindex from external battery limit (OSBL).

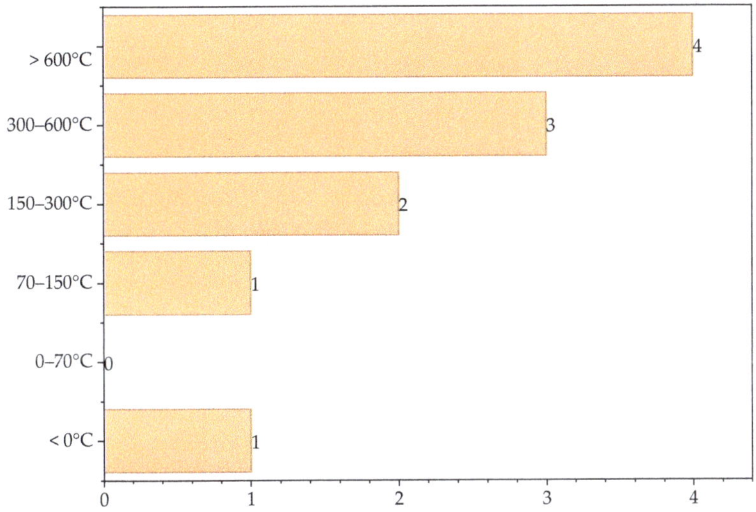

Figure 9. Temperature subindex (I_T).

Figure 10 represents the different maximum pressure ranges at which industrial processes operate. This is a very important indicator, as it allows us to identify the normal operating pressure and, in turn, estimate the optimal design pressure to which the equipment can be subjected. The pressure range is presented from 0.5 bar (0) to 1000 bar (4).

The equipment safety subindex or I_{EQ} (Figure 11) quantifies the main risks related to the equipment that is distributed across the different boundaries of the plant (ISBL and OSBL) and may represent a danger to the plant facilities, examples of which are high-pressure compressors, furnaces, reactors, storage tanks, etc.

Finally, the safe structure subindex (I_{ST}) is presented in the Figure 12, which allows for measuring how unsafe the industrial process is from the structure of the process itself and thus being able to describe the efficiency of the unit operations and other important elements that are within the processes; but for this, the bibliography referring to accidents and safety reports of similar production plants or those that include similar equipment and processes must be reviewed [22].

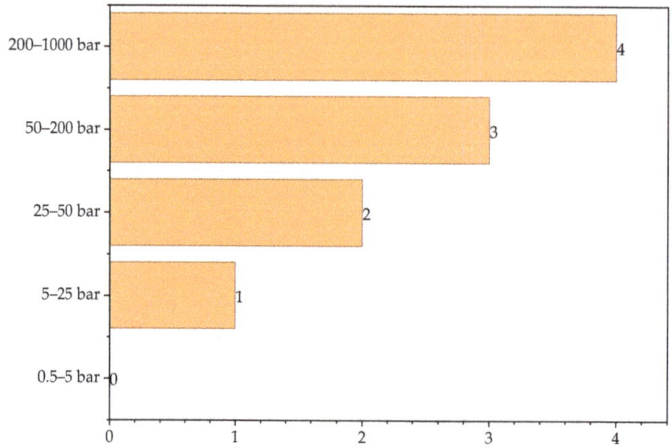

Figure 10. Pressure subindex (I_P).

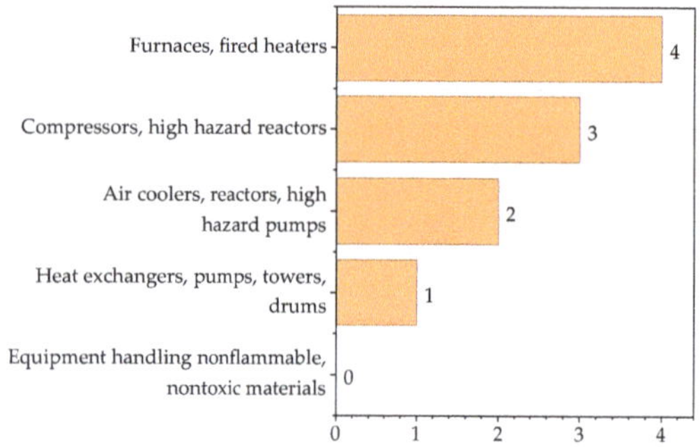

(a)

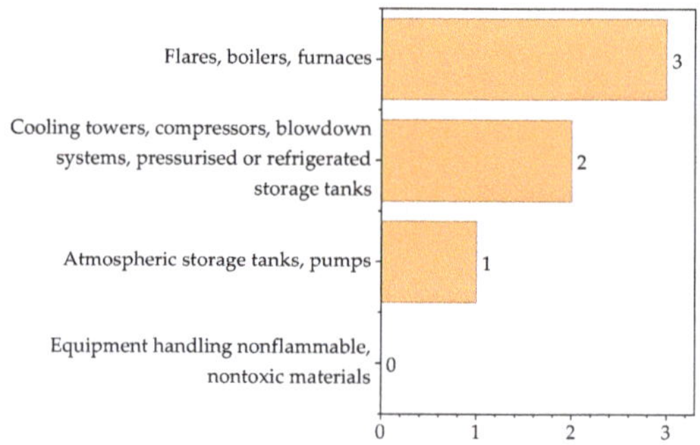

(b)

Figure 11. (**a**) Equipment safety subindex from the internal battery limit (ISBL); (**b**) equipment safety sub-index from external battery limit (OSBL).

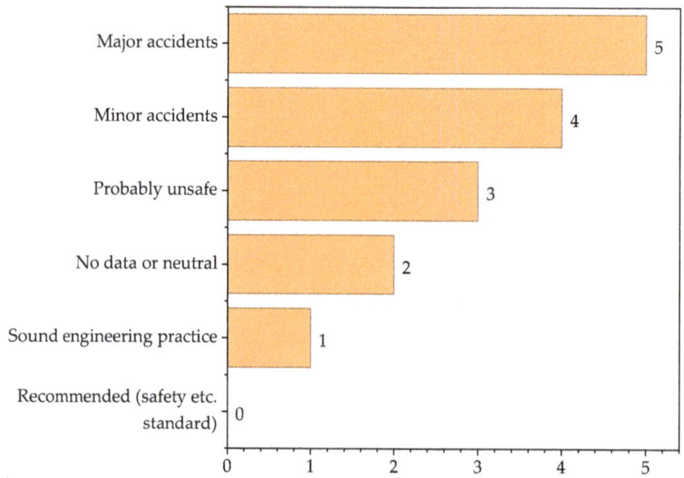

Figure 12. Secure structure subindex (I_{ST}).

3. Results and Discussion

3.1. Contribution of Chemical Process Indicators

The energy-integrated suspension production process for polyvinyl chloride faces significant challenges when it comes to assessing its intrinsic safety from the early stages of process design and sizing. This is evidenced by Figure 13, which represents all the contributions made by the physicochemical properties of the chemicals that interact in the different stages of the process. The first subscript analyzed is the main reaction subscript or $I_{RM,max}$, which reflects the enthalpy or heat released by the main chemical reaction, which corresponds to the polymerization of MVC occurring inside the R-101 reactor, with a ΔHr value of −1600 J/g. By comparing the previous heat of reaction with the ranges in Figure 13, it is concluded that the MVC polymerization reaction is strongly exothermic and would be given a score of 3. The United States Chemical Safety Board (CSB) lists strongly exothermic polymerization chemical reactions as a matter of concern, given the existence of thermal runaways, either generated by failures in the reactor cooling system or high concentrations of reactants, this being the cause of approximately 35% of accidents in polymerization reactors, so it is recommended to implement the design of control systems for reactor cooling [23].

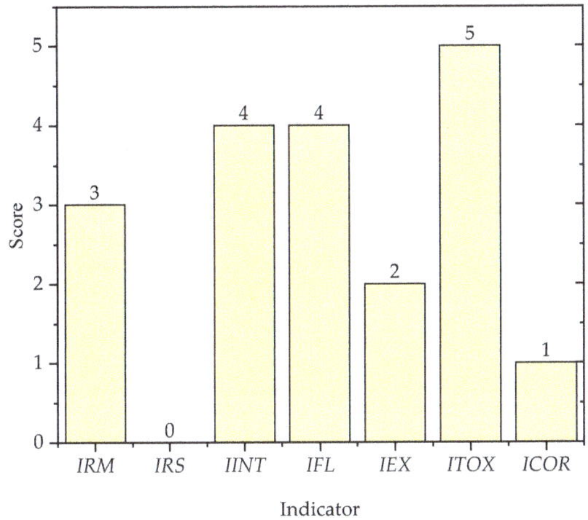

Figure 13. Indicators for the chemical subindexes of the energy-integrated PVC process.

However, since it is the polymerization of MVC, no secondary reactions are known, so there would be no heat released by any reaction other than the main one. Thus, it becomes a chemical risk with a score of 0 for the I_{RS} (secondary reaction subscript).

The other subindexes for the chemical part of the process are estimated through a search in bibliography or literature related to the properties of the substances used in the PVC production process. This literature was mostly technical sheets provided by the International Chemical Safety Cards (ICSCs) website and scientific articles.

Table 1 (supplementary materials) compiles the possible chemical interactions that substances may have throughout the process, that is, the possible reactions that would generate a hazard for the process. It is concluded that vinyl monochloride is the substance that would pose the greatest risk, with a score of 4 for the chemical interactions subindex (I_{INT}), because MVC when mixed with air, either in a leak or within the process itself, runs the risk of fire, poisoning, or explosion [24].

Table 1. Chemical interactions of substances.

Substance	Type of Interaction	Score I_{CI}
VCM	Explosion	4
H_2O	Does not interact	0
O_2	Does not interact	0
PVC	Explosion	4
PVA	Formation of toxic gas 1	2
N_2	Does not interact	0
Maximum score		4

From Table 2 (supplementary materials), you can see the cluster of flammability types of substances, according to their flash point, knowing that this concept is defined by the American Society for Testing and Materials (ASTM) as the lowest temperature at which an ignition source causes the vapors of a substance to ignite under specific conditions [25]. Additionally, a good indicator of flammability for fluids that do not have a flash point record is the boiling point of the substance [22]. Therefore, it is concluded that VCM is the substance with the highest risk of flammability, providing a score of 4 for I_{FL} due to the risk it represents, as it is highly flammable with a flash point of −78 °C. Given the existence of substances such as PVA and PVC that are solid and do not have a recorded flash point range, however, PVA is the only one that has a boiling point of 300 °C (considered combustible), if and only if it is in an aqueous solution, as is the case in the process in question.

Table 2. Flammability subindex.

Substance	Flash Point (°C)/Boiling Point (°C)	Flammability Type	Score I_{CI}
VCM	−78	Highly flammable	4
H_2O	-	Non-flammable	0
O_2	-	Non-flammable	0
PVC	-	-	0
PVA	300	Fuel	1
N_2	-	Non-flammable	0
	Maximum score		4

Given the relevance of preventing explosion risks from the design stage of the PVC production process by suspension with energy integration, it is required to quantify the explosiveness subindex, or I_{EX}, by subtracting the lower and upper explosive limits (UEL and LEL). These limits relate the minimum and maximum concentrations at which a substance or compound can burn in air (mainly oxygen) and maintain flame propagation [26]. Table 3 (supplementary materials) compiles the difference in limits for each substance, where again the VCM synthesizes the greatest explosive potential with an upper limit (UEL) of 33% and an LEL of 3.6%, thus denoting a difference of 29.4%. These values indicate that if we have a concentration of VCM in a mixture with air greater than 33%, the mixture would not be considered directly flammable due to the displacement of the combustible medium (O_2). Otherwise, if the mixture is less than 3.6%, there would be no room for a flame to burn for a long time.

The remaining substances, such as water, oxygen, and nitrogen, are not explosive when in contact with air. Therefore, they are considered non-explosive. In the case of PVC and PVA, this type of indicator would not apply, because they are mostly solid and do not contain information on technical data sheets. This leads the VCM to provide a score of 2 for the inherent safety indicator for the chemical part of the process.

Table 3. Explosivity subindex.

Substance	(UEL-LEL) %	Score I_{CI}
VCM	29.40	2
H_2O	Non-explosive	0
O_2	Non-explosive	0
PVC	-	0
PVA	-	0
N_2	Non-explosive	0
Maximum score		2

To quantify the toxicity indicator of substances, it is necessary to extract from the literature the TLVs, also known as toxicity threshold limit values, which express the limit concentrations in parts per million (ppm) to which an operator can be exposed without suffering damage. Generally, the American Conference of Governmental Industrial Hygienists (ACGIH) is responsible for providing this type of scientific guidance based on issues of hygiene, industrial safety, and health [27]. Table 4 (supplementary materials) lists the TLVs for each substance and their respective scores; therefore, MVC as a raw material and PVC powder have the same TLV of 1 ppm due to their potential hazard, and each is assigned a score of 5.

Table 4. Toxicity subindex.

Substance	TLV (ppm)	Score I_{CI}
VCM	1	5
H_2O	Non-toxic	0
O_2	Non-toxic	0
PVC	1	5
PVA	-	0
N_2	Non-toxic	0
Maximum score		5

However, when PVC comes into contact with high heat sources, such as fires, it can degrade into multiple substances that are within the range of carcinogenic or toxicological potential, such as benzene, chlorobenzene, carbon monoxide, methylene chloride, chloroform, and other chlorinated hydrocarbons that can cause other physiological effects [28].

However, the toxicological potential of PVC is greatly enhanced when exposed to high heat sources, in contrast to VCM, which is hazardous even under ambient temperature and pressure conditions. The fatality of vinyl monochloride is recorded, with three workers dying due to exposure to high concentrations of the monomer via the respiratory tract. They presented similar autopsies with congestion of internal organs, with priority given to the lungs and kidneys, in addition to blood clotting. Given the multiple occupational exposures that various workers in plants that handle VCM have had, they have been linked to a certain extent to Raynaud's phenomenon with pale and numb fingers, along with other complications such as seizures, low sexual performance, and cardiac irregularities [29]. Now, the selection of the substances with the greatest contribution to the chemical insecurity of the process is defined by the sum of the indicators I_{FL}, I_{EX}, and I_{TOX}, resulting in the substance with the highest risk of the process with the contribution of 11 points, which would be the VCM.

As the last subindex for the chemical part of the process, there is the corrosion indicator (I_{COR}), which requires the selection of a material capable of correctly containing the substance or compound with the highest score from the chemical points of view discussed previously, in addition to being able to withstand all the mechanical stresses (fatigue, scratches, compression, etc.) that will occur during the life of the plant. However, it is important to perform an additional review regarding the presence of components such as vinyl monochloride from a perspective other than toxicological, based on the decomposition of the material. Although VCM decomposes between 600 and 700 °C, it is important to take this into account in the inherent safety methodology given the prevention of internal leaks in the process or accidents related to combustion. According to the specialized literature on this type of industrial process, any type of combustion or flame could enhance the formation of hydrochloric acid (HCl), carbonyl chloride ($COCl_2$), and carbon monoxide (CO), which are dangerous substances, and even HCl causes strong structural damage if carbon steels are used [30].

Stainless steels such as AISI 304 and 316 are recognized as the preferred materials for this type of industrial plants, thanks to their high resistance to corrosion and good performance under mechanical stress [31]. Knowing the risks of the process, stainless steel is selected, preferably AISI 316 steel, as it is the most suitable material for working with VCM and derivatives, based on the conceptual design of a vinyl chloride production plant [32], which gives it a score of 1 for the chemical risks of the energy-integrated suspension PVC production process.

3.2. Contribution of Process Safety Indicator

Figure 14 shows the scores provided by each of the subindexes, where the ISBL and OSBL inventory subindexes were estimated by considering the capacity of the equipment known in engineering terms as containers, with a residence time of 1 h. To better understand the distribution of the PVC production plant by suspension with energy integration, Figure 14 is presented, which graphically describes the ISBL battery limits (area delimited by an orange border) and OSBL (area delimited by a green border). The ISBL inventory was taken as the inventory of the production process, which has a value of 1958.9 t/h, and for the OSBL inventory, the tons of raw materials fed to the process were considered, which are estimated at around 37.5 t/h. For the types of inventories, a score of 5 and 1 point is given, respectively, thus providing the highest score of 5 to the inventory subindex.

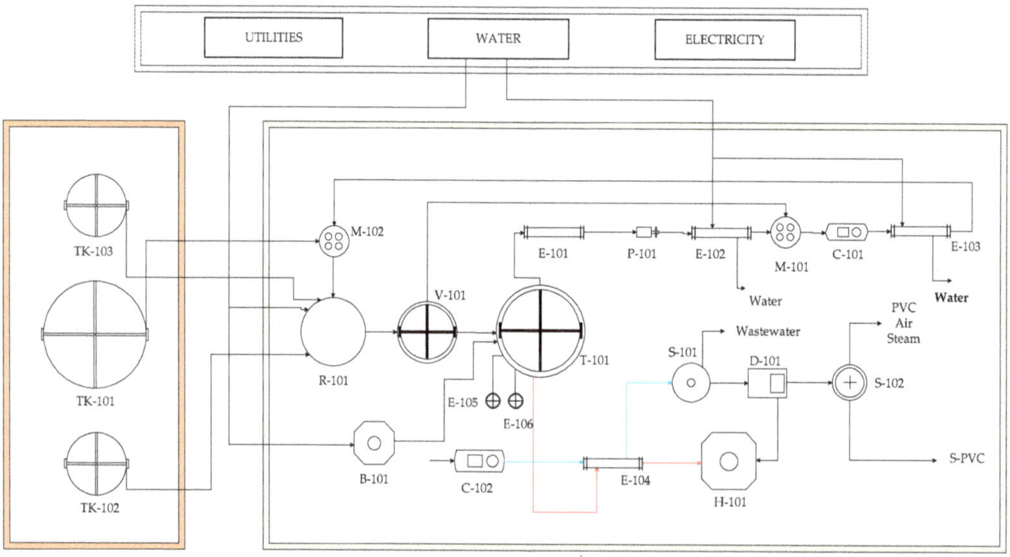

Figure 14. Layout of the energy-integrated PVC production plant according to ISBL and OSBL from a top view.

For the subindexes related to the process operating conditions such as temperature and pressure, maximum values of 250 °C and 13.7 bar are recorded, which translate into scores of 2 and 1, respectively. On the other hand, the safety subindex for equipment (I_{EQ}) obtains a score of 4 due to the presence of equipment that represents a high danger in the energy-integrated suspension PVC production process, of which the boiler stands out (B-101), as well as the burner (H-101) and compressors, which have potential temperatures and pressures. Finally, the safe structure subscript, or I_{ST}, the equipment location subindex, which considers the risks associated with the proximity of equipment to the plant core, gives a maximum score of 4. Finally, the safe process structure subindex is based on accidents at other PVC plants. Two significant incidents are the VCM explosion at Formosa Plastics in 2004, where the incorrect opening of a valve caused the release of VCM, which, upon entering into contact with the environment, generated flammable mixtures, resulting in an explosion and 5 dead workers [33]; and the Mexichem explosion in 2016, located at the petrochemical complex known as "Pajarito" in Coatzacoalcos, Mexico. Human error caused a leak in the feed to the polymerization reactor, leaving a total of 36 dead and approximately 100 injured [34]. These two accidents alone are sufficient to classify the plant as probably unsafe and assign a score of 3. However, other industrial accidents related to PVC production are found in the specialized literature, such as the partial explosion (sudden release of 4 tons of VCM) at a PVC production plant in Jouetsu, Japan [34]. Likewise, Ogle and collaborators recorded an explosion caused by the flashing of VCM sludge that entered a lower pressure tank under high pressure and temperature conditions [35]. Figure 15 allows to compile all the scores related to the various sub-indicators for the inherent safety part of the energy-integrated suspension PVC production process, denoting the process inventories that represent the greatest hazard in this case study.

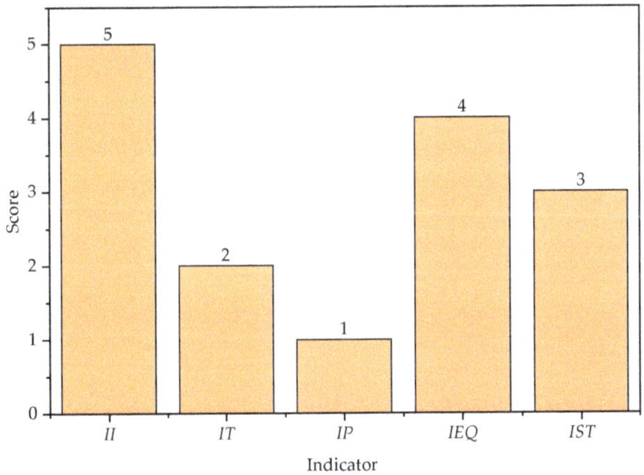

Figure 15. Indicators for the safety subindexes of the energy-integrated PVC process.

Figure 16 graphically represents the chemical and total safety risks of the energy-integrated suspension PVC production, which is considered intrinsically unsafe due to its total score in the inherent safety index of 34, as well as its base case for exceeding the regulatory limit imposed by the author of the methodology, with 24 points to be considered safe. Likewise, the chemical safety index obtained a value of 19, due to the presence of VCM in the process, this being the main risk of generating accidents. On the other hand, the process safety index presented a value of 15 points due to the presence of high inventory volumes that exceed 1900 t/h and history of inherently unsafe conditions.

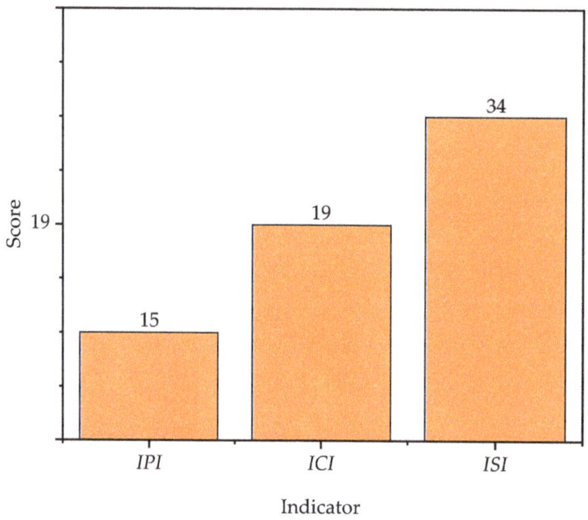

Figure 16. Total inherent safety index (I_{TI}) of the energy-integrated PVC production process.

The energy integration of the suspension PVC production process does not contribute to the improvement or reduction of the indicators of the inherent safety methodology developed by Heikkilä. However, process optimization is presented when analyzing natural gas consumption for heating services, that is, energy integration would play an important role in improving the energy efficiency of the process and, in turn, reducing the burning of natural gas that is normally used to meet the energy needs of certain equipment in the process. Consequently, the PVC production process would present an improvement in terms of its inherent safety, due to the fact of reducing natural gas inventories from 59.4 m^3/t to 52.5 m^3/t [8].

In a study conducted by Segovia et al., they also concluded that partial or few streams of energy integration in biodiesel and bioethanol production processes is a solution to address energy inefficiencies and increase the sustainability of the process from an economic and environmental point of view, with a 15.7% and 19.4% reduction in utility requirements for cooling and heating of bioethanol and biodiesel processes. On the other hand, the safety assessment does not show any changes in the overall risk of the processes; however, it is mentioned that the process inventory increases with the installation of new heat exchangers belonging to the energy integration network, but the natural gas inventories for heating decrease [36].

The search and implementation of new process control systems is recommended, with the aim of predicting leaks within the process equipment. Likewise, the importance of continuing to investigate process optimization, with the possible implementation of engineering resources such as heat pumps integrated into separation equipment, is highlighted, which, according to the reviewed bibliography, has allowed for a decrease of up to 44.97% in total annualized costs (TACs) and has enhanced the decarbonization of industrial processes [37]. In addition, research into new catalysts is recommended that allow for a higher conversion of reactants to products in a shorter time, thus allowing for the reduction of VCM inventories in the purification and recovery stages of said raw material.

4. Conclusions

From an engineering perspective, the inherent safety analysis demonstrates that the PVC production process by suspension with energy integration is considered unsafe due to its high score of 34 for the inherent safety indicator (ISI), thus exceeding the permissible limit of 24 for a process to be considered intrinsically safe. The high score is primarily due to the presence of vinyl chloride monomer (VCM), a highly toxic, flammable, and explosive substance, as well as the operation of critical equipment such as boilers, kilns, and dryers that present significant pressure and temperature conditions. Although energy integration improves thermal efficiency and reduces natural gas consumption (from 59.4 to 52.5 kg/t), it does not attenuate the inherent safety indices. A parametric sensitivity analysis of varying operating conditions or the implementation of alternative polymerization chemistries could bring information regarding behavior of safety indexes in smoothed conditions; however, since this research is based on a real-world process with operating conditions optimized and chemistry of polymerization well defined, that study will not provide relevant information to the industrial sector considering that the process is optimized. For that reason, variation of parameters is explicitly limited to quantifying the effect of energy integration on chemical and process safety indicators in PVC suspension polymerization. Any modification aimed at enhancing inherent safety would directly alter the predefined parameters of both the process simulation and the energy integration strategy.

Future research efforts should pursue a more comprehensive re-evaluation of the process design, incorporating a broader set of strategies to strengthen both safety and sustainability. Beyond conventional approaches, such as reducing hazardous inventories at the source and implementing advanced process control systems, several emerging technologies hold promise for enhancing both operational efficiency and inherent safety. For instance, industrial heat pumps could be employed to recover and reutilize low-grade waste heat from exothermic stages of PVC suspension polymerization. This not only contributes to significant reductions in external utility demands but also minimizes thermal accumulation within reactors, thereby lowering the likelihood of runaway scenarios. By stabilizing temperature profiles, heat pumps can indirectly enhance process safety while simultaneously advancing energy efficiency. Similarly, the use of high-conversion catalysts offers the potential to improve monomer utilization and reduce unreacted vinyl chloride inventories, which are the dominant hazard drivers in PVC production. By decreasing the concentration of hazardous intermediates and byproducts, such catalytic innovations directly contribute to inherent safety, while also improving process yields and reducing downstream purification loads. Another promising direction is the deployment of AI-enabled hazard detection systems, which leverage machine learning algorithms and real-time sensor data to identify early warning signals of unsafe operating conditions. These systems can enhance situational awareness, enable predictive maintenance, and support rapid decision-making in abnormal situations. By shifting from reactive to proactive risk management, AI-based approaches provide an additional safety layer that complements traditional inherent safety strategies. Finally, integrating techno-economic analyses with safety metrics represents a critical step toward holistic decision-making. Traditional evaluations often consider energy savings or risk mitigation independently, but a coupled framework allows for quantifying the trade-offs between operational efficiency, cost reduction, and hazard minimization. For industrial practitioners, such integration ensures that investments in energy efficiency or novel technologies are not only financially viable but also consistent with stringent safety requirements. Taken together, these approaches would provide a more robust framework for advancing inherent safety while ensuring the industrial feasibility of PVC production under evolving technological, environmental, and regulatory constraints.

Supplementary Materials: The following supporting information can be downloaded at: https://www.mdpi.com/article/10.3390/pr13092926/s1, Table S1: Chemical interactions of substances; Table S2: Flammability subindex; Table S3: Explosivity subindex; Table S4: Toxicity subindex.

Author Contributions: Conceptualization, Á.D.G.-D.; methodology, Á.D.G.-D.; software, A.M.-A. and J.M.D.-P.; validation, Á.D.G.-D.; formal analysis, A.M.-A. and J.M.D.-P.; investigation, A.M.-A., J.M.D.-P., and Á.D.G.-D.; resources, Á.D.G.-D.; data curation, A.M.-A. and J.M.D.-P.; writing—original draft preparation, A.M.-A. and J.M.D.-P.; writing—review and editing, Á.D.G.-D.; visualization, A.M.-A.; supervision, Á.D.G.-D.; project administration, Á.D.G.-D.; funding acquisition, Á.D.G.-D. All authors have read and agreed to the published version of the manuscript.

Funding: This research was funded by the Universidad de Cartagena through the projects "Optimization of the PVC production process on an industrial scale combining sustainability analysis and computer-assisted mass integration of processes", and "Optimization of the Industrial-Scale PVC Production Process by Combining Sustainability Analysis and Computer-Aided Process Energy Integration" approved by Resolution 01385 of 2021 and commitment acts No. 106 of 2021 and No. 049 of 2024.

Data Availability Statement: The data that support the findings of this study are available from the corresponding author, Á.D.G.-D., upon reasonable request.

Acknowledgments: The authors would like to thank the University of Cartagena for providing equipment and software to successfully conclude this work.

Conflicts of Interest: The authors declare no conflicts of interest.

Abbreviations

ISI	Inherent safety index
I_{CI}	Inherent safety index by chemicals
I_{PI}	Inherent process safety index
I_{RM}	Main reaction heat subindex, J/g
I_{RS}	Secondary reaction heat subindex, J/g
I_{INT}	Chemical interactions subindex
I_{FL}	Flammability subindex, °C
I_{EX}	Explosiveness subindex, %
I_{TOX}	Toxicity subindex, ppm
I_{COR}	Corrosivity subindex
I_I	Inventory subindex, t/h
I_T	Temperature subindex, °C
I_P	Pressure subindex, bar
I_{EQ}	Equipment safety subindex
I_{ST}	Safe structure level subindex
VCM	Vinyl chloride monomer
PVC	Polyvinyl chloride
PVA	Polyvinyl alcohol

References

1. Witlox, H.W.; Fernandez, M.; Harper, M.; Stene, J. Modelling and validation of atmospheric expansion and near-field dispersion for pressurised vapour or two-phase releases. *J. Loss Prev. Process Ind.* **2017**, *48*, 331–344. [CrossRef]
2. Hong, Y.; Pasman, H.J.; Sachdeva, S.; Markowski, A.S.; Mannan, M.S. A fuzzy logic and probabilistic hybrid approach to quantify the uncertainty in layer of protection analysis. *J. Loss Prev. Process Ind.* **2016**, *43*, 10–17. [CrossRef]
3. Dimian, A.C.; Bildea, C.S.; Kiss, A.A. Pinch point analysis. In *Computer Aided Chemical Engineering*; Elsevier: Amsterdam, The Netherlands, 2014; Volume 35, pp. 525–564. [CrossRef]
4. Bolt, H.M. Vinyl Chloride—A Classical Industrial Toxicant of New Interest. *Crit. Rev. Toxicol.* **2005**, *35*, 307–323. [CrossRef]
5. Nawaz, W.; Linke, P.; Koç, M. Safety and sustainability nexus: A review and appraisal. *J. Clean. Prod.* **2019**, *216*, 74–87. [CrossRef]
6. González-Delgado, Á.D.; Aguilar-Vásquez, E.; Ramos-Olmos, M. Chemical and Process Inherent Safety Analysis of Large-Scale Suspension Poly(Vinyl Chloride) Production. *Chemengineering* **2023**, *7*, 76. [CrossRef]
7. Park, S.; Xu, S.; Rogers, W.; Pasman, H.; El-Halwagi, M.M. Incorporating inherent safety during the conceptual process design stage: A literature review. *J. Loss Prev. Process Ind.* **2020**, *63*, 104040. [CrossRef]

8. Mendivil-Arrieta, A.; Aguilar-Vasquez, E.A.; Diaz-Perez, J.M.; Ramos-Olmos, M.; Gonzaléz-Delgado, Á.D. Energy Integration and WEP Technical Evaluation of a Large-Scale PVC Production Process. *Sci* **2025**, *7*, 41. [CrossRef]
9. Ahmad, S.I.; Hashim, H.; Hassim, M.H. A graphical method for assessing inherent safety during research and development phase of process design. *J. Loss Prev. Process Ind.* **2016**, *42*, 59–69. [CrossRef]
10. Chan, I.; Alwi, S.R.W.; Hassim, M.H.; Manan, Z.A.; Klemeš, J.J. Heat Exchanger Network Design Considering Inherent Safety. *Energy Procedia* **2014**, *61*, 2469–2473. [CrossRef]
11. Dunjó, J.; Fthenakis, V.; Vílchez, J.A.; Arnaldos, J. Hazard and operability (HAZOP) analysis. A literature review. *J. Hazard. Mater.* **2010**, *173*, 19–32. [CrossRef]
12. Marhavilas, P.K.; Filippidis, M.; Koulinas, G.K.; Koulouriotis, D.E. The integration of HAZOP study with risk-matrix and the analytical-hierarchy process for identifying critical control-points and prioritizing risks in industry—A case study. *J. Loss Prev. Process Ind.* **2019**, *62*, 103981. [CrossRef]
13. Sano, K.; Koshiba, Y.; Ohtani, H. Risk assessment and risk reduction of an acrylonitrile production plant. *J. Loss Prev. Process Ind.* **2020**, *63*, 104015. [CrossRef]
14. Evangelista Benites, G.; Loyola Carranza, W.; Ramírez Ruiz, R.; Aguilar Rojas, P. Optimización de redes de intercambiadores de calor en endulzamiento de gas natural vía tecnología pinch. *Sciéndo Ingenium* **2017**, *12*, 167–184.
15. Arunthavanathan, R.; Sajid, Z.; Amin, T.; Tian, Y.; Khan, F.; Pistikopoulos, E. Process safety 4.0: Artificial intelligence or intelligence augmentation for safer process operation? *AIChE J.* **2024**, *70*, e18475. [CrossRef]
16. Azizi, A. *Applications of Artificial Intelligence Techniques in Industry 4.0*; Springer: Singapore, 2019. [CrossRef]
17. Zhang, F.; Jan, N. Design and Implementation of Industrial Design and Transformation System Based on Artificial Intelligence Technology. *Math. Probl. Eng.* **2022**, *2022*, 1–9. [CrossRef]
18. Aguilar-Vásquez, E.; Ramos-Olmos, M.; González-Delgado, Á.D. A Joint Computer-Aided Simulation and Water-Energy-Product (WEP) Approach for Technical Evaluation of PVC Production. *Sustainability* **2023**, *15*, 8096. [CrossRef]
19. Mondal, S.K.; Uddin, M.R.; Paul, P.; Deb, A.; Azad, A. Minimization of the Process Loss in Condensate Fractionation Plant. *Procedia Eng.* **2014**, *90*, 524–529. [CrossRef]
20. Kletz, T.A. Inherently safer design: The growth of an idea. *Process Saf. Prog.* **1996**, *15*, 5–8. [CrossRef]
21. Kletz, T.A. Inherently safer plants. *Plant Oper. Prog.* **1985**, *4*, 164–167. [CrossRef]
22. Heikkilä, A.M. *Inherent Safety in Process Plant Design. An Index-Based Approach*; VTT Technical Research Centre of Finland: Espoo, Finland, 1999.
23. Cui, X.; Gui, X.; Hu, J.; Liu, J.; Zhou, R.; Gong, Z.; Li, W.; Yang, Y.; Dong, Y. Thermal safety and overall kinetics for methyl methacrylate solution polymerization via on-line process analytical technology. *Thermochim. Acta* **2023**, *730*, 179620. [CrossRef]
24. Tian, W.; Wu, H.; Liu, Z.; Liu, B.; Cui, Z. Intelligent prediction of incipient fault in vinyl chloride production process based on deep learning. *J. Clean. Prod.* **2024**, *472*, 143474. [CrossRef]
25. Bagheri, M.; Borhani, T.N.G.; Zahedi, G. Estimation of flash point and autoignition temperature of organic sulfur chemicals. *Energy Convers. Manag.* **2012**, *58*, 185–196. [CrossRef]
26. Giurcan, V.; Razus, D.; Mitu, M.; Oancea, D. Prediction of flammability limits of fuel-air and fuel-air-inert mixtures from explosivity parameters in closed vessels. *J. Loss Prev. Process Ind.* **2015**, *34*, 65–71. [CrossRef]
27. Lynch, H.N.; Prueitt, R.L.; Goodman, J.E. Critique of the ACGIH 2016 derivation of toluene diisocyanate Threshold Limit Values. *Regul. Toxicol. Pharmacol.* **2018**, *97*, 189–196. [CrossRef]
28. Chong, N.S.; Abdulramoni, S.; Patterson, D.; Brown, H. Releases of Fire-Derived Contaminants from Polymer Pipes Made of Polyvinyl Chloride. *Toxics* **2019**, *7*, 57. [CrossRef] [PubMed]
29. Todd, G.D.; Faroon, O.; Jones, D.; Lumpkin, M.H.; Stickney, J.; Citra, M.J. *Toxicological Profile for Vinyl Chloride*; Agency for Toxic Substances and Disease Registry (ATSDR) Toxicological Profiles: Atlanta, GA, USA, 2006.
30. O'Mara, M.M.; Grider, L.B.; Daniel, R.L. Combustion Products from Vinyl Chloride Monomer. *Am. Ind. Hyg. Assoc. J.* **1971**, *32*, 153–156. [CrossRef]
31. Veysi, A.; Roushani, M.; Najafi, H. Synthesis and evaluation of CuNi-MOF as a corrosion inhibitor of AISI 304 and 316 stainless steel in 1N HCl solution. *Heliyon* **2025**, *11*, e41296. [CrossRef]
32. Fàbregas i Oller, O.; Marín Merrouni, N.; Sánchez Martínez, A.; Sánchez Cano, S.; Serrano i Vallvé, M. Planta de producción de cloruro de vinilo. 2018. Available online: https://ddd.uab.cat/record/199194 (accessed on 1 June 2025).
33. U.S. Chemical Safety and Hazard Investigation Board. *Investigation Report—Vinyl Chloride Monomer Explosion (5 Dead, 3 Injured, and Community Evacuated)*; U.S. Chemical Safety and Hazard Investigation Board: Washington, DC, USA, 2007.
34. Aquino-Gaspar, H.M.; Díaz-Ovalle, C.O.; López-Molina, A.; Conde-Mejía, C.; Valenzuela-Gómez, L.M. Incident analysis of the "Pajaritos" petrochemical complex. *J. Loss Prev. Process Ind.* **2021**, *70*, 104404. [CrossRef]
35. Ogle, R.A.; Megerle, M.V.; Morrison, D.R.; Carpenter, A.R. Explosion caused by flashing liquid in a process vessel. *J. Hazard. Mater.* **2004**, *115*, 133–140. [CrossRef]

36. Hernández, J.G.S.; Gómez-Castro, F.I.; Romero-Izquierdo, A.G.; Conde-Mejía, C.; López-Molina, A. Partial energy integration between biofuels production processes: Effect on costs, CO_2 emissions and process safety. *Process Saf. Environ. Prot.* **2022**, *159*, 918–930. [CrossRef]
37. Zhu, J.; Chen, L.; Liu, Z.; Hao, L.; Wei, H. Synergy of electrification and energy efficiency improvement via vapor recompression heat pump and heat exchanger network to achieve decarbonization of extractive distillation. *Sep. Purif. Technol.* **2022**, *293*, 121065. [CrossRef]

processes

MDPI

Article

The Design of an Intensified Process and Production Plant for Cosmetic Emulsions Using Amazonian Oils

Laura Scalvenzi [1,*], Estela Guardado Yordi [1], Edgar Wilfrido Santamaría Caño [1], Ibeth Nina Avilez Tolagasi [1], Matteo Radice [1], Reinier Abreu-Naranjo [2], Lianne León Guardado [3], Luis Ramón Bravo Sánchez [1] and Amaury Pérez Martínez [1,*]

1 Facultad de Ciencias de la Tierra, Universidad Estatal Amazónica, Puyo 160150, Ecuador; e.guardadoy@uea.edu.ec (E.G.Y.); ueaedgarsantamaria95@outlook.com (E.W.S.C.); ibethnina2599@gmail.com (I.N.A.T.); mradice@uea.edu.ec (M.R.); lbravo@uea.edu.ec (L.R.B.S.)
2 Facultad de Ciencias de la Vida, Universidad Estatal Amazónica, Puyo 160150, Ecuador; rabreu@uea.edu.ec
3 Independent Researcher, Miami, FL 33012, USA; liannegleon@gmail.com
* Correspondence: lscalvenzi@uea.edu.ec (L.S.); amperez@uea.edu.ec (A.P.M.)

Abstract: The cosmetic industry in the Ecuadorian Amazon region faces the challenge of competitively integrating locally sourced plant-based raw materials into efficient and sustainable production processes. This study proposes the design of a pilot plant for the production of a cosmetic emulsion (CE), using oils extracted from Morete (*Mauritia flexuosa*) and Ungurahua (*Oenocarpus bataua*), with a focus on process intensification to reduce both capital investment and resource consumption. Process design methodologies and computational simulation (SuperPro Designer V10) were applied, along with Systematic Layout Planning (SLP) principles to optimize spatial configuration. The intensified scheme enabled the integration of extraction lines, reducing the number of major equipment units from 12 to 9 and lowering the investment from USD 1,016,000 to USD 719,000. Energy and environmental indicators showed consumption levels of 5.86 kWh and 48.4 kg of water per kg of cream, which are lower than those reported for other natural cosmetics plants. The intensified design achieved a Net Present Value (NPV) of USD 577,000 and a payback period of 3.93 years. Furthermore, solid by-products were valorized through circular economy principles. This approach offers a feasible, viable, and sustainable solution for the utilization of these Amazonian oils in the cosmetic industry.

Keywords: technological process; vegetable oils; SuperPro Designer V10; SketchUp web 2022; enhanced technology

1. Introduction

In recent years, the emulsions industry has been in a constant state of flux, and by the year 2020, this market was valued at USD 341.1 billion. It is expected to reach USD 560.5 billion by 2030, with a compound annual growth rate of 5.1%, between 2021 and 2030 [1].

The emulsions industry in Ecuador represents 1.6% of the GDP, producing 1100 million dollars a year and growing annually by 10%, which has led to the generation of many job opportunities [2]. The industry is placing greater emphasis on individuals aged 12 to 25, because this age group constitutes the primary consumer base for emulsion products such as cosmetic emulsion [3].

Cosmetic emulsion (EC) refers to homogeneous, semi-solid preparations intended for skin application consisting of opaque emulsion systems [4]. The consistency and properties of these creams vary depending on the type of emulsion and the raw materials used. These raw materials are primarily vegetable oils—substances produced by the metabolism of certain plants [5]. Therefore, it is necessary to use plant oils as raw materials. These oils not only serve sensorial and functional roles in the formulation, but they may also exhibit desirable depigmenting activity in certain cosmetic products [6]. They can also enhance oxidative stability, the bioavailability of bioactive compounds, and skin compatibility, which is key in the design of differentiated and sustainable products. In cosmetic production, the use of plant oils and the analysis of their triacylglycerol composition are essential to formulate sustainable products. These oils not only reduce the environmental footprint, but also act as (i) natural emollients, which improve skin flexibility and resilience, (ii) strengthen the skin barrier through their hydrophobic nature, and (iii) provide antioxidant benefits that enhance the overall quality of the cosmetic product [7].

When applied to the skin, the water available in the cream evaporates and creates a cooling sensation, while the oil creates a protective barrier. Creams with a higher amount of oil, or oily phase, are ideal for dry, sensitive skin or skin prone to atopic dermatitis, as they provide superior hydration and nourishment [8].

ECs are used for skin care, moisturizing and slowing down the aging process [9]. Many consumers prefer to use products containing plant-based components, which has led to research into alternatives that meet these requirements. Plant oils are also used to make soaps, medicines, foodstuffs, and other products [10]. There are a variety of plant oils; however, the most traditional are olive, avocado, and coconut oil [11]. In the Amazonian forest, promising oils have been extracted from fruits such as Morete (*Mauritia flexuosa*) and Ungurahua (*Oenocarpus bataua*). Amazonian oils are distinguished by their high content of essential fatty acids (such as oleic and linoleic acids), phytosterols, and antioxidant compounds, making them high-value functional raw materials for cosmetic formulations with both ecological appeal and sensorial benefits [12].

Studies have shown that ECs, formulated with these oils, exhibited properties such as skin softening, as well as enhancing skin radiance and firmness. Other fruits, including Sacha Inchi (*Plukenetia volubilis*), Chontaduro (*Bactris gasipaes*), and Ginger (*Zingiber officinale*), showed similar properties but few studies are available [13]. Proaño et al. [14] developed an exfoliating cream using passion fruit oil and its seeds as an alternative raw material, addressing the significant waste generated by passion fruit seeds. Similarly, Rivera et al. [15] formulated an exfoliating cream based on Morete peels, highlighting its potential as a valuable contribution to the development of new emulsion-based formulations by Proaño et al. [14].

The utilization of plant by-products in cosmetics opens the door to circular economy strategies, which can be incorporated into the plant design to minimize waste, reduce raw material costs, and add value to local agro-industrial processes [16–19].

A study reports that the production of Morete and Ungurahua-based cream involves two distinct phases, each with a specific technological process tailored to meet defined criteria. These phases incorporate key unit operations—heating, mixing, agitation, homogenization, and cooling—which must be precisely controlled to ensure the final product's physical stability, sensory quality, and functional performance [20].

Technological advancements in emulsion production have progressed significantly, and a variety of equipment and processing techniques are now available for manufacturing diverse cosmetic emulsion formulations [21]. Process design methodologies, such as the one proposed by Cerda Mejía et al. [22] for hydroalcoholic gel production, have been successfully applied to the development of products analogous to emulsion-based creams.

In this case, simulation and computational modeling tools—such as process flow diagrams, Aspen Plus-type simulators, and energy consumption estimation—were applied to facilitate the scaling of processes from the laboratory to the pilot plant level, incorporating criteria of sustainability and operational efficiency.

Beltrán Chacón & Aguayo Carvajal [23] mention that it should be taken into account that the investment for the start-up of an agro-industrial plant is significant, as the acquisition of equipment represents one of the biggest expenses within a company. For this reason, a well-planned and designed plant should favor the efficient use of the resources within it, thus contributing to environmental sustainability. The process should also be optimized to minimize complexity and waste while enhancing overall efficiency. Additionally, the consideration of worker safety and ergonomics is essential to mitigate potential future costs related to compensation, regulatory fines, or other liabilities.

To reduce investment and acquisition costs, process intensification can be considered. According to [24], process intensification represents one of the most promising areas for industrial development. This approach involves modifying conventional processes or developing novel technologies to lower energy consumption, enhance yields, and improve product quality. Specifically, it aims to increase efficiency and production benefits, improve processing quality and safety, minimize the size of both primary and auxiliary equipment, and reduce waste and energy demands through the adoption of more sustainable technologies [25].

Research on the oil properties of Morete and Ungurahua has been carried out at laboratory level (basic research), and cosmetic emulsions have been produced in small quantities [20]. However, in the Amazonian context, the problem is that there is no technological process or plant designed to obtain EC from Morete and Ungurahua oils at a pilot or industrial level. This reveals a technological gap that currently limits industrial-scale production, due to the absence of well-defined parameters such as plant capacity, emulsion yield, energy consumption, material compatibility, and standardized operating conditions. In response, this study aims to design a pilot plant for the production of a cosmetic emulsion formulated with Amazonian plant oils, by applying process simulation tools and principles of process intensification to develop an efficient, scalable, and environmentally sustainable manufacturing system.

2. Materials and Methods

The design of an industrial plant for the production of EC was carried out following the methodology proposed by Dimian [26], which comprises four stages. These stages include the definition of requirements, conceptual design, and basic design, which collectively form the core of the process design. Additionally, detailed engineering was incorporated to develop the plant layout, ensuring a well-structured facility capable of producing high-quality cosmetic emulsion with efficiency and sustainability [26]. The complete procedures for fruit selection, oil extraction, emulsion formulation, final product measurement, and material balance calculations were described in detail in Guardado et al. [20].

2.1. Proposal for the Design of the Technological Process

The design of the technological process of an EC was carried out using the methodology proposed by Pérez-Martínez et al. [27]. This phase includes product identification, technology selection, and definition of the technological scheme. Production capacity, macro-location, and mass and energy balances are assessed. Raw material availability, environmental compatibility, and equipment design and costs are evaluated. Process control is implemented, followed by investment and production cost analysis to identify optimized, viable alternatives. Finally, the integration of emerging technologies is considered.

The process intensification strategies employed included equipment integration as proposed by Stankiewicz and Moulijn [28], utility integration based on the approach in [29,30], and by-product valorization within a circular economy framework as suggested by Frosch and Gallopoulos [31]. These techniques were selected to achieve the following intensification objectives: (a) reducing the number of equipment units by leveraging similarities in the extraction processes of Morete and Ungurahua oils; (b) minimizing energy and material consumption through steam reuse; and (c) decreasing environmental impact by implementing a valorization strategy for the generated waste.

2.2. Plant Distribution Strategy for the Production of Emulsion Creams

As a complement to the process design, the simulation methodology proposed by Dimian et al. [32] was applied, comprising four stages: data analysis, input, simulation execution, and result evaluation. Initially, relevant data is collected and analyzed, then entered the simulator to configure process parameters. The simulation was executed to model system behavior under various conditions. Finally, the results were assessed to optimize process design and operation [32].

To simulate the design of an EC manufacturing plant, the SuperPro Designer V10.0 (Intelligen, Freehold, NJ, USA) simulator was used. The simulation considered a 7% discount rate and a 20-year analysis horizon for the calculation of dynamic economic indicators. Additionally, the breakdown of operating costs implemented in SuperPro Designer V10 was considered.

Plant layout was developed using Richard Muther's Systematic Layout Planning (SLP) methodology (1968). This approach supports efficient design by systematically considering material flow, accessibility, safety, and optimal space utilization in the cosmetic emulsion manufacturing plant [33,34].

This method minimizes material handling costs, reduces production time, and improves workflow by strategically organizing the workstation, departments, equipment, and other elements within a facility; the nature of this distribution can vary depending on the type of industry, production processes, workflow needs, and other factors [35]. Computerized software, specifically SketchUp Web 2022, was used to visualize and optimize the distribution and sizing of areas and equipment.

3. Results

3.1. Proposal for the Design of the Technological Process

3.1.1. Product in Demand

The production of EC requires the extraction of oils from Morete and Ungurahua fruits. Once obtained, the fatty phase (oils and cocoa butter) and the aqueous phase (purified water) were prepared. The emulsifier was then added and mixed, followed by the incorporation of the aqueous into the fatty phase. Finally, a preservative is added, and the mixture stored.

3.1.2. Technology Selection

Figure 1a,b illustrate the processes to produce EC using Morete and Ungurahua fruit oils characterized by unit operations. Two technologies with similar characteristics are used in the traditional method (Figure 1a), while the intensified technology (Figure 1b) evaluates the economic feasibility of a single extraction line for both oils. In the proposed process, both oils are extracted using a single technology; when Morete oil is not being extracted, the line is cleaned and prepared for Ungurahua oil extraction, and vice versa. The first step involves selection and washing, where fruits with bruises or poor conditions are discarded based on ripeness, ensuring cleanliness. The fruits are then softened at 100 °C for 1 h, facilitating pulping and allowing for easier oil extraction.

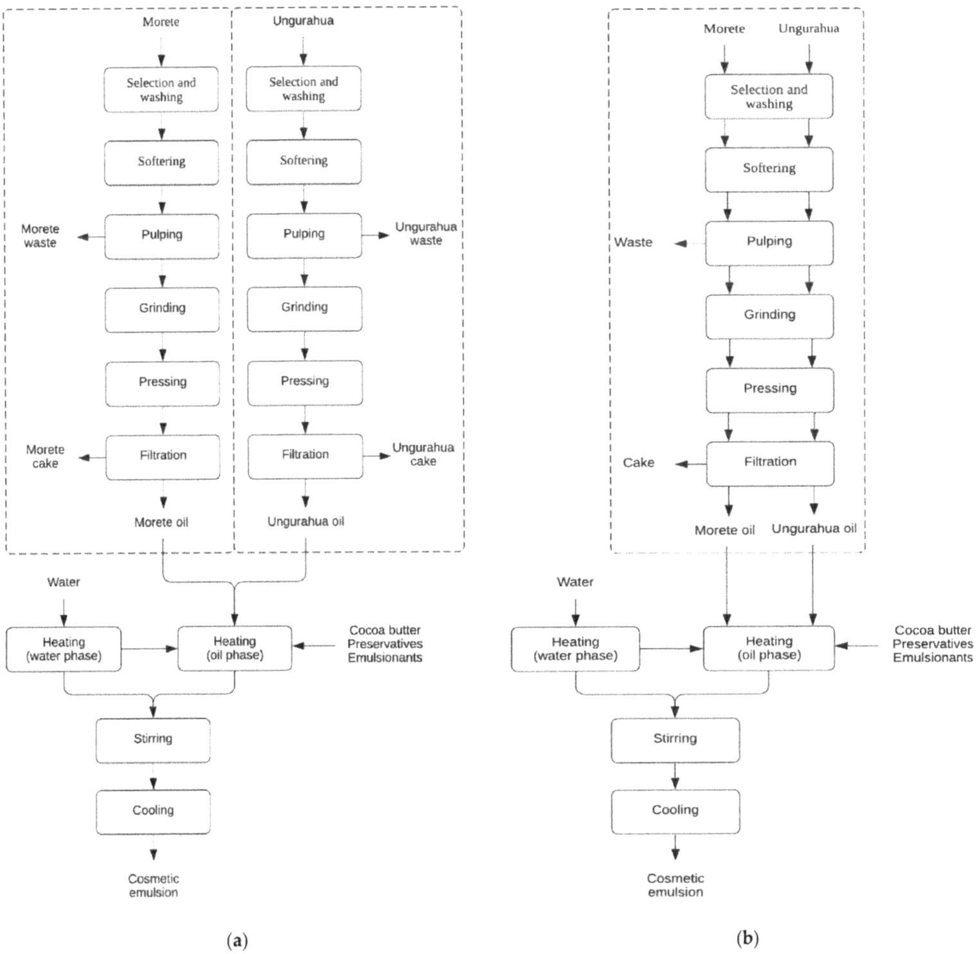

Figure 1. A block diagram illustrating the process of obtaining Morete and Unguarahua oil and emulsion with (**a**) traditional technology [20]; (**b**) intensified.

All of the processes mentioned above fit the Gantt chart, as summarized in Figure 2a,b.

3.1.3. The Technological Scheme

Figure 3a,b present the process flow diagrams for traditional and intensified technologies. It can be observed that the vegetable oil production line is streamlined, with a single technology employed, leading to a more efficient work organization as shown in the Gantt chart in Figure 2. In the intensified technology (Figure 3b), after softening and progression through each unit operation, the equipment can be cleaned and reused for the alternate extraction process once the first extraction is completed.

3.1.4. Production Capacity Estimation

To estimate the production capacity of cosmetic emulsion from Morete and Ungurahua, 2.5 kg of Morete and 10.5 kg of Ungurahua were used to produce a total of 18.98 kg of cosmetic emulsion, with 13 kg coming from the main ingredients, and the production ratio was calculated by dividing the amount of cream produced by the total ingredients, resulting in a production rate of 1.46 kg of cream per kilogram of ingredients.

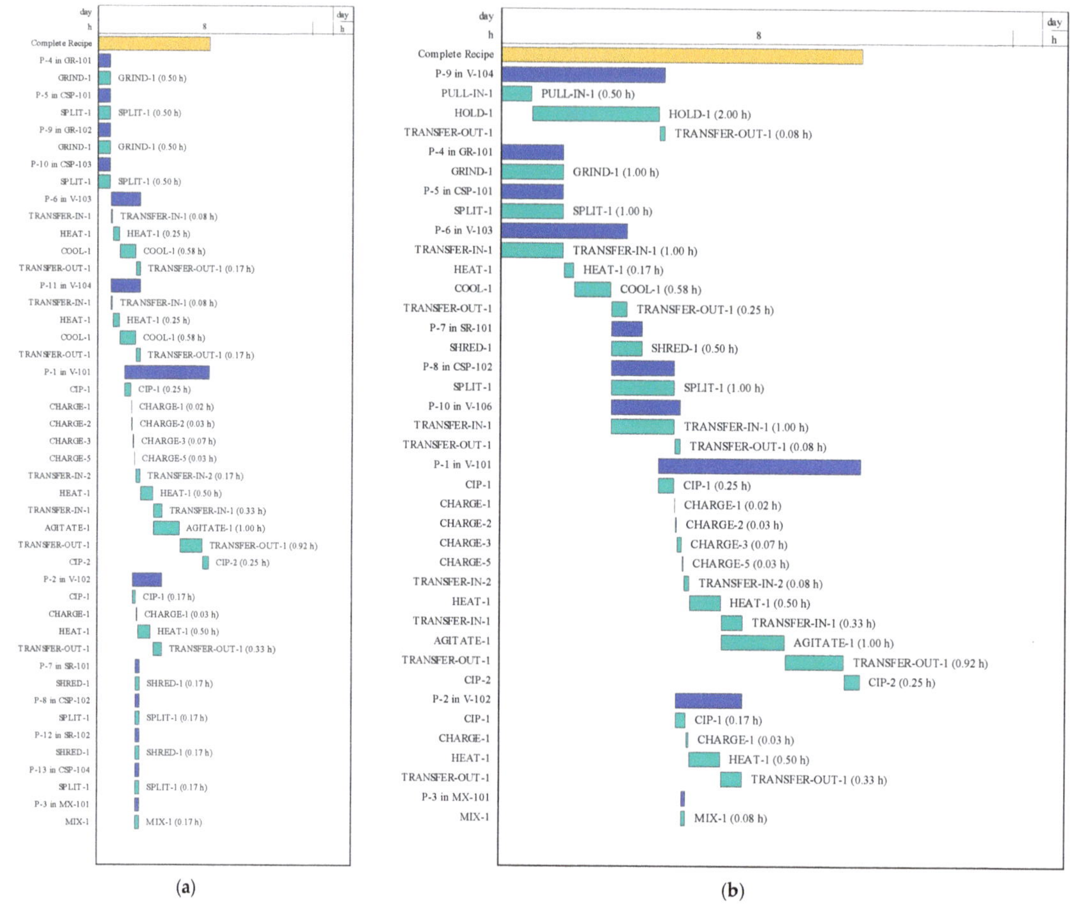

Figure 2. Gantt chart (**a**); traditional [20]; (**b**) intensified. The key stages are represented, including grinding (GRIND), separation (SPLIT), heating (HEAT), agitation (AGITATE), material transfer (TRANSFER-IN and TRANSFER-OUT), and cleaning (CIP), allowing for the visualization of the duration and sequence of each operation within the process.

3.1.5. Location

Due to the availability of the raw material, the processing plant for the extraction and production of EC will be located in the province of Napo, Tena Canton, in the Muyuna parish, as shown in Figure 4.

3.1.6. Mass and Energy Balances, and Environmental Compatibility

Table 1 details the environmental indicators associated with the annual production of 4717.48 kg, representing 260 batches of cosmetic creams for both traditional and intensified technologies.

Furthermore, in terms of energy consumption, traditional plants of the same size reported an expenditure varying between 8 and 10 kWh/kg of cream and an estimated carbon footprint of 3.5–4.0 kg CO_2e/kg product [36]. However, the intensified scheme reduced energy consumption to 5.86 kWh/kg and limits emissions to around 2.3–3.0 kg CO_2e/kg, thanks to the shared use of steam for heating and the aqueous phase, as well as the optimization of equipment distribution. These results demonstrate a 25–30% improvement in energy efficiency and emission reduction.

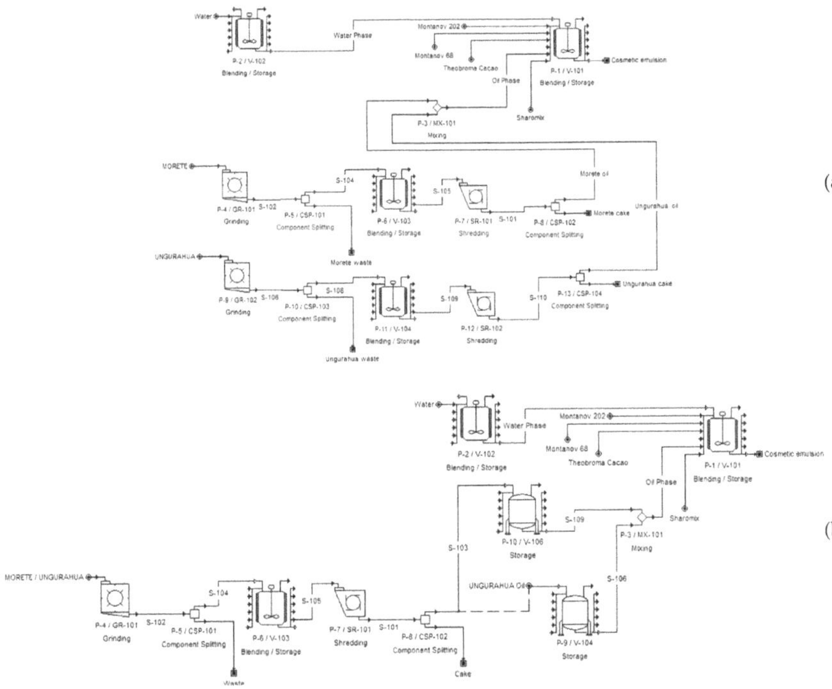

(a)

(b)

Figure 3. Process flow diagram (**a**); traditional [20]; (**b**) intensified. GR-101, GR-102 (grinding); CSP-101, CSP-102, CSP-103, CSP-104 (component splitting); SR-101, SR-102 (shredding); V-101, V-102, V-103, V-104 (blending/storage); P-102, P-103, P-104 (transfer pumps); M-103 (final mixing); Montanov 202, Montanov 68b, Theobroma cacao, Sharomix (ingredients for the oil phase of the emulsion); cosmetic emulsion (final product).

Table 1. Comparison of extraction methods, unit operations, and equipment for Morete and Ungurahua oils.

Environmental Indicator	Input/Output Current	Amount		Unit
		Traditional Technology	Intensified Technology	
Raw material consumption	Montanov 68	0.011	0.011	kg/kg
	Montanov 202	0.036	0.036	kg/kg
	Morete fruit	0.136	0.136	kg/kg
	Sharomix	0.011	0.011	kg/kg
	Cocoa butter	0.111	0.111	kg/kg
	Ungurahua fruit	0.563	0.563	kg/kg
Water consumption	Water	48.411	48.411	kg/kg
Energy consumption	Power consumption	5.86	5.86	kW·h/kg
	Steam consumption	10	10	kg/kg
	Refrigerated water	260	260	kg/kg
Discharge	Of gases	-	-	-
	Of liquids	-	-	-
	Of solids	0.56	0.56	kg/kg
Cosmetic emulsion		4717.48	4717.48	kg/yr

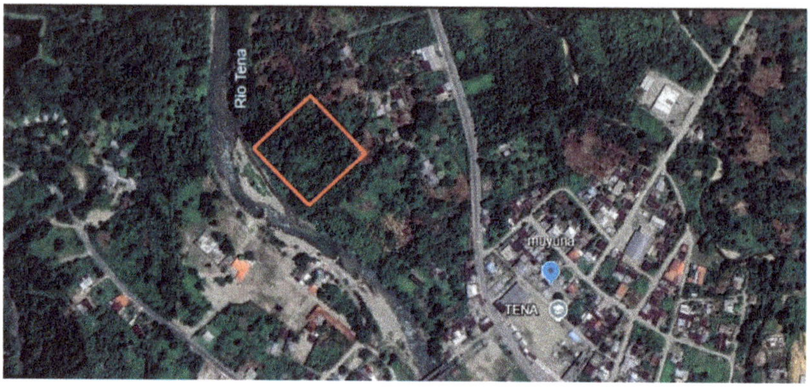

Figure 4. The location of the processing plant. The red box indicates the possible location of the plant.

3.1.7. Sizing of Equipment and Cost of Acquisition

To determine the equipment size and calculate acquisition costs, it is crucial to define the entire manufacturing process for both traditional and intensified technologies. Table 2 lists the equipment used in the processes of extracting plant oils and preparing EC, along with their design parameters, quantities, and purchasing costs. The total cost to purchase equipment for the traditional technology is USD 126,000.00, while the cost for the intensified technology is USD 88,000.00, reflecting a reduction in the amount of equipment.

Table 2. Equipment acquisition cost.

Quantity	Name	Design Parameter	Cost (USD)	
			Traditional Technology	Intensified Technology
1	Turbo-emulsifier	Tank volume = 22.47 L	20,000	20,000
1	Turbo-emulsifier	Tank volume = 14.66 L	20,000	20,000
1	Pulper	Nominal Yield = 2.55 kg/h	14,000	14,000
1	Pulper	Nominal Yield = 10.58 kg/h	14,000	
1	Jacketed tank	Tank volume = 2.62 L	10,000	10,000
1	Jacketed tank	Tank volume = 8.95 L	10,000	
1	Shredder	Nominal Yield = 2.55 kg/h	1000	6000
1	Shredder	Nominal Yield = 2.16 kg/h	1000	
1	Press	Nominal Yield = 12.98 kg/h	6000	
1	Press	Nominal Yield = 45.82 kg/h	6000	
1	Storage tank	Tank volume = 1.11 L	-	1000
1	Storage tank	Tank volume = 2.58 L	-	1000
	Equipment not listed		25,000	18,000
	Total		126,000	88,000

3.1.8. Economic Analysis and Feasibility

The Total Plant Direct Cost (TPDC) of the intensified design (Table 3) demonstrated an approximate 31% reduction, compared to conventional technology. This reflects the impact of the decreased number and size of equipment, optimized layout, and streamlined installation processes on this cost. This reduction in investment expenses results in an approximate 29% overall decrease in total investment cost. Consequently, the intensified process offered an economic advantage by requiring significantly less capital for plant investment.

Table 3. Estimated investment costs of traditional vs. intensified technology.

Cost Items	Cost (USD) Traditional Technology	Intensified Technology
3A. Total Plant Direct Cost (TPDC)		
1. Equipment Purchase	126,000	88,000
2. Installation	51,000	34,000
3. Process Piping	44,000	31,000
4. Instrumentation	50,000	35,000
5. Insulation	4000	3000
6. Electrical	13,000	9000
7. Buildings	57,000	40,000
8. Yard Improvement	19,000	13,000
9. Auxiliary Facilities	50,000	35,000
TPDC	414,000	287,000
3B. Total Plant Indirect Cost (TPIC)		
10. Engineering	103,000	72,000
11. Construction	145,000	100,000
TPIC	248,000	172,000
3B. Total Plant Indirect Cost (TPIC)		
3C. Total Plant Cost (TPC = TPDC + TPIC)		
TPC	662,000	459,000
3D. Contractor's Fee and Contingency (CFC)		
12. Contractor's Fee	33,000	23,000
13. Contingency	66,000	46,000
CFC = 12 + 13	99,000	69,000
3E. Direct Fixed Capital Cost (DFC = TPC + CFC)		
A. DFC	761,000	528,000
B. Working Capital	217,000	165,000
C. Startup Cost	38,000	26,000
D. Up-Front R&D	0	0
E. Up-Front Royalties	0	0
F. Total Investment (A + B+C + D+E)	1,016,000	719,000
G. Investment Charged to This Project	1,016,000	719,000

After the intensification process, the total annual operating cost is reduced from USD 441,000 to USD 324,000 (Table 4). Most of the savings result from a relevant decrease in costs depending on the plant and the elimination of waste treatment expenses. Although staff costs still account for nearly half of the total budget, process intensification reduces the need for facilities and inputs, thereby lowering operating costs without compromising product quality.

Figure 5a shows that for traditional technology, the investment cost for 260 batches is USD 1,016,000.00, while the annual production cost is USD 441,000.00. In contrast, for intensified technology (Figure 5c), the investment cost for 260 batches is USD 747,000.00, and the annual production cost is USD 357,000.00.

Both traditional and intensified technologies for producing emulsion cream are cost-effective, but intensified technology provides greater economic benefits. While traditional technology has a Net Present Value (NPV) of USD 216,000.00 (Figure 5b), intensified technology achieves an NPV of USD 577,000.00 (Figure 5d), indicating a significantly higher return on investment in a shorter time.

Table 4. Estimated production costs in US dollars: Traditional vs. intensified technology.

Cost Items	Traditional Technology (USD)	Percent	Intensified Technology (USD)	Percent
Raw Materials	27,000	6.12	27,000	8.33
Labor-Dependent	217,000	49.21	161,000	49.69
Facility-Dependent	161,000	36.51	112,000	34.57
Laboratory/QC/QA	33,000	7.48	24,000	7.41
Consumables	0.00	0.00	0.00	0.00
Waste Treatment/Disposal	3000	0.68	0.00	0.00
Utilities	0.00	0.00	0.00	0.00
Transportation	0.00	0.00	0.00	0.00
Miscellaneous	0.00	0.00	0.00	0.00
Advertising/Selling	0.00	0.00	0.00	0.00
Running Royalties	0.00	0.00	0.00	0.00
Failed Product Disposal	0.00	0.00	0.00	0.00
Running Royalties	0.00	0.00	0.00	0.00
Failed Product Disposal	0.00	0.00	0.00	0.00
Total	441,000	100.00%	324,000	100.00%

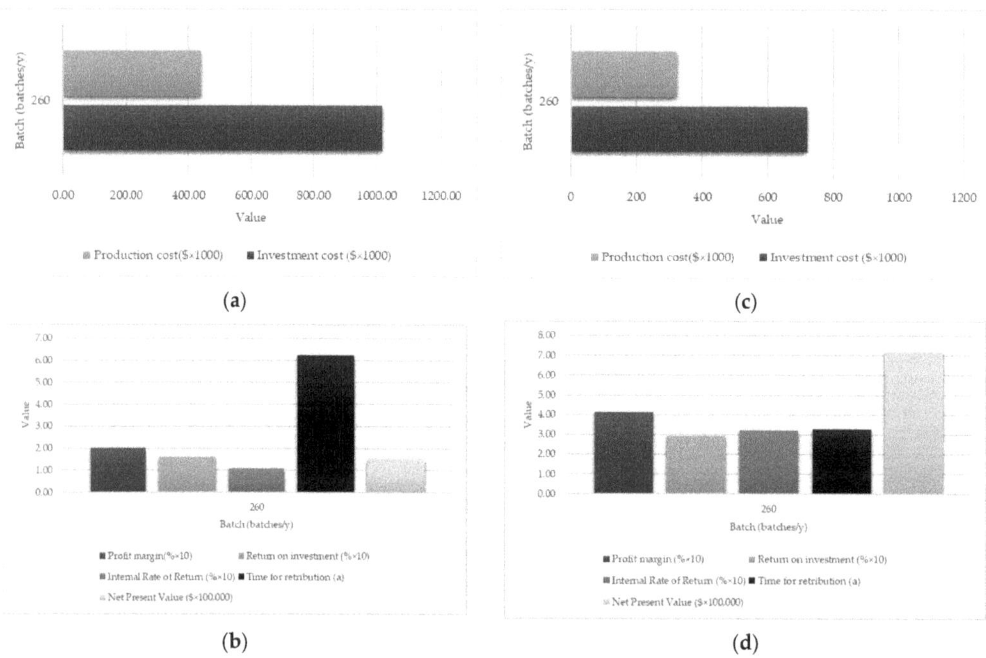

Figure 5. The results of the economic analysis; investment and production cost: (**a**) traditional [20]; (**c**) intensified; (**b**) dynamic economic and profitability indicators. (**b**) Traditional [20]; (**d**) intensified.

3.2. Plant Layout

The plant layout is the result of applying the Systematic Layout Planning (SLP) in its qualitative form. Priority was given to proximity relationships and functional flow between areas, without relying on distance or travel time metrics. Thus, the processes are grouped and sequenced in a logical manner, despite the absence of specific numerical indicators of operational efficiency.

The proposed layout for the ECC production plant, illustrated in Figure 6, begins at the unloading zone, followed by the raw material reception area (Z1), which includes designated sections for Morete and Ungurahua fruits. The production process initiates with the extraction of plant oils, represented by yellow arrows, and includes the following unit operations: selection (A), washing (B), softening (C), pulping (D), and pressing and filtration (E). Conveyor belt systems, shown with brown arrows, are integrated into pulping and pressing to facilitate the removal of solid waste.

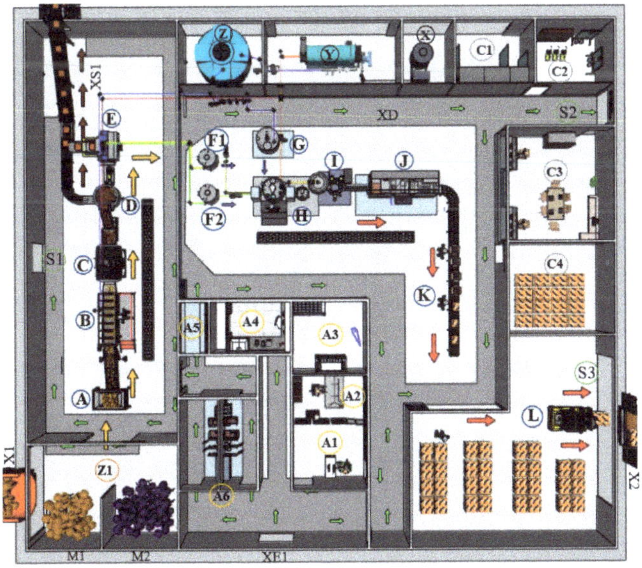

Figure 6. The distribution of the plant for producing emulsion creams. Production area: A. Selection; B. Washing; C. Softening; D. Pulping; E. Pressing and filtering; F1. Morete oil; F2. Ungurahua oil; G. Turbo-emulsifier aqueous phase; H. Turbo-emulsifier oil phase; I. Packaging machine; J. Labeling; K. Packaging; L. Storage; M1. Morete fruits; M2. Ungurahua fruits. Administration area: A1. Secretary; A2. Administrator; A3. Inputs and ingredients; A4. Laboratory; A5. Disinfection chamber; A6. Dressing rooms. Maintenance and control area: C1. Electrical systems; C2. Maintenance warehouse; C3. Control room; C4. Container and label warehouse. Complementary areas: X. Boiler fuel; X1. Discharge area; X2. Discharge area of finished products; XE1. Main entrance; XD. Staff movement area; XD. Waste exit; Y. Boiler; Z, Water storage. Emergency exits: S1., S2., S3. Discharge area: Z1. Initial disposal of the raw material. Cargo area.

After oil extraction, the oils are stored in dedicated tanks (F1) for Morete oil and (F2) for Ungurahua oil. The oil phase is then prepared in the turbo-emulsifier (H), and the aqueous phase (G) is added based on defined operational parameters. This sequence is indicated by blue arrows. The final processing stages include packaging (I), labeling (J), and boxing (K), concluding with final storage and a designated loading area (L). The production flow progresses linearly from (A) to (L), ensuring a streamlined, non-redundant workflow throughout the plant.

3.2.1. Principle of Integration

Specific areas are established for the movement of workers, marked in gray with green arrows, thus keeping all the following areas separate: production, administration, complementary systems, and a control and maintenance area.

Exclusive personnel routes were established to strategically group the production, administrative, and maintenance areas, minimizing interference between activities and ensuring a continuous, continuous process flow.

3.2.2. Principle of the Minimum Distance Traveled

Five strategic points are identified in the process: (1) placement of raw materials (Z1); (2) and (3) an analysis of oil samples (F1, F2) and cream (H) in the laboratory (A4); (4) the addition of inputs (A3) into the turbo-emulsifier for the fatty phase (H); and (5) the supply of materials from (C4) to the packaging (I), labeling (J), and final packing stations (K). By arranging these points in a logical sequence, unnecessary movements are removed, as each activity directly receives inputs from the previous stage without intersecting paths.

3.2.3. Material Flow

The production area begins with the oil extraction, involving unit operations A through E, indicated by yellow arrows. This constitutes the first operational zone in the process sequence. The extracted oils (F1 for Morete and F2 for Ungurahua) are stored, after which the turbo-emulsifier is initiated: first, the aqueous phase (G) is prepared and subsequently incorporated into the fatty phase (H) to form the emulsion. This progression is represented by blue arrows. The process then advances to the packaging unit (I), labeling station (J), and final packing and storage (K and L), as indicated by red arrows.

Additionally, this flow principle applies to the disposal of by-products from the pulping (D) and pressing (E) stages. These residues are transported out of the facility via conveyor belts, illustrated with brown arrows in Figure 6, ensuring efficient waste management without interfering with the main production line.

This sequential configuration ensures a continuous and unidirectional flow of materials and waste across all areas, by positioning extraction, emulsification, and packaging as contiguous stages, thereby eliminating cross-traffic.

3.2.4. Cubic Space Principle

Water flow is supplied to both the washing (B) and softening (C) stages during the oil extraction process. For cream preparation, filtered water is specifically allocated to the aqueous phase (G). Superheated steam is available in the extraction area to facilitate softening (C), while in the cream formulation stage, it is used both to heat the aqueous phase (G) and to regulate the temperature of the oil phase (H).

Through the designation of dedicated water and steam supply points for each stage—washing, softening, and formulation—pipeline overlap is eliminated, and spatial utilization is optimized without the need for volumetric calculations.

3.2.5. Principle of Satisfaction and Security

The administrative area is organized into distinct sections, including secretary (A1), administrator (A2), supply and material warehouse (A3), laboratory (A4), disinfection chamber (A5), and separate dressing rooms for men and women (A6), ensuring both staff satisfaction and product safety. This structured approach extends to the control and maintenance department (C3). The oil extraction and cream production processes are managed from a central control room, supervised by qualified staff. Additional dedicated spaces are provided for the electrical control system, maintenance storage, and the storage of labels and containers. In the complementary systems area, spaces are physically separated by solid walls to prevent heat transfer to the water (Z) and fuel (X) storage areas during operation, thereby minimizing the risk of accidents. In the case of an accident at the plant, three emergency exits were designed (S1, S2, S3).

The well-defined separation of offices, laboratories, and control areas reduces functional conflicts and enhances safety, as staff move through designated zones without interfering with critical operations.

3.2.6. Principle of Flexibility

The production area, comprising both the oil extraction and cream manufacturing processes, is designed with sufficient space to facilitate maintenance and accommodate the integration of additional, mobile, and easily removable equipment. The layout also incorporates the administration, complementary systems, and control and maintenance areas. This systematic and organized approach minimizes operational delays, enhances spatial efficiency, and supports smooth plant operation. Incorporating space for maintenance and movable equipment enables the plant design to adapt to future changes without requiring a complete layout reconfiguration, thereby ensuring operational continuity.

4. Discussion

The application of process intensification principles to the design of a pilot plant for cosmetic emulsion (CE) production using Morete and Ungurahua oils has demonstrated the efficient utilization of available raw materials [20]. The extraction and processing of these traditionally underutilized oils have been optimized to maximize cream production yield per kilogram of input, achieving 1.46 kg of CE/kg. This result confirms the feasibility of converting local seasonal fruits into high value-added products while strengthening supply chains in the Amazon region [20]. Locating the plant in Tena (Ecuador) and establishing supply agreements with local associations or communities is expected to ensure a steady flow of raw materials despite the seasonality of harvests.

Moreover, this study demonstrated that the use of local raw materials is not only applicable but also improves the final product by introducing elements of differentiation and sustainability [20]. Morete and Ungurahua oils, rich in essential fatty acids and antioxidants, provide superior cosmetic properties (hydration, repair, and skin barrier protection) that allow the CE to be positioned competitively in both regional and national markets, while also generating employment opportunities [18].

The integration of circular economy principles into the design enables the repurposing of pressing by-products into exfoliant ingredients or raw materials for biofertilizers, thereby closing the production loop and minimizing solid waste generation [33]. A major finding of this study is the relevant reduction in capital investment, driven by technological enhancements and strategic operational planning. By unifying the extraction lines for both oils with intermediate cleanings, the number of main equipment units was reduced from 12 to 9, and CAPEX (capital expenditure) decreased from USD 126,000 to USD 88,000. Simulation using SuperPro Designer V10 indicated a NPV of USD 577,000 and a payback period of 3.93 years—parameters that confirm the economic feasibility of an intensified scheme over a conventional design [34,35]. The reduction in fixed capital investment leads to decreased financial risk and a shorter payback period—key factors in attracting investment for sustainable agro-industrial initiatives. In addition, the study offers a comprehensive and well-structured representation of the plant layout, developed using the Systematic Layout Planning (SLP) methodology. The linear arrangement of processing areas—from raw material reception and extraction to turbo-emulsification and final packaging—reduces internal movement by 15%, minimizes downtime, and facilitates maintenance without interrupting production. The strategic zoning of thermal, humidity, and auxiliary systems, along with the incorporation of three emergency exits and service corridors, ensures compliance with international safety and ergonomic standards for pilot-scale operations. This schematic representation provides a solid foundation for the future construction of the pilot facility and serves as a valuable tool for training operational personnel.

The analysis of resource consumption and waste generation indicates the use of 48.4 kg of water, 10 kg of steam, and 5.86 kWh of electricity per kilogram of cream produced, along with the generation of 0.56 kg of solid waste per kilogram of cosmetic emulsion (CE). The water consumption results presented in the intensified design of this study were lower than those reported by Nydrioti et al. [37] which were 81.6 kg/kg of product in a natural cosmetics plant. Furthermore, in terms of energy consumption, traditional plants of the same size reported an expenditure varying between 8 and 10 kWh/kg of cream and an estimated carbon footprint of 3.5–4.0 kg CO_2e/kg product [36].

These figures reflect competitive environmental performance, remaining within acceptable limits for small-scale cosmetic manufacturing processes [37]. Furthermore, the valorization of press cake offers promising opportunities for integrating circular economy principles—for instance, through the extraction of residual phenolic compounds for cosmetic formulations or the fermentation of pulp to produce high-value biofertilizers [36].

Studies of chemical characterization of pressing cakes (e.g., argan, sunflower, and sesame) have shown total phenolic contents in the range of 3–10 mg GAE/g DM and DPPH antioxidant activities exceeding 15–78%, identifying them as rich sources of bioactive compounds [38].

Furthermore, analyses of commercial cosmetic formulations have reported that anti-aging and sunscreen products (13.2% and 5.2%, respectively) incorporate phenolics such as resveratrol, ferulic acid, or chrysin, leveraging their photoprotective and antioxidant properties to mitigate solar damage and oxidative stress [39].

These findings indicate that pressing cakes contain bioactive compounds which, if extracted, could serve as raw materials for formulating antioxidant tonics, anti-aging creams, or sunscreens of renewable origin—thus closing the production cycle within the framework of the circular economy and providing more affordable and sustainable ingredients for the cosmetic industry.

5. Conclusions

The proposed design of the CE production plant optimizes material flow and space utilization while ensuring operational safety for plant personnel. The layout of the plant is divided into several key areas: production, which includes plant oil extraction and cream formulation processes, discharge and loading zones, administration, supporting systems, and areas for control and maintenance. The process design was initially defined, followed by the application of integration principles such as minimizing material travel distances, ensuring efficient flow, optimizing cubic space, and prioritizing the safety and well-being of plant personnel interacting with the technology.

Additionally, the proposal for an intensified process in plant oil extraction and EC production reduces the amount of equipment, thus lowering both capital expenditure and overall investment. This streamlined approach demonstrates superior efficiency and profitability, resulting in a NPV of USD 577,000.00, a profit margin of 35.48%, and a reduced payback period of just 3.93 years.

Future research should explore emerging technologies such as ultrasound-assisted extraction and microwave treatments, which have the potential to increase yields while reducing processing times. The implementation of a digital twin, supported by a mathematical assistant and real-time sensor data to monitor operational parameters, would enable the predictive optimization of critical variables and facilitate preventive maintenance, thereby ensuring consistent CE quality. This holistic approach not only strengthens the competitiveness of the Amazonian cosmetic agro-industry but also establishes a foundation for future sustainable innovation and the valorization of the region's endogenous resources.

Author Contributions: Conceptualization, A.P.M. and E.G.Y.; methodology, E.W.S.C., L.L.G. and I.N.A.T.; software, A.P.M. and R.A.-N.; formal analysis, L.S., M.R. and L.R.B.S.; investigation, E.G.Y., L.L.G. and L.R.B.S.; writing—original draft preparation, R.A.-N. and L.S.; writing—review and editing, M.R. and E.G.Y.; supervision, A.P.M. All authors have read and agreed to the published version of the manuscript.

Funding: This study was funded by Universidad Estatal Amazónica in Puyo, Ecuador, and has been completed as part of the project: Desarrollo de Nuevos Productos Agroindustriales de Alto Valor Agregado a Partir de Aceites Fijos, Esenciales y Extractos de Plantas Ricos en Metabolitos Antioxidantes o Antimicrobianos [Development of New Agro-Industrial Products with High Added Value from Fixed Oils, Essential Oils, and Plant Extracts Rich in Antioxidant or Antimicrobial Metabolites].

Data Availability Statement: The original contributions presented in this study are included in the article. Further inquiries can be directed to the corresponding authors.

Acknowledgments: The authors wish to thank Helen Pugh for proofreading the article.

Conflicts of Interest: The authors declare no conflicts of interest.

References

1. Ferreira, M.; Matos, A.; Couras, A.; Marto, J.; Ribeiro, H. Overview of Cosmetic Regulatory Frameworks around the World. *Cosmetics* **2022**, *9*, 72. [CrossRef]
2. Ruilova Accini, P.V.; Sempertegui Seminario, C.A.; Guerrero Muñoz, M.K. Calidad Del Servicio de Las Empresas Asociadas a La Industria Cosmética En El Ecuador. *Soc. Tecnol.* **2019**, *4*, 298–311. [CrossRef]
3. Mancheno Saá, M.; Gamboa Salinas, M.J. El Branding Como Herramienta Para El Posicionamiento En La Industria Cosmética. *Univ. Soc.* **2018**, *10*, 82–88.
4. Basurto Jimbo, E.; García Mir, V.; Rueda Rodríguez, E.; Noles Ramón, K. Elaboración de Una Crema Cosmética a Partir de Extractos *Coriandrum sativum* L. (Culantro). *Publicación Cuatrimest.* **2021**, *6*, 153–166.
5. Cobos Yanez, D.B. Elaboración de Una Crema Nutritiva Facial a Base de La Pulpa de Chirimoya (Annona Cherimola, Annonaceae). Master's Thesis, Universidad Politécnica Salesiana, Quito, Ecuador, 2015.
6. Capp Zilles, J.; Vallenot Lemos, M.A.; Anders Apel, M.; Kulkamp-Guerreiro, I.C.; Rigon Zimmer, A.; Vidor Contri, R. Vegetable Oils in Skin Whitening—A Narrative Review. *Curr. Pharm. Des.* **2025**, *31*, e13816128361413. [CrossRef]
7. Jašek, V.; Figalla, S. Vegetable Oils for Material Applications—Available Biobased Compounds Seeking Their Utilities. *ACS Polym. Au* **2025**, *5*, 105–128. [CrossRef]
8. Pupiales Martínez, S.A.; Torres Cando, T.E. Obtención de Aceites Esenciales a Partir de Pino (Pinus), Eucalipto (Eucalyptus), Menta (Mentha), Caléndula (Caléndula Officinalis), y Su Aplicación En La Elaboración de Una Crema Con Fines Terapéuticos Fines Terapéuticos. Bachelor's Thesis, Universidad Estatal de Bolívar, Guaranda, Ecuador, 2023.
9. Madurga, M. El Papel de La Cosmética: Excipientes y Conservantes. *Rev. De Pediatría De Atención Primaria* **2009**, *XI*, 81–100. [CrossRef]
10. Montalván, M.; Malagón, O.; Cumbicus, N.; Tanitana, F.; Gilardoni, G. Análisis Químico de Aceites Esenciales Amazónicos de Una Comunidad Shuar Ecuatoriana. *Granja* **2023**, *38*, 32–44. [CrossRef]
11. Pons, G.A. Aceites Vegetales, Hacia Una Producción Sostenible. *Hombre Máquina* **2015**, *46*, 9–19.
12. Guardado Yordi, E.; Radice, M.; Scalvenzi, L.; Pérez Martínez, A. Diseño Del Proceso Sostenible Para La Obtención de Una Emulsión Cosmética Desde Un Enfoque de Biocomercio. *Rev. Politécnica* **2024**, *54*, 35–46. [CrossRef]
13. Mosquera, T.; Noriega, P.; Tapia, W.; Pérez, S.H. Evaluación de La Eficacia Cosmética de Cremas Elaboradas Con Aceites Extraídos de Especies Vegetales Amazónicas: *Mauritia flexuosa* (Morete), Plukenetia Volubilis (Sacha Inchi) y Oenocarpus Bataua (Ungurahua). *La Granja* **2012**, *16*, 14. [CrossRef]
14. Proaño, J.; Rivadeneira, F.; Moncayo, P.; Mosquera, E. Aceite de Maracuyá (Passiflora Edulis): Aprovechamiento de Las Semillas En Productos Cosméticos. *Enfoque UTE* **2020**, *11*, 119–129. [CrossRef]
15. Rivera, J.; Luna, S.; Rodríguez, N.; Dahua, R. Evaluación de Las Propiedades Antioxidantes y Físicas de Una Crema Exfoliante Desarrollada a Partir de La Cáscara de *Mauritia flexuosa* L. (Morete). *Polo Conoc.* **2024**, *9*, 491–510.
16. Campos, D.A.; Gómez-García, R.; Vilas-Boas, A.A.; Madureira, A.R.; Pintado, M.M. Management of Fruit Industrial By-products—A Case Study on Circular Economy Approach. *Molecules* **2020**, *25*, 320. [CrossRef]

17. Del Rio Osorio, L.L.; Flórez-López, E.; Grande-Tovar, C.D. The Potential of Selected Agri-Food Loss and Waste to Contribute to a Circular Economy: Applications in the Food, Cosmetic and Pharmaceutical Industries. *Molecules* **2021**, *26*, 515. [CrossRef] [PubMed]
18. Machado, M.; Silva, S.; Costa, E.M. Byproducts as a Sustainable Source of Cosmetic Ingredients. *Appl. Sci.* **2024**, *14*, 10241. [CrossRef]
19. Mondello, A.; Salomone, R.; Mondello, G. Exploring Circular Economy in the Cosmetic Industry: Insights from a Literature Review. *Environ. Impact Assess. Rev.* **2024**, *105*, 107443. [CrossRef]
20. Guardado Yordi, E.; Guambuguete Guaman, I.S.; Freire Fuentes, M.E.; Radice, M.; Scalvenzi, L.; Abreu-Naranjo, R.; Bravo Sánchez, L.R.; Pérez Martínez, A. Conceptual Design of the Process for Making Cosmetic Emulsion Using Amazonian Oils. *Processes* **2025**, *13*, 1770. [CrossRef]
21. Romero, D.; Aillón, F.; Freire, A.; Radice, M. Design of an Industrial Process Focused on the Elaboration of Cosmetics from Amazonian Oils: A Biotrade Opportunity. *Mol2Net* **2016**, *2*, 1–5. [CrossRef]
22. Cerda-Mejía, V.; González-Suárez, E.; Guardado-Yordi, E.; Cerda-Mejía, G.; Pérez Martínez, A. Producción de Gel Hidroalcohólico En Tiempos de COVID-19, Oportunidad Para Diseñar El Proceso Que Garantice La Calidad. *Cent. Azúcar* **2021**, *48*, 88–97.
23. Beltrán Chacón, J.P.; Aguayo Carvajal, V.R. Estudio Técnico: Localización y Diseño de Plantas Agroindustriales. *Braz. J. Bus.* **2022**, *4*, 1951–1960. [CrossRef]
24. Rodríguez Cortina, J. Contribución al Estudio de La Intensificación Del Proceso de Secado de Tomillo (Thymus Vulgaris l.): Aplicación de Ultrasonidos de Potencia y Secado Intermitente. Ph.D. Thesis, Universitat Politècnica de València, Valencia, Spain, 2013.
25. Rodriguez Barragan, O.A. Intensificacion de Procesos de Transferencia de Materia Mediante Ultrasonidos de Potencia. Aplicacion al Secado Convectivo y a La Extraccion Con Fluidos Supercriticos. Ph.D. Thesis, Universidad de les Illes Balears, Illes Balears, Spain, 2014.
26. Dimian, A.C. *Integrated Design and Simulation of Chemical Processes*; Gani, R., Ed.; Elsevier: Amsterdam The Netherlands, 2003; Volume 13, ISBN 978-0-444-62700-1.
27. Pérez-Martinez, A.; Cervantes-Mendieta, E.; Julián-Ricardo, M.C.; González-Suárez, E.; Gómez-Atanay, A.; Oquendo-Ferrer, H.; Galindo-Llanes, P.; Ramos-Sánchez, L. Procedimiento Para Enfrentar Tareas de Diseño de Procesos de La Industria Azucarera y Sus Derivados. *Rev. Mex. Ing. Quim.* **2012**, *11*, 333–349.
28. Stankiewicz, A.I.; Moulijn, J.A. Process Intensification: Transforming Chemical Engineering. *Chem. Eng. Prog.* **2000**, *96*, 22–34.
29. Linnhoff, B.; Akinradewo, C.G. Linking Process Simulation and Process Integration. *Comput. Chem. Eng.* **1999**, *23*, S945–S953. [CrossRef]
30. Linnhoff, B.; Townsend, B.W. Designing Total Energy Systems. *Chem. Eng. Prog.* **1982**, *78*, 7.
31. Frosch, R.A.; Gallopoulos, N.E. Strategies for Manufacturing. *Sci. Am.* **1989**, *261*, 144–153. [CrossRef]
32. Dimian, A.C.; Bildea, C.S.; Kiss, A.A. Chapter 2—Introduction in Process Simulation. In *Computer Aided Chemical Engineering*; Elsevier: Amsterdam The Netherlands, 2014; Volume 35, pp. 35–71.
33. Muther, R. *Planificación y Proyección de La Empresa Industrial: (Método S.P.L., Sistematic Layout Planning)*; Carreras Fontseré, L., Ed.; Editores Técnicos Asociados, S.A.: Kansas City, MO, USA, 1968; Volume 1.
34. Suhardini, D.; Septiani, W.; Fauziah, S. Design and Simulation Plant Layout Using Systematic Layout Planning. *IOP Conf. Ser. Mater. Sci. Eng.* **2017**, *277*, 012051. [CrossRef]
35. Álvarez Arias, D.; De Ávila Moore, J.; Hurtado Rivera, J. Aplicación de Metodología SLP Para Redistribución de Planta En Micro Empresa Colombiana Del Sector Marroquinero: Un Estudio de Caso. *Boletín Innovación Logística Oper.* **2022**, *4*. [CrossRef]
36. Rocca, R.; Perossa, D.; Fumagalli, L. Analysis and Modelling for Industrial Energy Efficiency in the Cosmetics Industry: A Real Industrial Case in an Italian Manufacturing Company. *Cosmetics* **2024**, *11*, 161. [CrossRef]
37. Nydrioti, I.; Moutsaki, M.-M.; Leounakis, N.; Grigoropoulou, H. Implementation of the Water Footprint as a Water Performance Indicator in Industrial Manufacturing Units Located in Greece: Challenges and Prospects. *Environ. Sci. Pollut. Res.* **2024**, *31*, 803–819. [CrossRef]
38. Hallouch, O.; Ibourki, M.; Asbbane, A.; Devkota, K.; Giuffrè, A.M.; Majourhat, K.; Gharby, S. Exploring the Bioactive Potential of Argan Oil Cake: A Comprehensive Physicochemical Comparison with Various Seeds Cakes. *Curr. Res. Nutr. Food Sci. J.* **2025**, *13*, 77–100. [CrossRef]
39. Jesus, A.; Ratanji, S.; Cidade, H.; Sousa, E.; Cruz, M.T.; Oliveira, R.; Almeida, I.F. Phenolics as Active Ingredients in Skincare Products: A Myth or Reality? *Molecules* **2025**, *30*, 1423. [CrossRef] [PubMed]

processes

MDPI

Article

Conceptual Design of the Process for Making Cosmetic Emulsion Using Amazonian Oils

Estela Guardado Yordi [1,*], Irma Sofia Guambuguete Guaman [2], Mayra Elizabeth Freire Fuentes [2], Matteo Radice [1], Laura Scalvenzi [1], Reinier Abreu-Naranjo [3], Luis Ramón Bravo Sánchez [1] and Amaury Pérez Martínez [1]

1 Facultad de Ciencias de la Tierra, Universidad Estatal Amazónica, Pastaza 160150, Ecuador; mradice@uea.edu.ec (M.R.); lscalvenzi@uea.edu.ec (L.S.); lbravo@uea.edu.ec (L.R.B.S.); amperez@uea.edu.ec (A.P.M.)

2 Carrera de Agroindustria, Facultad de Ciencias de la Tierra, Universidad Estatal Amazónica, Pastaza 160150, Ecuador; sofiaguambu2001@gmail.com (I.S.G.G.); mayritafreiree@gmail.com (M.E.F.F.)

3 Facultad de Ciencias de la Vida, Universidad Estatal Amazónica, Pastaza 160150, Ecuador; rabreu@uea.edu.ec

* Correspondence: e.guardadoy@uea.edu.ec; Tel.: +593-32892-118

Abstract: In recent years, there has been a growing interest in natural and sustainable cosmetic ingredients, particularly those derived from Amazonian plant oils. The present research focuses on the creation of a prototype cosmetic emulsion from two Amazonian oils, morete oil (*Mauritia flexuosa* L.f.) and ungurahua oil (*Oenocarpus bataua* Mart). The aim of the study was to develop a conceptual design of the process for making cosmetic emulsion using Amazonian oils. The methodology consisted of observational data collection, definition of unit operations and equipment, and process simulation. The design was simulated using SuperPro Designer V10.0. Experimental data, unit operations, equipment, and operation time confirmed the feasibility of a conceptual process design for scaling up. In the conceptual design, an operation time of 4.25 h was estimated, which would allow the production of two or more batches per day, depending on the demand, and the initial investment was expected to be recovered within 6.24 years. This study highlights the potential application of Amazonian oils in the cosmetic industry, promoting financially viable, natural, and ecologic products. Future research should analyze extraction yields, alternative strategies for efficient scale-up, and the long-term stability of emulsions under different storage conditions.

Keywords: cosmetic emulsions; process design; process scale-up; process simulation; unit operations; vegetable oils

1. Introduction

The cosmetics industry is a dynamic and constantly evolving sector, with global prominence in key markets such as the European Union, the United States, China, Brazil, and Japan [1]. Today, the industry continues to develop and produce innovative and successful products. Consumers can therefore select cosmetic creams on the basis of performance and efficacy [2].

In Ecuador, the consumption of cosmetics for personal care is of great significance, representing 1.6% of the Gross Domestic Product (GDP) and experiencing an annual growth of 10% [3]. Based on recent research, Gordillo López et al. [4] mentioned that the country consumes approximately 51.5 million beauty products per year, equivalent to an average of 3.09 units per person.

In the cosmetic industry, Amazonian vegetable oils have gained relevance due to their emollient, nourishing, and antioxidant properties, which make them key ingredients in the formulation of skin and hair care products [5]. A representative example is ungurahua oil (*Oenocarpus bataua*), extracted from the fruits of a palm tree native to the Amazon. This oil is highly valued for its richness in essential fatty acids, tocopherols, and phytosterols, fundamental components in cellular metabolism that favor hydration, protection, and hair and skin repair. Traditionally, the Amazonian Shuar and Achuar peoples have used this oil in hair treatments to strengthen hair, add shine, and prevent hair loss. This knowledge has aroused the interest of the cosmetic industry in terms of incorporating innovative and sustainable formulations [6].

Emulsions play a crucial role in the formulation of cosmetic products, as they enhance product stability, improve the delivery of active ingredients, and provide desirable sensory properties. They are fundamental in creams, lotions, and other skincare formulations due to their ability to hydrate and protect the skin. From a technical perspective, a cosmetic emulsion may be defined as a semi-solid system composed of two distinct phases: an aqueous phase and an oil phase, which are kept stable by the addition of an emulsifying agent [7]. As emulsions are thermodynamically unstable, energy is required for their formation [8]. Their basic composition is enriched by the presence of active ingredients, preservatives, fragrances, and flavorings, among other components [9].

However, cosmetic emulsions are classified into several groups, the most representative of which are water-in-oil (W/O), where the water is dispersed in a continuous oil phase, and oil-in-water (O/W), the most commonly used formulation in which the continuous phase is aqueous and the oil is dispersed into it [10]. These emulsions have the function of softening the skin and making it supple [11]. In addition, the most important properties include viscosity, color, stability, ease of dilution, and formation [12].

Increasing market interest in formulated products (emulsions) has driven the advancement of innovative approaches to their design. Today, products are scaled up using trial-and-error methods based on modeling [13]. According to Ruiz and Álvarez [14], this process is traditionally performed according to dimensional analysis, geometric similarity, and empirical relationships from a data set. Scaling up from the laboratory to the industrial environment is therefore a critical and decisive step during process design [15]. Broadly speaking, Newtonian fluids are simpler to scale up [16]. In contrast, non-Newtonian or, in this case, emulsions are more complex due to changes in their properties, such as viscosity and flow conditions [17]. In general, the process of scaling up involves obtaining data at different levels; on a laboratory scale, it allows us to take data to design another plant of a different size. It is therefore crucial that a product made in small quantities must present the same properties and characteristics as one produced in larger series [18].

A study by Türedi and Acaralı [19] argues that scaling up an emulsion technology depends on the correct choice of stirrer speed, mixing time, and process temperature. Meanwhile, research by Burakova et al. [18] suggests that to scale up, it is necessary to consider the risks that can lead to the production of heterogeneous and unstable creams. The latter authors developed a technology to produce emulsions based on dry extracts of bergenia or "elephant's ear" (*Bergenia crassifolia*) under laboratory conditions. In this regard, they used three pilot series for production, considering possible risks such as mixer speed, mixing time, temperature, etc., where they obtained a stable cosmetic product. Likewise, Campos Prada [20] proposed the scaling up of the mixing process of concentrated O/W emulsions in order to study their dynamics under controlled hydrodynamic conditions. Restrepo Jimenez [21] also demonstrated that it is possible to scale up emulsification processes, supporting the feasibility of scaling up cosmetic emulsions through multiscale design and controlled operating parameters. Moreover, May-Masnou et al. [17] maintain that the quality and final properties of emulsions are linked to various process factors. Even small changes in the agitation speed, the way in which the components are added, or the size of the container can cause variations in the product in addition to the loss of raw material, time, and economic resources. Therefore, it is essential to perform a scaling analysis of these procedures and to study the impact of the variables to predict their behaviors and optimization at the industrial level. These analyses would save resources and time in inefficient trials.

Although several attempts have been made to carry out pilot laboratory scale-ups of certain technological processes for emulsions, they are not sufficient due to the lack of information on experimental data in their designs. For this reason, the aim of the study was to develop a conceptual design of the process for making a cosmetic emulsion using Amazonian oils.

2. Materials and Methods

2.1. Study Design

This study developed a conceptual design based on a case study to analyze the extraction of vegetable oils from morete (*Mauritia flexuosa* L.f.) and ungurahua (*Oenocarpus bataua* Mart) fruits obtained in the Local Market, Puyo Ecuador, and their application in the production of a cosmetic emulsion. The information used came from the observation and analysis of experiments carried out by other researchers that have not yet been published. The study was divided into three phases (Figure 1):

- Phase 1: Information retrieval and observational data collection. This focused on collecting data on vegetable oil extraction and the formulation of cosmetic emulsions through observation, measurement, recording, and analysis.
- Phase 2: Identification and definition of unit operations and processes. This involved identifying, categorizing, and selecting appropriate unit operations for oil extraction and emulsion production based on industry standards and observed procedures.
- Phase 3: Process simulation and diagram construction. This was designed to integrate process data into simulation models and visual representations, ensuring a structured and scalable workflow.

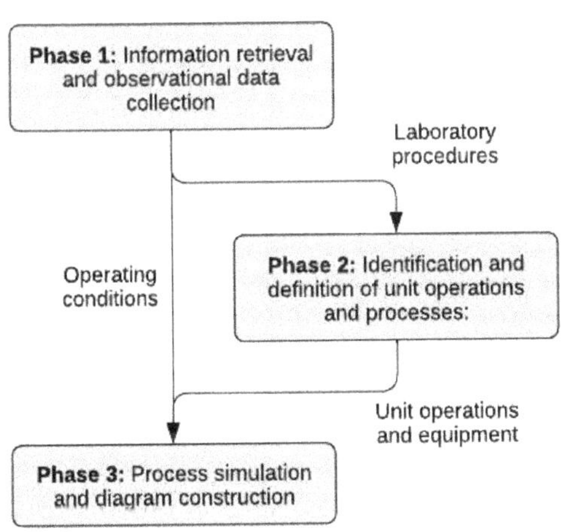

Figure 1. Methodological phases used in the conceptual design of the process for obtaining the cosmetic emulsion.

This study was conducted based on the observation of an ongoing, unpublished experimental process focused on data documentation rather than the direct execution of experiments. Observations were systematically recorded to register processing data, operational parameters, and material flows. Findings were contrasted by reviewing the literature on vegetable oil extraction and cosmetic formulation.

2.1.1. Phase 1: Information Retrieval and Observational Data Collection

The first phase of the study involved the systematic observation and analysis of unpublished laboratory experiments on oil extraction and emulsion formulation, which were previously conducted by other researchers. These observations served as the basis for the development of the conceptual design and the scaling up of the process to the artisanal level.

From the observation and recording of these experimental data, operational parameters were identified. The observed procedures were then transformed into a process design that is adaptable to a larger scale. The objective was to collect data for the development of a conceptual process design. The parameters recorded included the following:

- Processing conditions: temperature, time, and sequence of the operations.
- Composition of raw materials: type and quantity of ingredients used in oil extraction and emulsion formulation; these data were subsequently entered into the simulation software.
- Unit operations: identification of essential steps in the vegetable oil extraction and formulation process.
- Material flows: documentation of inputs and outputs at each stage of the process.

2.1.2. Phase 2: Identification and Definition of Unit Operations and Processes

In the second phase, the conceptual design of the technological process (extraction of vegetable oils and production of cosmetic emulsions) began by selecting the extraction method, identifying its unitary operations, and deciding upon the equipment.

First, the extraction method was selected based on laboratory and bibliographic information. This enabled the proposal and analysis of technological alternatives for the extraction method based on the nature of the raw material, its compatibility with traditional practices, and the purity and stability of the final product.

Next, the data collected in Phase 1 were analyzed and converted into unit operations. To achieve this, it was necessary to adopt the heuristic method based on reasoning, which is based on the application of practical rules and previous experiences for the efficient resolution of design problems, as stated by López-Arévalo et al. [22]. Within this approach, the equipment and operating conditions were also chosen.

As part of the methodological approach adopted in this study, heuristic rules geared toward the conceptual design of the process were established. These rules were formulated based on technical criteria and previous experience in the analysis of similar processes and served as a guide for the selection of unit operations and equipment. The heuristic rules proposed were as follows:

1. The process scalability rule: If a unit operation is feasible on a small scale but involves critical conditions (such as temperature, pressure, or residence time), then its scalability should be evaluated with phenomenological models before its industrial implementation.
2. The material and equipment compatibility rule: The construction material of the equipment must be compatible with the chemical and physical properties of the processed product in order to avoid product and equipment degradation.
3. The energy consumption minimization rule: Whenever possible, production methods should be selected that minimize energy consumption without compromising product quality.

Since the technological process was conceived as a discontinuous production, its design was structured by considering the availability of raw materials in the Amazon and the synchronization of batch operations, as proposed in Guardado Yordi et al. [5].

2.1.3. Phase 3: Process Simulation and Diagram Construction

The data obtained in the initial phases of the study were used to define the parameters required for the simulation of the cosmetic cream production process. For this purpose, an artisanal scale was used in order to adapt the design to the production conditions of the Amazon region. The simulation integrated the information of the oil extraction process with the unitary operations and equipment necessary for the emulsion formulation.

This phase focused on process scale-up under a process modeling and simulation approach, as proposed by Yazdanpanah [23]. The block diagram for the transformation of raw materials into the final product was created, as well as the Gantt chart, both of which allowed the conformation of the process flow diagram and the simulation.

Analysis and Economic Feasibility

SuperPro Designer V10.0 (Intelligen, Freehold, NJ, USA) software was used to simulate the process. In addition, an analysis of its technical and economic feasibility was carried out according to the proposal of Pérez-Martínez et al. [24]. The input data for the simulation included experimental values obtained from the literature and data based on the results observed in Phase 1. The economic dynamic indicators calculated were as follows: net present value (NPV), internal rate of return (IRR), return on investment (ROI), payback period, and gross margin. The economic evaluation horizon was set at 10 years, with a discount rate of 7%, which took into account raw material and operating costs [5].

3. Results

3.1. Phase 1: Information Retrieval and Observational Data Collection

3.1.1. Extraction of Vegetable Oil from Morete (*Mauritia flexuosa* L.f.) and Ungurahua (*Oenocarpus bataua* Mart)

The following are the results of the information gathered by the authors by observing the experimental procedure of other investigators at a laboratory scale for both fruits:

(a) The morete fruits were selected and separated from those showing any damage. Subsequently, 35 kg of fruit was weighed, cleaned, and washed with 12.5 L of water to remove any impurities, such as soil. Then, the fruits were softened with 20 L of water at a temperature of 60 °C for two hours to facilitate the removal of the seed. The rind and pulp of the seed were then separated from the fruit by hand. As a result of this procedure, 8 kg of pulp and 27 kg of residue were obtained. The pulp was subjected to a drying process for a period of 24 h at a temperature of 60 °C, resulting in 3000 g of dry pulp. The oil was then extracted using the decoction method. At this stage, the pulp was boiled to extract the oil contained in it, obtaining 325 mL or 280.82 g of the product. The percentage yield at this stage was 9.36%, which is the proportion of oil in relation to the weight of the dehydrated pulp obtained after the drying process.

(b) The ungurahua fruits were selected and separated from those showing any damage. 3498.30 g of fruit was received and washed to remove molds and impurities. The fruits were then softened by boiling them in 6996.6 mL of water. After boiling, the fruits were left for a period of two hours to allow softening and pulp extraction. The husk and pulp were then ground. After obtaining 1097.53 g of ground pulp, the decoction process was carried out to extract the oil. This procedure resulted in obtaining a total of 19 mL of oil, equivalent to 17.16 g with a yield of 0.6%.

3.1.2. Emulsion Production

Below is a description of the information gathered by observing the experimental procedure at a laboratory scale to obtain the cosmetic emulsion:

(a) Table 1 shows the formulation used to make 1 kg of cosmetic cream as well as the ingredients and quantities used.

(b) After obtaining the raw material in optimal conditions, the ingredients to produce 1 kg of the final product were weighed in order to create the cream. This process was divided into two parts: an aqueous phase, consisting of 645 g of purified sterile water, and an oil phase, containing 3 g of Montanov 202, 10 g of Montanov 68 (emulsifiers), 155 g of cocoa butter, 44 g of morete oil, 102 g of ungurahua oil, and 10 g of preservatives. Previously, the mixtures were subjected to a water bath at a temperature of 75 °C for 20 min to achieve liquid homogeneity across all ingredients (Figure 2). Once the desired temperature was reached and the ingredients were ready, they were transferred to the homogenizer/emulsifier at 7000 rpm for 40 min, where the water was added slowly to the oil phase to achieve a uniform fluid.

Table 1. Formulation for 1 kg of cosmetic cream.

Ingredient	Vendor Location	Amount (g)
Montanov 202 (emulsifier 1)	(Formulator Sample Shop, Lincolnton, NC 28092, USA)	34
Montanov 68 (emulsifier 2)	(Formulator Sample Shop, Lincolnton, NC 28092, USA)	10
Cocoa butter	(Local Market, Puyo, Ecuador)	155
Morete oil	(Local Market, Puyo, Ecuador)	44
Ungurahua oil	(Local Market, Puyo, Ecuador)	102
Preservatives	Essential oils were obtained in our laboratory by steam distillation Sharomix (Hebbe cosmetics, Cuernavaca, Mexico)	10
Water	Distilled in our laboratory	645

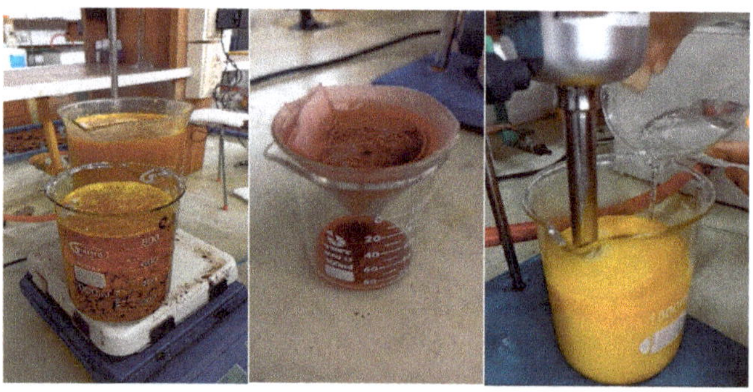

Figure 2. Experimental plant for obtaining vegetable oils and cosmetic cream.

3.2. *Phase 2: Identification and Definition of Unit Operations and Processes*

Four methods of extraction of morete (*Mauritia flexuosa* L.f.) and ungurahua (*Oenocarpus bataua* Mart) oils were compared by evaluating their unit operations and the equipment required. The methods analyzed in the conceptual design were decoction, solvent extraction, cold pressing, and hot pressing. Each of them was different in terms of raw material preparation, oil yield, and operating conditions. However, when analyzing the technological feasibility, cold pressing was selected. Table 2 presents a summary of the unit operations involved in each method, together with the equipment used for each alternative evaluated.

Table 2. Comparison of extraction methods, unit operations, and equipment for morete and ungurahua oils.

Process Stage	Method: Option 1 (Decoction)	Method: Option 2 (Solvent Extraction)	Method: Option 3 (Cold Pressing)	Method: Option 4 (Hot Pressing)	Equipment Used
Softening of material	Heating in water at 60 °C	Maceration in the solvent	Heating in water at 60 °C	Heating in water at 60 °C	Jacketed tank
Grinding/ Pulping	Manual separation	Manual separation	Ground with a machine	Ground with a machine	Grinding mill or pulper
Drying	24 h at 60 °C	24 h at 60 °C	24 h at 60 °C	24 h at 60 °C	Tray dryer
Oil extraction	Boiling and decanting	Solvent extraction	Cold pressing	Hot pressing	Oil press machine or extraction reactor
Filtration	Gravity filtration	Solvent evaporation and filtration	Mechanical filtration	Mechanical filtration	Plate filter

As for the production of the cosmetic emulsion, the unit operations shown in Table 3 were used. The turbo emulsifier was the most suitable piece of equipment since all operations can be carried out in it and it helps to guarantee the stability of the final product.

Table 3. Unit operations and equipment for the production of cosmetic emulsion.

Process Stage	Unit Operation	Equipment Used
Raw material preparation	Addition of raw materials	Turbo emulsifier
Heating	Water phase heating	Turbo emulsifier
Heating	Oil phase heating	Turbo emulsifier
Mixing	Homogenization of phases	Turbo emulsifier
Cooling	Controlled cooling	Cooling system

3.3. Phase 3: Process Simulation and Diagram Construction

The block diagram (Figure 3A) represents the interconnection of the main operations of the process, identifying the stages from the input of raw materials to obtaining the final product. The simulation results indicated that the process requires the sequence of operation units for oil extraction and emulsification, ensuring a continuous flow of the oil extraction and subsequent obtaining of the cosmetic emulsion.

The simulation showed that the total processing time for the production of one batch of cosmetic cream at the artisanal level is 4.25 h (Figure 3B). Given that the Gantt chart organizes the sequence of operations represented in the block diagram, it facilitated the planning and coordination of the technological process. In the Gantt chart (Figure 3B), the progress of the activities and the logical sequence for carrying out both phases are graphically summarized, given their interdependence. For this, the aqueous phase was prepared and then the lipid phase since it is a W/O emulsion. Each activity is listed vertically, with its start time and duration indicated by a horizontal line along a time scale [25].

Figure 4 shows the process flow diagram, where the distribution of the equipment and the sequence of the transformation of the raw materials into the cosmetic emulsion can be observed. The simulation made it possible to evaluate the operating efficiency of the industrial scale-up, showing that the technological configuration used in the laboratory can be adapted to larger-scale production without altering the operating conditions for extracting the vegetable oils and obtaining the emulsion.

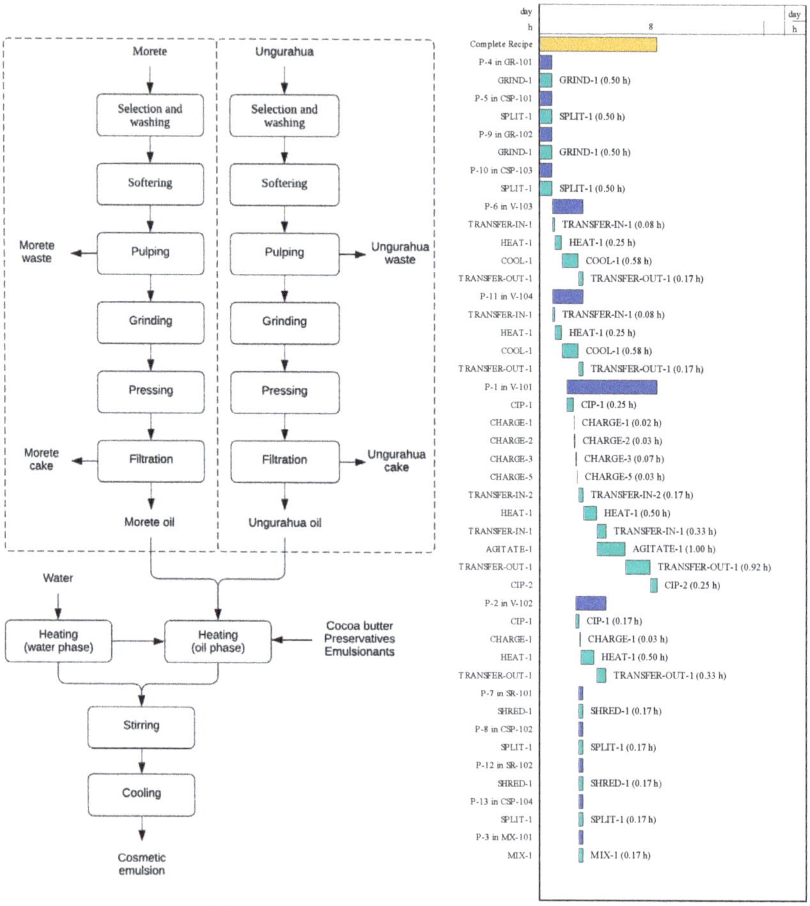

(A) (B)

Figure 3. Procedure for obtaining cosmetic cream. (**A**) Block diagram. Continuous lines (——) represent the main flow of the process, indicating the sequence of unit operations from the selection of raw materials to the finalization of the product. Dashed lines (- - - - - -) mark out the stages of the process, separating the extraction of the vegetable oils (morete and ungurahua) from the production of the cosmetic emulsion. They also indicate the relationship between the processed raw materials and their integration in the final formulation. (**B**) Gantt chart of the vegetable oil extraction and cosmetic cream production process. The key stages are represented, including grinding (GRIND), separation (SPLIT), heating (HEAT), agitation (AGITATE), material transfer (TRANSFER-IN and TRANSFER-OUT), and cleaning (CIP), allowing the visualization of the duration and sequence of each operation within the process.

As a result of observing other investigators carry out experiments, it was evident that the technological process for the extraction of vegetable oils from morete and ungurahua uses various technologies. First, the raw materials were selected and meticulously washed. The fruit was then softened at a temperature of 100 °C for one hour to facilitate pulping, which separates the pulp from the fruit and separates the seed and peel as residues. The resulting pulp was crushed to facilitate subsequent pressing. Once the oil was obtained, filtration was carried out to obtain a final product free of impurities and residues that can be used to produce cosmetic cream.

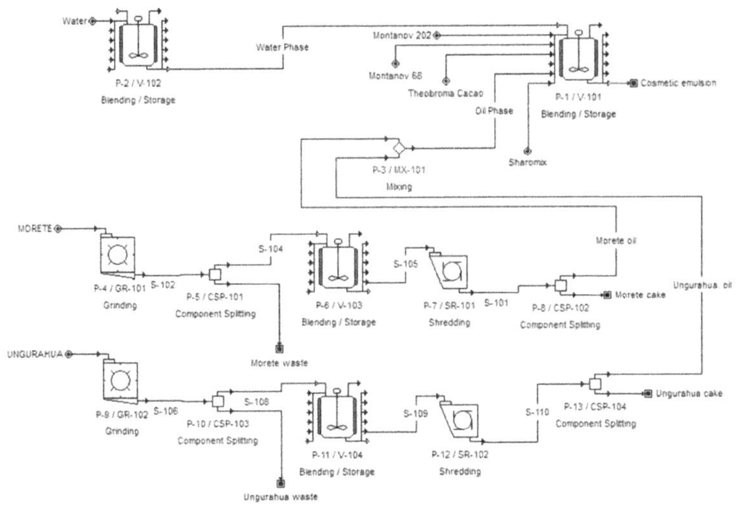

Figure 4. Process flow diagram for obtaining vegetable oils and making cosmetic cream. GR-101, GR-102 (grinding); CSP-101, CSP-102, CSP-103, CSP-104 (component splitting); SR-101, SR-102 (shredding); V-101, V-102, V-103, V-104 (blending/storage); P-102, P-103, P-104 (transfer pumps); M-103 (final mixing); Montanov 202, Montanov 68b, *Theobroma cacao*, Sharomix (ingredients for the oil phase of the emulsion); cosmetic emulsion (final product).

The production of the cosmetic cream began with the simultaneous incorporation of the two phases, oil and aqueous. The first phase involved heating a combination of cocoa butter, emulsifiers (Montanov 68, 202), oils, and preservatives (Sharomix), while the second phase comprised only water. This procedure was carried out at a temperature of 70–80 °C for a period of 40 min.

Then, both phases were mixed at the end of the heating process, and by constant stirring at 7000 rpm, the aqueous phase was incorporated into the oil phase. Finally, once the desired emulsion was achieved, it was cooled to room temperature.

The above-mentioned procedures coincide with the Gantt Chart (Figure 3B) for the extraction of morete and ungurahua oils. Once obtained, both oils passed simultaneously to the heating phase of the aqueous and oil phases in separate equipment, both starting at the same temperature (75 °C) and time. At the end of this process, the aqueous phase was combined with the oil phase to homogenize and form the desired emulsion. The total duration of the process to produce cosmetic cream was 4.25 h.

In the process flow diagram (Figure 4), one can see the technology consisting of two turbo emulsifiers with a capacity of 10 kg. The first one is used to prepare the aqueous phase, and the second one is used for the oil phase to obtain the emulsion. This process followed detailed operations (Figure 3) to obtain the cosmetic cream.

In the same way, Figure 5 depicts the process flow diagram for obtaining morete oil and ungurahua oil. The process began with the input of fruits into the pulper to separate the seeds and peels from the fruit. Subsequently, the fruits were cooked to soften them and obtain the condensate as a residue. Once the fruits had a smooth texture, they were crushed and subjected to cold pressing to extract the oil, and as a residue the morete cake and ungurahua cake. The oil obtained was filtered to eliminate the particles present, resulting in the final product, i.e., vegetable oils.

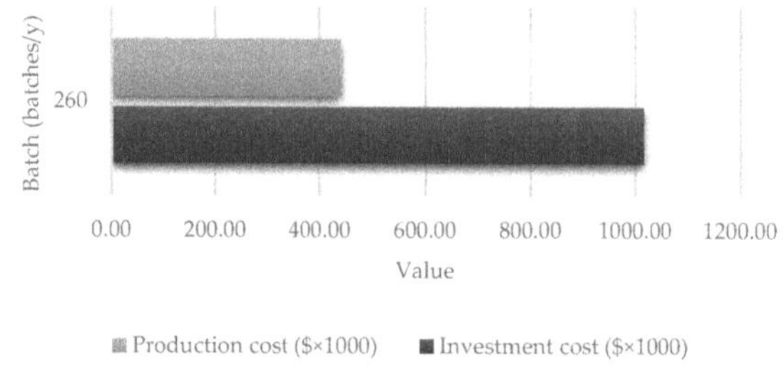

(A)

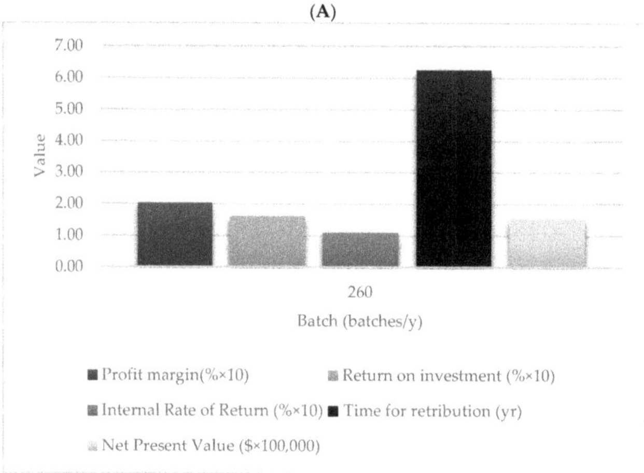

(B)

Figure 5. Results of the economic analysis: (**A**) investment and production costs; (**B**) dynamic economic and profitability indicators.

3.3.1. Mass and Energy Balance, Consumption vs. Availability of Raw Materials, and Environmental Compatibility of Technology

Table 4 presents a comprehensive analysis of the consumption of environmental indicators linked to the annual production of 4717.48 kg of cosmetic cream. This analysis provides a detailed overview of the consumption of raw materials, water, and energy, as well as the amount of waste generated from the initial waste and the residual cake resulting from the morete and ungurahua pressing process. The data presented provides a clear and accurate picture of the environmental footprint associated with the production of cosmetic cream, allowing for a comprehensive technical assessment of its environmental impact.

Table 4. Environmental indicators * for the artisanal creation of cosmetic emulsion.

Environmental Indicator	Input/Output Current	Amount	Unit
Raw material consumption	Montanov 68	0.011	kg/kg
	Montanov 202	0.036	kg/kg
	Morete fruit	0.136	kg/kg
	Sharomix	0.011	kg/kg
	Cocoa butter	0.111	kg/kg
	Ungurahua fruit	0.563	kg/kg
Water consumption	Water	48.411	kg/kg

Table 4. *Cont.*

Environmental Indicator	Input/Output Current	Amount	Unit
Energy consumption	Power consumption	5.86	kW·h/kg
	Steam consumption	10	kg/kg
	Refrigerated water	260	kg/kg
Discharge	Of gases	-	-
	Of liquids	-	-
	Of solids	0.56	kg/kg
Cosmetic emulsion		4717.48	kg/yr

* Calculations according to Pérez-Martínez et al. [24].

3.3.2. Equipment Sizing and Procurement Cost

For the sizing and acquisition cost of the equipment, it is essential to establish the entire manufacturing process of the technologies. Table 5 shows the equipment involved in the processes of obtaining vegetable oils and cosmetic cream, the design parameter that characterizes each one of them, and the quantity and acquisition cost of each one of them, the latter being USD 126,000.00.

Table 5. Equipment specifications and acquisition cost for the production of cosmetic emulsion.

Quantity	Equipment	Design Parameter	Unit Cost (USD)	Cost (USD)
1	Turbo emulsifier	Tank volume = 22.47 L	20,000	20,000
1	Turbo emulsifier	Tank volume = 14.66 L	20,000	20,000
1	Pulper	Nominal Yield = 2.55 kg/h	14,000	14,000
1	Pulper	Nominal Yield = 10.58 kg/h	14,000	14,000
1	Jacketed tank	Tank volume = 2.62 L	10,000	10,000
1	Jacketed tank	Tank volume = 8.95 L	10,000	10,000
1	Crusher	Nominal Yield = 2.55 kg/h	1000	1000
1	Crusher	Nominal Yield = 2.16 kg/h	1000	1000
1	Press	Nominal Yield = 12.98 kg/h	6000	6000
1	Press	Nominal Yield = 45.82 kg/h	6000	6000
	Unlisted equipment		25,000	25,000
		Total		126,000

3.3.3. Analysis and Economic Feasibility

The investment cost (Figure 5A) for 260 batches is USD 1,016,000.00, while the production cost is lower at USD 44,100.00 per year. The NPV determines the different costs and benefits of technological investment, which, to produce the cosmetic cream, was positive for the number of batches at USD 216,000.00. This value indicates that it is possible to recover the investment. The profit margin and return on investment show positive values of 20.22% and 16.04%, respectively. The venture is also economically feasible, which leads to an increase in profitability (Figure 5B). Indeed, the IRR is positive, implying higher profitability. The only drawback is the long payback time, which stands at 6.24 years. Therefore, the operation appears to be profitable and able to generate profits that exceed the initial capital.

4. Discussion

The extraction yield of morete using the decoction method was 9.36% relative to the dehydrated pulp. Rivera et al. [26] suggested that the most efficient method for morete oil extraction is by using the pulp under cold pressing, with a pre treatment at 85 °C for a period of 10 min, generating a yield of 56.77%. In contrast, Rivera Chasiquiza [27] reported the oil content in morete pulp by machine pressing to be 59.42% when heat treatment was applied and the rindless fruit was used at 85 °C for 10 min. Paredes Amasifuen [28] found that by applying heat treatment prior to oil extraction, a high fat percentage of more than 19.0% was achieved. This process involves heating, crushing, extraction with a manual press, and separation by decantation and filtration. Furthermore, another study by Adrianzén et al. [29] commented that the amount of oil extracted is directly related to the heating temperature of the pulp. They also showed that this percentage decreases when using the pulp with peel during pre-treatment prior to pressing.

Applying the decoction method to dried ungurahua pulp produced a yield of 0.6%. This figure is significantly below the results reported by various other authors who used different techniques during pulp softening and extraction methods, which could contribute to their higher yields. The procedures used to obtain oil from ungurahua are similar to those reported by other authors [30,31], who agree on the seed softening time, set at 2 h. Peña et al. [32] obtained a yield of 19.06% using the pressing method. Unlike other studies, Chaves Yela et al. [33] did not report the percentage yield of the extracted oil, although they did describe in detail the artisanal process and extensively characterized its physicochemical properties and lipid profile. The process began with the harvesting and storage of ripe fruits for 24 h, followed by washing, selection, softening, pulping, and filtration at 130 °C. Emphasis was placed on the process of filtering with a cloth as a guarantee of the oil's purity, and proper storage ensured that its properties were preserved and a high-quality product was obtained.

The low oil recovery observed in the present study raises concerns regarding the economic feasibility of using decoction as the main extraction method. While the method aligns with traditional practices, alternative techniques such as cold pressing or supercritical fluid extraction (SFE) should be considered to enhance yield. SFE, particularly with CO_2, has been explored in other vegetable oil extractions, demonstrating improved oil purity and higher efficiency while eliminating the risk of solvent contamination [34]. Future research should evaluate the implementation of SFE or enzymatic-assisted extraction to optimize oil recovery without compromising environmental and safety standards.

The process for the preparation of the cosmetic cream involved heating the oil and aqueous phases separately. Once the components of the oil phase reached a liquid state and the required temperature, the aqueous phase was combined with the oil phase to obtain the desired cosmetic emulsion. This coincides with the phase inversion method, also known as the indirect method, used by previous researchers [35,36]. In this method, the oil phase is heated separately from the aqueous phase, and through continuous stirring, the aqueous phase is gradually incorporated into the oil phase until the desired emulsion is achieved.

The study carried out by Rivera et al. [26] highlights that cold pressing, complemented by preheating at 85 °C for 10 min, represents the most efficient option in terms of yield, with a production of over 56.77%. This method preserves the functional properties of the product during extraction, unlike hot pressing, which prevents the loss of volatile components observed in decoction extraction methods. In addition, it is noted that this technique does not cause potential skin irritation associated with the use of hexane or other organic solvents, making it a safer and more effective alternative.

The equipment selected for the extraction of oils from both morete and ungurahua is the same because these two fruits share similar characteristics in terms of their softening, pulping, and oil extraction. We based this choice on the information provided by Aliaga Zumaeta and Quispe Alarcon [37], who used a pulper designed to separate the pulp from the fibrous material, pips, and skin of various fruits. This equipment, made of stainless steel, consists of brushes and nylon that rotate at high speeds, which facilitates the breaking of the fruit. It has a processing capacity of 1200 kg per hour. Finally, a pressure and temperature regulator was used. It has a capacity of 370 kg/h. The pressure applied helps to raise the temperature of the pulp, thus helping to obtain a high-quality oil.

In order to select the technology, we were guided by the methodology proposed by Mosquera et al. [36], which involves the creation of a W/O cosmetic emulsion and rapid agitation and a cooling process with slow agitation.

For the selection of the necessary equipment, we relied on the work of Romero et al. [38], who suggest the use of an emulsifier made of stainless steel. This equipment is designed to heat up and withstand both external and internal pressures, as well as vacuum. In addition, it has the capacity to mix at different agitation speeds, adapting to the viscosity of the emulsion. Finally, the device has a cooling system composed of a double chamber through which water and steam circulate. For these reasons, this equipment was seen as the most suitable for carrying out the cosmetic cream production process.

The time required to produce the cosmetic cream was 4.25 h. Therefore, it is feasible to produce two or more batches per day. In comparison, in a research project carried out by Aguilar [39] for the production of 10 kg of cosmetic cream, the total time was 0.52 h. In the heating phase, Zurita Acosta and López Pérez [40] used a jacketed mixing tank at 65–75 °C for 20 min. Furthermore, Chauhan and Gupta [41] used a melting kettle for heating at 90 °C for 10 to 15 min until the oils and fats were melted. In the mixing and melting process, Celeiro et al. [42,43] reported that it should be kept running for 15 to 20 min until a homogeneous mixture is obtained.

The raw materials used in this context were renewable, so the technology used is environmentally friendly. In addition, a minimal amount of solid waste was generated, as detailed in Table 5. The small amounts of waste, together with the efficient use of raw materials and energy, as well as the implementation of sustainable practices in the production and collection of these raw materials, ensure that the proposed technology complies with the recommendations set out by Bom et al. [34] and Rocca et al. [44].

The values obtained in the production of 260 batches/year, evaluated through dynamic economic indicators, demonstrate that the process is economically viable and that the recovery of the investment is feasible, which is in line with the research by Cerda et al. [45,46]. What is more, both product quality and market demand suggest the possibility of increasing the quantity of batches produced, resulting in an increase in revenue and a reduction in the time required to recover the investment, as noted by Cerda et al. [47].

5. Conclusions

With this research, it has been possible to prove that, to carry out the conceptual design of a technological process, it is essential to obtain experimental data that facilitate its subsequent scaling up. The unit operations, the equipment, and the operating time of the case study designed in this research should be confirmed or modified during such an experiment.

In the conceptual design for obtaining cosmetic cream, an operating time of 4.25 h was estimated, which would allow the production of two or more batches per day, depending on demand. Furthermore, the initial investment was expected to be recovered within 6.24 years.

The results obtained indicate that the extraction process of Amazonian vegetable oils and their incorporation into cosmetic emulsions have potential for scalability, provided that the appropriate processing conditions are maintained to preserve the essential physicochemical properties of the commercial formulations. The simulation of the process using SuperPro Designer V10.0 has made it possible to evaluate the technical feasibility, optimize operational parameters, and estimate economic feasibility based on dynamic indicators.

From an industrial perspective, this study shines a light on the potential application of Amazonian oils in the cosmetic industry, promoting the development of sustainable formulations aligned with the growing market interest in natural and ecological products. The proposed process is framed within the current trends of green chemistry and circular economy. This makes it a viable option for companies seeking to integrate regional biodiversity into innovative formulations, adding value to both the industry and local communities.

In addition, the methodological approach presented in this study can serve as a reference for future industrial projects, particularly those aimed at scaling up bioproducts derived from natural resources. The combination of traditional extraction techniques with modern process simulation tools offers a comprehensive strategy that balances productive efficiency, environmental sustainability, and economic viability, favoring the application of this strategy in broader industrial contexts.

To strengthen the applicability of the process at the industrial level, future research should focus on optimizing extraction yields, evaluating alternative strategies for efficient scale-up, and analyzing the long-term stability of emulsions under different storage conditions. Furthermore, validating the process at a pilot scale and integrating advanced emulsification technologies will be key steps to consolidate its implementation in the cosmetic industry.

This study establishes a technical and economic basis for the industrialization of cosmetic emulsions from Amazonian oils, confirming that process conceptualization, simulation, and economic analysis are essential for the development and scale-up of formulations with industrial viability and market potential.

Author Contributions: Conceptualization, A.P.M. and E.G.Y.; methodology, I.S.G.G. and M.E.F.F.; software, A.P.M. and R.A.-N.; formal analysis, L.S., M.R. and L.R.B.S.; investigation, E.G.Y. and L.R.B.S.; writing—original draft preparation, R.A.-N. and E.G.Y.; writing—review and editing, M.R. and L.S.; supervision, A.P.M. All authors have read and agreed to the published version of the manuscript.

Funding: This study was funded by Universidad Estatal Amazónica in Puyo, Ecuador, and has been completed as part of the project: Desarrollo de Nuevos Productos Agroindustriales de Alto Valor Agregado a Partir de Aceites Fijos, Esenciales y Extractos de Plantas Ricos en Metabolitos Antioxidantes o Antimicrobianos [Development of New Agro-Industrial Products with High Added Value from Fixed Oils, Essential Oils, and Plant Extracts Rich in Antioxidant or Antimicrobial Metabolites].

Data Availability Statement: All relevant data are included within the article.

Acknowledgments: The authors wish to thank Helen Pugh for proofreading the article.

Conflicts of Interest: The authors declare no conflicts of interest or potential conflicts of commercial interest.

References

1. Bermond, C.; Cherrad, S.; Trainoy, A.; Ngari, C.; Poulet, V. Real-time qPCR to evaluate bacterial contamination of cosmetic cream and the efficiency of protective ingredients. *J. Appl. Microbiol.* **2021**, *132*, 2106–2120. [CrossRef] [PubMed]
2. Gómez Guarguati, I.C. Diseño Integrado Multiescala de Emulsiones Directas: Relación Entre Propiedades Reológicas y Texturales. Master's Thesis, Universidad de Los Andes, Bogota, Colombia, 2020.
3. Laura, R.; Javier, O.; Alejandro, H.; Bladimir, G. *La Cadena de Valor de los Ingredientes Naturales del Biocomercio en las Industrias Farmacéutica, Alimentaria y Cosmética-FAC*; Editorial Tadeo Lozano: Bogota, Colombia, 2012.
4. Gordillo López, R.C.; Romero Moya, E.A.; Romero, M.E. Optimización del Capital de Trabajo de una Empresa de la Industria Cosmética por Medio de un Esquema de Incentivos a la Fuerza de Ventas. Master's Thesis, Faculty of Social Sciences and Humanities FCSH-ESPOL, Guayaquil, Ecuador, 2020.
5. Guardado Yordi, E.; Radice, M.; Scalvenzi, L.; Pérez Martínez, A. Diseño del Proceso Sostenible para la Obtención de una Emulsión Cosmética desde un Enfoque de Biocomercio. *Rev. Politécnica* **2024**, *54*, 35–46. [CrossRef]
6. Asociación de Municipalidades Ecuatorianas. La Selva y Sus Componentes Naturales Para Embellecer. Available online: https://ame.gob.ec/2020/10/16/la-selva-y-sus-componentes-naturales-para-embellecer/ (accessed on 16 March 2025).
7. Torres, Y. Elaboración de una Crema con Actividad Exfoliante con Cáscara de Cacao (*Theobroma cacao* L.), Proveniente de la Provincia de Manabí. Ph.D. Thesis, Universidad Central del Ecuador, Quito, Ecuador, 2017.

8. Lendínez Gris, M. Estudio de Emulsiones Altamente Concentradas de Tipo W/O: Relación Entre Tamaño de Gota y Propiedades. Ph.D. Thesis, Universitat de Barcelona, Barcelona, Spain, 2015.
9. Torres Taipe, K.V. Estudio de Factibilidad para la Elaboración de Una Crema Hidratante a Base de Cáscaras de Huevo en La ciudad de Ambato, Provincia de Tungurahua. Licentiate Thesis, Universidad Técnica de Ambato, Ambato, Ecuador, 2021.
10. Salvador, A.; Chisvert, A. *Analysis of Cosmetic Products*; Elsevier: Cambridge, MA, USA, 2011.
11. Milan, A.L.K.; Milão, D.; Souto, A.A.; Corte, T.W.F. Estudo da Hidratação da Pele por Emulsões Cosméticas para Xerose e sua Estabilidade por Reologia. *Rev. Bras. Ciências Farm.* **2018**, *43*, 649–657. [CrossRef]
12. Venkataramani, D.; Tsulaia, A.; Amin, S. Fundamentals and applications of particle stabilized emulsions in cosmetic formulations. *Adv. Colloid Interface Sci.* **2020**, *283*, 102234. [CrossRef]
13. Suaza Montalvo, A. Desarrollo de Una Estrategia de Escalamiento para Procesos de Producción de Emulsiones. Master's Thesis, Universidad Nacional de Colombia, Bogota, Colombia, 2020.
14. Ruiz, Á.A.; Álvarez, H. Escalamiento de procesos químicos y bioquímicos basado en un modelo fenomenológico. *Inf. Tecnol.* **2011**, *22*, 33–52. [CrossRef]
15. Eraso Lasso, S.L. Aproximación al Proceso de Escalado de Emulsiones Concentradas Desde el Diseño Multiescala. Chemical Engineering Thesis, Universidad de Los Andes, Bogota, Colombia, 2015.
16. Schramm, L. *Emulsions, Foams, and Suspensions*; Wiley-VCH: Hoboken, NJ, USA, 2005.
17. May-Masnou, A.; Porras, M.; Maestro, A.; González, C.; Gutiérrez, J.M. Scale invariants in the preparation of reverse high internal phase ratio emulsions. *Chem. Eng. Sci.* **2013**, *101*, 721–730. [CrossRef]
18. Burakova, M.A.; Abrosimova, O.N.; Ladutko, Y.M.; Smekhova, I.E. Transfer of Cosmetic Emulsion Cream Technology from Laboratory to Pilot Phase. *Drug Dev. Regist.* **2022**, *11*, 59–67. [CrossRef]
19. Türedi, E.; Acaralı, N. Evaluation of cosmetic creams containing Black cumin (Nigella sativa)-Lemon balm (*Melissa officinalis* L.)-Aloe vera (Aloe barbadensis miller) essences by modeling with Box Behnken method in Design Expert. *Ind. Crops Prod.* **2022**, *187*, 115303. [CrossRef]
20. Campos Prada, D. Estudio de Correlaciones Experimentales para una Emulsión Aceite en Agua (O/W) Comercial. Licentiate Thesis, Universidad de los Andes, Bogota, Colombia, 2018.
21. Restrepo Jiménez, D. Aproximación al Diseño Multiescala en el Proceso de Escalado de Emulsiones Concentradas-Parámetro de Escalado. Licentiate Thesis, Universidad de los Andes, Bogota, Colombia, 2014.
22. López-Arévalo, I.; Bañares-Alcántara, R.; Aldea, A.; Rodríguez-Martínez, A.; Jiménez, L. Generation of process alternatives using abstract models and case-based reasoning. *Comput. Chem. Eng.* **2007**, *31*, 902–918. [CrossRef]
23. Yazdanpanah, N. Process simulation and mathematical modelling for process scale-up and technology transfer: Development and manufacturing of active pharmaceutical ingredients. *Chim. Oggi-Chem. Today* **2020**, *38*, 1–7.
24. Pérez-Martínez, A.; Cervantes-Mendieta, E.; Julián-Ricardo, M.C.; González-Suárez, E.; Gómez-Atanay, A.; Oquendo-Ferrer, H.; Galindo-Llanes, P.; Ramos-Sánchez, L. Procedimiento para enfrentar tareas de diseño de procesos de la industria azucarera y sus derivados. *Rev. Mex. Ing. Quím.* **2012**, *11*, 333–349.
25. Gallegos, J.d.C. Análisis del riesgo en la administración de proyectos de tecnología de información. *Ind. Data* **2006**, *9*, 104–107.
26. Rivera, M.; Ramos, M.; Silva, M.; Briceño, J.; Álvarez, M. Efecto de la temperatura previa a la extracción en el rendimiento y perfil de ácidos grasos del aceite de morete (*Mauritia flexuosa* LF). *LA GRANJA. Rev. Cienc. Vida* **2022**, *35*, 98–111. [CrossRef]
27. Rivera Chasiquiza, M. Efecto de la Temperatura de Extracción en el Rendimiento y Perfil de Ácidos Grasos del Aceite de Morete (*Mauritia flexuosa Lf*). Licentiate Thesis, Universidad Técnica de Ambato, Ambato, Ecuador, 2019.
28. Paredes Amasifuen, J.A. Determinación del Rendimiento y Características Fisicoquímicas del Aceite Obtenido Mediante Extracción Mecánica en Frío de Tres Ecotipos de Aguaje (*Mauritia flexuosa* L.) en la Región de Ucayali. Licentiate Thesis, Universidad Nacional de Ucayali, Pucallpa, Peru, 2021.
29. Adrianzén, N.; Rojas, C.; Luján, G.L. Efecto de la temperatura y tiempo de tratamiento térmico de las almendras trituradas de Sacha Inchi (*Plukenetia volubilis* L.) sobre el rendimiento y las características físico-químicas del aceite obtenido por prensado mecánico en frío. *Agroind. Sci.* **2011**, *1*, 46–55.
30. Ocampo-Duran, Á.; Fernández-Lavado, A.; Castro-Lima, F. Aceite de la palma de seje *Oenocarpus bataua Mart.* por su calidad nutricional puede contribuir a la conservación y uso sostenible de los bosques de galería en la Orinoquia Colombiana. *Orinoquia* **2013**, *17*, 215–229. [CrossRef]
31. Giacopini, M.I.; Guerrero, O.; Moya, M.; Bosch, V. Estudio comparativo del consumo de aceite de oliva virgen o seje sobre el perfil lipídico y la resistencia a la oxidación de las lipoproteínas de alta densidad (HDL) del plasma de rata. *Arch. Latinoam. Nutr.* **2011**, *61*, 143.
32. Peña, L.F.; Carrillo, M.P.; Giraldo, B.; Castro, S.Y.; Cardona, J.; Díaz, R.; Mosquera, L.E.; Hernández, M.S. *Desarrollo Tecnológico para el Aprovechamiento Sostenible de Frutos de las Palmas Asaí (Euterpe precatoria), Seje (Oenocarpus bataua), Moriche (Mauritia flexuosa)*; Instituto Amazónico de Investigaciones Científicas SINCHI: Leticia, Colombia, 2018; p. 95.

33. Chaves Yela, J.A.; Ortiz Tobar, D.P.; Bahos Ordoñez, E.M.; Ordoñez Forero, G.A.; Villota Padilla, D.C. Análisis del perfil de ácidos grasos y propiedades fisicoquímicas del aceite de palma de mil pesos (*Oenocarpus bataua*). *Perspect. Nutr. Hum.* **2020**, *22*, 175–188. [CrossRef]
34. Khattab, R.; Rempel, C.; Suh, M.; Thiyam, U. Quality of canola oil obtained by conventional and supercritical fluid extraction. *Am. J. Anal. Chem.* **2012**, *3*, 966–976. [CrossRef]
35. Bom, S.; Jorge, J.; Ribeiro, H.M.; Marto, J. A step forward on sustainability in the cosmetics industry: A review. *J. Clean. Prod.* **2019**, *225*, 270–290. [CrossRef]
36. Mosquera, T.; Noriega, P.; Tapia, W.; Pérez, S.H. Evaluación de la eficacia cosmética de cremas elaboradas con aceites extraídos de especies vegetales Amazónicas: *Mauritia flexuosa* (Morete), *Plukenetia volubilis* (Sacha Inchi) y *Oenocarpus bataua* (Ungurahua). *La Granja* **2012**, *16*, 14–22. [CrossRef]
37. Aliaga Zumaeta, E.; Quispe Alarcon, A. Estudio de Prefactibilidad para la Implementación de una Planta Productora de Mascarillas de Tela Hidratante a Base de Camu Camu (*Myrciaria dubia*). Licentiate Thesis, Universidad de Lima, Lima, Peru, 2022.
38. Romero, D.P.; Freire, A.; Aillon, F.E.; Radice, M. Design of an industrial process focused on the elaboration of cosmetics using Amazonian vegetal oils: A biotrade opportunity. In *MOL2NET'16, Conference on Molecular, Biomed., Comput. & Network Science and Engineering*, 2nd ed.; MDPI: Basel, Switzerland, 2022. [CrossRef]
39. Aguilar, C. Optimización del Proceso de Fabricación de Productos de Tocador y Limpieza en una Industria Cosmética de Ventas por Catálogo. Licentiate Thesis, Universidad de San Carlos de Guatemala, Guatemala City, Guatemala, 2011.
40. Zurita Acosta, N.; López Pérez, A.M. *Elaboración de Emulsiones Cosméticas con Ingredientes de Origen Natural*; Universidad de los Andes: Bogota, Colombia, 2021.
41. Chauhan, L.; Gupta, S. Creams: A Review on Classification, Preparation Methods, Evaluation and its Applications. *J. Drug Deliv. Ther.* **2020**, *10*, 281–289. [CrossRef]
42. Celeiro, M.; Garcia-Jares, C.; Llompart, M.; Lores, M. Recent Advances in Sample Preparation for Cosmetics and Personal Care Products Analysis. *Molecules* **2021**, *26*, 4900. [CrossRef] [PubMed]
43. Quillupangui, L.; Arroyo, F. Mejoramiento de la eficiencia general del equipo mediante la simulación de eventos discretos. estudio de caso en la industria cosmética. *Espacios* **2021**, *42*, 18–28. [CrossRef]
44. Rocca, R.; Acerbi, F.; Fumagalli, L.; Taisch, M. Sustainability paradigm in the cosmetics industry: State of the art. *Clean. Waste Syst.* **2022**, *3*, 100057. [CrossRef]
45. Cerda, V.R.; González, E.; Guardado, E.; Cerda, G.L.; Pérez, A. Producción de gel hidroalcohólico en tiempos de COVID-19, oportunidad para diseñar el proceso que garantice la calidad. *Cent. Azúcar* **2021**, *48*, 88–97.
46. Costa, V.B.F.d.; Valério, V.E.d.M.; Miranda, R.d.C. Economic analysis of a cosmetic initiative addressing stochastic aspects and risk quantification. *Acta Scientiarum. Technol.* **2023**, *45*, e59725. [CrossRef]
47. Cerda, V.R.; Guardado, E.; Cerda, G.L.; Vinocunga, R.; Pérez, A.; González, E. Procedure for the determination of operation and design parameters considering the quality of non-centrifugal cane sugar. *Entre Cienc. Ing.* **2022**, *16*, 43–50. [CrossRef]

processes

MDPI

Article

A Study of the Kinetics, Structure, and Morphology of the Effect of Organic Additives on Barium Sulfate Precipitation Reactions in Propan-1-ol–Water and Ethanol–Water Mixture Solutions

Lassaad Mechi [1,2,*], Khalid S. K. Alshammri [1], Abdulmohsen K. D. Alsukaibi [1], Hanen Azaza [3], Fathi Alimi [1], Fekhra Hedhili [4] and Younis Moussaoui [3]

1 Department of Chemistry, College of Science, University of Hail, P.O. Box 2440, Ha'il 81451, Saudi Arabia; kha.saadi@uoh.edu.sa (K.S.K.A.); a.alsukaibi@uoh.edu.sa (A.K.D.A.); f.alimi@uoh.edu.sa (F.A.)
2 Laboratoire des Matériaux et de l'Environnement pour le Développement Durable LR18ES10, Université Tunis El Manar, Tunis 1006, Tunisia
3 Faculty of Sciences of Gafsa, University of Gafsa, Gafsa 2112, Tunisia; azaza.hanen@yahoo.fr (H.A.); y.moussaoui2@gmail.com (Y.M.)
4 Department of Physics, College of Science, University of Hail, P.O. Box 2440, Ha'il 81451, Saudi Arabia
* Correspondence: l.mechi@uoh.edu.sa

Abstract: Barium sulfate precipitation in production industrial facilities and in petroleum reservoir systems is a dangerous operational problem. The solvent acts as a second component in the system during the onset of crystallization from solution, significant impacting the kinetics. Few studies have investigated the influence of organic solvents on barium sulfate precipitation. In this study, we examine the precipitation reaction of barium sulfate in mixed propan-1-ol–water and ethanol–water solvents at 303.15 K. The temporary conductivity variation is determined to follow the kinetics of the precipitation reaction and the germination time of barium sulfate crystals. A large variation is found in the precipitation reaction rate and induction time due to differences in physical parameters such as polarity and dielectric constants between water and organic solvents. This difference in physical properties leads to a stronger variation in intermolecular interaction between the solute and the solvent, especially in hydrogen bonds. The solid phase obtained at the end of the precipitate reaction is characterized through FTIR, XRD, and SEM techniques, demonstrating an important difference in the structure, morphology, and agglomeration phenomena of the precipitate obtained in water–ethanol and water–propan-1-ol mixtures compared to pure water solutions.

Keywords: barium sulfate; precipitation; organic solvent; kinetic; morphology

1. Introduction

The phenomenon of precipitation is a fundamental process of chemistry, often encountered in industry, especially when working in aqueous environments where water is one of the main constituents of the system. All thermodynamic and kinetic parameters of the precipitation process are related to the solubility of the solute in the solvent. The properties of the solute and solvent influence the interaction between salts and solvents. Solvents are identified by the Debye–Hückel technique based on their physical characteristics, including density, dielectric constant, viscosity, relative permittivity, and miscibility [1]. Since solvent mixtures are used in many industrial processes and laboratory operations, the solutes' solubility in mixed solvents is crucial from a practical standpoint. In the petroleum industry, the precipitation of barium sulfate in pipelines during the production phase is a notable example of scale formation in a mixed solvent. Indeed, studies have shown that the aqueous phase in oil slicks is rich in organic material due to the solubility of gases in water; contact between crude oil and formation water occurs [2,3] during water extraction in petroleum production.

Extensive studies have involved barium sulfate precipitation and co-precipitation phenomena in aqueous solutions [4–14]. The study of organic solvent effects on barium sulfate precipitation has received minimal experimental attention. In 2008, Jons et al.'s studies show that in the methanol–water mixture solution, the solubility of barium sulfate decreases, the crystal growth and nucleation times are faster, and a large difference in the morphology occurs when the amount of methanol increases [15]. In 2016, Esam A. G.'s study confirmed that the solubility of barium sulfate decreases in an ethanol–water mixture compared to a pure water solution [16]. Contrary to previous studies, in the case of calcium sulfate, Gomis et al. demonstrated that the solubility of calcium sulfate increases in the presence of ethanol [17].

It is well understood that in barium sulfate, previous studies have confirmed the effect of ethanol and methanol on the barium sulfate precipitation process.

However, studying the effects of adding these organic solvents requires more attention and greater synchronization between the physical properties of the solvents and the precipitation process. To achieve this goal, we propose studying the effect of two solvents with different physical properties: ethanol as a total miscible solvent and propan-1-ol as a partially miscible solvent with water (Table 1). In this paper, we present a kinetic, structural, and morphological study divided into two parts. In the first part—the solution study—we conduct a conductivity analysis to identify the effect of organic solvents on the kinetics of nucleation and crystal germination during the precipitation reaction. In the second part—the solid study—we present the characterization of the solid phase obtained using FTIR, XRD, and SEM techniques in order to determine the effect of the presence of organic solvents on the structure and morphology of the barite crystals.

Table 1. Physical properties of different solvents.

Solvent	Dipole Moment (D)	Dielectric Constant	Miscibility with Water
Water	1.85	78.5	---
Ethanol	1.69	24	Total
Propan-1-ol	1.68	20	Partial

2. Experimental Section

2.1. Experimental Unit

Figure 1: 1: Conductivity cell using JENWAY 4520 (Bibby Scientific Ltd., Stone, Staffs, UK); 2: electrode conductivity; 3: magnetic stirrer; 4: heating head; 5: reactor of 500 mL; and 6: thermostatic bath.

2.2. Chemical Reagents

Analytical-grade $BaCl_2$ and Na_2SO_4, ethanol, and propan-1-ol were supplied by SIGMA-ALDRICH (Germany), FLUKA (Honeywell International Inc.), and Lab-Scan (Ireland).

2.3. Experimental Procedure

To monitor the precipitation of barium sulfate, 100 mL of Na_2SO_4 solution and a 100 mL of $BaCl_2$ with a volume V (10 mL or 50 mL) of the organic solvent were introduced into a cylindrical reactor designed to resemble pipeline geometry under magnetic steering

(500 tr/min). We use a very high stirring speed to quickly obtain a homogeneous mixture between the organic and aqueous phases. Subsequently, the temperature for the reaction is set at the working temperature (at T = 303.15 K) using a bath equipped with a thermostat, since the different parameters of the precipitation reaction can change if the temperature is modified. We chose to work at temperatures near 303 K and at atmospheric pressure to ensure the environment closely resembled the precipitation conditions found at the surface of oil wells, in distribution pipes, or within the pipes of desalination units. In addition, we compared our results to the majority of previous work related to the precipitation of barite in the mixture phase [15–17]. At the end of each precipitation reaction, the solution was filtered under a Buchner system to recover the solid phase. The precept obtained was dried in an oven at a temperature equal to 105 degrees for 24 h to eliminate all solvent molecules, until the weight of the powder no longer decreases. This result is supported by the absence of any signal related to the solvent molecule in the infrared spectrum. At the start time, 100 mL of a $BaCl_2$ solution, prepared at the working temperature, was added to 100 mL of a Na_2SO_4 solution to initiate the precipitation reaction. The conductivity of the solution was measured at different times to monitor the precipitation reaction at T = 303.15 K and pH = 6.7 (in the presence of 50 mL ethanol, pH = 6.6, and in the presence of 50 mL propanol, pH = 6.4). Us SO_4^{-2} is an inactive base; the literature shows that within the range of 3–9, barite nucleation and growth are not affected by pH variation due to the addition of an organic solvent [18]. The pH must not exceed 7 to prevent the precipitation of $BaCO_3$ or $Ba(OH)_2$. The composition of all working solution was illustrated in Table 2.

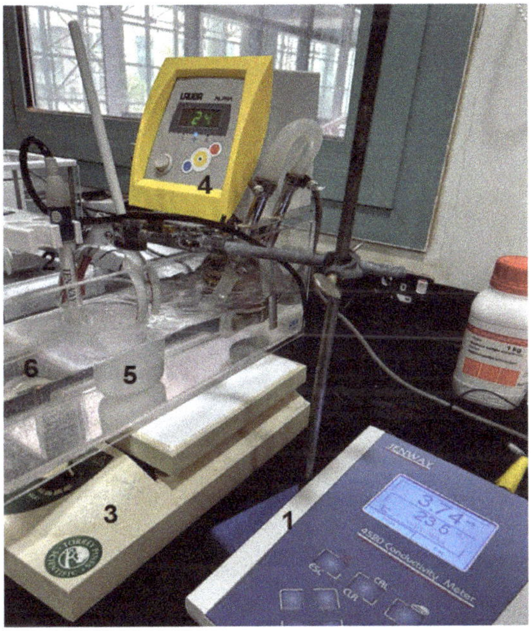

Figure 1. Experimental unit.

Table 2. Composition of working solutions.

Solution \ Composition	V of $BaCl_2$ (mL) (5×10^{-3} M)	V of Na_2SO_4 (mL) (5×10^{-3} M)	V (mL) of Add Organic Solvent	Molarity of Added Organic Solvent (M)	Mass of Precipitate
Solution S0	100	100	0	0	0.2131
Solution S1	100	100	10 mL of Ethanol	0.68	--
Solution S2	100	100	50 mL of Ethanol	3.43	0.1940
Solution S3	100	100	10 mL of Propan-1-ol	0.53	--
Solution S4	100	100	50 mL of Propan-1-ol	2.66	0.1882

All experiments were performed in triplicate; all conductivity data are expressed as the mean ± standard deviation in Figures 2 and 3.

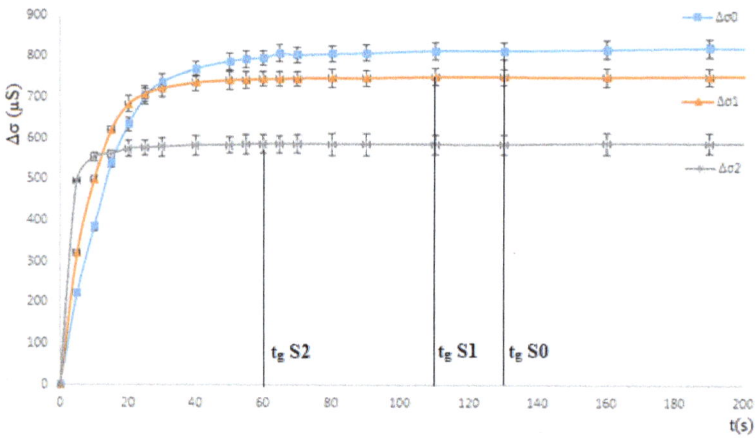

Figure 2. Temporal delta conductivity variation ($\Delta\sigma = \sigma_0 - \sigma_t$) in barium sulfate precipitation at T = 30 °C for S0, S1 (10 mL ethanol), and S2 (50 mL ethanol).

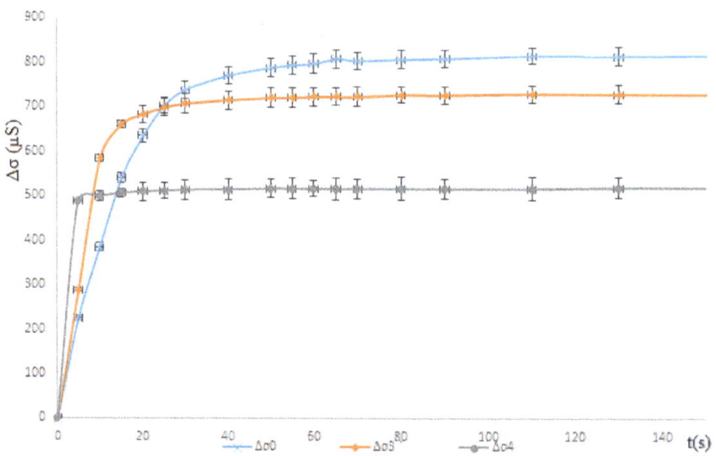

Figure 3. Temporal delta conductivity change ($\Delta\sigma = \sigma_0 - \sigma_t$) in barium sulfate precipitation at T = 30 °C for S0, S3 (10 mL propan-1-ol), and S4 (50 mL propane).

2.4. Theoretical Background

The value of barium sulfate supersaturation can be expressed by the following equation:

$$\Omega_{BaSO4} = \frac{\gamma_{Ba^{+2}}\left[Ba^{+2}\right]\gamma_{SO_4^{-2}}\left[SO_4^{-2}\right]}{k_{sp,BaSO4}} \quad (1)$$

The $k_{sp,BaSO_4} = 1.14 \times 10^{-10}$ at T = 303 K in pure water [19].

The specific activity coefficient can be calculated according to the extended Debye–Hückel equation. The Davies equation is an empirical extension of the Debye–Hückel theory, which can be used to calculate activity coefficients of electrolyte solutions at concentrations higher than 0.001 M [20].

$$\log \gamma_i = AZ_i^2\left(\frac{\sqrt{I}}{1+\sqrt{I}} - 0.31\right) \quad (2)$$

$$\mathrm{I} = \frac{1}{2}\sum\nolimits_{ions} m_i Z_i^2 \quad (3)$$

$A = 1.82 \times 10^6\ (\varepsilon T)^{-3/2} = 0.4961\ \mathrm{mol}^{-1/2}\ \mathrm{kg}^{1/2}$ at T = 303 K.

$\gamma = 0.9991$ (In dilute solutions, the activity coefficient is almost equal to 1);

$\Omega_{BaSO4} = 13{,}682$ in our synthetic solutions.

2.5. Analysis Techniques

At ambient temperature, the solid phase was analyzed using XRD, FTIR, and SEM techniques. XRD was performed using Cu Kα radiation (λ = 0.15418 nm) and a Philips X'PERTPRO diffractometer in step scanning mode. The scanning range for the XRD patterns was 2 h = 5–90°. A fixed counting period of 4 s and a tiny angular step of 2 h = 0.017° were employed. Software "Fullproof" [21] and HighScore Plus (version 3.0) were used to calculate the XRD reflection positions and for the solid phase matching. Infrared spectra of the samples in KBr pellets were obtained through diffuse reflectance, accumulating 40 scans on an Affinity-1C Schimadzu spectrophotometer, within the range of 400–4000 cm^{-1} at a resolution of 4 cm^{-1}. Scanning electron microscopy (SEM) images were obtained using a Philips FEI Quanta 250 model SEM device at an accelerating voltage of 30 KV.

3. Results and Discussions

This study is devoted to the analysis of barium sulfate precipitation reactions in the presence of certain organic fluids (ethanol and propan-1-ol) (Table 2). This investigation is based on conductivity measurements in the liquid phase, in addition to a morphological and spectroscopic exploration of the solid phase obtained at the end of these reactions.

3.1. Solution Study

Given that solution composition differs for each experiment, in order to compare results, it is more effective to present the $\Delta\sigma$ conductivity variation instead of the solution conductivity curves. Delta conductivity ($\Delta\sigma$) is the difference between the initial conductivity and the conductivity at time t: $\Delta\sigma = \sigma_0 - \sigma_t$.

Therefore, we investigated the effects of two organic solvents with differing miscibility in aqueous solution (ethanol and propan-1-ol) on the reaction involving barium sulfate precipitation. We showed their effects one by one. Indeed, the precipitation rate of barium sulfate was investigated using the conductimetric technique, where the supersaturation is larger than 1. The rate of linear growth of barium sulfate crystals is limited by a process occurring at the crystal–solution interface through the following reaction:

$$Ba^{2+}(aq) + SO_4^{2-}(aq) \rightarrow BaSO_{4(s)}$$

3.1.1. Ethanol Effect: Total Miscibility

The effect of ethanol on barium sulfate precipitation is assessed by monitoring the conductivity measurements in synthetic solutions during the precipitation reaction. The temporal variation of $\Delta\sigma$ curves in the various solutions S0, S1, and S2 is shown in Figure 2.

Figure 2 shows that ethanol influences the kinetics and thermodynamic of barite precipitation. All curves are distinguished by the existence of two zones. The first corresponds to a nonlinear variation in the conductivity as a function of time, corresponding to nucleation and to crystalline growth evolution (t_{ind} + tg). The second step, which relates to the linear part of the curve, corresponds to the equilibrium state (end of the reaction). As the supersaturation coefficient is higher in our case ($\Omega_{BaSO4} = 13{,}682$), the induction time is very small, which is why the induction step is not detectable [22].

On one hand, it is understood that ethanol added in different volumes affects the kinetics and thermodynamic of the barite precipitation reaction. Thus, when we increase the volume of ethanol, the total $\Delta\sigma$ variation decreases (233 $mS{\cdot}cm^{-1}$ between S0 and S2). Therefore, the presence of ethanol decreases the mass of the precipitate obtained (m_0 = 0.2131 g, m_2 = 0.1940 g), which implies an increase in solubility. This result was expected due to the decrease in the dielectric constant and the polarity of the mixture (Table 1), as well as the difference in the value of the free energy of solvation [15–17]. This difference in polarity and dielectric constant leads, at the microscopic scale, to variations in the hydrogen bonds associated with water and ethanol molecules. Consequently, these factors directly affect the precipitation phenomenon. Some of the hydrogen bonds separating the molecules of water are disrupted when an ethanol molecule is added to the water. Although there are new attractions that occur between ethanol and water molecules, the structure of the water is significantly altered due to these new attractions differing from the ones that are broken.

On the other hand, for the same reason, Figure 2 illustrates that the kinetics of barite crystallization in ethanol–water mixtures for the supersaturated solution are affected. In the first step of the precipitation reaction (the crystal growth step), the rate of the precipitation reaction increases as the volume of the added ethanol increases. In addition, the crystal germination time, tg, in S1 (tg = 110 s) and S2 (tg = 60 s) is noted to be less than in S0 (tg = 130 s). In this respect, the results of our study indicate that the dielectric environment can play a critical role in determining the relative stability of the crystalline phases (the nucleation process). These results imply that both nucleation and growth occur more quickly in ethanol than in water, which can also affect the morphology of barite particles. These results align with the precipitation of barite in the presence of methanol. Jones et al. linked this modification to the variation in the surface tension factor of barium sulfate particles [15]. The conductivity measurements show that the water–ethanol solutions exhibit both faster nucleation and crystal growth. It is anticipated that adding ethanol will alter the surface tension of the barite particles. The Gibbs–Thomson equation, the basis of classical nucleation theory, states that surface tension can influence the nucleation rate J by

$$J = v_D C_N \tag{4}$$

where v_D is the rate of impingement of ions on the nuclei, and C_N is the concentration of critical nuclei.

$$C_N = Ce^{\frac{\Delta G}{K_B T}} \tag{5}$$

$$\Delta G^c = \frac{16\,\pi\,\gamma^3\,V_0^2}{3\,k_B^3\,T^3\,Ln\,(S^*)^2} \tag{6}$$

where γ is the surface tension, C is the solution concentration, $S^* = C/C_{eq}$ is the supersaturation, and V_0 is the volume of a unit cell.

Referring to Equations (5) and (6), factors that can significantly affect the nucleation rate in water and water–ethanol mixtures at the same temperature and supersaturation levels are the variations in surface tension γ and solubility [15]. On one hand, as demonstrated in a different study [23], surface tension decreases in the ethanol–water mixture compared to that of pure water. On the other hand, solubility increases [15], directly implying an increase in the nucleation rate, in agreement with our experiment results.

3.1.2. Propan-1-ol Effect: Partial Miscible

In the case of propan-1-ol addition, Figure 3 shows the same phenomenon observed with the addition of ethanol. When the volume of propan-1-ol increases, the total $\Delta\sigma$ variation decreases (307 mS.cm^{-1} between S0 and S4). Therefore, the presence of propan-1-ol decreases the mass of the precipitate (m_0 = 0.2131 g, m_4 = 0.1882 g). Propan-1-ol demonstrates a greater effect compared to the addition of ethanol due to the significant difference in the dielectric constant and polarity between pure water and propan-1-ol (Table 1). These results imply that both nucleation and growth occur more quickly in the presence of propan-1-ol (the nucleation process) than in pure water, which can also affect the morphology of barite particles obtained at the end of the reaction [15–17]. These variations can be attributed to the difference in solubility and in surface tension γ (Equations (4)–(6)).

3.2. Solid Study

The solid phase obtained was characterized by FTIR, XRD, and SEM techniques. We chose to characterize the solid phase recovered from the solutions S0, S2, and S4.

3.2.1. FTIR

The infrared spectra of barium sulfate precipitate obtained from solutions S0, S2, and S4 (Figures 4–6) show several peaks. Peak assignments were made based on the literature data [15,24].

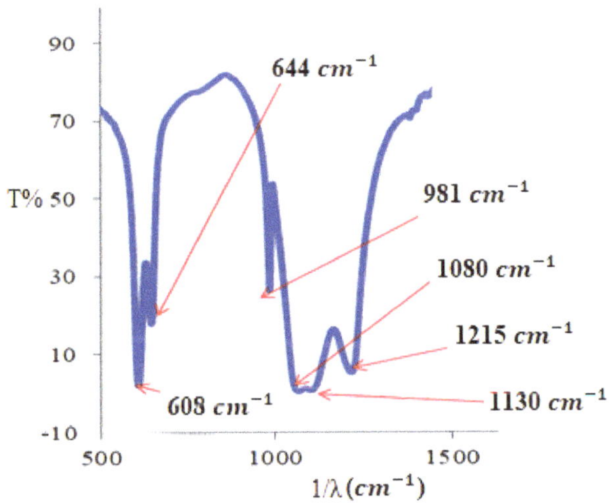

Figure 4. FTIR transmittance spectrum of pure $BaSO_{4(s)}$ obtained in pure water (S0).

Figure 4 shows the FT-IR spectra of the pure $BaSO_4$ obtained from solution S0. The literature states that the sulfate group has three fundamental vibrational modes (T_d molecular point group). There is one nondegenerate mode (V1) at 981 cm^{-1} assigned to the symmetric stretching vibration of the SO_4^{2-} group (mode (V2) is inactive); one doubly degenerate mode (V4) in the low frequency domain at 608 cm^{-1} and 644 cm^{-1}, corresponding to deformation vibration; and one triply degenerate mode (V3) at 1080 cm^{-1}, 1130 cm^{-1}, and 1215 cm^{-1} assigned to the antisymmetric stretching vibration of the SO_4^{2-} group [24].

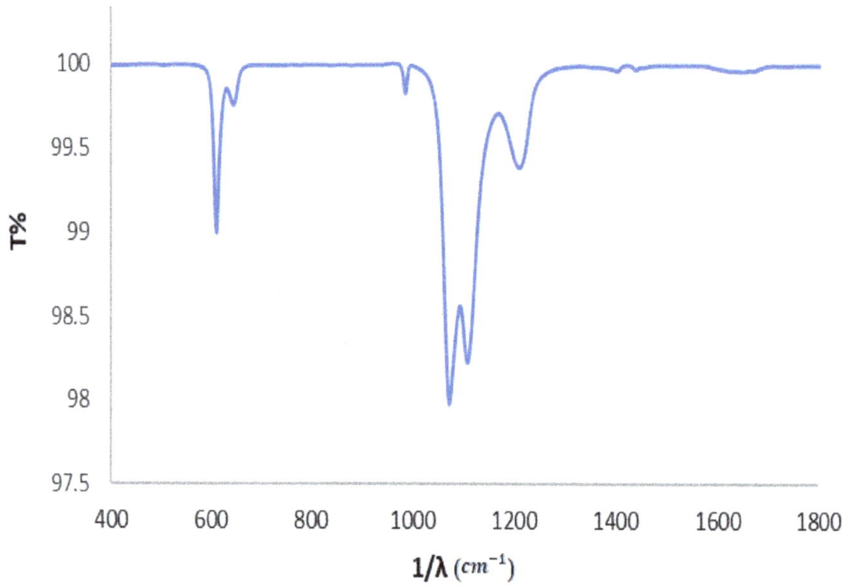

Figure 5. FTIR transmittance spectrum of pure $BaSO_{4(s)}$ obtained in the presence of ethanol (S2).

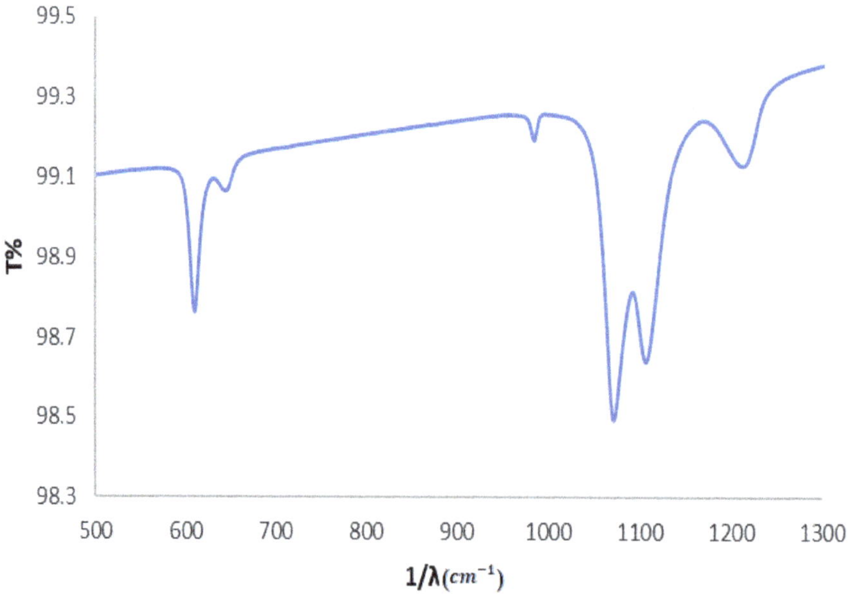

Figure 6. FTIR transmittance spectrum of $BaSO_{4(s)}$ obtained in the presence of propan-1-ol (S4).

The comparison of the three spectra in Figures 4–6 shows that the presence of ethanol and propan-1-ol leads to a difference in the antisymmetric vibration frequencies (V3). This difference can be attributed to a structural difference in the crystal lattice attributed to the presence of organic solvents [15,24]. That indicates a modification in morphology and in the lattice parameters. Given the presence of all the pics related to the vibrations of the sulfate group in the barite network, we can confirm that the solid phase obtained from the S2 and S4 solutions is barium sulfate. To confirm these results, we examined the solid deposits obtained using the X-ray diffraction technique to characterize the structure and the electron microscopy technique to analyze the morphology.

3.2.2. XRD

The identification of the solid phase obtained from S2 and S4 was carried out by matching it with highScore Plus, identified as the barium sulfate ICSD pattern-code 01-080-0512 [25]. Figures 7 and 8 confirm the $BaSO_4$ structure for both solid phases obtained from S2 and S4.

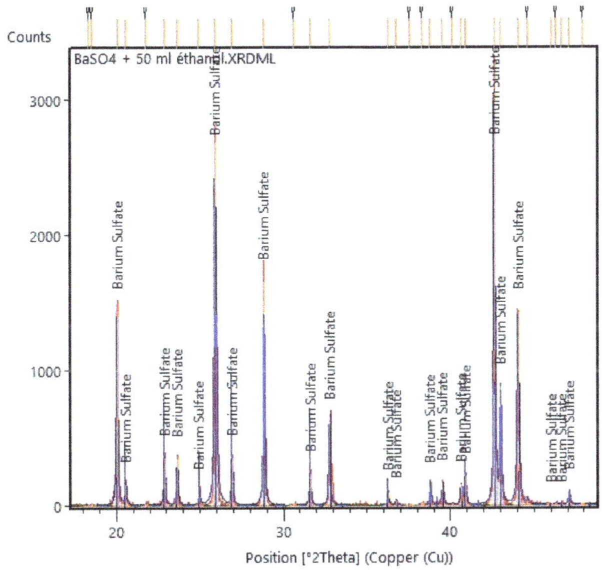

Figure 7. Qualitative characterization of the solid obtained from S2 via HighScore plus software.

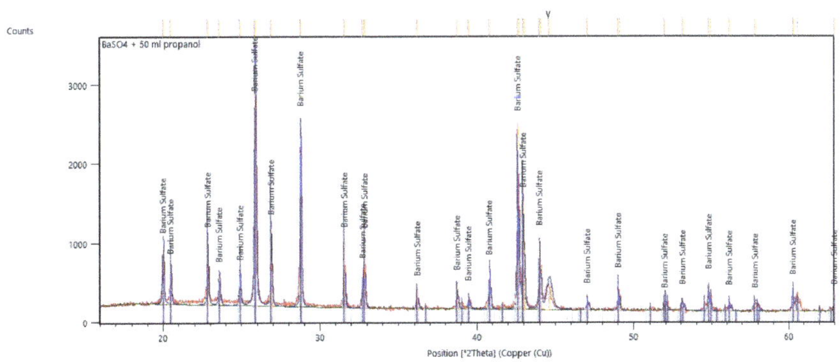

Figure 8. Qualitative characterization of the solid obtained from S4 via HighScore plus software.

Figure 9 shows that the presence of an organic solvent causes a slight shift in the XRD peaks to higher 2θ angles [9]. The peak shift arises from lattice distortions involving a slight compression of the crystal lattice, which results in a decrease in the unit cell volume. In addition, we can observe a modification in the position of the principal peak. These results allow us to predict that the morphology of barite will change in the solutions S2 and S4 because the main orientation of germination will be modified due to a modification in the electrostatic field [15,26]. Indeed, XRD results confirm the FTIR results.

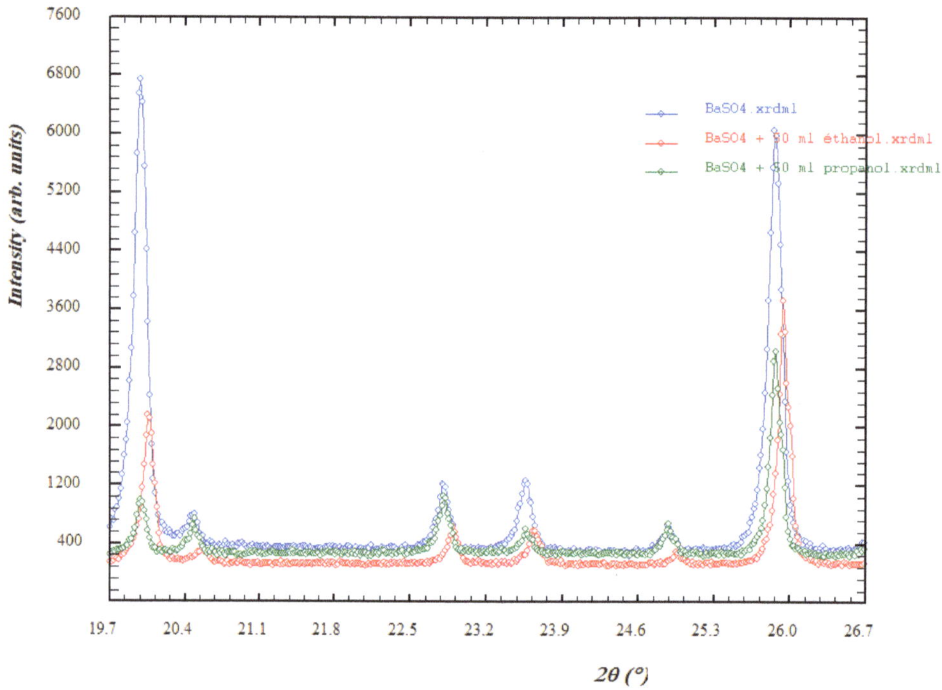

Figure 9. Superposition of XRD patterns of barite obtained from S0, S2, and S4.

3.2.3. SEM

The solid phase obtained from solutions S0, S2, and S4 was also examined using the SEM technique to confirm our FTIR and XRD results related to morphology interpretation.

SEM images depicted in Figures 10–12 indicate that the morphologies of solid barite obtained from S2 and S4 are different compared to S0. We observed a strongly anisotropic growth of two-dimensional nuclei [5]. The variations in the solvent surface contacts of polar crystals must be linked to a noticeable differential in growth rate at their opposing hemihedral faces. According to a specially designed, tailor-made inhibitor theory, a solvent acting as an adsorbed additive would inhibit the regular deposition of incoming molecular layers and hence prevent crystal formation at that face [27]. Thus, the difference in interaction is attributed to the difference in crystal growth direction.

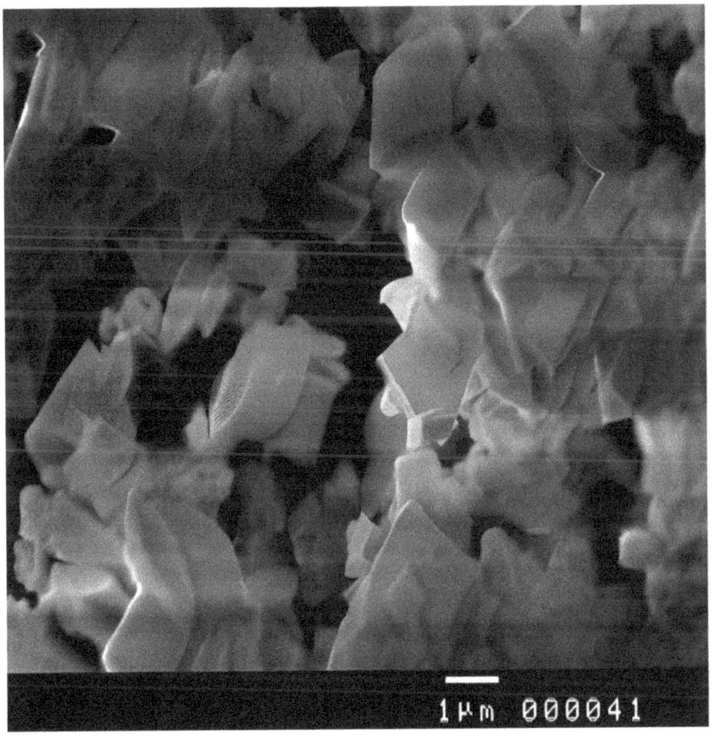

Figure 10. SEM image of a barite solid obtained from S0.

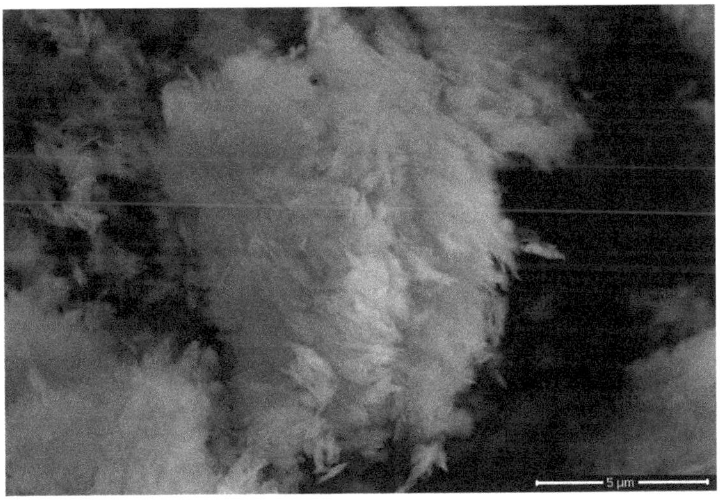

Figure 11. SEM image of a barite solid obtained from S2.

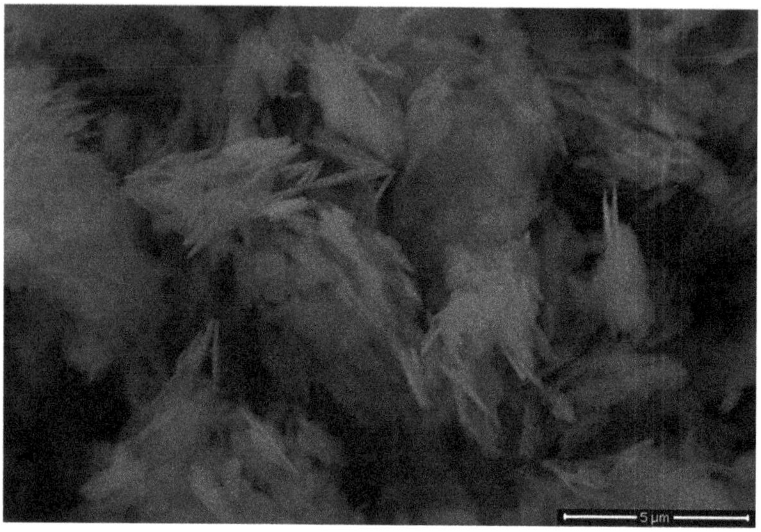

Figure 12. SEM images of a barite solid obtained from S4.

The agglomeration of solid barite is more pronounced in S2 and S4 than in S0. This result can be attributed to differences in crystal–crystal interactions in various solutions (dynamics of collisions), which affect the development of crystalline bridges and interparticle consolidation during the agglomeration of barite due to differences in crystal growth rates (Figures 2 and 3). Crystal agglomeration and aggregation disturbances depend on crystal growth rates [10,28,29].

SEM images illustrated in Figures 11 and 12 show that in the presence of ethanol, a homogeneous morphology can be achieved from S2 (total miscibility of solvent), while a heterogeneous morphology can be achieved from S4 (partial miscibility of solvent). This result can be attributed to the difference in miscibility between ethanol and propan-1-ol in aqueous solution.

All solid characterization techniques confirm that there is a structural and morphological difference attributed to the presence of organic solvents, according to the conductivity study.

4. Conclusions

This work explores the influence of adding organic solvents (ethanol and propanol-1-ol) into barium sulfate precipitation in an aqueous medium. The difference in physical parameters, such as polarity and dielectric constant, between water and these organic solvents provides a perturbation in the intermolecular interaction between solute and solvent, especially the hydrogen bond. Further analysis of the conductivity variation in the saturated solution of barium sulfate shows that stronger variations in intermolecular interactions between the solute and the solvent affect the kinetics of the nucleation process and the mass of the precipitate obtained. It can be seen that the water–ethanol and water–propanol solutions exhibit faster nucleation and crystal growth. In addition, when the volume of ethanol increases, the total $\Delta\sigma$ variation decreases (indicated by a decrease in the mass of the precipitate obtained), implying an increase in barite solubility. Solid phase analyses using FTIR, XRD, and SEM techniques confirm the conductivity results. For the solid phase obtained, FTIR and XRD spectra illustrate a slight difference in water–ethanol and water–propan-1-ol mixtures compared to pure water. Both techniques confirm the formation of barite in all solvent mixtures. SEM images confirm all previous analyses and show a significant difference in morphology and agglomeration phenomena due to the presence of organic solvent. The difference in morphology between the solids obtained from S2 and S4 arises from the differing miscibility with water of ethanol and propan-1-ol.

Author Contributions: Conceptualization, L.M. and K.S.K.A.; Data curation, L.M. and K.S.K.A.; Formal analysis, K.S.K.A. and H.A.; Funding acquisition, L.M.; Investigation, A.K.D.A.; Methodology, L.M. and A.K.D.A.; Project administration, L.M.; Resources, A.K.D.A.; Software, F.H.; Supervision, L.M.; Validation, H.A. and F.A.; Writing—original draft, L.M. and Y.M.; Writing—review and editing, L.M. and F.H. All authors have read and agreed to the published version of the manuscript.

Funding: This research has been funded by the Scientific Research Deanship at the University of Ha'il, Saudi Arabia, through project number <RG-23 229>.

Data Availability Statement: The data used to support the findings of this study are available from the corresponding author upon request.

Conflicts of Interest: The authors declare no conflicts of interest.

References

1. Robinson, R.A.; Stokes, R.H. *Electrolytes Solutions*; Butterworth & Co. (Pulishers) Ltd.: Devon, UK, 2002.
2. Gene Collins, A. *Geochemistry of Oilfield Waters*, 1st ed.; Elsevier Scientific Publishing Company: Amsterdam, The Netherlands, 1975; pp. 195–201.
3. Wang, S.Y.; Mark, B.; Alice, M.B.; Aila, M.; Leena, S.; Donald, M. The water solubility of crude oils and petroleum products. *Oil Chem. Pollut.* **1990**, *7*, 57–84.
4. Bosbach, D.; Hall, C.; Putnis, A. Mineral Precipitation and Dissolution in Aqueous Solution: In-Situ Microscopic Observations on Barite (001) with Atomic Force Microscopy. *Chem. Geol.* **1998**, *151*, 143–160. [CrossRef]
5. Bracco, J.N.; Gooijer, Y.; Higgins, S.R. Hydrothermal atomic force microscopy observations 478 of barite step growth rates as a function of the aqueous barium-to-sulfate ratio. *Geochim. Cosmochim. Acta* **2016**, *183*, 1–13. [CrossRef]
6. Pina, C.M.; Putnis, C.V.; Becker, U.; Biswas, S.; Carroll, E.C.; Bosbach, D.; Putnis, A. An atomic force microscopy and molecular simulations study of the inhibition of barite growth by phosphonates. *Surf. Sci.* **2004**, *553*, 61–74. [CrossRef]
7. Pina, C.M.; Becker, U.; Risthaus, P.; Bosbach, D.; Putnis, A. Molecular-scale mechanisms of crystal growth in barite. *Nature* **1998**, *395*, 483–486. [CrossRef]
8. Bin Merdhah, A.B. Inhibition of barium sulphate scale at high-barium formation water. *J. Petrol. Sci. Eng.* **2012**, *90–91*, 124–130. [CrossRef]
9. Azaza, H.; Doggaz, A.; Mechi, L.; Optasanu, V.; Tlili, M.; Ben Amor, M. Synthesis of intermediate crystal $Ba_{1-x}Ca_xSO_4$ system via co-precipitation of $BaSO_4$-$CaSO_4$ and partial hindrance of gypsum formation. *Desalin. Water Treat.* **2017**, *66*, 80–87. [CrossRef]
10. Azaza, H.; Mechi, L.; Doggaz, A.; Optasanu, V.; Tlili, M.; Ben Amor, M. Enhancement of calcite formation in presence of sulfate bariyum: Kinetic & morphological studies. *Arab. J. Geosci.* **2017**, *10*, 1–9.
11. Wu, D.; Liu, D.; Luo, H.; Wang, J.; Zhao, H.; Dong, Y. Studies on the dissolution mechanism of barium sulfate by different alkaline metal hydroxides: Molecular simulations and experperiments. *J. Mol. Liq.* **2025**, *418*, 126708. [CrossRef]
12. de Freitas Dam, R.S.; dos Santos, M.C.; Salgado, W.L.; da Cruz, B.L.; Schirru, R.; Salgado, C.M. Prediction of fluids volume fraction and barium sulfate scale in a multiphase system using gamma radiation and deep neural network. *Appl. Radiat. Isot.* **2023**, *201*, 111021.
13. Li, L.; He, X.; Zhang, X.; Wang, S.; Guo, S.; Tang, N.; Wang, X. A facile method to control the morphologies of barium sulfate particles by using carboxylic carbon quantum dots as a regulator. *Colloid. Surf. A* **2021**, *631*, 127668. [CrossRef]
14. Van Der Leeden, M.C.; Kashchiev, D.; Van Rosmalen, G.M. Precipitation of Barium Sulfate: Induction Time and the Effect of an Additive on Nucleation and Growth. *J. Colloid. Interface Sci.* **1992**, *152*, 338–350. [CrossRef]
15. Jones, F.; Piana, S.; Gale, J.D. Understanding the Kinetics of Barium Sulfate Precipitation from Water and Water–Methanol Solutions. *Cryst. Growth Des.* **2008**, *8*, 817–822. [CrossRef]
16. Gomaa, A. Solubility and Solvation Parameters of Barium Sulphate in Mixed Ethanol-Water Mixtures at 301.15 K. *Int. J. Mater. Chem.* **2012**, *2*, 16–18. [CrossRef]
17. Gomis, V.; Saquete, M.D.; García-Cano, J. $CaSO_4$ solubility in water–ethanol mixtures in the presence of sodium chloride at 25 °C application to a reverse osmosis process. *Fluid Ph. Equilib.* **2013**, *360*, 248–252. [CrossRef]
18. Ruiz-Agudo, C.; Putnis, V.C.; Ruiz-Agudo, E.; Putnis, A. The influence of pH on barite nucleation and growth. *Chem. Geol.* **2015**, *6*, 7–18. [CrossRef]

19. Monnin, C. A thermodynamic model for the solubility of barite and celestite in electrolyte solutions and seawater to 200 °C and to 1 kbar. *Chem. Geol.* **1999**, *153*, 187–209. [CrossRef]
20. Davies, C.W. *Ion Association*, 1st ed.; Butterworths: London, UK, 1962; pp. 37–52.
21. Rodriguez-Carvajal, J. FULLPROF: A Program for Rietveld Refinement and Pattern Matching Analysis. In Proceedings of the Satellite Meeting on Powder Diffraction of the XV Congress of the IUCr, Toulouse, France, 16–19 July 1990; p. 127.
22. Mersmann, A.; Eble, A.; Heye, C. *Cristallization Technology Handbook*, 1st ed.; Marcel Dekker: New York, NY, USA, 1994; pp. 85–104.
23. Nassif, A.G.; Ibrahim, S.S.; Majdi, H.S.; Alsalhy, Q.F. Ethanol Separation from an Ethanol–Water Solution Using Vacuum Membrane Distillation. *Membranes* **2022**, *12*, 807. [CrossRef]
24. Ramaswamy, V.; Vimalathithan, R.; Ponnusamy, M.V. Synthesis and characterization of $BaSO_4$ nano particles using micro emulsion technique. *Adv. Appl. Sci. Res.* **2010**, *1*, 197–204.
25. Degen, T.; Sadki, M.; Bron, E.; König, U.; Nénert, G. The HighScore suite. *Powder Diffr.* **2014**, *29* (Suppl. S2), S13–S18. [CrossRef]
26. Jones, F.; Jones, P.; Ogden, M.I.; Richmond, W.R.; Rohl, A.L.; Saunders, M. The interaction of EDTA with barium sulphate. *J. Colloid. Interf. Sci.* **2007**, *316*, 553–561. [CrossRef] [PubMed]
27. Meir, L.; Leslie, L. The effect of solvent on crystal growth and morphology. *Chem. Eng. Sci.* **2001**, *56*, 2245–2253.
28. Brunsteiner, M.; Jones, A.G.; Pratola, F.; Price, S.L.; Simons, S.J.R. Toward a Molecular Understanding of Crystal Agglomeration. *Cryst. Growth Des.* **2005**, *5*, 3–16. [CrossRef]
29. Wójcik, J.A.; Jones, A.G. Particle disruption of precipitated $CaCO_3$ crystal agglomerates in turbulently agitated suspensions. *Chem. Eng. Sci.* **1998**, *53*, 1097–1101. [CrossRef]

processes

MDPI

Article

Porous Zn Nano-Wafer Aerogels for Asymmetric Supercapacitors: Synthesis, Structural Engineering, and Performance

Ramya Ramkumar [1,†], Ganesh Koyyada [1,†], Md Riad Al Rabbi Abir [1], Thirumala Rao Gurugubelli [2], Woo Kyoung Kim [1,*] and Jae Hong Kim [1,*]

1 School of Chemical Engineering, Yeungnam University, Gyeongsan 38541, Republic of Korea; ramya.iitm@gmail.com (R.R.); ganeshkoyyada@gmail.com or ganeshkoyyada@ynu.ac.kr (G.K.); riad13842@gmail.com (M.R.A.R.A.)
2 Department of Physics, School of Sciences & Humanities, SR University, Warangal 506371, Telangana, India; thirumalaphy@gmail.com
* Correspondence: wkim@ynu.ac.kr (W.K.K.); jaehkim@ynu.ac.kr (J.H.K.)
† These authors contributed equally to this work.

Abstract: Transition metal oxide aerogels (AGLs) have attracted considerable attention in recent years due to their exceptional properties, including high surface area, significant porosity, and ultralow density. In this study, we report the first-time synthesis of zinc oxide nano-wafers and zinc aerogels for application as supercapacitor electrodes. The aerogels were synthesized via a novel one-pot hydrolysis method using $NaBH_4$ as a reducing agent and subsequently annealed at 200 °C ($Zn_{AGL(200)}$) and 450 °C ($Zn_{AGL(450)}$) to investigate the influence of temperature on their electrochemical properties. Structural and morphological characterizations were conducted using XRD, FTIR, BET, XPS, SEM, and TEM analyses. Among the fabricated electrodes, the aerogel annealed at 200 °C ($Zn_{AGL(200)}$) exhibited superior energy storage performance, attributed to its amorphous, continuous network structure, which enhanced its surface area and reduced its density compared to both the as-synthesized ($Zn_{AGL(RT)}$) and 450 °C-annealed ($Zn_{AGL(450)}$) counterparts. A two-electrode device demonstrated excellent cycling stability over 10,000 cycles, achieving an energy density of 7.97 Wh/kg and a power density of 15 kW/kg. These findings highlight the potential of zinc aerogels as materials for next-generation lightweight energy storage systems, with promising applications in industrial, mechanical, and aerospace technologies.

Keywords: zinc oxide; aerogels; supercapacitor; nickel foam

1. Introduction

The global demand for efficient energy storage has highlighted the limitations of present technologies, such as capacitors, batteries, and fuel cells, in meeting the needs of a growing population [1,2]. Supercapacitors (SCs) have emerged as a viable option due to their high power density, short charge–discharge times, and excellent cycle stability [3]. However, there are certain shortcomings, the most noticeable of which is their higher rates of self-discharge when compared to lithium-ion batteries, which can result in significant energy loss over time [4,5]. Studies suggest that a high surface area plays a crucial role in enhancing the electrochemical performance of pseudocapacitive supercapacitors by offering more Faradaic active sites [6,7]. Additionally, larger pore volume facilitates ion transport within the electrode, thereby improving the rate capability [8].

Aerogels (AGLs) have recently sparked widespread interest because of their unusual structure-dependent optical, mechanical, electrical, and magnetic capabilities [9,10]. Their high porosity, huge surface area, and ultralightweight properties make them suitable scaffolds for high-performance electrode materials in energy storage applications [11,12]. Notably, their exceptionally low density offers a significant advantage over traditional nanoscale materials. Initially, aerogel research concentrated on carbon-based matrices like graphene, with metals utilized as conductive and capacitive components [13]. However, recent advances have moved beyond carbon frameworks to investigate the potential of metal oxide aerogels as freestanding electrode materials, widening their applicability in next-generation supercapacitors and energy storage devices [14,15].

Among many transition metals, zinc oxide (ZnO) is a low-cost metallic oxide with sufficient electrochemical activity (an energy density of 650 A g^{-1}) [16]. ZnO's high theoretical capacitance, eco-friendliness, and stability make it a promising contender for supercapacitor electrodes [17–19]. Recent research has investigated the combination of ZnO with graphene-based materials to improve electrochemical performance. Das et al. used waste biomass-derived 3D graphene aerogels (GAs) as cathode materials for zinc-ion hybrid supercapacitors (ZHSCs), reaching a specific capacitance of 353.1 F g^{-1} at 0.1 A g^{-1} and ~84.2% capacity retention over 10,000 cycles at 10 A g^{-1} [19]. Their porous structure enabled efficient charge storage and ion transport, making them promising for energy storage applications. Ghazitabar et al. successfully synthesized an N-doped graphene aerogel/Co_3O_4/ZnO ternary nanocomposite, which demonstrated improved electrical conductivity and enhanced electrochemical properties with a high specific capacitance of 543 F g^{-1} [16]. Hassan et al. reported a specific capacitance of 108.95 mV/s for graphene aerogel integrated with ZnO materials [20]. Despite these promising advances, the synthesis and application of ZnO-based aerogel nanocomposites in electrochemical energy storage remain underexplored. While numerous studies have concentrated on producing ZnO aerogels for a variety of applications, their potential as high-performance supercapacitor electrodes has yet to be fulfilled.

In this study, we devised a one-pot synthesis technique for zinc aerogels and investigated their structural and electrochemical properties by annealing at 200 °C and 450 °C, respectively. These aerogels were used as electrode materials in supercapacitor applications, and the 200 °C-annealed sample ($Zn_{AGL(200)}$) demonstrated improved electrochemical performance, with a maximum energy density of 7.97 Wh/kg and a power density of 15 kW/kg. This improved performance is due to its amorphous nanocrystalline, continuous network structure, which provides a large surface area and ultralow density when compared to the as-synthesized ($Zn_{AGL(RT)}$) and 450 °C-annealed ($Zn_{AGL(450)}$) counterparts. These findings emphasize zinc aerogels' potential for enhanced energy storage as well as other industrial and therapeutic uses.

2. Materials and Methods

The detailed characterizations of aerogels, electrochemical analysis, and device fabrications are provided in the Electronic Supplementary Materials.

2.1. Materials

Zinc nitrate ($Zn(NO_3)_2$, 99%), sodium borohydride ($NaBH_4$, 99%), sodium sulfate (Na_2SO_4, 99%), and potassium hydroxide (KOH, 99%) were purchased from Sigma-Aldrich. Ethanol, iso propyl alcohol, and acetone were purchased from Alfa Aesar. Carbon black was purchased from Merck Chemicals. The nitrogen gas cylinder was purchased from a local dealer (Republic of Korea). All experiments were performed with deionized water, and the temperature was maintained at 25 °C, unless otherwise specified.

2.2. Preparation of $Zn_{AGL(RT)}$, $Zn_{AGL(200)}$, and $Zn_{AGL(450)}$ Aerogels

Zinc aerogels were synthesized by dissolving $Zn(NO_3)_2$ in a mixture of ethanol and deionized water, followed by nitrogen bubbling for 20 min. A 0.5 M $NaBH_4$ solution in ethanol was then added, leading to an instant color change to pale white, indicating aerogel formation. The resulting hydrogels were washed multiple times with DI water and ethanol and then freeze-dried for two days. The obtained Zn aerogels were stored in a desiccator. To prepare ZnO aerogels, the Zn aerogels were annealed at 200 °C and 450 °C for 2 h at a heating rate of 10 °C/min. Amorphous aerogels exhibited higher solubility in ethanol than their crystalline counterparts.

3. Results and Discussion

The SEM images of the as-prepared zinc aerogel samples ($Zn_{AGL(RT)}$) and annealed samples ($Zn_{AGL(200)}$ and $Zn_{AGL(450)}$), shown in Figure 1a–c, reveal thin wafer-like flaky nanoporous structures. The $Zn_{AGL(RT)}$ samples show significantly large flakes with sharp edges and a highly porous nature, as observed from the SEM studies, and when annealed at 200 °C, the resultant $Zn_{AGL(200)}$ samples show more open flaky structures with nanoparticle formation resulting from annealing. The $Zn_{AGL(450)}$ samples resulting from annealing the aerogel at 450 °C show more nanoparticle nature and less aggregation of nanoflakes. The EDS (Figure 1d) of the zinc aerogels annealed at 200 °C shows the presence of zinc and no impurities (the carbon and oxygen obtained from the background). Although the SEM images appear similar, the TEM analysis reveals significant differences. The HR-TEM analysis of the as-synthesized $Zn_{AGL(RT)}$, $Zn_{AGL(200)}$, and $Zn_{AGL(450)}$ is presented in Figure 2a,c,e and Figure 2b,d,f, respectively. The HR-TEM images of the as-synthesized $Zn_{AGL(RT)}$ (Figure 2c,d) confirm the presence of nanoflake structures with edge widths ranging from 5 to 10 nm, incorporating aggregated zinc nanoparticles within the nanostructured framework. Upon annealing at 200 °C, the nanoflakes exhibit a more interconnected and continuous morphology, suggesting the fusion of nanoparticles into a well-developed network. This transformation is likely driven by water evaporation and the subsequent filling of void spaces by zinc moieties, facilitated by thermal energy. In contrast, the 450 °C-annealed samples display significant aggregation of nanoflakes, leading to the formation of distorted aerogel structures. The SAED analysis further supports these structural transitions, with diffuse rings observed in the as-synthesized aerogel ($Zn_{AGL(RT)}$) indicating an amorphous nature, while the $Zn_{AGL(200)}$ exhibits distinct diffraction spots in a ring-like pattern, suggesting the presence of nanocrystalline domains with some degree of structural order. The $Zn_{AGL(450)}$ aerogel presents well-defined diffraction rings with bright spots, confirming its highly crystalline nature. The measured d-spacing corresponding to the (103) plane of ZnO further substantiates the crystalline phase transformation occurring at elevated temperatures.

The specific surface area, pore volume, and average pore diameter of the $Zn_{AGL(RT)}$ and the annealed aerogel samples $Zn_{AGL(200)}$ and $Zn_{AGL(RT)}$ were analyzed using nitrogen adsorption studies, as illustrated in Figure 3a,b. All samples exhibited type II isotherms, indicating monolayer formation and suggesting a predominantly macroporous structure. The marked point in Figure 3 signifies the completion of monolayer formation. The absence of hysteresis further confirmed that adsorption and desorption occurred on a non-porous or macroporous surface. The as-synthesized zinc aerogels ($Zn_{AGL(RT)}$) demonstrated the highest BET surface area of 90.5 m^2/g with a pore volume of 0.45 cm^3/g. Upon annealing, the surface area decreased to 63.8 m^2/g for the $Zn_{AGL(200)}$ sample and 14.3 m^2/g for the $Zn_{AGL(450)}$ sample, following the typical trend where increasing annealing temperatures lead to a reduction in BET surface area.

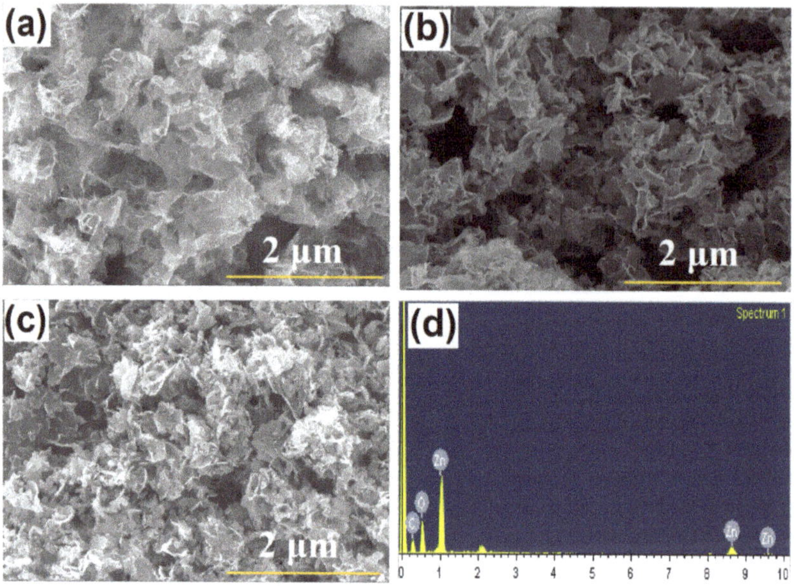

Figure 1. FESEM images of (**a**) $Zn_{AGL(RT)}$, (**b**) $Zn_{AGL(200)}$, (**c**) $Zn_{AGL(450)}$, and (**d**) EDS spectrum for sample $Zn_{AGL(RT)}$.

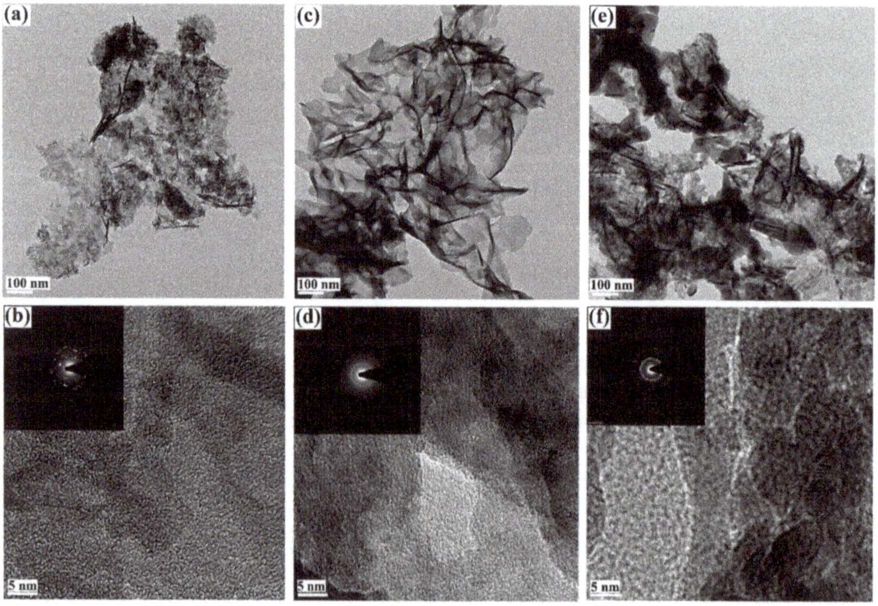

Figure 2. TEM and HRTEM images of (**a**,**b**) $Zn_{AGL(RT)}$, (**c**,**d**) $Zn_{AGL(200)}$, and (**e**,**f**) $Zn_{AGL(450)}$. The inset shows the corresponding SAED patterns of (**b**,**d**,**e**).

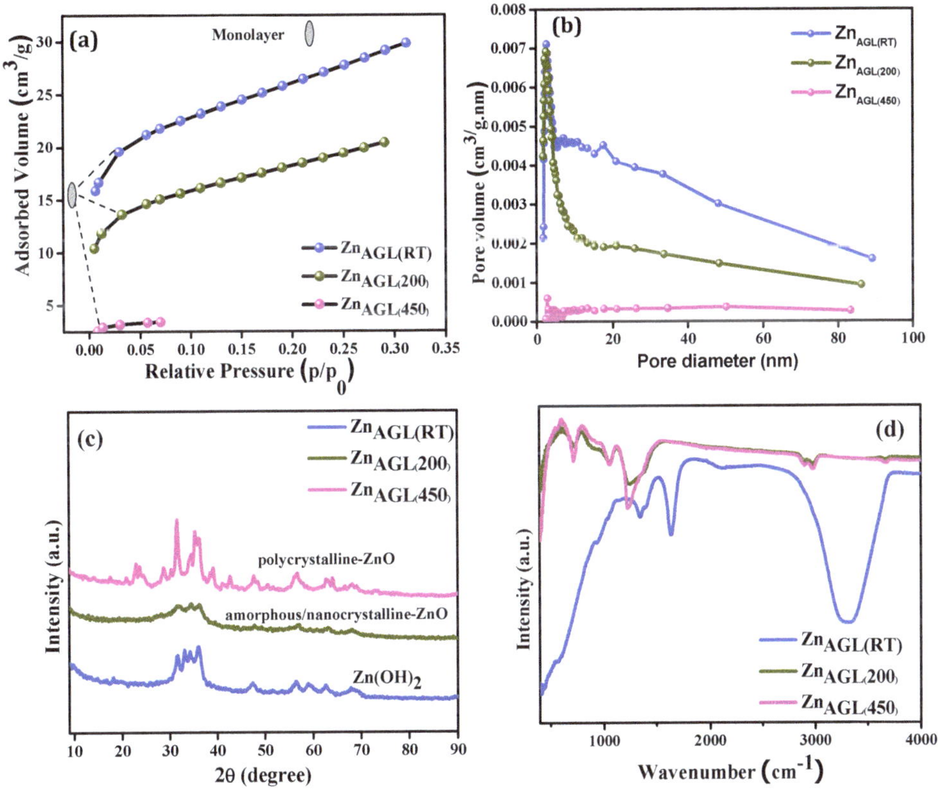

Figure 3. (**a**) BET absorption graph and (**b**) pore volume of as-synthesized zinc aerogels ($Zn_{AGL(RT)}$), $Zn_{AGL(200)}$ and $Zn_{AGL(450)}$, (**c**) XRD, and (**d**) FTIR of ($ZnA_{GL(RT)}$), $Zn_{AGL(200)}$, and $Zn_{AGL(450)}$.

The XRD and FTIR of the zinc aerogels are given in Figure 3c,d, respectively. The XRD of the as-synthesized samples revealed an amorphous nature for the as-synthesized zinc aerogels ($Zn_{AGL(RT)}$) and the annealed sample $Zn_{AGL(200)}$. The annealed sample at 450 °C showed more crystalline peaks, as also confirmed by HR-TEM analysis. The $Zn_{AGL(RT)}$ showed peaks corresponding to zinc metal, and the annealed samples $Zn_{AGL(200)}$ and $Zn_{AGL(450)}$ showed that for zinc hydroxide and oxides, respectively. The peak at 33.3° corresponding to the (002) face of zinc was the preferred orientation for the as-synthesized sample, whereas the strong crystalline peak at 62.4° for the annealed sample at 450 °C corresponded to the (103) plane of the zinc oxide aerogel. The annealing of the as-synthesized sample at 200 °C produced largely amorphous nature aerogels, as also confirmed by the HR-TEM analysis in Figure 2c,d.

Materials' FTIR spectra are useful in determining the functional groups present in them. The FTIR of the as-synthesized zinc aerogels showed peaks at 1397 cm^{-1}, 1639 cm^{-1}, and 3250–3350 cm^{-1}. The three peaks present in the as-synthesized samples are characteristic of zinc aerogels. The bandwidth from 1500 to 600 denotes the fingerprint region for zinc oxide materials. The peaks present for the annealed samples at 720, 1051, 1230, 2900, and 2985 cm^{-1} indicated the C-H, C=O, C-H, CH_2, and CH_3 vibrations, respectively, occurring due to the presence of carbon groups during the annealing process (200 and 450 °C). The Zn-O peaks appeared below 500 cm^{-1} in $Zn_{AGL(200)}$ and $Zn_{AGL(450)}$ samples and were more pronounced in both annealed samples.

Table 1. Comparison of various zinc ion and aerogel-based material electrodes and their performances for supercapacitor applications.

System	Electrolyte	Sp. Capacitance(F/g)	ED//PD (Wh/kg//kW/kg)	Ref.
ZHSC	$Zn(CF_3SO_3)_2$	540(0.1 A/g)	188/49	[18]
MXene/ZHSC	$ZnSO_4$	-	55/3	[21]
TI2CTx-MXene/ZISC	-	233 (1 A/g)	130/1	[22]
GA/ZHSC	$ZnSO_4$	353 (1 A/g)	77/15	[19]
Zn/chitosan aerogels	KOH	230 (0.5 A/g)	4.67/5	[17]
ZnO/CA	KOH	375 (75 mA/cm^2)	-	[23]
Zn-Co-S aerogel	KOH	820 (1 A/g)	47/0.7	[24]
$Zn_{AGL(200)}$	KOH	288 (1 A/g)/	8/15	This work

The XPS studies were carried out for the as-synthesized ($Zn_{AGL(RT)}$) and the annealed aerogels $Zn_{AGL(200)}$ and $Zn_{AGL(450)}$ in order to deduce the elemental composition and purity of the samples, and the results are shown in Figure 4a–f. The Zn 2p spectra showed two distinct peaks related to the Zn $2p_{1/2}$ and Zn $2P_{3/2}$, revealing Zn^{+2} in the prepared AGL compounds [25]. For the $Zn_{AGL(RT)}$, Zn $2p_{1/2}$ and Zn $2P_{3/2}$ were observed at 1044.7 to 1021.5 eV, respectively, with a spin–orbit splitting ratio (ΔBE) of 23.04 eV. In the $Zn_{AGL(200)}$ aerogel, the peaks slightly shifted to 1044.9 and 1021.8 eV, with a ΔBE of 23 eV, suggesting an enhanced defect density and hydroxylation due to increased oxygen vacancies [26]. The 450 °C-annealed AGL ($Zn_{AGL(450)}$) showed peaks at 1021.5 and 1044.6 eV, with a ΔBE of 23.1 eV, revealing a reduced defect density and improved crystallinity. The O1s spectra of AGL samples were deconvoluted into three distinct peaks, representing the various chemical states of oxygen elements on the AGL surface. The deconvolution of the O 1s XPS spectra revealed three unique peaks, each representing a different chemical state of oxygen on the Zn aerogel surface. The signal at 530.0–530.5 eV is due to lattice oxygen (O_L), suggesting that oxygen elements are linked within the Zn-O crystal lattice. The second peak at 531.0–531.5 eV is linked to defect-related oxygen (O_D) or oxygen vacancies, indicating non-stoichiometry and structural defects in the ZnO lattice [27]. The third peak, which ranges from 532.0 to 533.5 eV, represents adsorbed oxygen species or hydroxyl groups (OH) formed by surface hydroxylation or physiosorbed water. The $Zn_{AGL(RT)}$ had an O_H/O_L ratio of 0.53, indicating considerable surface defects and hydroxylation. This ratio increased to 0.89 for the $Zn_{AGL(200)}$ sample, indicating greater enrichment of oxygen vacancies and hydroxylation [28]. The $Zn_{AGL(450)}$ sample showed a lower O_H/O_L ratio of 0.36 after higher temperature annealing, indicating enhanced crystallinity and decreased defect density and surface hydroxylation.

Initially, to estimate the comparative energy storage capacity of the $Zn_{AGL(RT)}$, $Zn_{AGL(200)}$, and $Zn_{AGL(450)}$ aerogels, cyclic voltammetry (CV) was implemented using a three-electrode arrangement. The setup consisted of Ni-foam working electrodes loaded with the prepared samples, a Ag/AgCl reference electrode, and a Pt counter electrode in an aqueous 1 M KOH solution. The three zinc aerogel samples were subjected to electrochemical analysis, starting with cyclic voltammetry to measure the current generated at various scan rates after 200 stabilization cycles. The stabilization CV was carried out at 50 mV/s from 0 to 0.5 V. Figure 5a–c illustrate the change in the redox potentials of $Zn_{AGL(RT)}$, $Zn_{AGL(200)}$, and $Zn_{AGL(450)}$ at various scan rates from 5 mV/S to 100 mV/S at a potential window of 0 to 0.5 V. Enhanced current values were observed for $Zn_{AGL(200)}$ compared to $Zn_{AGL(RT)}$ and $Zn_{AGL(450)}$ (Figure 5j). The shape of the CV curves indicates the pseudocapacitive behavior of $Zn_{AGL(RT)}$, $Zn_{AGL(200)}$, and $Zn_{AGL(450)}$ [26], which is well established in most aerogel-based supercapacitors exhibiting capacitive behavior. Moreover, to understand the optimized materials loading and the effect of excess loading, we performed CV analysis for 2, 2.5, and 3 mg of $Zn_{AGL(200)}$ materials loading, and the obtained results are presented in Figure S1. Further, the specific capacity was calculated from the CV, and the obtained plots are displayed in Figure S2. After undergoing the CV tests, all the zinc aerogel samples were subjected to galvanostatic charge–discharge studies at various current densities, ranging from 1 to 20 A/g within a potential range of 0 to 0.4 V (Figure 5d,e). The curves also denoted pseudocapacitive behavior, which is consistent with the behavior typically observed in transition metal aerogel-based supercapacitor electrodes. Figure 5g–i present the specific capacitance of $Zn_{AGL(RT)}$, $Zn_{AGL(200)}$, and $Zn_{AGL(450)}$ across varying current densities (1–20 A/g), calculated using Equation (S1). Notably, $Zn_{AGL(200)}$ exhibited the highest specific capacity of 115 C/g (specific capacitance of 288 F/g), surpassing both $Zn_{AGL(RT)}$ and $Zn_{AGL(450)}$. This enhanced electrochemical performance can be attributed to their nanocrystalline network structures exhibiting unique defect-rich surfaces and the presence of oxygen vacancies, as confirmed by XPS analysis. These structural features facilitate improved charge storage, enhance ion diffusion kinetics, and contribute to superior electrochemical activity compared to the as-synthesized $Zn_{AGL(RT)}$ and highly crystalline $Zn_{AGL(450)}$ counterparts.

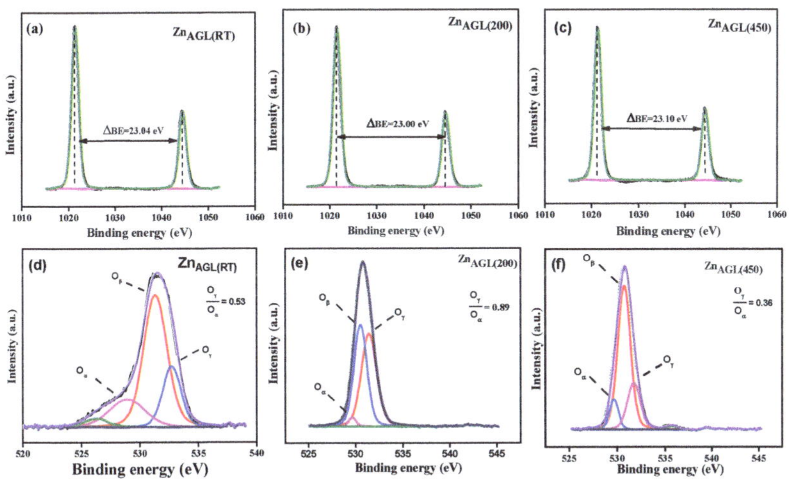

Figure 4. (**a–c**) Zinc 2p spectra of $ZnA_{GL(RT)}$, $Zn_{AGL(200)}$, and $Zn_{AGL(450)}$; (**d–f**) O 1s spectra of $ZnA_{GL(RT))}$, $Zn_{AGL(200))}$, and $Zn_{AGL(450)}$.

Impedance spectroscopy is an effective tool for analyzing various electrochemical parameters, including solution resistance, charge-transfer resistance, Warburg impedance, and double-layer capacitance, among others. Hence, in order to evaluate the effect of Zn aerogels in the presence of KOH electrolyte, Nyquist plots were generated at OCV for all samples, and the results were analyzed. The solution resistance was found to vary slightly, with 4, 2.4, and 0.8 ohms for the $Zn_{AGL(RT)}$, $Zn_{AGL(200)}$, and $Zn_{AGL(450)}$ electrodes. Also, the charge-transfer resistance values were 18 and 20 ohms for the $Zn_{AGL(RT)}$ and $Zn_{AGL(200)}$ aerogels. By contrast, in the $Zn_{AGL(450)}$ samples, the Rct resistance could not be determined due to the absence of a semicircle in the high-frequency region. Moreover, the performance of the $Zn_{AGL(200)}$ nanostructure electrode compared favorably against previously reported electrodes as shown in Table 1.

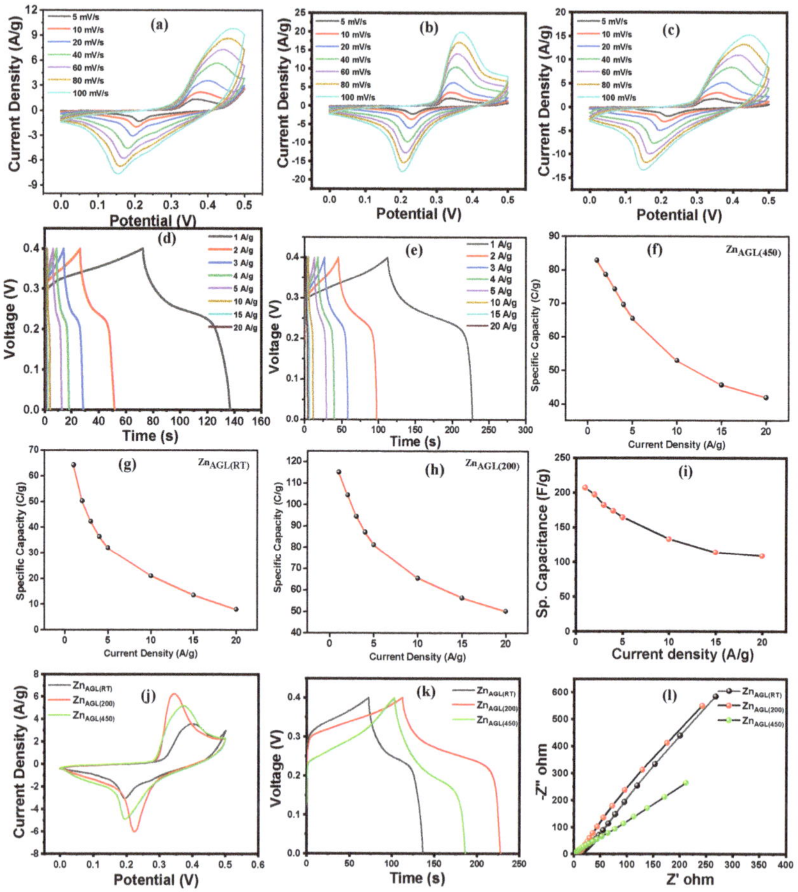

Figure 5. (**a**–**c**) CV curves, (**d**–**f**) GCD curves, and (**g**–**i**) the relationship between the specific capacitance and current density of $ZnA_{GL(RT)}$, $Zn_{AGL(200)}$, and $Zn_{AGL(450)}$ electrodes, respectively; (**j**) comparative CV curves, (**k**) comparative GCD, and (**l**) the EIS plots of $ZnA_{GL(RT)}$, $Zn_{AGL(200)}$, and $Zn_{AGL(450)}$ electrodes.

In order to evaluate the performance of the zinc aerogels in real-time applications, a two-electrode arrangement was constructed using Zn aerogels as positive electrodes and rGO as the negative counterparts. The mass loading of the electrodes was adjusted as per the following equation:

$$\frac{m_+}{m_-} = \frac{C^- \times V^-}{C^+ \times V^+} \tag{1}$$

where m_+ and m_- are the mass of the positive and negative electrodes; C^+ and C^- the specific capacitance; and V^+ and V^- the potential of the positive and negative electrodes, respectively. The mass loading for the positive electrode was 1.6 mg, and that for the negative electrode was 3 mg, respectively.

The CV for the device was carried out from 0 to 1.5 V within scan rates of 5–100 mV/s (Figure 6a). The device exhibited a pseudocapacitive behavior, and the current increased with increasing scan rates. The peak current increase at fast scan rates indicates the capacitance of the redox reactions. The galvanostatic charge–discharge curves were then generated in order to determine the real-time capacitance properties of the zinc aerogel electrode materials (Figure 6b). The specific capacitance was calculated to be from ~50 F/g to 26 F/g when the current density varied from 1 to 20 A/g (Figure 6c). Figure 6d displays the relationships between ED, PD, and discharge time, along with Ragone plots for the fabricated device. Notably, the $Zn_{AGL(200)}$//AC device achieved an energy density of 8 Wh/kg at a power density of 15,000 W/kg and maintained an energy density of 2.1 Wh/kg at a power density of 1760 W/kg while operating at a potential of 1.5 V. In addition, to understand the stable potential window of the devices, they were employed using various voltages ranging from 1.2 to 1.6 V (Figure 6e), revealing the broad operational potential of the device.

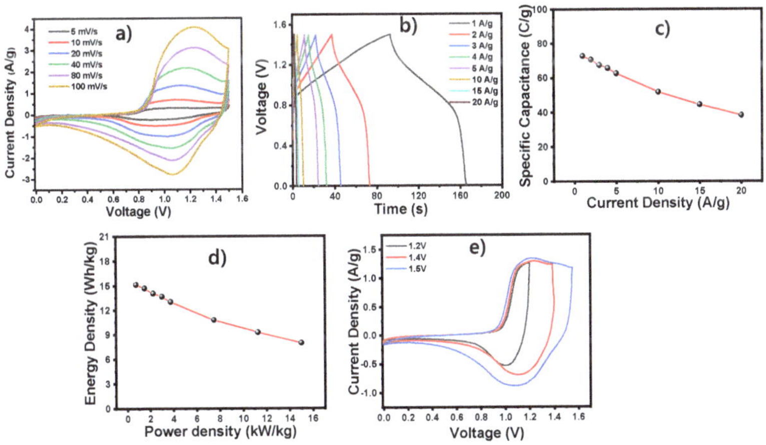

Figure 6. (**a–c**) $Zn_{AGL(200)}$//Ac device: (**a**) CV profile with various scan rates; (**b**) GCD profile at various current densities; (**c**) specific capacitance; (**d**) Ragone plot; (**e**) CV profile at various potentials.

The impedance spectra were also carried out for the device at an amplitude of 5 mV/s and a frequency range of 0.1 to 105 Hz. The EIS was run for the device before cycling, wherein the solution resistance and charge-transfer resistance values were found to be 1.1 and 91.9 ohms. The EIS resistance values for the device after cycling were found to be 73.6 and 292.5 ohms, respectively (Figure 7a). The increase in resistance after cycling may be due to the decreased activity of the material. Furthermore, to understand the stability of the constructed device, 10,000 cycles of consecutive GCD tests at 10 A/g current density were performed, and the obtained cyclic stability and columbic efficiency results are presented in Figure 7b. The device also showed excellent cyclability, up to 10,000 cycles with a Coulombic efficiency of 97%.

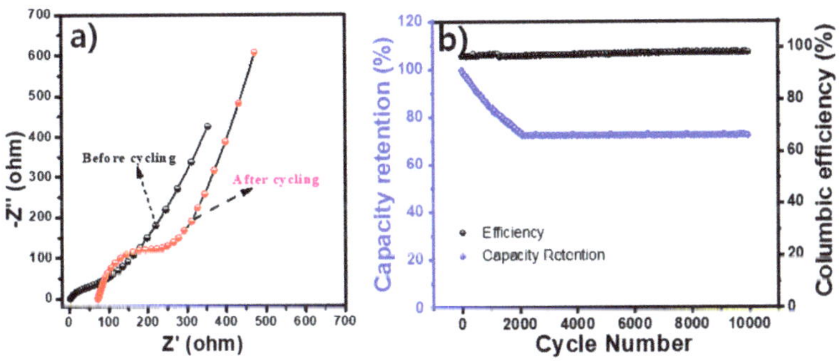

Figure 7. $Zn_{AGL(200)}$//Ac device: (**a**) EIS curves of the device before and after the cycling study; (**b**) cycling retention study.

The unique structural and chemical properties of $Zn_{AGL(200)}$ as a supercapacitor electrode are responsible for its superior electrochemical performance, which synergistically improves ion transport and charge storage. Initially, the amorphous nanocrystalline structure, which was verified by XRD (Figure 3c) and HR-TEM (Figure 2c,d), generated a continuous, interconnected nanoflake network with edge widths of 5–10 nm. This morphology provided a high density of active sites for Faradaic redox reactions, as demonstrated by the pseudocapacitive behavior observed in CV curves (Figure 5a–c). The amorphous nature of $Zn_{AGL(200)}$ minimized lattice constraints, enabling greater structural flexibility and ion accessibility during charge–discharge cycles, in contrast to the highly crystalline $Zn_{AGL(450)}$. Secondly, the XPS analysis (Figure 4d–f) revealed a high O_h/O_l ratio of 0.89 for $Zn_{AGL(200)}$, which suggested significant oxygen vacancies and surface hydroxylation. These oxygen vacancies functioned as defect sites, which facilitated the transfer of electrons between the Zn^{2+} and Zn^0 states, thereby enhancing electronic conductivity and promoting redox activity. The pseudocapacitive reactions in the KOH electrolyte were further facilitated by the presence of hydroxyl groups, as illustrated by the subsequent reaction:

$$Zn(OH)_2 + OH^- \leftrightarrow ZnOOH + H_2O + e^-$$

Thirdly, the BET surface area of 63.8 m^2/g and pore volume of 0.35 cm^3/g (Figure 3a,b) in $Zn_{AGL(200)}$ offered a substantial surface area for electrolyte ion adsorption and diffusion, thereby enhancing the rate capability and specific capacitance (288 F/g at 1 A/g). The efficient ion transport was ensured by the macroporous structure, as evidenced by type II isotherms, which mitigated the diffusion limitations observed in the more aggregated $Zn_{AGL(450)}$. Lastly, the enhanced electrochemical kinetics of $Zn_{AGL(200)}$ were confirmed by the low solution resistance (2.4 Ω) and charge-transfer resistance (20 Ω) in EIS measurements (Figure 5i), which were influenced by its interconnected morphology and defect-rich surface. Collectively, these factors enabled $Zn_{AGL(200)}$ to attain a high energy density of 7.97 Wh/kg and a power density of 15 kW/kg in the asymmetric supercapacitor configuration, rendering it a promising material for next-generation energy storage applications.

4. Conclusions

In summary, Zn aerogel materials enriched with oxygen vacancies and exhibiting ZnO defect chemistry were successfully synthesized in a sol–gel one-pot hydrolysis method using a borohydride. The resulting aerogels featured nano-wafer architectures composed of a Zn particle network with moderate porosity. XRD analysis confirmed that the annealed Zn aerogel samples maintained a predominantly amorphous nanocrystalline structure with embedded Zn polycrystalline domains. Electrochemical characterization, including cyclic voltammetry (CV), galvanostatic charge–discharge (GCD), and electrochemical impedance spectroscopy (EIS), demonstrated an exceptional highest specific capacity of 115 C/g (specific capacitance (C_{sp}) of 288 F/g) in a three-electrode configuration. Due to its superior electrochemical properties, $Zn_{AGL(200)}$ was selected for asymmetric supercapacitor (ASC) fabrication, employing reduced graphene oxide (rGO) as the negative electrode, yielding a specific capacitance (C_{sp}) of 49 F/g. The Ragone plot indicated an energy density (ED) of 7.97 Wh/kg and a power density (PD) of 15 kW/kg, underscoring its high-performance characteristics. Additionally, the unique morphology and lightweight properties of the aerogel, facilitated by the borohydride-assisted synthesis, make it an outstanding candidate for next-generation ultralight supercapacitors, addressing the growing energy storage demands of advanced technological applications.

Supplementary Materials: The following supporting information can be downloaded at: https://www.mdpi.com/article/10.3390/pr13051461/s1, General Procedures, Materials, Characterizations.

Author Contributions: Conceptualization, methodology, investigation, writing—original draft preparation, R.R.; software, validation, data curation, writing—review and editing, G.K.; formal analysis, M.R.A.R.A.; visualization, T.R.G.; supervision, funding acquisition, resources, W.K.K.; supervision, funding acquisition, J.H.K. All authors have read and agreed to the published version of the manuscript.

Funding: This research received no external funding.

Data Availability Statement: Data will be made available upon request.

Conflicts of Interest: The authors declare no conflicts of interest.

Abbreviations

The following abbreviations are used in this manuscript:

Csp	Specific capacitance
ED	Energy density
PD	Power density
ASC	Asymmetric supercapacitor
AGLs	Aerogels
EIS	Electrochemical impedance spectroscopy
CV	Cyclic voltammetry
GCD	Galvanostatic charge–discharge

References

1. Lim, J.M.; Jang, Y.S.; Van, T.; Nguyen, H.; Kim, J.S.; Yoon, Y.; Park, B.J.; Seo, D.H.; Lee, K.-K.; Han, Z.; et al. Advances in high-voltage supercapacitors for energy storage systems: Materials and electrolyte tailoring to implementation. *Nanoscale Adv.* **2023**, *5*, 615–626. [CrossRef] [PubMed]
2. Wan, J.; Lv, T.; Liu, Y.; Wang, X.; Yang, Y.; Chen, Z.; Qi, Y.; Cao, S.; Chen, T. Flexible Asymmetric Supercapacitors with Extremely Slow Self-Discharge Rate Enabled by a Bilayer Heterostructure Polymer Electrolyte. *Adv. Funct. Mater.* **2022**, *32*, 2108794. [CrossRef]
3. Shuja, A.; Khan, H.R.; Murtaza, I.; Ashraf, S.; Abid, Y.; Farid, F.; Sajid, F. Supercapacitors for energy storage applications: Materials, devices and future directions: A comprehensive review. *J. Alloys Compd.* **2024**, *1009*, 176924. [CrossRef]
4. Zhao, C.; Sun, X.; Li, W.; Shi, M.; Ren, K.; Lu, X. Reduced Self-Discharge of Supercapacitors Using Piezoelectric Separators. *ACS Appl. Energy Mater.* **2021**, *4*, 8070–8075. [CrossRef]
5. Šedajová, V.; Nandi, D.; Langer, P.; Lo, R.; Hobza, P.; Plachá, D.; Bakandritsos, A.; Zbořil, R. Direct upcycling of highly efficient sorbents for emerging organic contaminants into high energy content supercapacitors. *J. Colloid Interface Sci.* **2025**, *692*, 137481. [CrossRef]
6. Hou, L.; Yang, W.; Li, Y.; Wang, P.; Jiang, B.; Xu, C.; Zhang, C.; Huang, G.; Yang, F.; Li, Y. Dual-Template endowing N, O co-doped hierarchically porous carbon from potassium citrate with high capacitance and rate capability for supercapacitors. *Chem. Eng. J.* **2021**, *417*, 129289. [CrossRef]
7. Yogesh, G.K.; Nandi, D.; Yeetsorn, R.; Wanchan, W.; Devi, C.; Singh, R.P.; Vasistha, A.; Kumar, M.; Koinkar, P.; Yadav, K. A machine learning approach for estimating supercapacitor performance of graphene oxide nano-ring based electrode materials. *Energy Adv.* **2025**, *4*, 119–139. [CrossRef]
8. Pan, G.; Zhu, J.; Ma, S.; Sun, G.; Yang, X. Enhancing the electromagnetic performance of Co through the phase-controlled synthesis of hexagonal and cubic Co nanocrystals grown on graphene. *ACS Appl. Mater. Interfaces* **2013**, *5*, 12716–12724. [CrossRef]
9. Maleki, H.; Durães, L.; García-González, C.A.; del Gaudio, P.; Portugal, A.; Mahmoudi, M. Synthesis and biomedical applications of aerogels: Possibilities and challenges. *Adv. Colloid Interface Sci.* **2016**, *236*, 1–27. [CrossRef]
10. Ramkumar, R.; Suganthi, S.; Milton, A.; Park, J.; Shim, J.-J.; Oh, T.H.; Kim, W.K. MnO/Mn_2O_3 aerogels as effective materials for supercapacitor applications. *Energies* **2024**, *17*, 2258. [CrossRef]
11. Ramkumar, R.; Dhakal, G.; Shim, J.-J.; Kim, W.K. NiO/Ni nanowafer aerogel electrodes for high performance supercapacitors. *Nanomaterials* **2022**, *12*, 3813. [CrossRef] [PubMed]
12. Ramkumar, R.; Rajkumar, C.; Do, H.; Kim, H.; Kim, W.K. A remarkable oxygen vacancy-rich rare earth aerogel with high activity towards electro and catalytic reduction of 5-nitroquinoline. *J. Clean. Prod.* **2023**, *423*, 138683. [CrossRef]
13. Li, G.-R.; Feng, Z.-P.; Ou, Y.-N.; Wu, D.; Fu, R.; Tong, Y.-X. Mesoporous MnO_2/carbon aerogel composites as promising electrode materials for high-performance supercapacitors. *Langmuir* **2010**, *26*, 2209–2213. [CrossRef] [PubMed]

14. Huang, H.; Wang, X.; Tervoort, E.; Zeng, G.; Liu, T.; Chen, X.; Sologubenko, A.; Niederberger, M. Nano-Sized Structurally Disordered Metal Oxide Composite Aerogels as High-Power Anodes in Hybrid Supercapacitors. *ACS Nano* **2018**, *12*, 2753–2763. [CrossRef]
15. Zhang, Z.; Gao, Q.; Gao, H.; Shi, Z.; Wu, J.; Zhi, M.; Hong, Z. Nickel oxide aerogel for high performance supercapacitor electrodes. *RSC Adv.* **2016**, *6*, 112620–112624. [CrossRef]
16. Ghazitabar, A.; Naderi, M.; Fatmehsari Haghshenas, D.; Rezaei, M. Synthesis of N-doped graphene aerogel/Co_3O_4/ZnO ternary nanocomposite via mild reduction method with an emphasis on its electrochemical characteristics. *J. Alloys Compd.* **2019**, *794*, 625–633. [CrossRef]
17. Liu, L.; Du, B.; Liu, R.; Chen, X.; Song, H. N-Doped Hierarchically Porous Carbon Aerogels by Controlling the Zn–Chitosan Complex Ratio for High-Performance Supercapacitors. *Energy Fuels* **2022**, *36*, 5920–5927. [CrossRef]
18. Valentini, C.; Montes-García, V.; Ciesielski, A.; Samorì, P. Boosting Zinc Hybrid Supercapacitor Performance via Thiol Functionalization of Graphene-Based Cathodes. *Adv. Sci.* **2024**, *11*, 2309041. [CrossRef]
19. Das, G.S.; Jangir, L.K.; Raju, K.S.; Sharma, Y.C.; Tripathi, K.M. Waste biomass-based 3D graphene aerogels for high performance zinc-ion hybrid supercapacitors. *Chem. Commun.* **2024**, *60*, 10568–10571.
20. Hassan, K.; Hossain, R.; Sahajwalla, V. Recycled ZnO-fused macroporous 3D graphene oxide aerogel composites for high-performance asymmetric supercapacitors. *J. Am. Ceram. Soc.* **2022**, *105*, 7467–7478. [CrossRef]
21. Cui, H.; Mi, H.; Ji, C.; Guo, F.; Chen, Y.; Wu, D.; Qiu, J.; Xie, H. A durable MXene-based zinc ion hybrid supercapacitor with sulfated polysaccharide reinforced hydrogel/electrolyte. *J. Mater. Chem. A* **2021**, *9*, 23941–23954. [CrossRef]
22. Mateen, A.; Ansari, M.Z.; Hussain, I.; Eldin, S.M.; Albaqami, M.D.; Bahajjaj, A.A.A.; Javed, M.S.; Peng, K.-Q. Ti_2CTx–MXene aerogel based ultra–stable Zn–ion supercapacitor. *Compos. Commun.* **2023**, *38*, 101493. [CrossRef]
23. Kalpana, D.; Omkumar, K.; Kumar, S.S.; Renganathan, N. A novel high power symmetric ZnO/carbon aerogel composite electrode for electrochemical supercapacitor. *Electrochim. Acta* **2006**, *52*, 1309–1315. [CrossRef]
24. Kim, Y.; Parale, V.G.; Kim, T.; Kim, S.-H.; Choi, H.; Patil, U.M.; Kanamori, K.; Park, H.-H. Synthesis of Zn-Co-S nanowire bundle type aerogel electrodes for asymmetric supercapacitors. *Chem. Eng. J.* **2023**, *474*, 145875. [CrossRef]
25. Iaiche, S.; Djelloul, A. ZnO/$ZnAl_2O_4$ Nanocomposite Films Studied by X-Ray Diffraction, FTIR, and X-Ray Photoelectron Spectroscopy. *J. Spectrosc.* **2015**, *2015*, 836859. [CrossRef]
26. Guan, S.; Hao, L.; Murayama, M.; Xie, X.; Komuro, S.; Zhao, X. Influence of anneal temperature in air on surface morphology and photoluminescence of ZnO thin films. *IOP Conf. Ser. Mater. Sci. Eng.* **2019**, *522*, 012004. [CrossRef]
27. Chang, F.-M.; Brahma, S.; Huang, J.-H.; Wu, Z.-Z.; Lo, K.-Y. Strong correlation between optical properties and mechanism in deficiency of normalized self-assembly ZnO nanorods. *Sci. Rep.* **2019**, *9*, 905. [CrossRef]
28. Li, F.; Bu, Y.; Han, G.-F.; Noh, H.-J.; Kim, S.-J.; Ahmad, I.; Lu, Y.; Zhang, P.; Jeong, H.Y.; Fu, Z. Identifying the structure of Zn-N_2 active sites and structural activation. *Nat. Commun.* **2019**, *10*, 2623. [CrossRef]

processes

Article

Investigation of Sustainable Combustion Processes of the Industrial Gas Turbine Injector

Hafiz Ali Haider Sehole [1,2,*,†], Ghazanfar Mehdi [1,*,†], Rizwan Riaz [2,†] and Adnan Maqsood [2,†]

1 Department of Mechanical Engineering, School of Engineering, Aalto University, Otakaari 4, 02150 Espoo, Finland
2 School of Interdisciplinary Engineering and Sciences, National University of Sciences and Technology, Islamabad 44000, Pakistan
* Correspondence: ali.haider@aalto.fi (H.A.H.S.); ghazanfar.mehdi@aalto.fi (G.M.)
† These authors contributed equally to this work.

Abstract: This study investigates the combustion dynamics of methane in a dual swirl combustor, focusing on improving combustion efficiency and understanding flow features. Methane, as a conventional fuel, offers high energy content and relatively low carbon emissions compared to other hydrocarbons, making it a promising choice for sustainable energy solutions. Accurate numerical models are essential for the optimization of combustion processes, particularly in the design of combustion engines utilizing methane. In this work, we employ a partially premixed combustion model based on a mixture fraction and progress-variable approach to simulate methane combustion dynamics. Turbulent behavior is modeled using Detached-Eddy Simulation (DES), with the DLR dual swirl combustor serving as the geometric model. The simulations are performed at a global equivalence ratio of 0.65 for partially premixed methane. The results show good validation against experimental data, including time-averaged velocity components, turbulent fluctuations, mixture fraction, and temperature profiles. Additionally, the analysis of instantaneous flow features reveals the presence of a precessing vortex core. This study provides a robust numerical methodology, validated against experimental data, offering valuable insights into the combustion behavior of methane in dual swirl combustors and its industrial applicability.

Keywords: turbulence; DES; partially premixed combustion; shear flows

1. Introduction

The successful operation of modern gas turbines (GTs) is critical in meeting global energy demands while simultaneously reducing greenhouse gas emissions [1]. To achieve these goals, it is necessary that GT combustors operate with high efficiency and reliability, producing low emissions. This requires a comprehensive understanding of the complex processes within combustors, such as turbulent flow, heat transfer, and mass transfer. While experimental investigations provide valuable insights, they are often limited by practical constraints and can only partially capture the intricacies of combustion processes. Therefore, numerical simulations have become an indispensable tool, offering detailed insights that complement experimental findings. However, accurately simulating GT combustion remains challenging due to its inherent complexity, necessitating the ongoing development of mathematical and numerical models to enhance predictive capabilities and validate experimental results. This work contributes to this ongoing effort and aims

 https://doi.org/10.3390/pr13040960

to advance GT technology by providing critical insights into the combustion processes within combustors.

Recent research has focused on GT combustors operating under premixed conditions, with significant Large Eddy Simulation (LES) studies on the PRECCINSTA burner demonstrating good agreement with experiments [2–7]. However, most simulations have overlooked partial premixing despite its link to thermo-acoustic instabilities. The TECFLAM burner [8] has also provided valuable LES validation data with consistent results for various measurements. For non-premixed regimes, the MOLECULES combustor [9] has been investigated, offering insights into flow-field structures under high-pressure conditions. Multi-regime burner designs [10–12] have been investigated to produce flames with multi-regime characteristics and validate numerical models. Nonetheless, there is a lack of Detached-Eddy Simulation (DES) validation for partially premixed conditions, which pose modeling challenges due to complex turbulence–chemistry interactions. This work aims to bridge this gap by examining the DLR GT with its dual swirler design under partially premixed conditions.

A key challenge in GT combustor design is accurately modeling turbulence, especially in the presence of strong swirling flows. The DLR GT swirl injector consists of two swirler channels: the inner swirler and the outer swirler. Swirl is commonly applied to the main combustion air to create a vortex breakdown recirculation zone along the combustor's central axis, which enhances combustion efficiency and flame stability. However, strong swirling flows introduce additional complexity into turbulence modeling due to flow curvature and pressure gradient effects that increase anisotropy [13]. To address these challenges, this study employed DES to investigate reactive turbulent swirl flows within a GT combustor. Validation of turbulent flows, influenced by steep velocity and pressure gradients in conjunction with the combustion model, produces an independent study [14,15], requiring further investigation. DES utilizes the Strelets model, which combines the two-equation SST-RANS model with elements of the LES method [16]. This approach allows the model to apply the boundary-layer coverage of SST-RANS while transitioning to LES in regions where the turbulent length scale predicted by RANS is larger than the local grid spacing. The choice of DES over LES and DNS is made to reduce computational costs. LES is expensive in boundary-layer regions because it requires a fine mesh resolution along the wall. Since the accuracy of LES depends on grid resolution, Pope [17] recommends that the grid should resolve 80 percent of the turbulent kinetic energy away from the wall.

Simulating gas turbine combustion presents the challenge of accurately modeling the complex interaction between turbulence and chemistry. To tackle this issue, the DLR GT swirl combustor was analyzed using a partially premixed combustion model, which offers computational advantages over other models. Local mixtures (burned, unburned, or partially burned) are characterized by tracking the flame's propagation within the partially premixed model. The model treats burnt mixtures behind the flame similarly to diffusion flames, while cold mixtures represent the unburned sections ahead of the flame front. Thermo-chemistry calculations are pre-processed, and the interaction of turbulence and chemistry is accounted for using an assumed-shape Probability Density Function (PDF). A transport equation for the progress variable (C) is utilized to track the propagation of the flame front. The results of this study can provide useful insights into the performance of partially premixed combustion models in real-world gas turbine combustion systems. Although the model has been applied to several simple combustors, relatively less attention has been paid to its performance in existing combustion systems.

The combination of these advanced numerical methods and the focus on dual swirl combustor configurations aims to extend the understanding of combustion processes, ultimately contributing to the development of more efficient, reliable, and environmentally friendly gas turbine technologies.

While large eddy simulation (LES) has been widely used to investigate combustion dynamics in swirl-stabilized flames, there is a gap in understanding the specific effects of partially premixed combustion in these configurations, particularly in terms of its impact on combustion stability, efficiency, and flow dynamics. Previous studies have primarily focused on fully premixed or non-premixed flames, but partially premixed combustion, which is more representative of real-world conditions in practical combustors, has not been thoroughly explored in this context. This study aims to address this gap by employing a partially premixed combustion model in a dual swirl combustor setup, which is not commonly found in existing LES studies. Our approach focuses on both accuracy and computational efficiency, providing insights into methane combustion behavior in industrial applications while also highlighting the potential for a robust and computationally less expensive methodology. In summary, we believe this research offers valuable contributions to the field by investigating an underexplored aspect of swirl-stabilized flames and proposing an approach with practical applications in the design and optimization of combustion systems.

2. Experimental Setup

The experimental analysis was conducted by the German Aerospace Center (DLR) to investigate a dual swirl combustor that consist of a combustion chamber, a plenum, and a nozzle geometry. Dry air was supplied through an air inlet at room temperature and ambient pressure. The air was first directed through the plenum, then divided into two halves by two radial swirlers, as shown in Figure 1. The co-swirling air was then passed into the combustion chamber through a central nozzle (d_i = 15 mm) and an annular nozzle (d_i = 17 mm, d_o = 25 mm, curved to an outside diameter of d_o = 40 mm). The diameter and height of the plenum were 79 mm and 65 mm, respectively. The central (inside) and annular (outer) nozzles had 8 and 12 radial channels, respectively, each twisted at a predetermined angle.

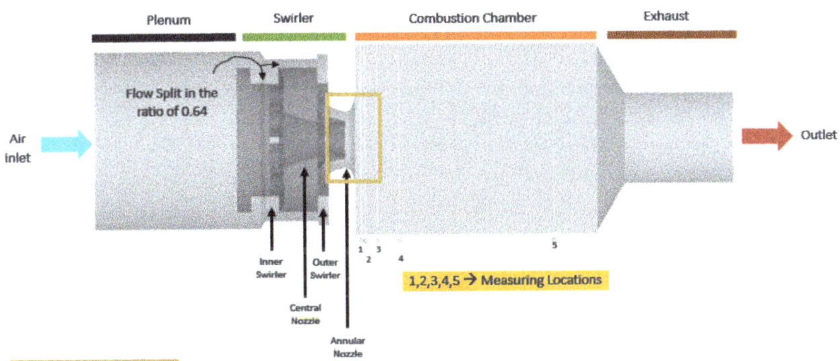

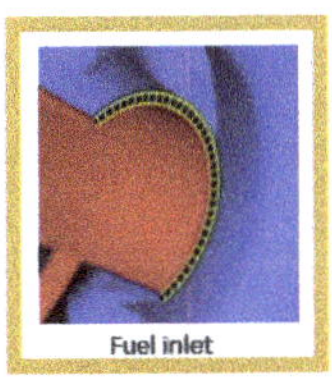

Name	Boundary	Value
Fuel Inlet	Mass Flow Inlet	0.000696 Kg/s
Air Inlet	Mass Flow Inlet	0.019 Kg/s
Outlet	Pressure Outlet	Static / Total Pressure
All others	Wall	Adiabatic

Figure 1. The numerical domain of the gas turbine model combustor encompasses both the boundary conditions and measurement locations.

The fuel was introduced through a non-swirling inlet consisting of 72 square segments, each with an area of 0.5×0.5 mm^2, positioned between the annular and central nozzles. The annular nozzle outlet and combustion chamber were positioned 4.5 mm above the central nozzle and fuel inlets. The combustion chamber was 114 mm high and had a surface area of 85×85 mm^2. The exhaust exit diameter was 40 mm.

The air mass flow rate was maintained at 0.019 kg/s, with an inlet temperature of 330 K. Pure methane was supplied through the fuel inlet at a mass flow rate of 0.000696 kg/s and a temperature of 330 K, yielding an equivalence ratio of 0.65 for the investigated flame. The swirl number, defined as the ratio of the maximum radial velocity to the bulk axial velocity, was calculated under the assumption of perfectly guided swirler channels and conserved angular momentum within the burner. This configuration resulted in an estimated swirl number of 0.96 at the burner nozzle exit.

The mass flow rate of air was 0.019 kg/s, and the temperature at the air inlet was set to 330 K. Pure methane was introduced at a mass flow rate of 0.000696 kg/s 330 K from the fuel inlet, which resulted in an equivalence ratio of 0.65 for the current flame under examination. The swirl number is calculated as the ratio of the maximum radial speed to the bulk axial velocity, assuming that the swirler channels are perfectly guided and the angular momentum inside the burner is maintained. An estimated swirl number of 0.96 at the burner nozzle exit was obtained.

All three velocity components were measured simultaneously using Laser Doppler Anemometry (LDA) systems, and Raman scattering was employed to measure the temperature and concentration of major species. Detailed information regarding the test rig and measurements can be found in Weigand et al. and Meier et al. [18,19].

3. Problem Formulation

3.1. Applied Mathematics and Numerical Modeling Overview

The turbulence model employed in this study is the detached-eddy simulation (DES) model, which does not rely on a specific statistical turbulence model. While Spalart proposed a DES method based on a single-equation RANS model [20], the present work utilizes the Strelets model [16]. This model combines the two-equation SST-RANS model with LES elements and accounts for the boundary layer in regions where the predicted turbulent length scale (L_t) is greater than the local grid spacing (Δ). Unlike the SST model, the turbulent length scale affects the $k - \omega$ equation's destruction term.

$$\frac{\partial(\rho k)}{\partial(t)} + \frac{\partial(\rho \bar{U}_j k)}{\partial x_j} = P_k - \beta^* \rho k w F_{DES} + \frac{\partial}{\partial x_j}\left[\left(\mu \frac{\mu_t}{k}\right)\frac{\partial k}{\partial x_j}\right] \tag{1}$$

The multiplier of the destruction term in Equation (1) is defined as the F_{DES} factor.

$$F_{DES} = \max\left(\frac{L_{t,SST}}{L_{t,DES}}, 1\right), \tag{2}$$

where

$$L_{t,SST} = \frac{\sqrt{k}}{\beta \omega} \tag{3}$$

and

$$L_{t,DES} = C_{DES}\Delta. \tag{4}$$

While the above approach has its benefits, it also has certain limitations, particularly in applications where flow separation in the boundary layer caused by the grid can pose challenges. When models rely on prediction of the turbulent length scale based on the local grid size, the issue of the LES mode being active in the boundary layer is a known concern.

To mitigate this problem, a zonal DES limiter is proposed, which incorporates the blending function of the SST turbulence model [21]. This technique helps to limit grid-induced separation and improve the accuracy of predictions in the boundary layer.

$$F_{DES} = max\left(\frac{L_{t,SST}}{L_{t,DES}}(1 - F_{SST}), 1\right) \tag{5}$$

The model's constants are given in Strelets et al.'s study [16]. As compared to other physical models, like LES and DNS, the Strelets model can face challenges in accurately resolving boundary-layer flows, particularly when grid-induced flow separation occurs. Local grid size influences the transition between RANS and LES modes, potentially activating the LES mode in boundary layers where RANS would be more appropriate, leading to less accurate predictions. Dependence on the turbulent length scale and grid resolution may result in under-resolved turbulence features in complex geometries. Zonal DES limiters help mitigate grid-induced separation but can add computational complexity and require careful tuning.

The simulations were conducted using ANSYS Fluent 16.1 commercial computational fluid dynamics (CFD) software. A coupled pressure-correction scheme was employed to resolve the velocity–pressure coupling. The linear system of equations was solved using a multi-grid method, while spatial discretization utilized a second-order scheme for most variables. For species and energy equations, a bounded high-resolution scheme with second-order accuracy was applied. Transient terms were discretized using a bounded second-order implicit formulation. Parallelization in Fluent follows the Single Program, Multiple Data (SPMD) architecture, where the computational domain is partitioned into tasks executed independently across processors. Inter-process communication is handled via the Message Passing Interface (MPI). Domain partitioning and memory allocation are automated, with RAM usage evenly distributed across all CPUs. The simulations were executed on a custom-built 11-node cluster (comprising head and compute nodes) interconnected via a 1 Gb Ethernet switch. The CentOS 7.9 operating system and Rocks Cluster distribution were used for cluster management. Performance limitations arise primarily from the 1 Gb Ethernet network, which may introduce bottlenecks in MPI communication during parallel computations. While memory allocation is balanced, memory-intensive cases risk exceeding available resources, potentially limiting scalability.

3.2. Combustion Model

Partially premixed combustion is a common combustion regime in which a portion of the fuel and oxidizer are premixed before entering the combustion chamber, while the remaining fuel is injected in a non-premixed manner. In ANSYS Fluent [22], partially premixed combustion is modeled using a mixture fraction-based approach, where a transport equation is solved for the mixture fraction (Z).

The mixture fraction is defined as the mass fraction of fuel in the combustion mixture and is expressed as follows:

$$Z = \frac{\rho_f}{\rho} \tag{6}$$

where ρ_f is the density of fuel and ρ is the density of the mixture. The transport equation for the mixture fraction is expressed as follows:

$$\frac{\partial(\rho Z)}{\partial t} + \nabla \cdot (\rho Z \mathbf{u}) = \nabla \cdot (\rho D_Z \nabla Z) + \dot{m}_f \tag{7}$$

where **u** is the velocity vector, D_Z is the diffusivity of the mixture fraction, and $\dot{m}_f$ is the mass injection rate of fuel. The mixture fraction is used to compute the local fuel–air equivalence ratio, a key parameter in the combustion process. The relationship between the mixture density and the mixture fraction is given by the following formula:

$$\rho = \rho_f Z + \rho_o (1 - Z) \tag{8}$$

where ρ_o is the density of the oxidizer [23].

The partially premixed combustion model in ANSYS Fluent also includes a transport equation for the progress variable (c), a scalar quantity representing the local extent of the combustion process. The transport equation for the progress variable is expressed as follows:

$$\frac{\partial(\rho c)}{\partial t} + \nabla \cdot (\rho c \mathbf{u}) = \nabla \cdot (\rho D_c \nabla c) + \dot{\omega}_c \tag{9}$$

where D_c is the diffusivity of the progress variable and $\dot{\omega}_c$ is the source term due to chemical reactions. The progress variable is used to track the location of the flame front, which separates the unburned reactants from the burned products.

To account for the effects of turbulence on the combustion process, ANSYS Fluent uses the Turbulent Flame Speed Closure (TFC) model, which relates the mean turbulent flame speed (U_t) to the local turbulence intensity and length scales. The mean turbulent flame speed is expressed as follows:

$$U_t = \frac{\alpha_T}{\alpha} S_L \tag{10}$$

where α_T is the turbulent diffusivity of the mixture fraction, α is the molecular diffusivity of the mixture, and S_L is the laminar flame speed. The TFC model allows for the influences of both turbulence and chemical kinetics on the combustion process.

In this study, the temperature and other thermodynamic properties are derived based on the mixture fraction (Z) and progress variable (C) using the partially premixed combustion model. The energy equation is not solved separately; instead, the temperature field is obtained from the combustion model, which utilizes chemical equilibrium tables to determine the thermodynamic state of the fluid. This approach effectively captures heat transfer and thermal dynamics through the interactions of (Z) and (C). The partially premixed combustion model in ANSYS Fluent uses a mixture fraction-based approach to model fuel–air mixing and includes transport equations for the mixture fraction and progress variable to track the combustion process. The turbulent flame speed closure model is used to account for the effects of turbulence on the combustion process.

The partially premixed combustion model is computationally less expensive, but it has limitations as compared to detailed chemical kinetics modeling. The mixture fraction-based approach assumes an equilibrium state or near-equilibrium condition, which may not capture transient or local non-equilibrium phenomena accurately. Simplifications in modeling the progress variable can fail to fully represent detailed chemical kinetics, particularly in highly reactive or non-premixed zones. The assumption of a predefined laminar flame speed (S_L) limits the ability to capture varying flame characteristics under different operating conditions. The TFC model relies on empirical correlations for turbulent diffusivity and flame speed, which may not be accurate for all turbulence and flame interaction regimes. Using precomputed equilibrium tables for thermodynamic properties limits flexibility in simulating cases with significant deviations from equilibrium.

3.3. Mesh Generation

The mesh resolution is a critical aspect of the computational setup, as it is essential to ensure that the simulation captures the relevant physical phenomena. In this study, the mesh resolution is determined based on the ratio of the integral length scale to the size of the grid cells (Δ). The integral length scale measures the size of the most significant turbulent structures in the flow and is calculated as the ratio of the kinetic energy (k) to the rate of dissipation (ϵ). The K-omega SST model is used to obtain values for the kinetic energy and dissipation rate, which are then used to calculate the integral length scale.

The integral length scale must be resolved within a few grid cells in each direction to ensure proper mesh resolution. A general guideline is to resolve at least 80% of the turbulent kinetic energy by capturing eddies with sizes larger than half the integral length scale. The mesh statistics are represented in Figure 2a, which shows a contour plot of the ratio of the integral length scale to the delta. The plot indicates the mesh resolution level, with higher values represents a well-resolved mesh. A maximum capture value of 5 or higher on the plot represents the cumulative turbulent kinetic energy against the length scale of eddies based on Kolmogorov's energy spectrum.

In this study, the mesh resolution was selected to ensure that the integral length scale is adequately resolved and that the turbulent kinetic energy is captured to a satisfactory level. The maximum value of (y^+) along the combustion chamber wall is 24.6, as shown in Figure 2b, which is considered appropriate for this kind of simulation where shear flows dominate inside the combustion chamber.

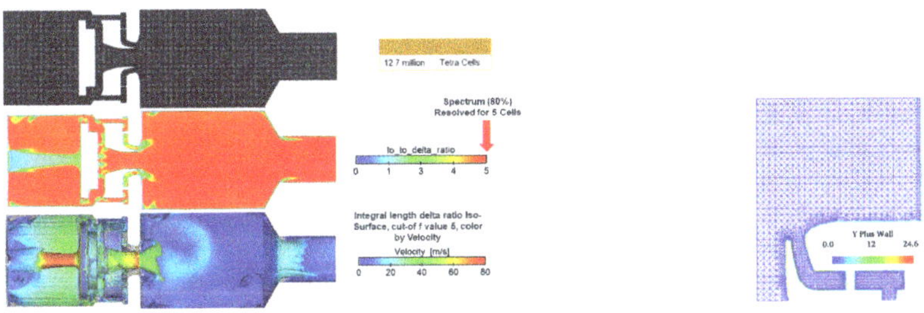

(a) (b)

Figure 2. (**a**) The top image depicts the grid, the middle image shows the ratio of the required length to the delta, and the bottom image displays the iso-surface of the integral length colored according to the velocity at a value of 5. (**b**) Wall y+ contour plot along the wall of the combustor.

3.4. Boundary Conditions

The numerical boundary conditions are illustrated in Figure 1. Air enters through the air inlet with a mass flow rate of 0.0176 kg/s and a temperature of 330 K. Pure methane is introduced from the fuel inlet at a mass flow rate of 0.000696 kg/s and a temperature of 330 K. The turbulent intensity at the air and fuel inlets is set to 5% (medium) and 15% (maximum), respectively. The eddy length scale at both inlets is 0.0005 m.

The wall boundary condition at the combustion chamber wall is set to 1050 K, while the bottom wall boundary condition is set to 600 K. All other wall boundary surfaces are assumed to be adiabatic.

4. Results and Discussions

4.1. Numerical Measurements of Mean Values and RMS Fluctuations

The reported results are based on time-averaged data collected after the combustion initialization process. The averaging process spans four residence times, with quantitative analysis performed after two residence times to ensure stability in the results.

Figure 3 depicts the time-averaged axial velocity field within the combustor, stabilized by enclosed swirl burners with concentric inflow. The two-dimensional contour plot and superimposed streamlines reveal the complex flow structure, characterized by distinct Internal and Outer Recirculation Zones (IRZ and ORZ, respectively) adjacent to the combustion chamber walls. Despite the square geometry of the chamber, the flow field retains approximately axial symmetry, though minor discrepancies between experimental and numerical results are evident. Both the IRZ and ORZ exhibit high turbulence levels, with periodic fluctuations in size and position over time. The region between these zones corresponds to the fresh gas inflow, acting as the primary pathway for unburned reactants. The figure underscores the dynamic nature of the flow, illustrating how recirculation zones govern flame stabilization and mixing processes. While the numerical model captures the overall flow topology, deviations in symmetry and turbulence dynamics highlight challenges in replicating experimental conditions.

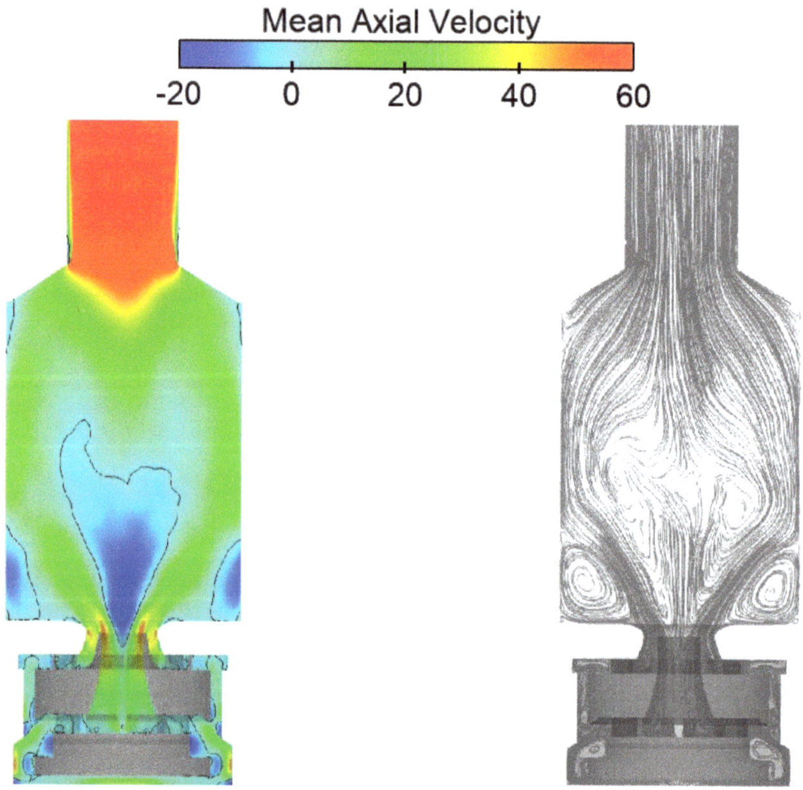

Figure 3. The figure represents the contour plot and streamlines of the mean axial velocity.

Figure 3 depicts a contour plot of the time-averaged axial velocity and corresponding streamlines. The solid black line marks the zero-axial-velocity contour, delineating the boundaries of the recirculation zones. Negative axial velocities at the center indicate the internal recirculation zone (IRZ) generated by vortex breakdown. The IRZ spans approximately 60 mm in length and 40 mm in width, extending roughly 4 mm into the combustor's primary and central air nozzles in the time-averaged flow field. Adjacent to the combustion-chamber corners, the outer recirculation zone (ORZ) forms, separated from the IRZ and the fresh inflow stream by shear layers. The IRZ exhibits high-velocity gradients and temporal fluctuations, rendering it dynamically unstable, with a time-dependent position and dimensions. A small recirculation bubble is also observed near the diffuser exit. The time-averaged flow separates approximately 2.5 mm below the burner mouth; however, due to flow unsteadiness and the absence of a sharp separation edge, this point fluctuates along the wall. Despite the combustion chamber's square geometry, the flow field retains approximately axial symmetry. Minor deviations from symmetry are evident in both experimental and numerical results, underscoring the challenges in replicating turbulent flow dynamics.

The air mass flow in the combustion chamber is split into two streams by passing through the swirlers in a fixed ratio of 0.64, which is not influenced by the choice of turbulence model. The division of the air mass flow rate is determined by the relative flow rate of air passing through the central (inner) swirler and that passing through the annular (outer) swirler. This fixed ratio ensures a stable and predictable combustion process, regardless of the turbulence level in the flow.

4.1.1. Comparison of Mean Velocity Profiles with Experimental and Other Numerical Models

Figures 4–6 present numerical results for the time-averaged and root mean square (RMS) velocity profiles in the axial, radial, and tangential directions, respectively. These are compared with experimental data at multiple heights within the combustion chamber to evaluate the accuracy of the numerical simulations. Each figure is divided into two parts: the first half displays the mean velocity profiles, while the second half illustrates the corresponding RMS fluctuations. In the mean velocity profiles of Figure 4 (axial direction), a positive peak velocity of approximately 30 m/s is observed at a height of 5 mm, corresponding to the incoming fresh gas stream. For the radial component (Figure 5), inwardly directed velocities in the region of $Y > 16$ mm signify the outer recirculation zone (ORZ), with maximum radial velocities reaching roughly half the magnitude of the axial component. The tangential velocity profiles (Figure 6) show relatively constant values within the ORZ, where maxima reflect contributions from the central and annular nozzle flows. However, the simulations fail to capture the minimum tangential velocity induced by the fuel nozzle and its wake in the ORZ in the range of 5 mm $\leq$ Y $\leq$ 20 mm.

Similarly, these results are compared with reference numerical data from the studies conducted by Widenhorn et al. [14] and Chen et al. [24]. Widenhorn et al. [14] implemented the Scale-Adaptive Simulation (SAS) method to simulate the flow, while Chen et al. used large eddy simulation (LES). In comparison to these reference numerical results, the present mean axial velocity profiles come much closer to predicting the axial velocity than those reported in the study by Chen et al. [24]. Widenhorn et al. [25] predicted significantly higher peak values for both the lower and upper peaks. This numerical pattern remains consistent across all mean axial velocity profiles from a height of 5 mm to 90 mm. The mean radial velocity profiles are more accurate compared to the experimental results. In comparison to the present study, the radial velocity exhibits a similar profile but is lower in magnitude near the injector at $h = 5$ mm when compared to that reported in the study by Chen et al. [24]. At a height of 20 mm, Chen et al. [24] predicted higher peak values of mean radial velocity compared to both Widenhorn et al. [25] and the present study. The mean tangential velocity profiles reported by Chen et al. [24] align more accurately with the experimental results, while the models proposed in the study by Widenhorn et al. [25] and in the present study also closely follow the experimental trends.

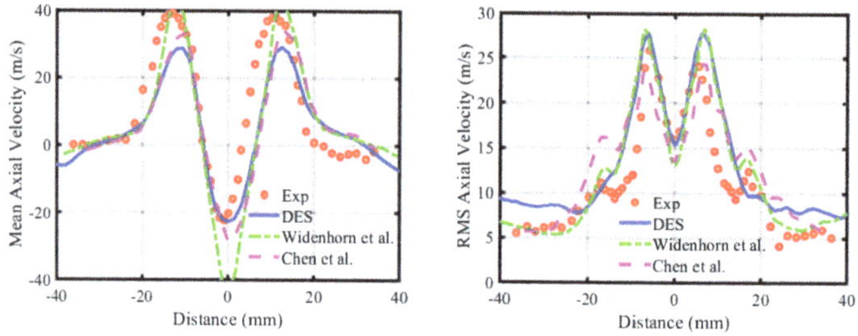

(**a**) Chamber height = 5 mm

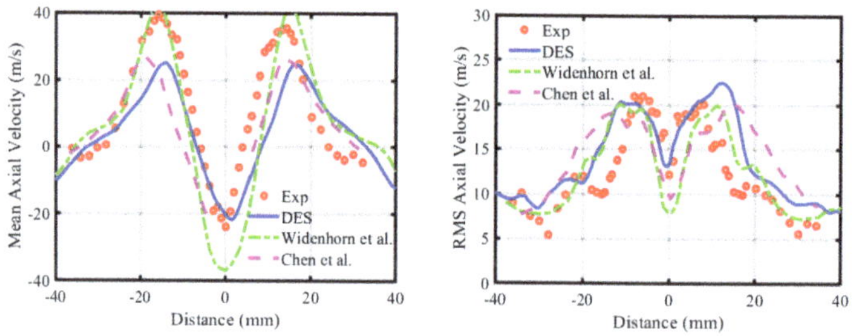

(**b**) Chamber height = 10 mm

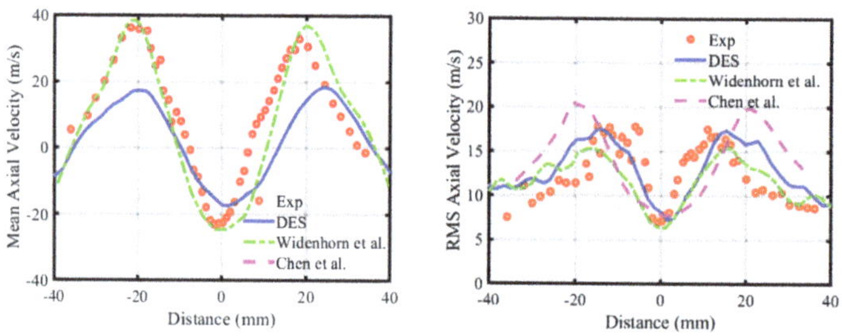

(**c**) Chamber height = 20 mm

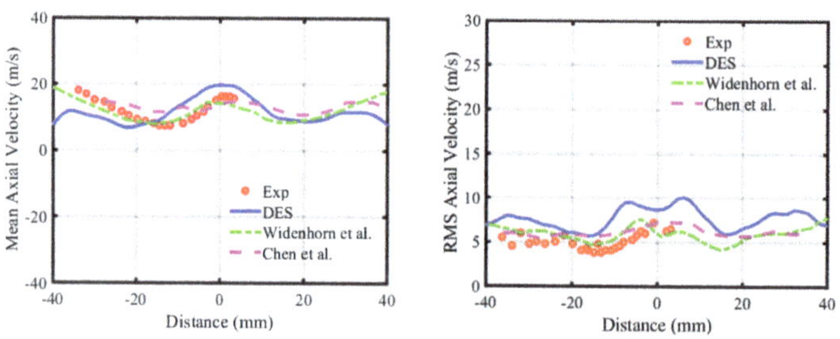

(**d**) Chamber height = 90 mm

Figure 4. Time-averaged axial velocity profiles (**left**) and root mean square values (RMS) of radial velocity profiles (**right**). The red dots represent the LDA measurements, and blue lines are numerical values (Widenhorn et al. [14] and Chen et al. [24]).

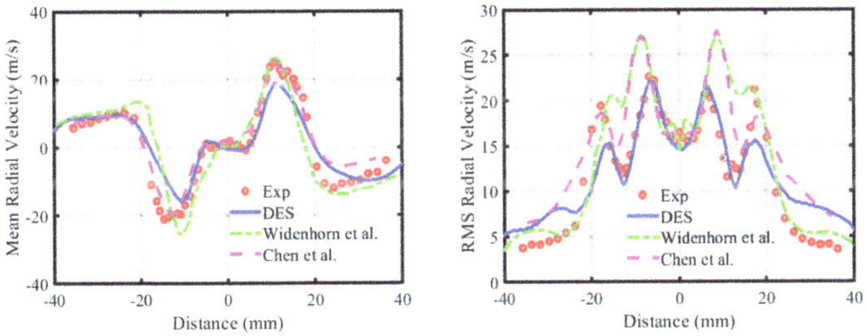

(a) Chamber height = 5 mm

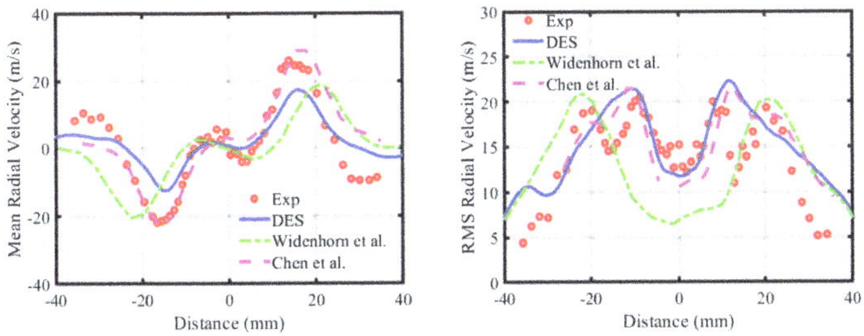

(b) Chamber height = 10 mm

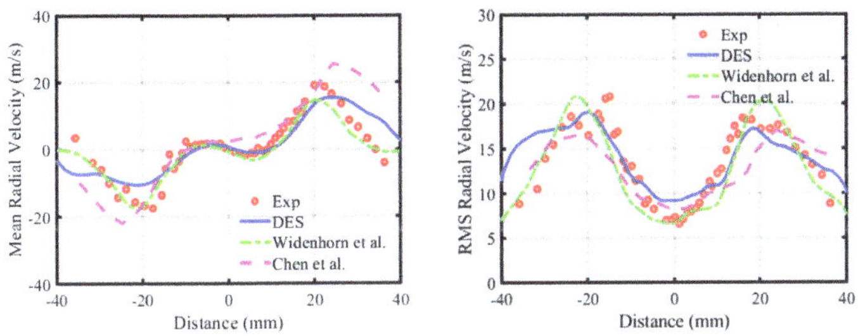

(c) Chamber height = 20 mm

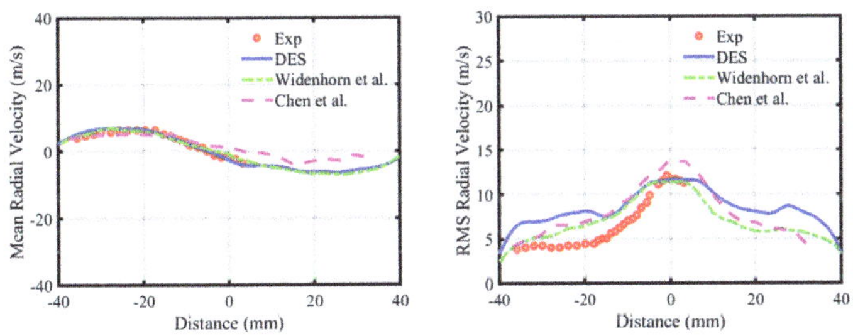

(d) Chamber height = 90 mm

Figure 5. Time-averaged radial velocity profiles (**left**) and root mean square values (RMS) of radial velocity profiles (**right**). The red dots represent the LDA measurements, and blue lines are numerical values (Widenhorn et al. [14] and Chen et al. [24]).

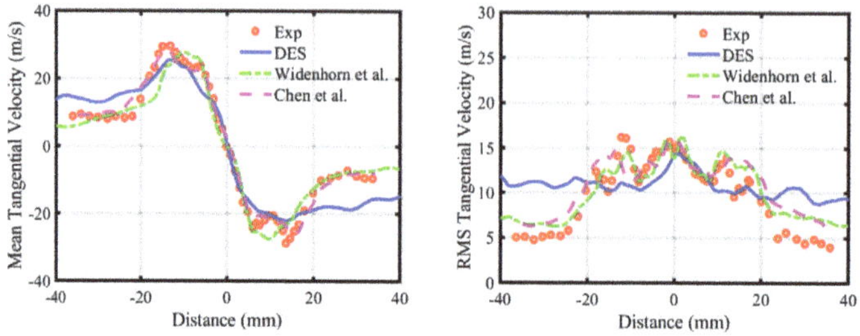

(**a**) Chamber height = 5 mm

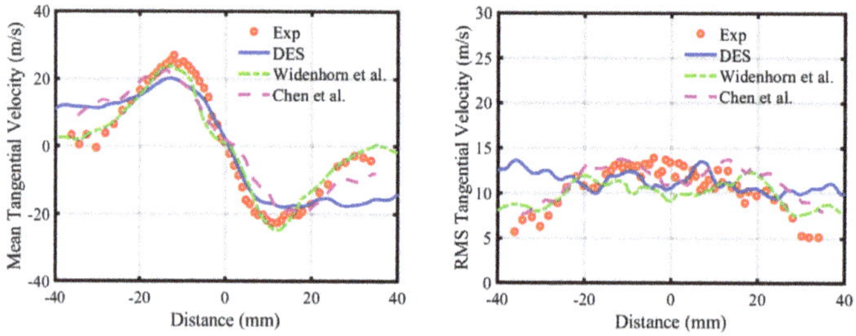

(**b**) Chamber height = 10 mm

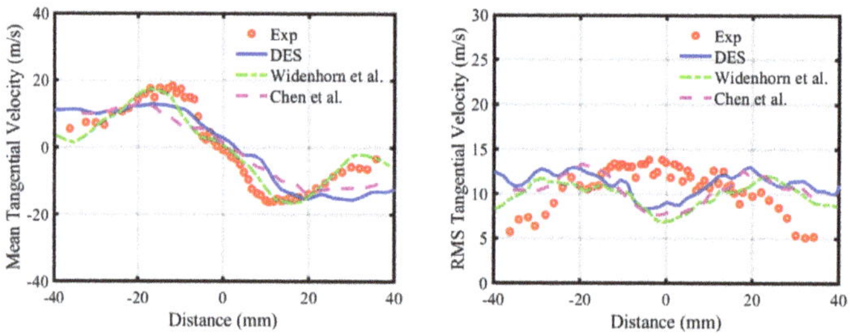

(**c**) Chamber height = 20 mm

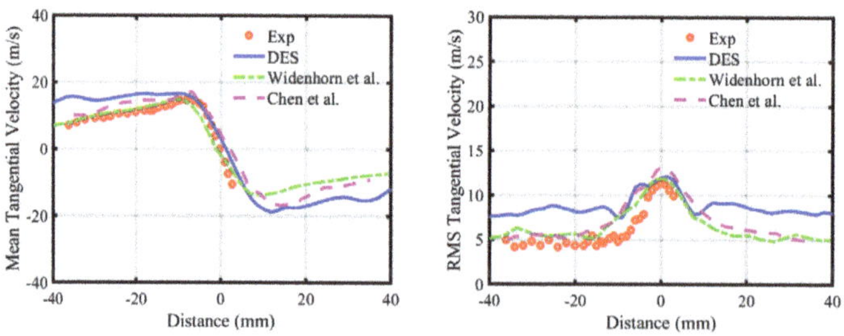

(**d**) Chamber height = 90 mm

Figure 6. The figure compares time-averaged tangential velocity profiles (**left**) and root mean square (RMS) tangential velocity profiles (**right**). Red dots denote experimental data from laser Doppler anemometry (LDA) measurements, while blue lines represent numerical simulation results (Widenhorn et al. [14] and Chen et al. [24]).

4.1.2. Comparison of RMS Velocity Profiles with Experimental Data and Other Numerical Models

The second panels of Figures 4–6 display the root mean square (RMS) profiles of the axial, radial, and tangential velocity components, respectively. The axial-velocity RMS profiles exhibit maximum fluctuations in the shear layers between the incoming fresh gas and the internal recirculation zone (IRZ), with peak values of 28 m/s 5 mm from the nozzle. These RMS values indicate that the IRZ is dynamically unstable, fluctuating predominantly in the axial direction, while the outer recirculation zone (ORZ) varies radially. At a height of 10 mm, the flow characteristics resemble those observed at 5 mm. However, at 20 mm, the RMS values align with measurements at the nozzle exit, albeit with a slight overestimation of the strength of the recirculation zone. The numerical results agree with experimental data for time-averaged axial velocity profiles, though turbulent peak values at 5 mm are marginally underestimated. For the radial velocity component, the maximum RMS values occur in the shear layers between the fresh gas inflow and the ORZ ($Y > 16$ mm). Broad peaks in turbulent fluctuations near $y = 6$ mm (axial direction) highlight shear-layer instabilities. While radial-velocity RMS profiles at the center line are accurately predicted at $h = 5$ mm and $h = 10$ mm, discrepancies in peak magnitudes persist. Notably, results at $h = 20$ mm and $h = 90$ mm show excellent agreement with experiments. The tangential-velocity RMS profiles prove more challenging to predict compared to axial and radial components. Accuracy is particularly reduced in the ORZ, whereas the IRZ exhibits strong agreement with experimental data across all measurement positions. This contrast underscores the limitations of the numerical model in resolving tangential dynamics within complex recirculation zones. The summary of peak values of numerical mean and RMS velocity components, in comparison with experimental values, is presented in Table 1.

The turbulent velocity fluctuations across axial, radial, and tangential components are summarized in the accompanying figures. These results highlight that the axial velocity component exhibits a maximum RMS value of approximately 26 m/s within the shear layers of the incoming fresh gas stream, located between the outer and internal recirculation zones (ORZ and IRZ, respectively). The radial component follows a comparable trend, with peak RMS values observed in both the fresh gas stream and ORZ. Elevated RMS levels in the shear layers near the air and fuel inlets suggest intense mixing dynamics. A sharp gradient in axial velocity fluctuations near the air–fuel nozzle implies instability in the local shear layers, challenging the assumption of a stable IRZ structure. While IRZ fluctuations predominantly occur in the axial direction, ORZ variations are concentrated radially. Turbulent activity diminishes toward the chamber center, contrasting with the highly dynamic behavior near the fresh gas inflow. At a height of 20 mm, axial and radial turbulence intensities decrease significantly, with flow characteristics remaining nearly consistent between 5 mm and 10 mm. By 90 mm, all three velocity components display uniform behavior, marked by minor RMS peaks at the rotational axis and chamber walls. These peaks likely arise from vortical structures (e.g., tornado-like flows) influencing the velocity field.

In comparison with the reference numerical results, the axial-velocity RMS profiles show some differences. At a height of 5 mm, Chen et al. [24] predicted lower peaks of axial-velocity RMS compared to Widenhorn et al. [25] and the present study. However, in comparison with the experimental results, all numerical results exhibit similar trends. At a height of 10 mm, the present study predicted lower values in the inner recirculation zone (IRZ) but higher peak values while still following a trend similar to that of the reference numerical results when compared to experimental data. At a height of 20 mm, Chen et al. [24] predicted higher peak values compared to the present work and other numerical studies. At a height of 90 mm, the present study predicted higher values than the reference numerical results. For the radial RMS profiles, the present study accurately captured the inner peaks of radial RMS at a height of 5 mm, whereas the reference numerical results overestimated these peaks. At a height of 10 mm, both Chen et al. [24] and the present study captured the IRZ or inner shear-layer fluctuations more accurately compared to Widenhorn et al. [25]. The remaining radial RMS profiles show similar trends. The tangential RMS profiles exhibit some fluctuations when compared with the reference numerical results but generally follow a trend similar to that of the experimental data.

Table 1. Comparison of peak time-averaged velocities and RMS values at different heights in the combustion chamber.

Height (mm)	Axial Velocity (m/s)	Radial Velocity (m/s)	Tangential Velocity (m/s)	RMS—Axial (m/s)	RMS—Radial (m/s)	RMS—Tangential (m/s)
5	**30 (Simulated)**	**19 (Simulated)**	**25 (Simulated)**	**27 (Simulated)**	**23 (Simulated)**	**14 (Simulated)**
	39 (Experimental)	12 (Experimental)	30 (Experimental)	26 (Experimental)	23 (Experimental)	16 (Experimental)
10	**25 (Simulated)**	**15 (Simulated)**	**20 (Simulated)**	**21 (Simulated)**	**22 (Simulated)**	**12 (Simulated)**
	35 (Experimental)	20 (Experimental)	20 (Experimental)	21 (Experimental)	21 (Experimental)	13 (Experimental)
20	**19 (Simulated)**	**15 (Simulated)**	**15 (Simulated)**	**17 (Simulated)**	**17 (Simulated)**	**13 (Simulated)**
	35 (Experimental)	19 (Experimental)	19 (Experimental)	17 (Experimental)	16 (Experimental)	14 (Experimental)
90	**20 (Simulated)**	**10 (Simulated)**	**17 (Simulated)**	**10 (Simulated)**	**11 (Simulated)**	**11 (Simulated)**
	19 (Experimental)	10 (Experimental)	17 (Experimental)	7 (Experimental)	11 (Experimental)	10 (Experimental)

4.2. Instantaneous Flow Structures

The time-averaged results only provide a general overview of the flow characteristics within the combustion chamber and do not capture the unsteady flow structures that are crucial to understanding the combustion process. Figure 7 shows the dominant unsteady flow structures in the chamber, characterized by a V-shaped incoming fresh stream of swirl gas. The surface also restricts streamlines in relationship with contour plots of instantaneous axial velocity, indicating the presence of small-scale, unstable vortices close to the inner and outer shear layers. These small structures, along with the high turbulent intensity between the shear layers, are vital in promoting the intense mixing of cold fresh gas and hot burning gases recirculating from the IRZ and ORZ, which aids in stabilizing the flame and contributing to the ignition process of fresh gases. The recirculation zone comprises small recirculation pockets represented by solid black lines rather than one large IRZ, as shown in Figure 3.

The highlighted vortices and the undulated inner shear layer are spatially offset, forming a staggered zig-zag pattern that widens with increasing distance from the center line toward the nozzle. This configuration suggests the presence of a Precessing Vortex Core (PVC), a hydrodynamic instability prevalent in both non-reacting and reacting flows at elevated swirl numbers. The precession frequency and amplitude depend critically on the swirl number, axial confinement, and boundary conditions. The time-averaged flow field inadequately resolves the zig-zag vortices and their helical trajectories. Furthermore, the helical structure dynamically shifts position over time, rendering steady-state simulations ineffective for accurate prediction. The PVC phenomenon involves the vortex core precessing around a mean axis while maintaining a helical shape, a behavior that profoundly influences combustion stability and emissions.

Figure 8A provides information on the time-averaged axial velocity and recirculation zones, showing a small recirculation bubble on the contour of the annular nozzle due to the unstable flow separation at the wall. A sharp edge does not cause this separation, as the flow is highly unstable in nature. However, the separation point fluctuates along the wall, as shown in Figure 8B–D. The size and shape of the ORZ are heavily dependent on time, and small vortices are generated during the separation and subsequently combine to form the ORZ.

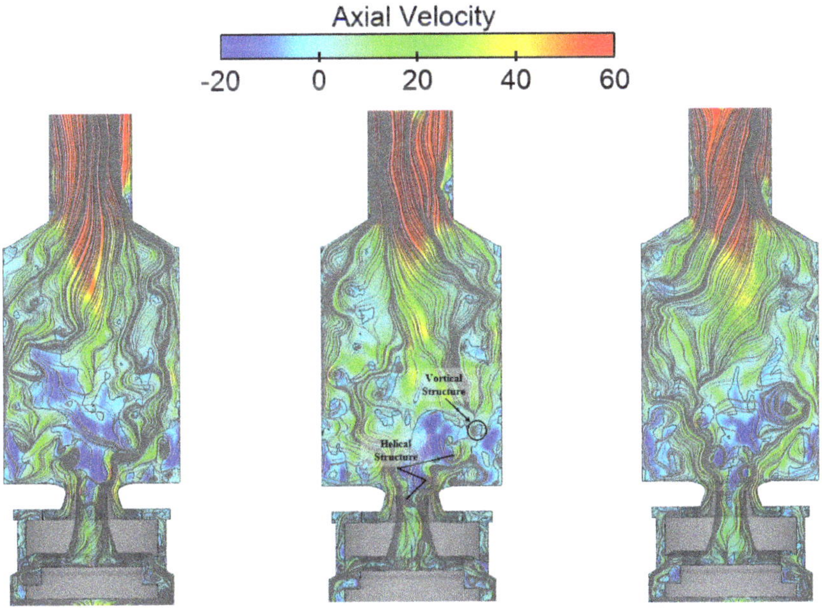

(a) t = 0.12000 s (b) t = 0.12930 s (c) t = 0.13410 s

Figure 7. Instantaneous axial-velocity contour plane at different time steps, visualized by streamlines and solid black lines indicating the zero-velocity location.

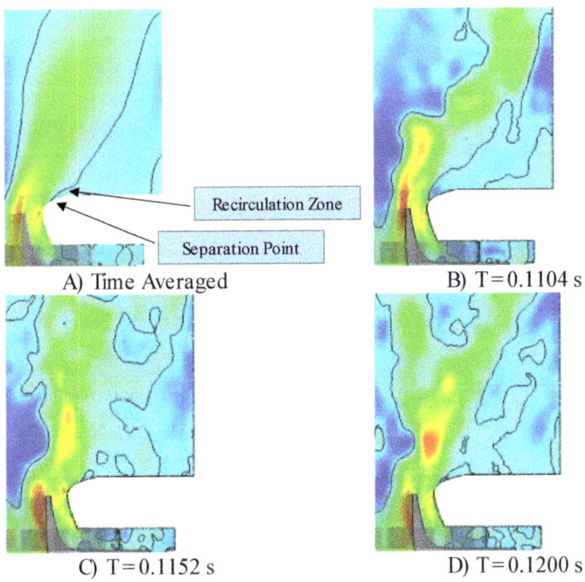

Figure 8. Mean and instantaneous axial-velocity planes at x = 0, representing re-circulation zones with black solid lines and the point of separation.

Figure 9 represents the continuous evolution of the PVC on different pressure iso-surfaces, colored according to axial velocity. Increasing the pressure causes the PVC to evolve and makes a smaller structure visible.

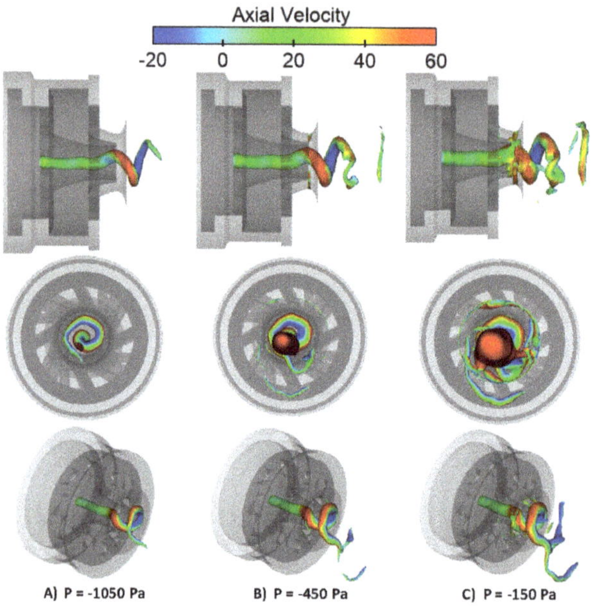

Figure 9. Variable-pressure iso-surfaces colored according to the axial velocity at a constant time step.

4.2.1. Precessing Vortex Core

The precessing vortex core (PVC) is a complex, irregular flow structure that rotates around the central axis and significantly influences combustion dynamics. Its formation and behavior depend on parameters such as the swirl number, equivalence ratio, and combustor geometry, as extensively analyzed by Syred et al. [26]. Numerical simulations conducted by Widenhorn et al. [14,25,27] confirm the presence of PVC across multiple load conditions in the current combustor design. Figure 10 visualizes the PVC using low-pressure iso-surfaces color-mapped according to axial velocity to capture its transient evolution. These iso-surfaces are shown at three distinct time instances, highlighting the intricate and unsteady nature of the PVC.

4.2.2. Vortical Structure

Figure 11 depicts a vortical structure in the upper combustion chamber, where an unsteady vortex core resides in the exhaust pipe. This tornado-like structure, experimentally investigated by Stopper et al. [28], arises from the combustion chamber's rapid radial contraction, which amplifies the swirling flow's angular velocity. The resulting precessing vortex core (PVC) migrates into the combustion chamber, altering the time-averaged shape of the inner recirculation zone (IRZ) and influencing the transport of recirculated gas to the combustor nozzle. As a common feature of swirling flows, the PVC precesses around its axis and interacts dynamically with other flow structures, including the IRZ and outer recirculation zone (ORZ). The PVC's significance in combustion systems stems from its ability to enhance turbulent mixing and stabilize combustion. By inducing strong axial and radial flow oscillations, the PVC improves fuel–air mixing, accelerates flame speed, and modifies time-averaged flow patterns, thereby reducing emissions and promoting combustion stability. Experimental studies highlight that PVC characteristics—such as size, precession frequency, and stability—are governed by parameters like the swirl number, combustor geometry, and operating conditions. For instance, higher swirl numbers intensify tangential momentum, directly affecting the PVC's evolution and interaction with recirculation zones.

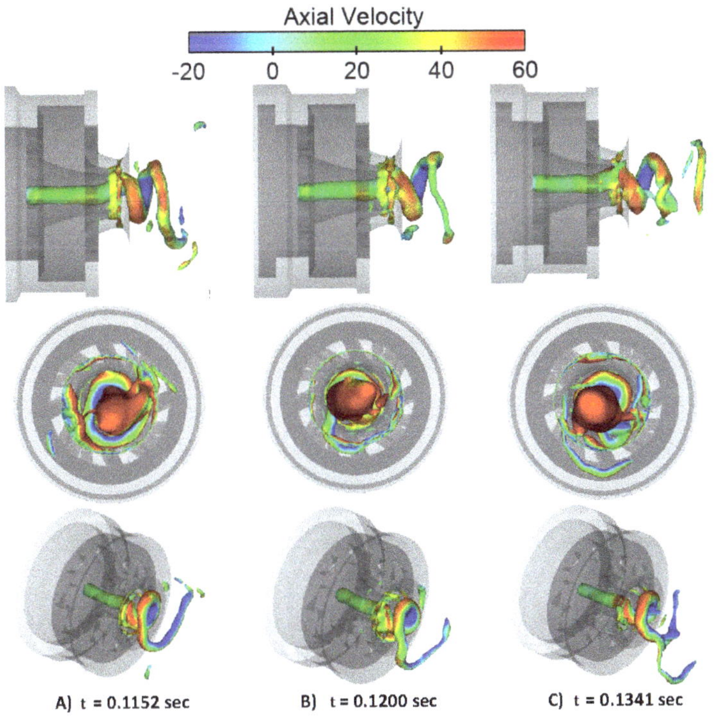

Figure 10. Pressure iso-surfaces colored according to the axial velocity at different time steps.

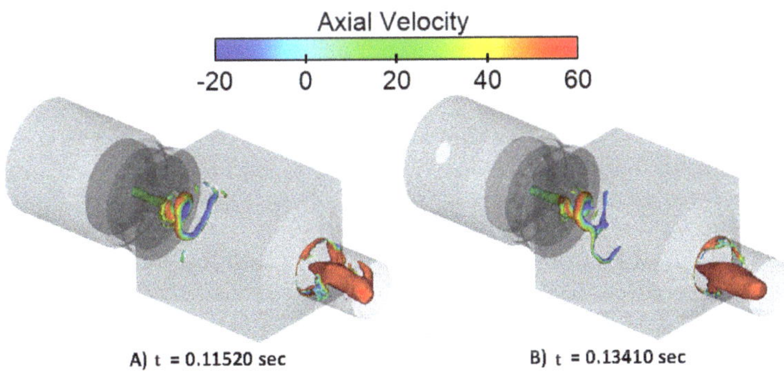

Figure 11. Vortical structure colored according to the axial velocity, representing the pressure on the iso-surface.

4.2.3. Vorticity

To clarify, there are four distinct reasons for the occurrence of vorticity in the combustion chamber. The first reason is the interaction of the helical structure with the inner shear layer, as previously mentioned. The second reason is the precessing vortex core (PVC), which rotates around the central axis of the combustion chamber, as shown in Figure 12. The third reason is the vortex breakdown phenomenon, which is depicted in a spiral shape as it approaches a stagnation point due to the geometric change between the fuel inlet and the conical part of the air nozzle at the combustion chamber entrance. This geometric change causes a sudden swirl increase, generating vorticity. The fourth reason is the occurrence of a vortical structure in the upper part of the chamber, as depicted in the figure. Vorticity can also occur due to a vortex core in the exhaust pipe.

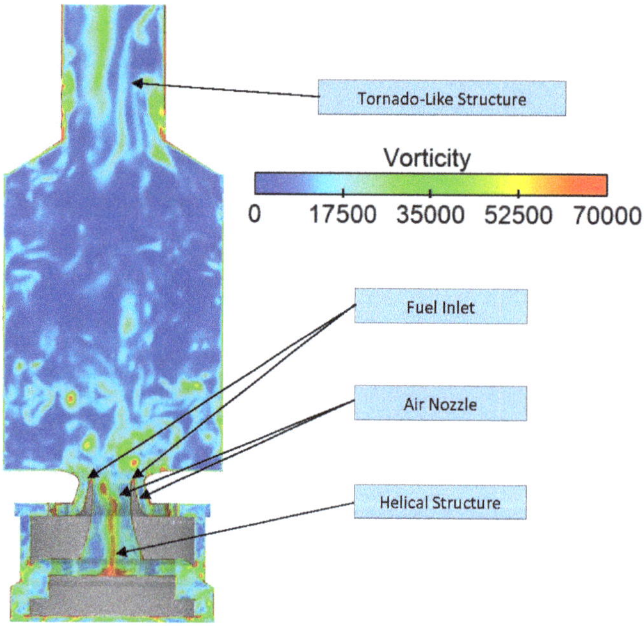

Figure 12. Vorticity plane at x = 0.

4.3. Temperature Field, Heat Release, and Mass Fractions

4.3.1. Time-Averaged Temperature Profiles

The temperature distribution in the combustion chamber is a critical parameter in understanding the combustion process. As shown in Figure 13A , the flame takes on a conical shape, a common characteristic of many combustion systems. The mean temperature is highest near the nozzle exit, gradually decreasing as it moves toward the combustor walls. The time-averaged flame root, which is the point where the flame is anchored to the nozzle exit, is approximately 15 mm above the nozzle exit. This position indicates that the flame is partially premixed before ignition, meaning that the fuel and air are partially mixed before combustion. The swirl motion of the air and fuel in the combustion chamber generates this partial mixing. The partially premixed flame structure is beneficial for reducing emissions and improving combustion efficiency, as it allows for more uniform mixing and better control of the combustion process.

The comparison of numerical and experimental time-averaged temperature profiles, shown in Figure 14, provides valuable insights into the simulation's accuracy and the flame's behavior. The distribution of mean temperatures reveals that the flame exhibits a conical shape, consistent with many combustion processes. At a height of 15 mm, corresponding to the flame root or anchoring point, the numerical center-line temperature is approximately 1800 K, which is recognized as a main combustion region. However, a significant discrepancy at a height of 10 mm in the combustion chamber is observed between the numerical and experimental data in the regions of the high-shear layer. The lowest simulated mean temperature is 600 K, which may indicate limitations in the simulation or measurement technique.

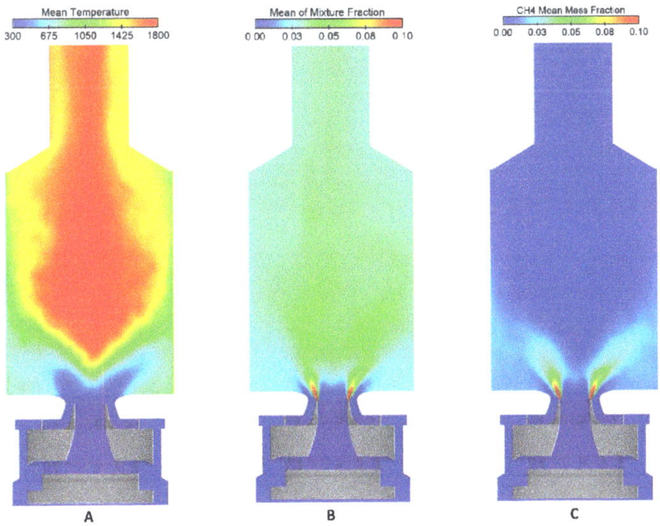

Figure 13. Two-dimensional x–y mean contour plane of (**A**) temperature, (**B**) mixture fraction, and (**C**) CH_4 fraction.

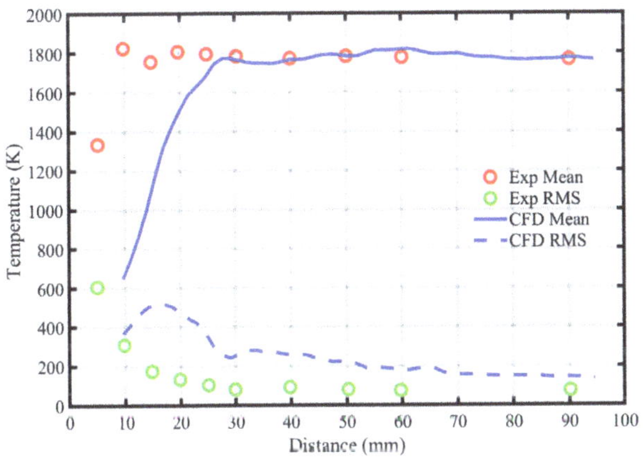

Figure 14. Numerical profiles of time-averaged and RMS temperature along the center line compared with experimental results of time-averaged and RMS profiles.

The turbulent fluctuations, quantified by the root-mean-square (RMS) temperature, are also compared between the numerical and experimental data. The results show that the turbulence intensity is higher in the numerical simulation than in the experiment, suggesting that the simulation may overpredict the turbulent mixing in the combustion chamber. Nonetheless, the comparison indicates a good agreement between the numerical and experimental data in the regions of low temperature, which are attributed to the approaching fresh gas stream.

The distribution of the time-averaged temperature provides valuable information about the combustion process and reveals the effects of mixing and heat transfer on the flame structure. Figure 14 shows that, for y > 10 mm, the mean temperature increases with height, primarily due to the mixing of the hot exhaust gas from the ORZ with the unburned gas. At h = 25 mm, the maximum mean temperature is achieved, indicating the location of the flame's peak temperature.

Within the IRZ, the maximum time-averaged mean temperature is T = 1827.6 K, which closely matches the experimental value of T = 1827 K. This region's mixing fraction (f) is higher than the global value, indicating that the IRZ is well-mixed and has a higher concentration of reactants. On the other hand, the ORZ has a lower temperature level compared to the IRZ. This can be attributed to the leaner mixture and heat losses to the ORZ wall.

The numerical results also capture the temperature gradients across the flame structure, with the highest temperatures occurring near the flame root and decreasing towards the flame tip. In addition, the turbulent fluctuations (RMS) of the temperature exhibit high values in the regions of the shear layers, where the mixing of the reactants and products is most intense. Overall, the numerical temperature profiles agree well with the experimental data and provide insights into the complex flame dynamics in the combustion chamber.

The time-averaged temperature profiles obtained through simulation are in good agreement with the experimental results, except for a slight deviation observed at a height of 5 mm, where the temperature near the center line is underestimated. The turbulent temperature fluctuation profiles obtained through simulation also agree with the experimental profiles, with peak values and overall shape closely resembling the measured data. However, at a height of 5 mm, the simulated turbulent temperature changes at the center line are slightly higher than the experimental values. Overall, these findings suggest that the simulation accurately captures the temperature behavior in the combustion chamber, except for a small discrepancy near the center line at 5 mm.

4.3.2. Mean Mixture Fraction

Figure 15 compares the numerical and experimental time-averaged mixture-fraction profiles. The mixture fraction reaches its maximum value above the fuel-nozzle exit, and the mean mixture fraction at the height of 5 mm is relatively low due to the nozzle configuration's rapid mixing. The maximum simulated mixture fraction is $f_{max} = 0.072$. The stoichiometric mixture fraction is reached at y = 5 mm and y = 10 mm, suggesting that the flame is not in equilibrium in these regions due to the low temperatures.

Interestingly, the mixture fraction in the IRZ is higher than the global value ($f_{global} = 0.036$), while the ORZ mixture fraction is equal to f_{global}. This difference implies that the increase in mixture fraction in the IRZ benefits ignition and flame stabilization, allowing temperatures above the global adiabatic flame temperature.

The time-averaged plots at h = 20 mm show a reduction in variation along the y-axis of the mixture fraction, indicating rapid mixing of the fuel stream. The broadened maximum of the mixture fraction suggests that the mixing process is enhanced. Finally, at h = 90 mm, the mixing is complete in the time-averaged plots, and the mixture fraction profile becomes uniform. Overall, the simulation and experimental results are in good agreement, except for the mixture fraction at a height of 5 mm, where the simulation underestimates the experimental values.

The IRZ, the region of the flame where combustion is mainly completed, exhibits higher temperature levels and a mixture fraction that exceeds the global value of $f_{global} = 0.036$. This is due to the efficient mixing of the fuel and air in this region, which allows for complete combustion and elevated temperatures. This is important for efficient energy conversion and reduced emissions in combustion systems.

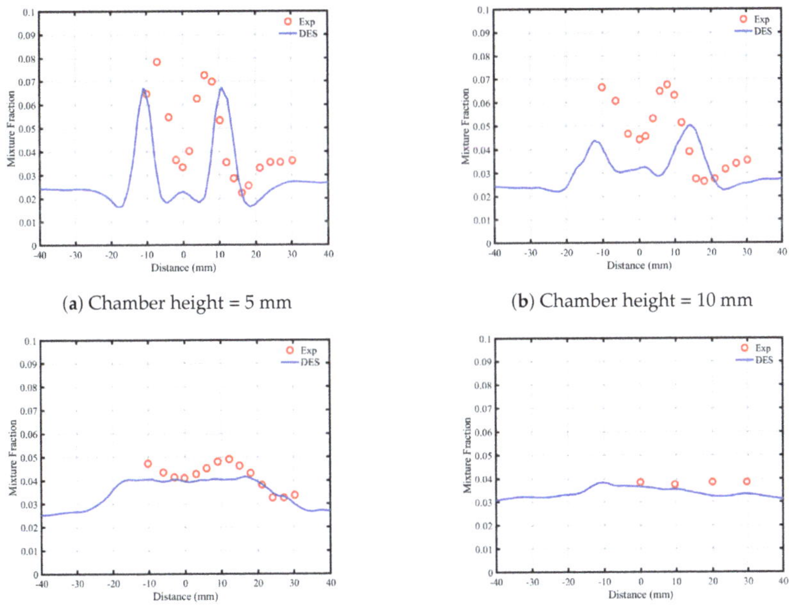

(**a**) Chamber height = 5 mm

(**b**) Chamber height = 10 mm

(**c**) Chamber height = 20 mm

(**d**) Chamber height = 90 mm

Figure 15. Blue lines are numerical profiles of the time-averaged mixture fraction, and the red dots are LDA measurements at different heights of chamber.

4.3.3. Methane Mass Fraction

Figure 13C shows the time-averaged distribution of the methane mass fraction. The numerical results presented in Figure 16 are in good agreement with the experimental data. The plots reveal that the highest CH_4 mass-fraction values are found above the fuel-nozzle exit, indicating the presence of unburned fuel in this region. At y > 15 mm, the methane mass fraction drops to approximately 1% or less in all axial positions. This decrease is due to the rapid mixing of the fresh methane stream with the hot combustion products. Notably, no CH_4 was detected in the exhaust gas region, indicating that the combustion process is efficient. Close to the nozzle, the mass-fraction fluctuations reach CH_4 = 0.075, a relatively high value, but rapidly decreases to CH_4 = 0.0 at greater heights. This behavior is consistent with the rapid mixing and combustion of the fuel in the IRZ, which is characterized by high temperatures and a mixture fraction that exceeds the global value.

The simulated time-averaged CH_4 mass fraction profiles agree with the experimental profiles at all positions. Similarly, the simulated turbulent mass-fraction fluctuation profiles generally match the experimental measurements, except for a slight overprediction at h = 20 mm. Notably, the distribution of other significant species, such as N_2, CO_2, and O_2, which are not represented here, also agrees well with the experimental results. Overall, these results demonstrate that the simulation accurately captures the behavior of the combustion process and provides valuable insights into the distributions and fluctuations of various chemical species.

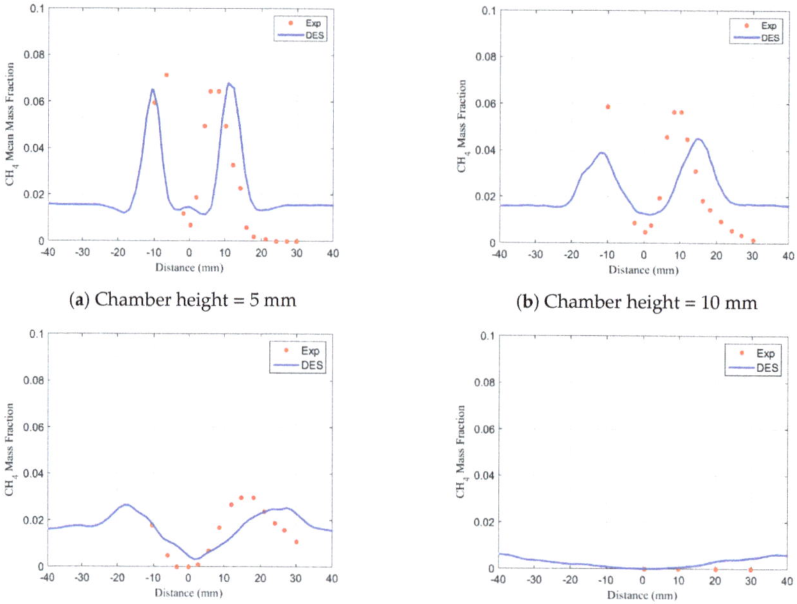

(**a**) Chamber height = 5 mm (**b**) Chamber height = 10 mm

(c) Chamber height = 20 mm (**d**) Chamber height = 90 mm

Figure 16. Blue lines are numerical profiles of the time-averaged mass fraction of CH_4, and the red dots are LDA measurements at different heights of chamber.

4.3.4. Instantaneous Temperature

Figure 17A represent the instantaneous temperature distribution inside the combustion chamber. The contour plot clearly shows that the inner recirculation zone (IRZ) is unstable and exhibits temperature fluctuations. The higher-temperature gases in the IRZ are susceptible to transport toward the central nozzle, which can have a detrimental effect on the combustion process, as unburned gases may mix with the burned gases before re-entering the combustion chamber.

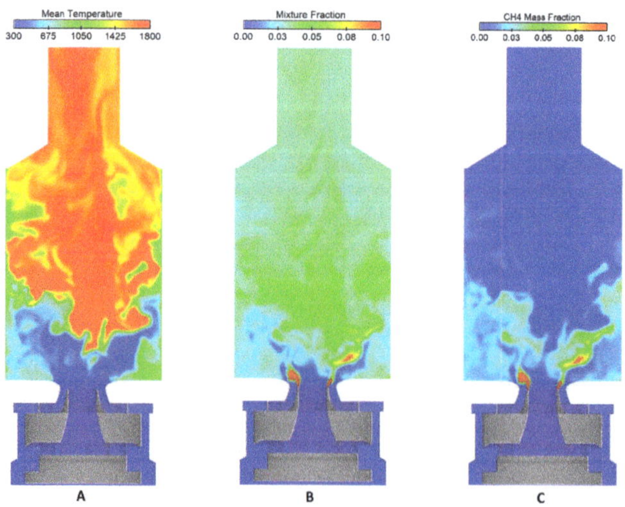

Figure 17. Two-dimensional x–y instantaneous contour plane of (**A**) temperature, (**B**) mixture fraction, and (**C**) methane mass fraction.

4.3.5. Instantaneous Methane Mass Fraction

The instantaneous mass fraction contour plot in Figure 17 illustrates the flow dynamics of methane in the combustion chamber. The vortices in the shear layers play a crucial role in mixing the hot, burned gases from the outer recirculation zone (ORZ) and inner recirculation zone (IRZ) with the cold, unburned incoming gases. As the vortices break down, they generate smaller eddies, increasing the mixing rate and promoting flame stabilization.

Figure 17 also shows that the methane mass fraction is highest near the fuel nozzle and decreases rapidly with distance from it. The maximum methane mass fraction occurs at the interface between the ORZ and IRZ, where burned gases from the ORZ mix with unburned incoming gases from the IRZ. This suggests that the combustion process strongly depends on the reactants' mixing rate and the transport of hot, burned gases into the incoming gas stream.

4.3.6. Instantaneous Heat Release

The combustion reaction primarily occurs in the inner and outer shear layers, where the burned gases from the outer recirculation zone (ORZ) and inner recirculation zone (IRZ) mix with the unburned incoming gas as represented in Figure 18. The reaction zones are highly dynamic and vary in both space and time. In this case, the mixture fraction in the ORZ is below the global value, leading to generally low reaction rates in this region. However, due to mixing with the hot exhaust gases from the IRZ, the ORZ can contribute to the overall reaction.

The reaction zone in the IRZ is characterized by a mixture fraction exceeding the global value, which promotes higher temperatures and reaction rates, resulting in more complete combustion. Nonetheless, the reaction zones in both the ORZ and IRZ exhibit significant instability, with substantial variations in reaction rates and flame fronts.

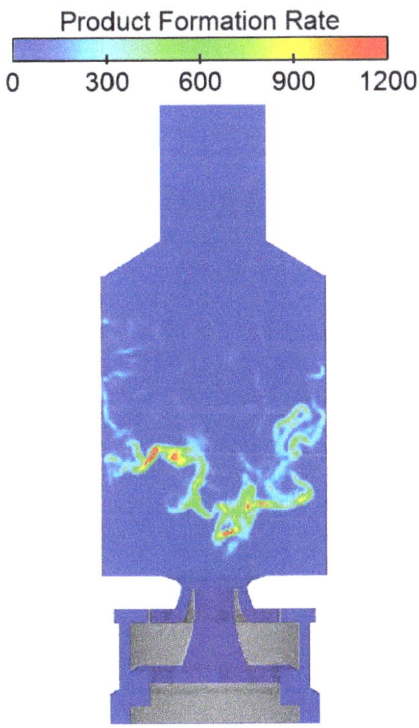

Figure 18. Two-dimensional x-y contour plane of the product formation rate.

4.4. Temperature–Mixture Fraction Correlation Analysis

The correlation between the temperature and mixture fraction of the flame at various heights (5 mm, 10 mm, and 15 mm) in the combustion chamber is represented in Figure 19. The different radial zones are color-coded, spanning from 0 to 30 mm in radius. The solid lines indicate the strained laminar counterflow diffusion calculations (yellow) and adiabatic equilibrium (black) results. The numerical simulation utilizes a partially premixed module that consists of mixture fractions and a progress variable. The probability density function (PDF) table includes 20 species with a flammability limit of 0.1.

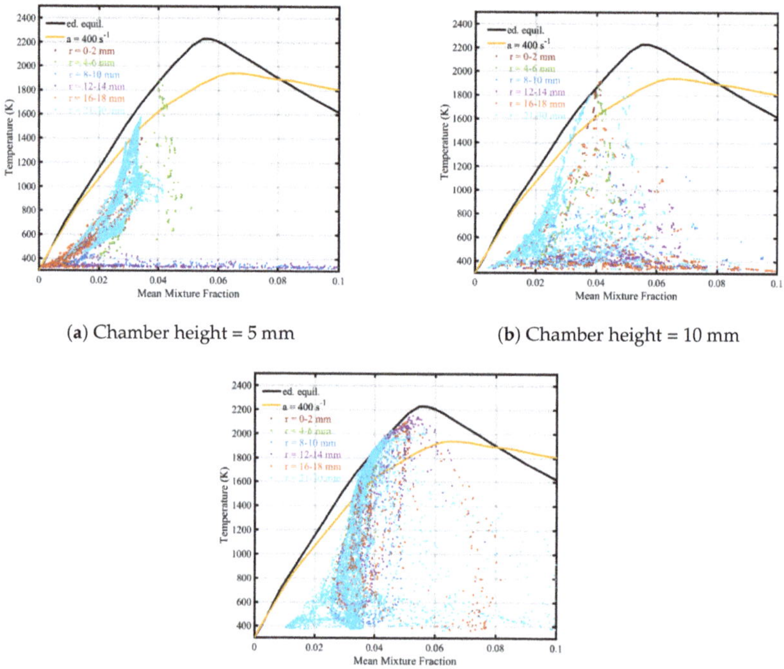

(**a**) Chamber height = 5 mm

(**b**) Chamber height = 10 mm

(**c**) Chamber height = 30 mm

Figure 19. Correlation between the temperature and mixture fraction of the flame at three different chamber heights. The colors represent different radial zones.

Although the investigation of partially premixed turbulent flames cannot be directly compared to counterflow diffusion flames, the calculated curves provide insight into the thermo-chemical state of the flames under examination. The mixture fraction disperses from $f = 0$ to $f = 0.2$ (equivalence ratio of $\Phi = 4.3$), with most samples between 0 and 0.1, indicating rapid mixing. At a height of 5 mm near the nozzle, the correlation between temperature and mixture fraction predominantly deviates from the equilibrium curve, indicating the absence of a well-defined mixture fraction in that region.

The maximum temperature in the outer recirculation zone (ORZ) reaches approximately 1400 K, while the peak value of the mixture fraction is around 0.03, which is well below the stoichiometric limit ($f_{\text{stoich}} = 0.055$). However, in the inner recirculation zone (IRZ), many samples are not yet ignited, with a significant number showing $T \approx 300$ K, even around $f_{\text{stoich}} = 0.055$. This observation indicates that the flames are likely to be classified as partially premixed.

At heights of 15 mm and 30 mm, the highest temperature samples are primarily from the IRZ and are scattered between $f \approx 0.04$ and $T = 1800$ K. These samples are located near the calculated curves, suggesting they are nearly completely burned. Furthermore, their mixture-fraction values exceed the global mixture fraction, indicating that fuel is more efficiently transported to the flame axes. This results in higher flame temperatures than the global adiabatic temperature for the global mixture fraction.

The IRZ plays a critical role in stabilizing swirl flames. Achieving a higher mixture fraction and temperature by adjusting the nozzle configuration can enhance the stabilization effect of the IRZ.

4.5. Species Mole Fraction

To a large extent, the species mole-fraction scatter plots agree with the scatter plots of temperature and the explanations provided above. The CH_4 and O_2 results are shown in Figure 20 as scatter plots at two different heights in the chamber (5 mm and 15 mm). A calculated curve representing the pure mixing of CH_4 and air is also included. Similar to the temperature scatter plots, the samples can be categorized into non-reacting, partially reacted, and fully reacted gas mixtures.

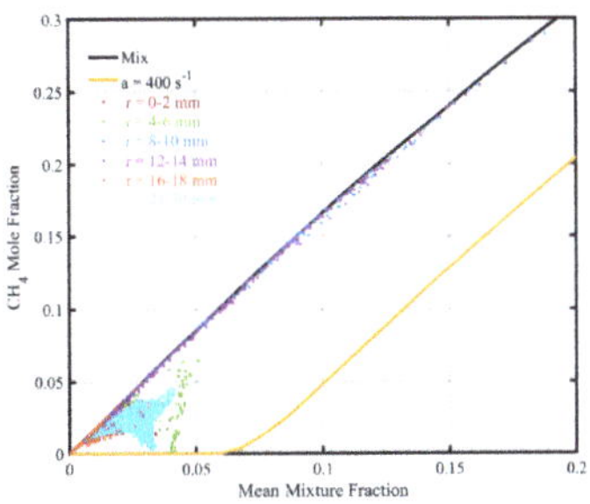

(**a**) Chamber height = 5 mm

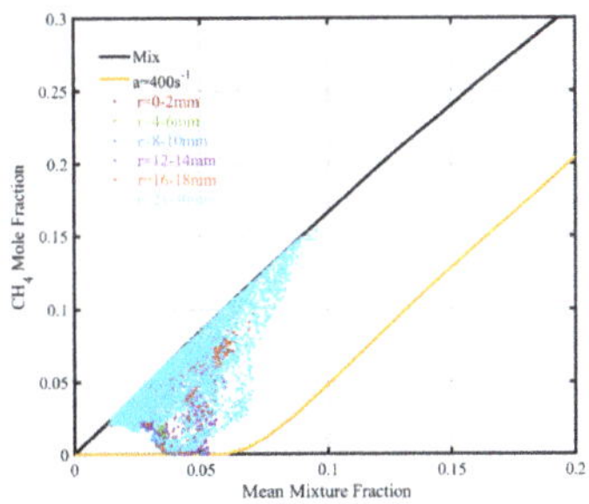

(**b**) Chamber height = 5 mm

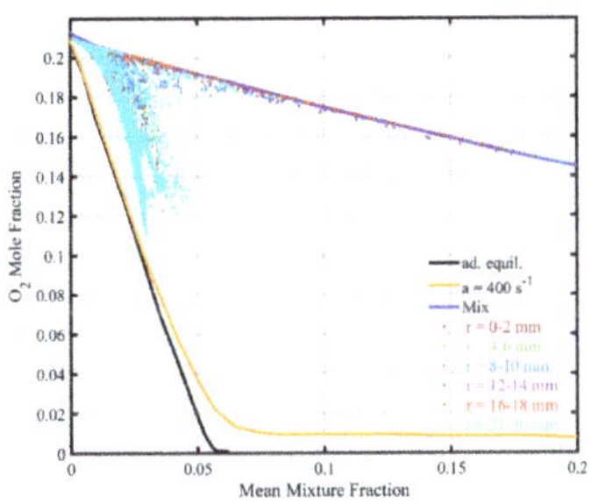

(**c**) Chamber height = 15 mm

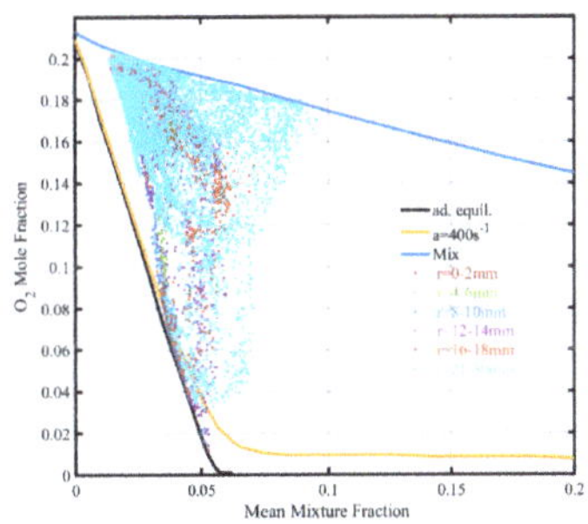

(**d**) Chamber height = 15 mm

Figure 20. Correlations between methane and mixture fraction and oxygen and mixture fraction at different heights.

The fuel-rich samples deviate from the calculated curve of counterflow diffusion flames and align closely with the "Mix" curve. The mixture fraction of CH_4 and O_2 further indicates that most samples from the radial region ($r \approx$ 4–14 mm) follow the "Mix" curve, demonstrating a high degree of premixing.

The correlation between methane and oxygen is presented in Figure 21, which directly illustrates the coexistence of fuel and air. Here, the samples with a methane mixture fraction of approximately zero are fully reacted, while all others follow the "Mix" curve, representing either pure mixing or partial reaction.

The correlation between temperature and carbon dioxide mole fraction at $h = 5$ mm and $h = 15$ mm is represented in Figure 22. The results clearly show that the inner recirculation zone (IRZ) and the adjacent shear layer are in sensible agreement with adiabatic equilibrium. However, the calculation based on counterflow diffusion exhibits much poorer agreement, particularly for high CO_2 mole fractions.

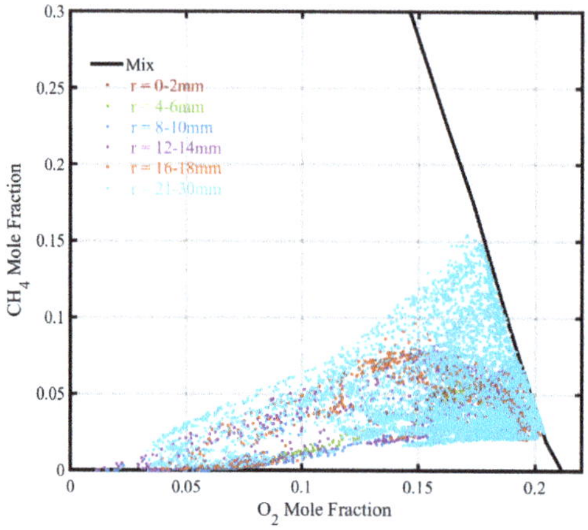

Figure 21. Correlation between methane and oxygen at different heights.

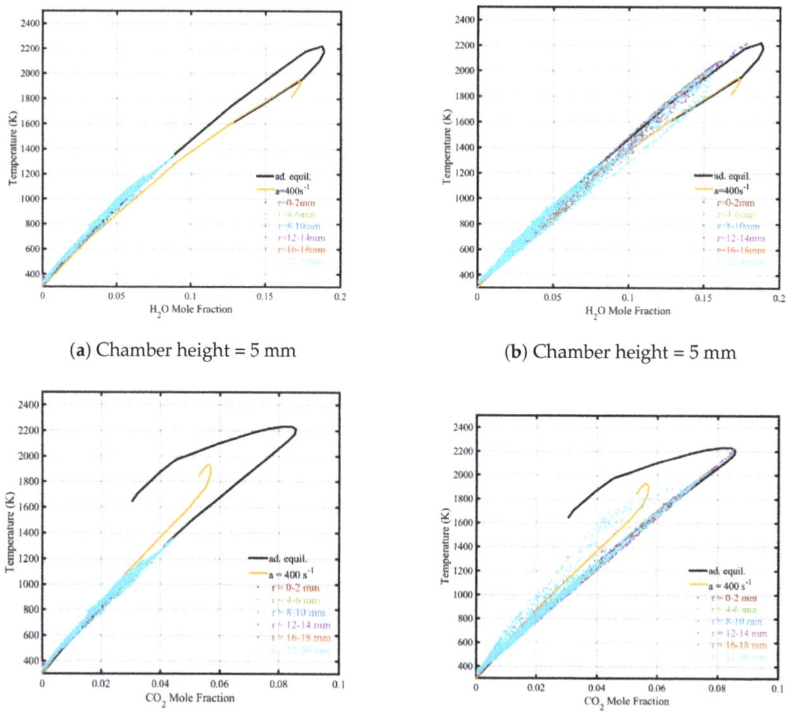

(**a**) Chamber height = 5 mm (**b**) Chamber height = 5 mm

(**c**) Chamber height = 15 mm (**d**) Chamber height = 15 mm

Figure 22. Correlations between water mole faction and temperature and between carbon dioxide mole fraction and temperature at different heights.

5. Conclusions

This study investigated partially premixed flames using a partially premixed combustion model coupled with a detached-eddy simulation (DES) approach, focusing on methane and air combustion at an equivalence ratio of 0.65. The research aimed to validate the model's ability to accurately simulate combustion dynamics in swirl-stabilized flames, a key feature of modern gas turbines. The numerical results were validated against experimental data, including time-averaged and root mean square velocity components, species profiles, mixture fractions, and temperature distributions. The comparison showed that the model captures the overall trends in the flow behavior, though minor discrepancies were observed, particularly in the adiabatic temperature region at lower mixture fractions. This indicates room for future improvements in the model, such as refinement of the PDF table values for more accurate predictions.

Additionally, the study provided insights into instantaneous flow structures and dynamic pressure changes, which deepen the understanding of the complexity and stability of the combustion process. The correlations between temperature, mixture fraction, and species concentrations were also explored, demonstrating the influence of these factors on combustion efficiency and stability.

One of the key contributions of this study is the significant reduction in computational cost. The proposed numerical setup is less computationally expensive than more detailed chemical mechanisms, offering a significant advantage in practical applications where rapid simulations are required. This reduction in computational cost represents a step towards sustainability, enabling faster design iterations and optimization without sacrificing essential accuracy. This is particularly relevant in the design and optimization of gas turbines, where computational efficiency is critical for real-time simulations and iterative design processes.

However, while the proposed model provides a good balance between accuracy and computational cost, there are limitations, particularly in the near-flame regions, where the model lacks the fine detail required for high-precision predictions. These discrepancies suggest that future studies should focus on improving the modeling of high-shear and near-flame regions, which could be addressed by refining the PDF values and exploring alternative turbulence–chemistry interaction models.

In short, this study presents a robust and computationally efficient methodology for simulating methane combustion in dual swirl combustors. While the model shows promise for gas turbine design and offers significant potential for sustainable engineering practices, further refinement is necessary for high-precision simulations in certain regions. Future work will aim to enhance model accuracy while maintaining computational efficiency, ultimately contributing to more sustainable and cost-effective design solutions in combustion engineering.

Author Contributions: Conceptualization, H.A.H.S., R.R. and A.M.; Methodology, G.M. and A.M.; Software, H.A.H.S.; Validation, H.A.H.S.; Formal analysis, H.A.H.S.; Resources, R.R.; Data curation, G.M.; Writing—original draft, H.A.H.S.; Writing—review and editing, G.M. and R.R.; Supervision, R.R.; Funding acquisition, G.M. All authors have read and agreed to the published version of the manuscript.

Funding: This research received no external funding.

Data Availability Statement: The original contributions presented in this study are included in the article. Further inquiries can be directed to the corresponding authors.

Acknowledgments: The author acknowledges the computational support provided by the Supercomputing Facility at SINES, NUST, Islamabad.

Conflicts of Interest: The authors declare no conflicts of interest.

References

1. Mehdi, G.; Fontanarosa, D.; Bonuso, S.; De Giorgi, M.G. Ignition thresholds and flame propagation of methane-air mixture: Detailed kinetic study coupled with electrical measurements of the nanosecond repetitively pulsed plasma discharges. *J. Phys. Appl. Phys.* **2022**, *55*, 315202.
2. Roux, S.; Lartigue, G.; Poinsot, T.; Meier, U.; Bérat, C. Studies of mean and unsteady flow in a swirled combustor using experiments, acoustic analysis, and large eddy simulations. *Combust. Flame* **2005**, *141*, 40–54.
3. Galpin, J.; Naudin, A.; Vervisch, L.; Angelberger, C.; Colin, O.; Domingo, P. Large-eddy simulation of a fuel-lean premixed turbulent swirl-burner. *Combust. Flame* **2008**, *155*, 247–266. [CrossRef]
4. Fiorina, B.; Vicquelin, R.; Auzillon, P.; Darabiha, N.; Gicquel, O.; Veynante, D. A filtered tabulated chemistry model for LES of premixed combustion. *Combust. Flame* **2010**, *157*, 465–475. [CrossRef]
5. Moureau, V.; Domingo, P.; Vervisch, L. From large-eddy simulation to direct numerical simulation of a lean premixed swirl flame: Filtered laminar flame-pdf modeling. *Combust. Flame* **2011**, *158*, 1340–1357.
6. Franzelli, B.; Riber, E.; Gicquel, L.Y.; Poinsot, T. Large eddy simulation of combustion instabilities in a lean partially premixed swirled flame. *Combust. Flame* **2012**, *159*, 621–637. [CrossRef]
7. Chikishev, L.M.; Sharaborin, D.K.; Lobasov, A.S.; Dekterev, A.A.; Tolstoguzov, R.V.; Dulin, V.M.; Markovich, D.M. LES simulation of a model gas-turbine lean combustor: Impact of coherent flow structures on the temperature field and concentration of CO and NO. *Energies* **2022**, *15*, 4362. [CrossRef]
8. Gregor, M.; Seffrin, F.; Fuest, F.; Geyer, D.; Dreizler, A. Multi-scalar measurements in a premixed swirl burner using 1D Raman/Rayleigh scattering. *Proc. Combust. Inst.* **2009**, *32*, 1739–1746.
9. Janus, B.; Dreizler, A.; Janicka, J. Experiments on swirl stabilized non-premixed natural gas flames in a model gasturbine combustor. *Proc. Combust. Inst.* **2007**, *31*, 3091–3098.
10. Fiorina, B.; Luu, T.P.; Dillon, S.; Mercier, R.; Wang, P.; Angelilli, L.; Ciottoli, P.P.; Hernández-Pérez, F.E.; Valorani, M.; Im, H.G.; et al. A joint numerical study of multi-regime turbulent combustion. *Appl. Energy Combust. Sci.* **2023**, *16*, 100221. [CrossRef]
11. Popp, S.; Hartl, S.; Butz, D.; Geyer, D.; Dreizler, A.; Vervisch, L.; Hasse, C. Assessing multi-regime combustion in a novel burner configuration with large eddy simulations using tabulated chemistry. *Proc. Combust. Inst.* **2021**, *38*, 2551–2558. [CrossRef]
12. Butz, D.; Hartl, S.; Popp, S.; Walther, S.; Barlow, R.S.; Hasse, C.; Dreizler, A.; Geyer, D. Local flame structure analysis in turbulent CH_4/air flames with multi-regime characteristics. *Combust. Flame* **2019**, *210*, 426–438.
13. Sloan, D.G.; Smith, P.J.; Smoot, L. Modeling of swirl in turbulent flow systems. *Prog. Energy Combust. Sci.* **1986**, *12*, 163–250. [CrossRef]
14. Widenhorn, A.; Noll, B.; Aigner, M. Numerical study of a non-reacting turbulent flow in a gas-turbine model combustor. In Proceedings of the 47th AIAA Aerospace Sciences Meeting Including the New Horizons Forum and Aerospace Exposition, Orlando, FL, USA, 5–8 January 2009; p. 647.
15. Benim, A.C.; Escudier, M.P.; Nahavandi, A.; Nickson, K.; Syed, K.J. DES Analysis of Confined Turbulent Swirling Flows in the Sub-critical Regime. In Proceedings of the Advances in Hybrid RANS-LES Modelling, Corfu, Greece, 17–18 June 2007; Peng, S.H., Haase, W., Eds.; Springer: Berlin/Heidelberg, Germany, 2008; pp. 172–181.
16. Strelets, M. Detached eddy simulation of massively separated flows. In Proceedings of the 39th Aerospace Sciences Meeting and Exhibit, Reno, NV, USA, 8–11 January 2001; p. 879.
17. Pope, S.B. Turbulent flows. *Meas. Sci. Technol.* **2001**, *12*, 2020–2021.
18. Weigand, P.; Meier, W.; Duan, X.R.; Stricker, W.; Aigner, M. Investigations of swirl flames in a gas turbine model combustor: I. Flow field, structures, temperature, and species distributions. *Combust. Flame* **2006**, *144*, 205–224.
19. Meier, W.; Duan, X.R.; Weigand, P. Investigations of swirl flames in a gas turbine model combustor: II. Turbulence–chemistry interactions. *Combust. Flame* **2006**, *144*, 225–236.
20. Spalart, P.R. Strategies for turbulence modelling and simulations. *Int. J. Heat Fluid Flow* **2000**, *21*, 252–263.
21. Noll, B.; Schütz, H.; Aigner, M. Numerical simulation of high-frequency flow instabilities near an airblast atomizer. In Proceedings of the Turbo Expo: Power for Land, Sea, and Air, New Orleans, LA, USA, 4–7 June 2001; American Society of Mechanical Engineers: New York, NY, USA, 2001; Volume 78514, p. V002T02A008.
22. Ansys Fluent. *Ansys Fluent Theory Guide*; Ansys Inc.: Canonsburg, PA, USA, 2011; Volume 15317, pp. 724–746.
23. Glassman, I.; Yetter, R.A.; Glumac, N.G. *Combustion*; Academic Press: Cambridge, MA, USA, 2014.
24. Chen, Z.X.; Langella, I.; Swaminathan, N.; Stöhr, M.; Meier, W.; Kolla, H. Large Eddy Simulation of a dual swirl gas turbine combustor: Flame/flow structures and stabilisation under thermoacoustically stable and unstable conditions. *Combust. Flame* **2019**, *203*, 279–300. [CrossRef]
25. Widenhorn, A.; Noll, B.; Stöhr, M.; Aigner, M. Numerical investigation of a laboratory combustor applying hybrid RANS-LES methods. In *Advances in Hybrid RANS-LES Modelling*; Springer: Berlin/Heidelberg, Germany, 2008; pp. 152–161.

26. Syred, N. A review of oscillation mechanisms and the role of the precessing vortex core (PVC) in swirl combustion systems. *Prog. Energy Combust. Sci.* **2006**, *32*, 93–161.
27. Widenhorn, A.; Noll, B.; Stöhr, M.; Aigner, M. Numerical characterization of the non-reacting flow in a swirled gasturbine model combustor. In *High Performance Computing in Science and Engineering07*; Springer: Berlin/Heidelberg, Germany, 2008; pp. 431–444.
28. Stopper, U.; Aigner, M.; Meier, W.; Sadanandan, R.; Stöhr, M.; Kim, I.S. Flow field and combustion characterization of premixed gas turbine flames by planar laser techniques. *J. Eng. Gas Turbines Power* **2009**, *131*, 021504.

processes

MDPI

Article

Synthesis of Polymeric Nanoparticles Using Fungal Biosurfactant as Stabilizer

Angélica Ribeiro Soares [1,2], Juliano Camurça de Andrade [2,3], Caroline Dutra Lacerda [2], Sidney Gomes Azevedo [4], Maria Tereza Martins Pérez [4,5], Lizandro Manzato [4,5], Sergio Duvoisin Junior [2] and Patrícia Melchionna Albuquerque [1,2,3,5,*]

1 Programa de Pós-Graduação em Biotecnologia e Recursos Naturais da Amazônia, Universidade do Estado do Amazonas, Manaus 69050-020, Brazil; angelsoares357@gmail.com

2 Grupo de Pesquisa Química Aplicada à Tecnologia, Escola Superior de Tecnologia, Universidade do Estado do Amazonas, Manaus 69050-020, Brazil; ju17camurca@outlook.com (J.C.d.A.); cdutralacerda@gmail.com (C.D.L.); sjunior@uea.edu.br (S.D.J.)

3 Programa Multicêntrico de Pós-Graduação em Bioquímica e Biologia Molecular, Universidade do Estado do Amazonas, Manaus 69050-020, Brazil

4 Laboratório de Síntese e Caracterização de Nanomateriais, Instituto Federal do Amazonas, Manaus 69075-351, Brazil; sidney.gomes@ifam.edu.br (S.G.A.); perezmariatereza@gmail.com (M.T.M.P.); lizandro@ifam.edu.br (L.M.)

5 Programa de Pós-Graduação em Biodiversidade e Biotecnologia da Rede Bionorte, Universidade do Estado do Amazonas, Manaus 69050-020, Brazil

* Correspondence: palbuquerque@uea.edu.br

Abstract: Polymeric nanoparticles (PNPs) are highly valuable across various industries due to their advantageous properties, including biocompatibility and enhanced release control, which are particularly important for pharmaceutical and cosmetic applications. Fungi, through secondary metabolism, are capable of producing biosurfactants (BSs)—amphiphilic molecules that reduce surface tension and can therefore substitute synthetic surfactants in PNP stabilization. In this study, we investigated the production of biosurfactants by the endophytic fungus *Aspergillus welwitschiae* CG2-16, isolated from the Amazon region, as well as its use as a PNP stabilizer. The fungus exhibited a 36% reduction in the surface tension of the culture medium during growth, indicative of BS production. The partially purified biosurfactant demonstrated an emulsification of 24%, a critical micelle concentration (CMC) of 280 mg/L, and an FTIR spectrum suggesting a lipopeptide composition. The biosurfactant was employed in the synthesis of poly-ε-caprolactone (PCL) nanoparticles via nanoprecipitation and emulsion/diffusion methods. Nanoprecipitation yielded spherical nanoparticles with a low polydispersity index (0.14 ± 0.04) and a high zeta potential (−29.10 ± 8.70 mV), indicating suspension stability. These findings highlight the significant role of biosurfactants in polymeric nanoparticle formation and stabilization, emphasizing their potential for diverse applications in pharmaceutical, cosmetic, and other industrial sectors.

Keywords: surface tension; nanoformulation; stabilization; PCL; fungi

1. Introduction

The synthesis of polymeric nanoparticles (PNPs) has attracted great interest in research involving nanomaterials due to their versatility in applications across areas such as medicine, agriculture, and engineering, among others [1,2]. Biodegradable polymers are preferred for obtaining nanoformulations as they offer advantages such as control over size, shape, and surface charge, in addition to being cost-effective, having low toxicity, and possessing good biocompatibility and biodegradability properties [3,4]. These characteristics enable their use in health and well-being applications, such as drug delivery, cosmetic formulations, and food products [5,6]. Poly-ε-caprolactone (PCL) is a semi-crystalline polymer that stands out in this context because, in addition to being approved by the

Food and Drug Administration (FDA) for use as a biomaterial, it is easy to process, has a prolonged degradation rate, and exhibits high biocompatibility [7–9].

The stability and functionalization of polymeric nanoparticles are critical aspects of their performance in specific applications [2,10]. The addition of surfactants—amphiphilic molecules—during the manufacture of nanoparticles has been considered of paramount importance since it contributes to the stabilization of the system [11]. Many synthetic surfactants may have low biodegradability and be toxic. Moreover, in most cases, their production does not meet the requirements of ecological synthesis [12,13]. As a more sustainable alternative, it is increasingly necessary to replace synthetic surfactants with biosurfactants, which are surfactants produced by microorganisms such as bacteria and fungi [14,15].

Fungi are diverse organisms known to exist in a wide range of morphologies, lifestyles, and development patterns and in various habitats, such as soil, water, air, animals, and plants, including environments with extreme conditions [16]. Such adaptive flexibility benefits them in terms of metabolite production, such as in the case of endophytic fungi—those associated with plant hosts and known for producing biologically active substances [17].

The production of fungal biosurfactants has been described in the literature, and many studies demonstrate the potential of using these microorganisms in the production of surfactant molecules [18,19]. Fungi produce a remarkable diversity of biosurfactants, including several unique to them, such as sophorolipids, mannosylerythritol lipids, polyol lipids, cellobiose lipids, and hydrophobins [20,21]. The distinct properties and versatility of these biosurfactants facilitate their application across various industries, including personal care, food production, agriculture, and pharmaceuticals [22–25]. However, studies on the production of biosurfactants from endophytic fungi remain scarce, highlighting the need to deepen the understanding of the relationship between these microorganisms and their host plants [26].

Some studies have investigated the efficiency of biosurfactants as substitutes in the production of metallic nanoparticles, demonstrating that they can be superior stabilizers compared to synthetic ones [27]. However, no studies have yet analyzed the behavior of biosurfactants during the synthesis of polymeric nanoparticles.

Therefore, this study aimed to investigate the synthesis of PNPs using the biosurfactant produced by an Amazonian endophytic fungus as a stabilizer. We determined the physicochemical properties of the fungal biosurfactant and performed a comparative analysis of the nanoprecipitation and emulsion/diffusion methods to produce PCL nanoparticles. The produced PNPs were characterized by dynamic light scattering (DLS), scanning electron microscopy (SEM) and transmission electron microscopy (TEM). The integration of fungal biosurfactants into the nanomaterials manufacturing process could represent a significant advance in materials science and enable the development of more sustainable formulations.

2. Materials and Methods

2.1. Production of Biosurfactants

For the production of the biosurfactant, the endophytic fungus *Aspergillus welwitschiae* CG2-16, deposited in the Central Microbiological Collection of the Amazonas State University (CCM/UEA), was used. This fungus was isolated in 2019 from the Amazonian species *Fridericia chica* [28]. The fungal identification details can be accessed in the GenBank database under the code PP336937.

To standardize the fungal inoculum, the culture, which had been preserved using the Castellani method [29], was reactivated on potato dextrose agar (PDA) to produce a suspension of asexual spores (conidia). Conidia were collected from fully sporulating colonies on a PDA plate, added to sterile distilled water, and standardized using a Neubauer chamber to achieve a concentration of 10^5 cells/mL. Experiments were conducted using conidia suspensions no older than one week [30].

The conidia suspension (400 μL) was transferred to 1 L Erlenmeyer flasks containing 400 mL of culture medium composed of 0.5 g/L of $MgSO_4$, 3.0 g/L of Na_2HPO_4, 1.0 g/L of KH_2PO_4, and 2.0 g/L of yeast extract. After autoclaving, soybean oil was added at 2.0 g/L, having been previously filtered through a membrane with a pore size of 0.22 μm. The flasks were incubated in a shaker under constant agitation at 170 rpm and 36 °C for 96 h [31].

After the cultivation period, the surfactant compounds were isolated from the cell-free culture medium using ethanol precipitation as the extraction method. The cell-free broth was mixed with cold ethanol (1:4 v/v) and kept at 4 °C for 48 h. The precipitate was collected via centrifugation at 5000 rpm for 20 min, treated with chloroform-methanol (2:1 v/v) to remove residual oils, and then dried at 60 °C until the weight remained constant [32].

2.2. Surface Tension Measurement

The Du Nouy ring method was used to determine the surface tension (ST) of the fungal culture medium using a semi-automatic force tensiometer (K20, Krűss GmbH, Hamburg, Germany). For each measurement, 25 mL of the cell-free supernatant was used. The equipment performed ten readings at a speed of 25%. Ultrapure water was used to calibrate the equipment [33].

2.3. Determination of CMC

To determine the critical micellar concentration (CMC) of the biosurfactant, a stock solution of 0.9 mg/mL was prepared. This solution was successively diluted with ultrapure water and analyzed using the tensiometer to determine the surface tension. The CMC was obtained from the plot of biosurfactant concentration versus surface tension, where the inflection point of the curve represents the CMC [34].

2.4. Emulsification Index

The analysis of emulsifying capacity was performed by calculating the emulsification index. For this, a mixture of 6 mL of kerosene and 4 mL of a solution containing 10 mg of the biosurfactant was mixed using a vortex for 2 min and then allowed to stand at 28 °C for 24 h [35]. The assays were performed in triplicate, and the synthetic surfactant sodium dodecyl sulfate (SDS) at 10% was used as a positive control. After the waiting period, the height of the emulsion layer and the total height were measured with the aid of a metal universal caliper (150 M, MTX, Suzano, Brazil), and the values were used to calculate E_{24} (Equation (1)).

$$\text{Emulsification index } (E_{24}) = \frac{\text{Emulsion layer height}}{\text{Total height}} \times 100 \quad (1)$$

2.5. Fourier-Transform Infrared Spectroscopy (FTIR)

The extracted biosurfactant was analyzed using a spectrophotometer (IRAffinity-1s, Shimadzu, Kyoto, Japan) to identify the main functional groups present in the fungal metabolite. The sample was analyzed with the aid of the attenuated total reflection (ATR) accessory, and the spectrum in the infrared region was obtained in the wavelength range of 400 to 4000 cm^{-1}, with a resolution of 1 cm^{-1} and an average of 70 scans.

2.6. Synthesis of Polymeric Nanoparticles

Two classical methods were used to obtain the PNPs: nanoprecipitation [7,36,37] and emulsion/diffusion [3,37,38]. The nanoparticle system was developed from two solutions: the organic phase and the aqueous phase. In both methods, analytical-grade reagents were used, which did not undergo additional purification. Poly-ε-caprolactone (PCL) was used as the wall material, Tween 80 was used as a non-ionic surfactant, and acetone was used for solubilization. At the end of the preparation of each formulation, the nanoparticle suspension was left overnight under constant agitation at room temperature until the complete removal of the organic solvents. The samples were coded as follows: NP—nanoparticles without biosurfactants; NPPB—nanoparticles containing the fungal biosurfactant, prepared using the nanoprecipitation method; and NPEB—nanoparticles prepared using the emulsion/diffusion method with the biosurfactant. Figure 1 summarizes the synthesis of nanoformulations I and II using nanoprecipitation or emulsion/diffusion.

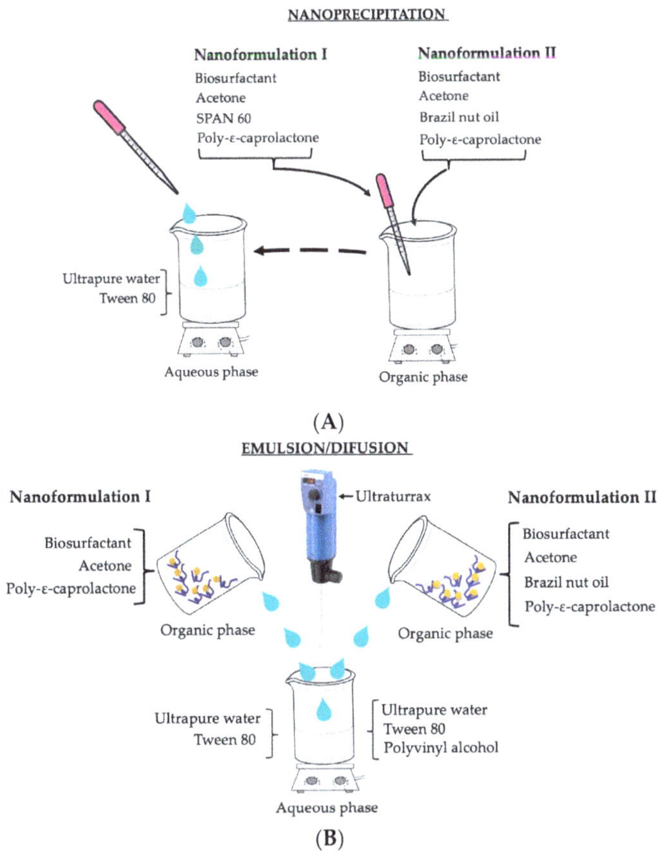

Figure 1. Illustration of the synthesis process of the nanoformulations prepared using the nanoprecipitation method (**A**) and the emulsion/diffusion method (**B**).

2.6.1. Nanoprecipitation Method—Nanoformulation I (NPPBI) and II (NPPBII)

For the preparation of the aqueous phase of nanoformulation I, 20 mg of Tween 80 was solubilized in 150 mL of ultrapure water. This phase was maintained under constant magnetic stirring at room temperature (28 ± 2 °C). The organic phase was prepared in three stages, using a magnetic stirrer (C-MAG HS 7, IKA, Campinas, Brazil) at 40 °C. Initially, 6 mg of the biosurfactant (BS) was solubilized in 700 μL of ultrapure water. Then, 10 mL of acetone was added, and the material was kept under stirring (solution I). In parallel, 60 mg of PCL was dissolved in 20 mL of acetone (solution II), and 40 mg of Span 60 was added to 10 mL of acetone (solution III). The preparation of the organic phase was completed by combining the three solutions. For nanoparticle formation, the organic phase was added to the aqueous phase dropwise with the aid of a Pasteur pipette.

For the preparation of nanoformulation II, the aqueous phase consisted of 20 mg of Tween 80 solubilized in 150 mL of ultrapure water. For the organic phase, 30 mg of PCL was added to 10 mL of acetone, and after solubilization, 25 mg of Brazil nut oil (BNO) was added (solution I). Solution II was prepared by dissolving 5 mg of the fungal biosurfactant in 10 mL of acetone. After solubilization, solution II was gently poured into solution I. Once the organic phase was completely solubilized, it was added to the aqueous phase dropwise with the aid of a Pasteur pipette.

2.6.2. Emulsion/Diffusion—Nanoformulation I (NPEBI) and II (NPEBII)

For the aqueous phase of nanoformulation I, 20 mg of Tween 80 was solubilized in 100 mL of ultrapure water. The mixture was kept under constant magnetic stirring until complete solubilization. For the preparation of the organic phase, all the solutions were kept under constant stirring at 40 °C until complete homogenization. Initially, 30 mg of PCL was added to 20 mL of acetone. After complete solubilization, 25 mg of BNO was added (solution I). Then, 5 mg of the BS was solubilized in 1 mL of soybean oil (solution II). After solubilization, solution II was gently added to solution I with the aid of a homogenizer (Ultra-Turrax, IKA, Campinas, Brazil), at 10,000 rpm for 30 s.

The preparation of the aqueous phase of nanoformulation II used two solutions. Initially, 20 mg of Tween 80 was solubilized in 50 mL of deionized water at 40 °C under constant stirring (solution I). Then, 100 mL of distilled water was added to 500 mg of polyvinyl alcohol (PVA) at 90 °C under slow stirring. After partial solubilization, the temperature was reduced to 40 °C, and the solution was placed in an ice bath so that the crystals could be macerated with the aid of a glass stick. Subsequently, the remaining material was stirred at 40 °C until complete solubilization (solution II). For the preparation of the organic phase, the solutions were kept under constant stirring at 40 °C until complete homogenization. The BS was solubilized in 10 mL of acetone (solution III), and 0.02 g of PCL was solubilized in 20 mL of acetone (solution IV). After the solubilization of solution IV, 25 mg of BNO was added to the phase with PCL, and solution III was poured into solution IV. The organic phase was then poured into the aqueous phase with the aid of a homogenizer (Ultra-Turrax, IKA, Campinas, Brazil), at 10,000 rpm for 30 s.

2.7. Characterization of Polymer Nanoparticles

2.7.1. Particle Size Measurement by Dynamic Light Scattering (DLS) and Zeta Potential (ζ)

The average particle diameter and polydispersity index (PDI) were measured using the dynamic light scattering (DLS) technique on a nanoparticle analyzer (SZ-100-Z, Horiba Scientific, Tokyo, Japan). The analysis was performed at 25 °C at an angle of 90° to the laser. In the same equipment, the zeta potential was measured via electrophoretic mobility using the Zeta-Meter system at a temperature of 25 ± 2 °C.

To measure the mean particle diameter and PDI of the samples, 1 mL of each sample was diluted in 3 mL of deionized water. For the analysis of nanoparticles containing the BS, 200 μL of the formulation was diluted in 5 mL of deionized water. For the analysis of nanoparticles without the BS, 200 μL of the formulation was diluted in 4 mL of deionized water. The final solution of each sample was filtered through a membrane with a pore size of 0.45 μm. Subsequently, the solution was inserted into a cuvette, and five readings were taken on the DLS equipment.

To characterize the surface charges of the nanoparticles using the ζ-potential, double capillary cuvettes were used. The samples were inserted individually using a 1 mL syringe and analyzed at a voltage of 34 mV, positioned at an angle of 90° with respect to the laser beam. The intensity-weighted mean value was measured, and the average was calculated from three distinct measurements.

2.7.2. Scanning Electron Microscopy (SEM)

The nanoformulation was prepared by placing a drop of the NPPBII suspension onto a watch glass and spreading it evenly. The suspension was then dried in an oven at 40 °C until fully dry, forming a thin film. This nanoparticle film was attached to a metal stub using double-sided carbon tape, coated with a 10 nm layer of platinum using a vacuum sputter coater (EM ACE600, Leica Microsystems, Wetzlar, Germany), and subsequently examined with a scanning electron microscope (JSM-IT500H, Jeol Ltd., Tokyo, Japan) in secondary electron mode.

2.7.3. Transmission Electron Microscopy (TEM)

The sample was subjected to sonication for 5 min, and subsequently, 5 μL was deposited onto copper grids (300 mesh) coated with Formvar/Carbon. The grids were left to dry at room temperature for 2 h. The images were acquired using a transmission electron microscope (JEM 1400Flash, Jeol Ltd., Tokyo, Japan) operating at 120 kV.

2.8. Statistical Analysis

Statistical analysis was performed to compare the results of particle size, PDI, and ζ-potential of the various formulations. The data were presented as mean and standard deviation. All readings were performed in triplicate using independently prepared samples. The analyzed data were compared using a one-way ANOVA, followed, in cases of differences, by the Tukey test ($p < 0.05$), with the aid of SigmaPlot 15.0 (Systat Software, San Jose, CA, USA).

3. Results

3.1. Production and Characterization of the Fungal Biosurfactant

After 96 h of growth of the fungus *Aspergillus welwitschiae* CG2-16, the maximum reduction in the surface tension of the culture medium was observed, which was 36%, resulting in 36.0 mN/m. After the extraction and partial purification of the fungal biosurfactant, a yield of 0.87 mg/mL was obtained. The biosurfactant extracted from the culture medium showed an emulsification index of 24% and a CMC of 280 mg/L (Figure 2).

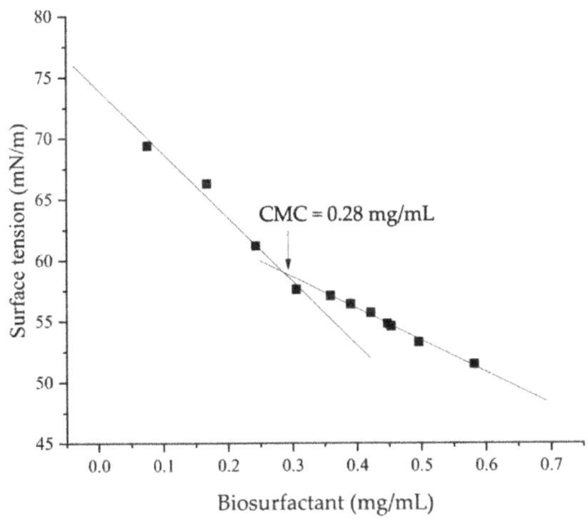

Figure 2. Variation of surface tension as a function of the concentration of the biosurfactant produced by the endophytic fungus *Aspergillus welwitschiae* CG2-16. The inflection point indicates the critical micellar concentration.

The FTIR spectrum of the fungal biosurfactant (Figure 3) revealed important structural characteristics of this metabolite. A low-intensity band is observed between 2960 and 2850 cm^{-1}, which corresponds to the aliphatic C-H bond; a broad and intense band is observed at 3400 cm^{-1} that indicates the asymmetric elongation of N-H bonds in secondary amides; and a characteristic peak is observed at 1650 cm^{-1} for the amide C=O bond [39].

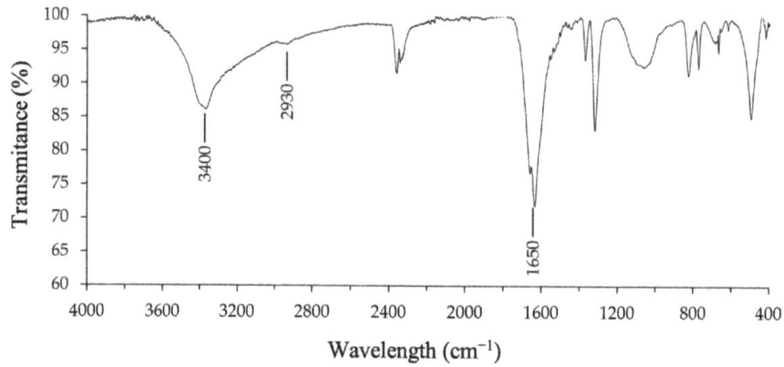

Figure 3. FTIR spectrum of the biosurfactant produced by the endophytic fungus *Aspergillus welwitschiae* CG2-16.

3.2. Production and Characterization of the Nanoformulations

The average particle diameter, PDI and zeta potential values of the nanoformulations produced via nanoprecipitation and emulsion/diffusion methods are shown in Table 1.

Table 1. Average particle diameter, polydispersity index (PDI) and zeta potential of nanoformulations produced by nanoprecipitation and emulsion/diffusion methods, with two different compositions (I and II), containing the biosurfactant produced by the fungus *Aspergillus welwitschiae* CG2-16. Data are expressed as mean and standard deviation.

Nanoformulation	Average Particle Diameter (nm)	PDI	Zeta Potential (mV)
NPPI	237.6 ± 9.3	0.12 ± 0.07	−48.50 ± 3.42
NPPII	-	-	-
NPEI	-	-	-
NPEII	-	-	-
NPPBI	247.8 ± 12.2 ^{a}	0.11 ± 0.08 ^{a,b}	−45.00 ± 1.13 ^{a}
NPPBII	206.9 ± 1.9 ^{a}	0.14 ± 0.04 ^{a}	−29.10 ± 8.67 ^{b}
NPEBI	177.8 ± 12.8 ^{a,b}	0.27 ± 0.06 ^{b}	−43.39 ± 7.40 ^{a}
NPEBII	147.6 ± 2.7 ^{b}	0.32 ± 0.09 ^{b}	−21.90 ± 2.50 ^{b}

NPP = Nanoparticles without biosurfactant, formulated using the nanoprecipitation method. NPE = Nanoparticles without biosurfactant, formulated using the emulsion/diffusion method. B = with biosurfactant. Different letters indicate a significant difference ($p < 0.05$) between variables in the same column, according to the Tukey test.

The synthesis process of the nanoformulations without the biosurfactant, composed only of Tween 80 (NPPII, NPEI, and NPEII), prevented the formation of nanoparticles, as the analysis via DLS indicated that the average size of the particles present was greater than the measurement limit of the equipment (10 μm). NPPI had a mean diameter of 237.6 ± 9.3 and was the only nanoformulation without the biosurfactant that resulted in the formation of nanoparticles. However, in this formulation, the surfactant Span 60 was added, which acted to stabilize the nanosystem.

The mean diameters of the nanoparticles with biosurfactants (NPPBI and NPPBII) were compared with the value obtained for NPPI (the formulation without the BS). It is observed that the nanoformulations prepared with the same methodology did not show a significant difference between them ($p > 0.05$) regarding the average diameter of the particles. In addition, it can be noted that the method selected for the synthesis influences the size of the nanoparticles (Figure 4). This idea is supported by the significant difference between the average particle size in the NPEBII nanoformulation and the particle sizes in the NPPBI and NPPBII nanoformulations. The NPEBII nanoformulation resulted in the smallest nanoparticle size among the nanoformulations.

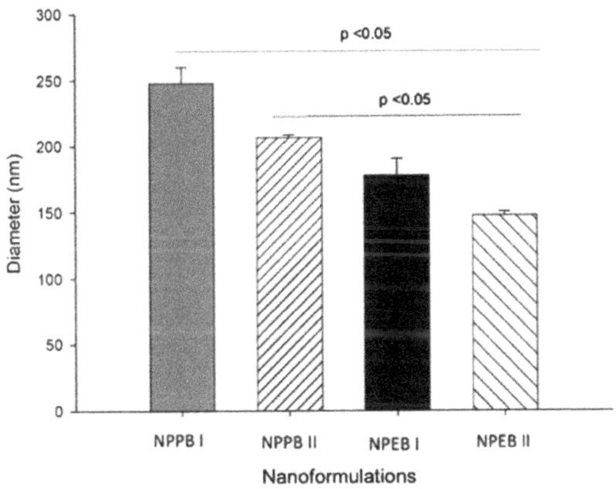

Figure 4. Average particle diameter in the nanoformulations prepared using the nanoprecipitation (NP) and emulsion/diffusion (ED) methods, with two different compositions (I and II), containing the biosurfactant produced by the fungus *Aspergillus welwitschiae* CG2-16. Data are expressed as mean and standard deviation. A significant difference ($p < 0.05$) in indicated, according to the Tukey test.

Figure 5 shows the PDI of the nanoformulations. The NPPBI and NPPBII samples presented a PDI of 0.11 ± 0.08 and 0.14 ± 0.04, respectively, indicating a homogeneous distribution of the particles. On the other hand, the formulations prepared using the emulsion/diffusion method, with and without the biosurfactant, showed a higher PDI, with NPEBI and NPEBII ranging from 0.27 ± 0.06 to 0.32 ± 0.09.

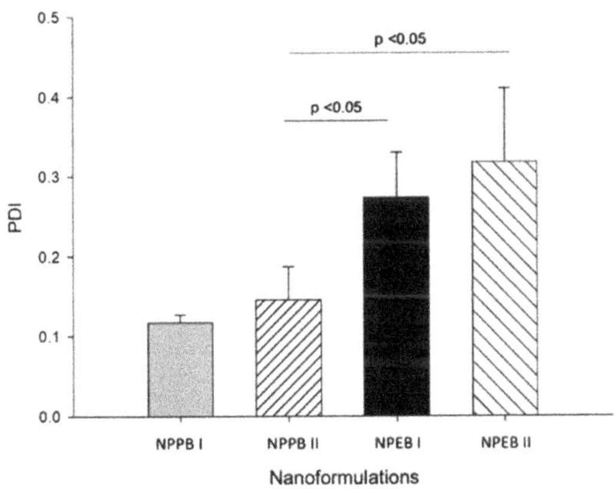

Figure 5. Polydispersity index (PDI) of the nanoformulations prepared using the nanoprecipitation (NP) and emulsion/diffusion (ED) method, with two different compositions (I and II), containing the biosurfactant produced by the fungus *Aspergillus welwitschiae* CG2-16. Data are expressed as mean and standard deviation. A significant difference ($p < 0.05$) in indicated, according to the Tukey test.

For the zeta potential, it is observed that the nanoformulations prepared with the same methodology presented significant differences among themselves (Figure 6), ranging from −29.10 to −45.00 mV for the NP nanoformulations and from −21.90 to −43.39 mV for those prepared using ED. In addition, significant differences were observed between NPPBI and NPEBII and between NPPBII and NPEBI ($p < 0.05$). The NPPBI and NPPBII formulations presented zeta potentials of −45.00 ± 1.10 mV and −29.10 ± 8.67 mV, respectively. In comparison, NPPI showed a zeta potential of −48.50 ± 3.42 mV.

The nanoparticle prepared using the nanoprecipitation method containing the fungal biosurfactant (NPPBII) was investigated by SEM and TEM. The micrographs are shown in Figures 7 and 8, respectively. The SEM image reveals a spherical shape, which is a known characteristic of PCL nanoparticles. The diameter size of the spheres ranged between 179 and 181 nm.

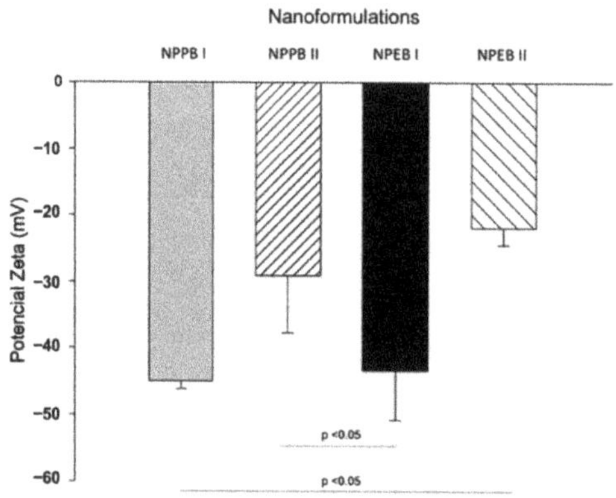

Figure 6. Zeta potential (mV) of the nanoformulations prepared using the method of nanoprecipitation (NP) and emulsion/diffusion (ED), with two different compositions (I and II), containing the biosurfactant produced by the fungus *Aspergillus welwitschiae* CG2-16. Data are expressed as mean and standard deviation. A significant difference ($p < 0.05$) in indicated, according to the Tukey test.

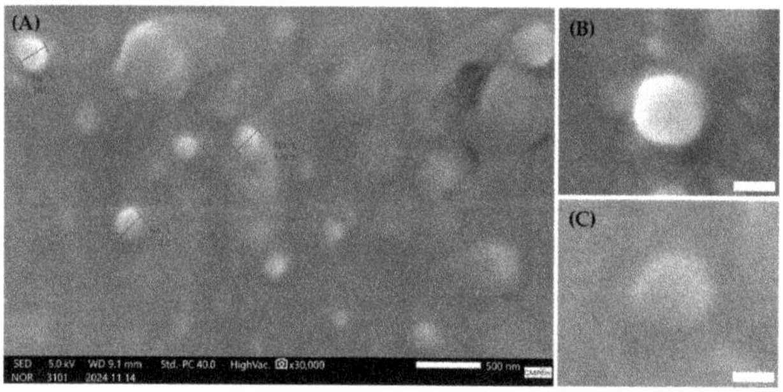

Figure 7. Morphology of the NPPBII nanoparticles, determined by SEM (**A**). Isolated particles at higher magnification (**B**,**C**). Bar: 500 nm (**A**), 100 nm (**B**,**C**).

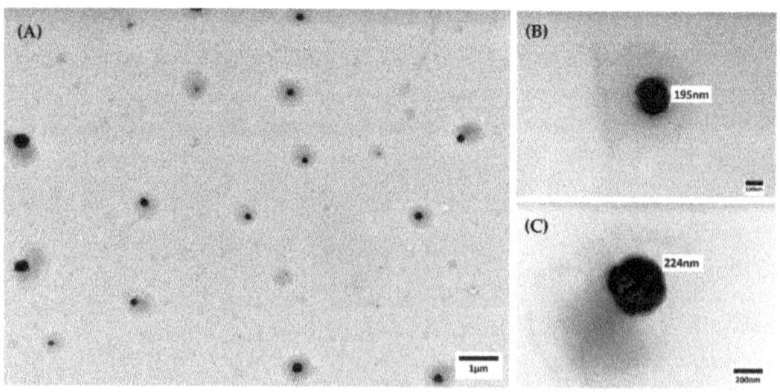

Figure 8. Morphology of the NPPBII nanoparticles, determined by TEM (**A**). Isolated particles at higher magnification (**B**,**C**). Bar: 1 μm (**A**), 100 nm (**B**) and 200 nm (**C**).

TEM analysis confirmed the size and morphology of the nanoparticles produced using the nanoprecipitation method, incorporating the fungal biosurfactant (NPPBII). The representative TEM image (Figure 8) reveals distinct spherical nanoparticles, uniformly distributed without signs of aggregation or adhesion—characteristic features of PCL nanoparticles. The particle diameters ranged from 156 to 228 nm, consistent with the SEM analysis (Figure 7).

4. Discussion

The surface tension reduction and emulsification index are screening tests frequently used to determine the presence of surfactants in culture media [40]. The 36% reduction in surface tension demonstrates the potential of the biosurfactant produced by the fungus *A. welwitschiae* CG2-16. This result not only confirms the effectiveness of the fungus in producing biosurfactants but also indicates its potential for applications in processes that require the reduction of ST, such as in the cleaning, cosmetics, and pharmaceutical industries [34]. In addition, the production of BSs in only 96 h of cultivation represents an important result, especially for a fungal metabolite, which generally produces these compounds in longer cultivation times. The endophytic fungus *Aspergillus niger*, isolated from the *Piper hispidum* plant, for example, which also led to a 36% reduction in the surface tension of the culture medium, obtained this result only after 8 days [26].

The biosurfactant produced by *A. welwitschiae* CG2-16 can be considered a promising surfactant when considering the CMC value (280 mg/L)—a crucial parameter that indicates the efficiency of the biosurfactant in practical applications, as it defines the minimum concentration required for the formation of micelles. Other biosurfactants have CMC values in the same range, and some are even lower than synthetic surfactants [41,42], which is one of the advantages of using biosurfactants. In addition, the BS obtained from *A. welwitschiae* CG2-16 presented an emulsification index of 24%, which demonstrates its ability to stabilize emulsions. However, considering the low E_{24} value, it can be suggested that its main application is as a surfactant and not as a bioemulsifier [43,44].

The results obtained from the FTIR analysis allow us to suggest that the biosurfactant extracted from *A. welwitschiae* CG2-16 belongs to the class of lipopeptides [39,45]. This class of biosurfactants is commonly found in fungi [18] and consists of a fatty acid chain linked to a peptide moiety. Lipopeptides are among the most popular biosurfactants, with high structural diversity and various functional activities [42]. Due to the intensity of the bands observed, the BS obtained from *A. welwitschiae* CG2-16 is possibly composed of a major peptide chain and a small lipid portion. The low intensity of the C-H bond bands indicates the presence of a small hydrophobic portion, while the characteristic bands of peptide bonds have a high intensity. According to Mnif et al. [42], the variation in the composition of the fatty acid component, as well as the type, quantity, and arrangement of amino acids within the peptide chain, contributes significantly to the structural diversity of lipopeptides. Moreover, each lipopeptide family, defined by a consistent peptide core, can be further subdivided into different isoforms based on variations in the length of the fatty acid chain.

The fungal biosurfactant proved to be essential for the formation of polymeric nanoparticles from the nanoformulations tested in the present study, which were prepared using two different methods. The emulsion/diffusion method produced nanoparticles with a smaller diameter (147.6 and 177.8 nm) when compared to the nanoprecipitation method (206.9 and 247.8 nm). This size difference between the nanoparticles prepared using different methodologies has also been observed in other studies. Abriata et al. [46] developed PNPs with PCL via the emulsion/diffusion method for loading paclitaxel and obtained a mean particle diameter of 140 nm and a PDI of 0.1. On the other hand, PCL nanoparticles containing the essential oil of palmarosa (*Cymbopogon martinii*) and the monoterpene geraniol, prepared using the nanoprecipitation method, presented an average size of 282.1 and 289.3 ± 2 nm, respectively, with a PDI below 0.14 [7]. These results are in accordance with those found in the present study.

The results for the PDI are important for determining the degree of homogeneity of the particle diameters present in the suspension: the closer the value is to zero, the more homogeneous the system. Values below 0.1 represent a monodisperse system [47]. The type and concentration of the oil used in the formulation may interfere with the PDI [48]. In the present work, two types of oils were used: soybean oil for the solubilization of the biosurfactant in NPEII and Brazil nut oil for the greater stability of the organic phase in NPPII, NPEI, and NPEII. NPPI was the only nanoformulation in which no oil was used, and it presented the lowest PDI value, corroborating the fact that the PDI can be affected by the use of oils.

The PDI values of the nanoformulations obtained show that the nanoprecipitation method, especially when combined with the biosurfactant, produces nanoparticles with a more uniform size distribution, which is corroborated by the SEM findings. This conclusion is also supported by data from the literature, which demonstrate that nanoprecipitation is an effective method for producing homogeneous nanoparticles [49].

The zeta potential is related to the surface charge of the nanoparticles—an important parameter for evaluating the stability of the colloidal suspension and the interaction between the nanoparticles. Dispersions with zeta potential values greater than 30 mV (in modulus) are considered highly stable [50]. The nanoformulations obtained in our study have high negative ζ-potential values, indicating that they are stable systems. The NPPBI formulation stood out for having a zeta potential of -45.00 ± 1.13 mV and is thus a promising system for future applications. Negative values of ζ-potential indicate the presence of negative charges on the nanoparticle surface and can lead to an increase in solubility, as observed by Bouallegue et al. [51]. A less negative value for the ζ-potential was observed for the NPPBII formulation, which suggests that the introduction of the biosurfactant can alter the surface charge of the nanoparticles, potentially influencing their interaction with the surrounding environment. Studies have shown that biosurfactants can alter the surface of nanoparticles, modulating their zeta potential and, consequently, their stability and biological interaction [27,52,53].

With the exception of the NPPI formulation, it was not possible to define the particle size, PDI, and zeta potential of the other formulations without the biosurfactant using the DLS technique. The particles present in these formulations must have a diameter greater than 10 μm, which is the maximum limit that the equipment can evaluate. In contrast, the NPPBI formulation presented a size of 247.8 nm, a PDI of 0.11, and a zeta potential of −45.00, thus demonstrating the importance of the biosurfactant in stabilizing the nanoformulation.

The SEM image of NPPBII revealed that the PCL nanoparticles containing the fungal biosurfactant were homogeneously distributed and had a spherical shape, with diameters ranging around 180 nm. Comparing these results with those obtained from DLS, an inevitable difference in size is observed, which can be explained by the different approaches and conditions of each technique. SEM provides a direct analysis of particle size, without the influence of the solvent, observing the actual particle size. On the other hand, DLS measures the hydrodynamic size of the particles, considering the solvent layer or the interaction of the nanoparticles with the molecules of the dispersing medium, which increases the apparent particle size [54], as observed in our study.

TEM (transmission electron microscopy) generates images by transmitting an electron beam through a sample. This technique is especially valuable for characterizing polymeric nanoparticles, as it offers sub-nanometer resolution, providing detailed insights into nanoparticle morphology [38]. TEM micrographs complement the findings of SEM and DLS analyses, revealing spherical nanoparticles that are uniformly distributed, free from aggregation, and approximately 200 nm in diameter.

The biosurfactant produced by the fungus *A. welwitschiae* CG2-16 assisted in the stabilization and uniformity of the synthesized nanoparticles, probably by decreasing the surface tension, thereby facilitating the formation of smaller and more uniform spherical nanoparticles [55–57], as corroborated by SEM and TEM images. Surfactants have been widely used for this purpose and are commonly employed as stabilizers to prevent the agglomeration of colloidal suspensions and allow for the acquisition of well-structured nanosystems. In addition, these surface-active molecules have the advantage of allowing the reduction of ST and increasing the affinity of lipid structures [58]. Some of these compounds have even demonstrated the ability to reduce the diameter of nanoparticles [59].

According to Vecino et al. [53], biosurfactants reduce the formation of aggregates and facilitate a uniform morphology of the nanoparticles. SEM and TEM images of NPPBII show a uniform spherical shape of the PCL nanoparticle formed with the use of the *A. welwitschiae* CG2-16 biosurfactant, without agglomeration. On the other hand, the FTIR analysis suggests that the *A. welwitschiae* CG2-16 BS is a lipopeptide. Therefore, it can be inferred that the lipid structure of the BS interacts with the apolar moiety of the PCL, stabilizes the surface by reducing charges, and leads to a uniform spherical nanoparticle.

The use of biosurfactants as stabilizers has already been evaluated in the synthesis of metal nanoparticles as a way of developing more sustainable nanosystems with lower risks to health. The use of a rhamnolipid extracted from *Pseudomonas aeruginosa* for coating silver nanoparticles applied in enhanced oil recovery has been reported. The silver nanoparticles based on the biosurfactant were non-toxic and obtained greater stability than chemically synthesized nanoparticles [52]. In another study, in addition to the greater stability, silver and iron nanoparticles coated with biosurfactants showed reduced cell adhesion by modifying the hydrophobicity of the surface and, because of this, demonstrated excellent antibiofilm activity [60].

The presence of the fungal biosurfactant was crucial for the composition of the NPPBII and NPEBII nanoformulations. These did not have any other surfactant in their composition besides the nonionic surfactant Tween 80, which was considered inefficient for the stability of these nanoformulations without the presence of the biosurfactant. NPPI showed the formation of stable nanoparticles because it was composed of Span 60 and Tween 80. Thus, it is suggested that the interaction between Tween 80 and the biosurfactant was able to keep the other nanoformulations stable. The results obtained in this research revealed a promising perspective on the use of fungal biosurfactants in combination with poly-ε-caprolactone (PCL) for the synthesis of polymeric nanoparticles.

PCL is recognized for its easy accessibility, biodegradability, and high biocompatibility and has become a material of interest in several areas of study [61]. The efficacy of PCL nanoparticles was demonstrated for loading *Nigella sativa* oil and applying it in the treatment of leishmaniasis, which evidences the ability of nanoparticles to provide a continuous and enhanced release of oil molecules and result in a significant inhibition of the growth of *Leishmania infantum* [62]. In addition, according to Morsy [63], stabilizers are key in the preparation of polymeric nanoparticles, which shows the importance of the choice and proper concentration of components in the formulation.

Due to the physicochemical characteristics of polymer nanoparticles stabilized with biosurfactants, they could be used for various applications. In the area of drug delivery, nanoparticles with reduced sizes and improved colloidal stability are ideal for the controlled release of drugs since they allow for constant and safe administration and improve therapeutic efficacy. This system can be particularly useful in the treatment of chronic and infectious diseases, where continuous and controlled administration is crucial [64,65]. In nanocosmetics, the stabilizing properties of biosurfactants can be used in the formulation of products such as photoprotective and anti-aging creams and lotions, which require prolonged stability and the uniform distribution of active ingredients.

The biodegradability of biosurfactants also meets the growing demand for products that generate fewer environmental impacts [15,48]. Nanopesticides have been studied as an option to enable the use of biopesticides and thus reduce the environmental impacts caused by synthetic agrochemicals [66]. Essential oils are considered an advantageous alternative to pesticides, and the nanoencapsulation of these could increase availability and enhance their efficiency [67–69]. In this sense, biosurfactants can be used to stabilize nanoparticles containing essential oils and increase the efficiency of the use of these natural resources [70].

The ability of biosurfactants to reduce surface tension can also be explored in the remediation of contaminated soils and waters, facilitating the degradation and removal of pollutants [71,72]. Stabilized nanoparticles can be employed for the targeted delivery of remediation agents to improve the efficiency of environmental cleanup processes [73]. Therefore, polymeric nanoparticles stabilized with biosurfactants present themselves as an interesting solution for diverse applications in different areas, such as pharmaceuticals (controlled drug release), cosmetics (active compound delivery), agriculture (biopesticide dispersion), environmental (the remediation of contaminated sites), and food (the encapsulation of volatile compounds), among many others.

5. Conclusions

The biosurfactant produced by the Amazonian endophytic fungus *A. welwitschiae* CG2-16 can be used in the synthesis of polymer nanoparticles with PCL, ensuring the stability of the nanoformulations. It was observed that the methodology used in the preparation of the nanoformulations influences the size of the PNPs, with the smallest particle diameters obtained using the emulsion/diffusion method, while the nanoformulation produced using the nanoprecipitation method presented a higher zeta potential. The application of biosurfactants not only improves the properties of the nanoparticles but also contributes to the expansion of the use of this class of biomolecules.

The vast application potential of these formulations opens the way for future research projects and technological development to further explore the benefits of fungal biosurfactants as an alternative material that causes fewer environmental impacts than synthetic surfactants. However, further studies are needed to fully characterize these polymeric nanoparticles and explore their potential applications. Limitations include the need to optimize the synthesis processes and further investigate the long-term stability and environmental impact of these PNPs. Nonetheless, these biosurfactants offer a sustainable route for developing advanced materials with reduced ecological footprints.

Author Contributions: Conceptualization, P.M.A. and A.R.S.; methodology, A.R.S., M.T.M.P. and S.G.A.; validation, A.R.S., J.C.d.A. and S.G.A.; formal analysis, A.R.S. and S.G.A.; investigation, A.R.S., S.G.A., M.T.M.P., C.D.L. and J.C.d.A.; resources, P.M.A., S.D.J. and L.M.; data curation, A.R.S. and C.D.L.; writing—original draft preparation, A.R.S., S.G.A. and C.D.L.; writing—review and editing, P.M.A. and J.C.d.A.; supervision, P.M.A. and L.M.; project administration, P.M.A.; funding acquisition, P.M.A., S.D.J. and L.M. All authors have read and agreed to the published version of the manuscript.

Funding: This research was funded by Fundação de Amparo à Pesquisa do Estado do Amazonas (FAPEAM) (grant numbers 01.02.016301.00568/2021-05 and 01.02.016301.00101/2024-08) and by Coordenação de Aperfeiçoamento de Pessoal de Nível Superior (CAPES) (grant nunber 88881.510151/2020-01—PDPG Amazônia Legal and finance code 001).

Data Availability Statement: The original contributions presented in the study are included in the article, further inquiries can be directed to the corresponding author.

Acknowledgments: The authors gratefully acknowledge Universidade do Estado do Amazonas—UEA, Instituto Federal do Amazonas—IFAM, Sistema Nacional de Laboratórios em Nanotecnologias—SisNANO, Centro Multiusuário para Análise de Fenômenos Biomédicos—CMABIO, FAPEAM and CAPES for supporting this research.

Conflicts of Interest: The authors declare no conflict of interest.

References

1. Altammar, K.A.A. Review on nanoparticles: Characteristics, synthesis, applications, and challenges. *Front. Microbiol.* **2023**, *14*, 1155622. [CrossRef] [PubMed]
2. Zielinska, A.; Carreiró, F.; Oliveira, A.M.; Neves, A.; Pires, B.; Nagasamy Venkatesh, D.; Durazzo, A.; Lucarini, M.; Eder, P.; Silva, A.M.; et al. Polymeric nanoparticles: Production, characterization, toxicology and ecotoxicology. *Molecules* **2020**, *25*, 3731. [CrossRef] [PubMed]
3. Azevedo, S.G.; Rocha, A.L.F.; de Aguiar Nunes, R.Z.; da Costa Pinto, C.; Ţălu, Ş.; da Fonseca Filho, H.D.; de Araújo Bezerra, J.; Lima, A.R.; Guimarães, F.E.G.; Campelo, P.H.; et al. Pulsatile controlled release and stability evaluation of polymeric particles containing *Piper nigrum* essential oil and preservatives. *Materials* **2022**, *15*, 5415. [CrossRef]
4. Begines, B.; Ortiz, T.; Pérez-Aranda, M.; Martínez, G.; Merinero, M.; Argüelles-Arias, F.; Alcudia, A. Polymeric nanoparticles for drug delivery: Recent developments and future prospects. *Nanomaterials* **2020**, *10*, 1403. [CrossRef]
5. Krishnaswamy, K.; Orsat, V. Sustainable delivery systems through green nanotechnology. In *Nano- and Microscale Drug Delivery Systems: Design and Fabrication*; Grumezescu, A.M., Ed.; Elsevier: Amsterdam, The Netherlands, 2017; pp. 17–32. [CrossRef]
6. Parupudi, A.; Mulagapati, S.H.R.; Subramony, J.A. Nanoparticle technologies: Recent state of the art and emerging opportunities. In *Nanoparticle Therapeutics: Production Technologies, Types of Nanoparticles, and Regulatory Aspects*; Kesharwani, P., Singh, K.K., Eds.; Elsevier: Amsterdam, The Netherlands, 2022; pp. 3–46. [CrossRef]
7. Jummes, B.; Sganzerla, W.G.; da Rosa, C.G.; Noronha, C.M.; Nunes, M.R.; Bertoldi, F.C.; Barreto, P.L.M. Antioxidant and antimicrobial poly-ε-caprolactone nanoparticles loaded with *Cymbopogon martinii* essential oil. *Biocatal. Agric. Biotechnol.* **2020**, *23*, 101499. [CrossRef]
8. MacCraith, E.; O'Brien, F.J.; Davis, N.F. Biodegradable materials for surgical management of stress urinary incontinence: A narrative review. *Eur. J. Obstet. Gynecol. Reprod. Biol.* **2021**, *259*, 153–160. [CrossRef]
9. Mulinti, P.; Brooks, J.E.; Lervick, B.; Pullan, J.E.; Brooks, A.E. Strategies to improve the hemocompatibility of biodegradable biomaterials. In *Hemocompatibility of Biomaterials for Clinical Applications: Blood-Biomaterials Interactions*; Siedlecki, C.A., Ed.; Elsevier: Amsterdam, The Netherlands, 2017; pp. 253–278. [CrossRef]
10. Pulingam, T.; Foroozandeh, P.; Chuah, J.A.; Sudesh, K. Exploring Various techniques for the chemical and biological synthesis of polymeric nanoparticles. *Nanomaterials* **2022**, *12*, 576. [CrossRef]
11. Cortés, H.; Hernández-Parra, H.; Bernal-Chávez, S.A.; Del Prado-Audelo, M.L.; Caballero-Florán, I.H.; Borbolla-Jiménez, F.V.; González-Torres, M.; Magaña, J.J.; Leyva-Gómez, G. Non-ionic surfactants for stabilization of polymeric nanoparticles for biomedical uses. *Materials* **2021**, *14*, 3197. [CrossRef] [PubMed]
12. Badmus, S.O.; Amusa, H.K.; Oyehan, T.A.; Saleh, T.A. Environmental risks and toxicity of surfactants: Overview of analysis, assessment, and remediation techniques. *Environ. Sci. Pollut. R.* **2021**, *28*, 62085–62104. [CrossRef]
13. Johnson, P.; Trybala, A.; Starov, V.; Pinfield, V.J. Effect of synthetic surfactants on the environment and the potential for substitution by biosurfactants. *Adv. Colloid Interface Sci.* **2021**, *288*, 102340. [CrossRef]
14. Drakontis, C.E.; Amin, S. Biosurfactants: Formulations, properties, and applications. *Curr. Opin. Colloid Interface Sci.* **2020**, *48*, 77–90. [CrossRef]
15. Santos, A.C.; Morais, F.; Simões, A.; Pereira, I.; Sequeira, J.A.D.; Pereira-Silva, M.; Veiga, F.; Ribeiro, A. Nanotechnology for the development of new cosmetic formulations. *Expert Opin. Drug Deliv.* **2019**, *16*, 313–330. [CrossRef] [PubMed]
16. Gautam, A.K.; Verma, R.K.; Avasthi, S.; Sushma, B.Y.; Devadatha, B.; Niranjan, M.; Suwannarach, N. Current insight into traditional and modern methods in fungal diversity estimates. *J. Fungi* **2022**, *8*, 226. [CrossRef]
17. Gurgel, R.S.; de Melo Pereira, D.Í.; Garcia, A.V.F.; Fernandes de Souza, A.T.; Mendes da Silva, T.; de Andrade, C.P.; Lima da Silva, W.; Nunez, C.V.; Fantin, C.; de Lima Procópio, R.E.; et al. Antimicrobial and antioxidant activities of endophytic fungi associated with *Arrabidaea chica* (Bignoniaceae). *J. Fungi* **2023**, *9*, 864. [CrossRef]
18. Sanches, M.A.; Luzeiro, I.G.; Alves Cortez, A.C.; Simplício de Souza, É.; Albuquerque, P.M.; Chopra, H.K.; Braga de Souza, J.V. Production of biosurfactants by Ascomycetes. *Int. J. Microbiol.* **2021**, *2021*, 6669263. [CrossRef]
19. Silva, A.C.S.; Santos, P.N.; Silva, T.A.L.; Andrade, R.F.S.; Campos-Takaki, G.M. Biosurfactant production by fungi as a sustainable alternative. *Arq. Inst. Biol.* **2018**, *85*, e0502017. [CrossRef]
20. Abdel-Mawgoud, A.M.; Stephanopoulos, G. Simple glycolipids of microbes: Chemistry, biological activity and metabolic engineering. *Synth. Syst. Biotechnol.* **2018**, *3*, 3–19. [CrossRef] [PubMed]
21. Garay, L.A.; Sitepu, I.R.; Cajka, T.; Xu, J.; Teh, H.E.; German, J.B.; Pan, Z.; Dungan, S.R.; Block, D.E.; Boundy-Mills, K.L. Extracellular fungal polyol lipids: A new class of potential high value lipids. *Biotechnol. Adv.* **2018**, *36*, 397–414. [CrossRef]
22. Bae, I.; Lee, E.S.; Yoo, J.W.; Lee, S.H.; Ko, J.Y.; Kim, Y.J.; Lee, T.R.; Kim, D.; Lee, C.S. Mannosylerythritol lipids inhibit melanogenesis via suppressing ERK-CREB-MiTF-tyrosinase signalling in normal human melanocytes and a three-dimensional human skin equivalent. *Exp. Dermatol.* **2019**, *28*, 738–741. [CrossRef]
23. Maniglia, B.C.; Laroque, D.A.; Andrade, L.M.; Carciofi, B.A.M.; Tenório, J.A.S.; Andrade, C.J. Production of active cassava starch films; effect of adding a biosurfactant or synthetic surfactant. *React. Funct. Polym.* **2019**, *144*, 104368. [CrossRef]
24. Shah, V.; Daverey, A. Effects of sophorolipids augmentation on the plant growth and phytoremediation of heavy metal contaminated soil. *J. Clean. Prod.* **2021**, *280*, 124406. [CrossRef]
25. Chuo, S.C.; Ahmad, A.; Mohd-Setapar, S.H.; Mohamed, S.F.; Rafatullah, M. Utilization of green sophoro-lipids biosurfactant in reverse micelle extraction of antibiotics: Kinetic and mass transfer studies. *J. Mol. Liq.* **2019**, *276*, 225–232. [CrossRef]

26. Silva, M.E.T.; Duvoisin, S., Jr.; Oliveira, R.L.; Banhos, E.F.; Souza, A.Q.L.; Albuquerque, P.M. Biosurfactant production of *Piper hispidum* endophytic fungi. *J. Appl. Microbiol.* **2021**, *130*, 561–569. [CrossRef]
27. Nitschke, M.; Marangon, C.A. Microbial surfactants in nanotechnology: Recent trends and applications. *Crit. Rev. Biotechnol.* **2022**, *42*, 294–310. [CrossRef]
28. De Melo Pereira, D.Í.; Gurgel, R.S.; de Souza, A.T.F.; Matias, R.R.; de Souza Falcão, L.; Chaves, F.C.M.; da Silva, G.F.; Martínez, J.G.; de Lima Procópio, R.E.; Fantin, C.; et al. Isolation and identification of pigment-producing endophytic fungi from the Amazonian Species *Fridericia chica*. *J. Fungi* **2024**, *10*, 77. [CrossRef]
29. Castellani, A. The viability of some pathogenic fungi in sterile distilled water. *J. Trop. Med. Hyg.* **1939**, *42*, 225–226.
30. Wen, G.; Cao, R.; Wan, Q.; Tan, L.; Xu, X.; Wang, J.; Huang, T. Development of fungal spore staining methods for flow cytometric quantification and their application in chlorine-based disinfection. *Chemosphere* **2020**, *243*, 125453. [CrossRef]
31. Soares, A.R. Produção de Biossurfactantes Fúngicos e Aplicação No Desenvolvimento de Nanopartículas Poliméricas. Master Thesis, Amazonas State University, Manaus, Brazil, 24 June 2024.
32. Monteiro, A.S.; Bonfim, M.R.Q.; Domingues, V.S.; Corrêa, A.; Siqueira, E.P.; Zani, C.L.; Santos, V.L. Identification and characterization of bioemulsifier-producing yeasts isolated from effluents of a dairy industry. *Bioresour. Technol.* **2010**, *101*, 5186–5193. [CrossRef]
33. Pereira, D.D.F.; Duvoisin Junior, S.; Albuquerque, P.M. Study of biosurfactants production by Amazon fungi. *J. Eng. Exact Sci.* **2017**, *3*, 688–695.
34. Makkar, R.S.; Cameotra, S.S. Biosurfactant production by a thermophilic *Bacillus subtilis* strain. *J. Ind. Microbiol. Biotechnol.* **1997**, *18*, 37–42. [CrossRef]
35. Pornsunthorntawee, O.; Wongpanit, P.; Chavadej, S.; Abe, M.; Rujiravanit, R. Structural and physicochemical characterization of crude biosurfactant produced by *Pseudomonas aeruginosa* SP4 isolated from petroleum contaminated soil. *Bioresource Technol.* **2008**, *99*, 1589–1595. [CrossRef]
36. Noronha, C.M.; Granada, A.F.; de Carvalho, S.M.; Lino, R.C.; Matheus, M.V.; Barreto, P.L.M. Optimization of α-tocopherol loaded nanocapsules by the nanoprecipitation method. *Ind. Crops Prod.* **2013**, *50*, 896–903. [CrossRef]
37. Costa, Í.C.; Azevedo, S.G.; Sanches, E.A.; da Fonseca Filho, H.D. Characterization of polymeric nanoparticles filled with *Piper nigrum* essential oil by atomic force microscopy. *Matéria* **2021**, *26*, e12981. [CrossRef]
38. Crucho, C.I.C.; Barros, M.T. Polymeric nanoparticles: A study on the preparation variables and characterization methods. *Mater. Sci. Eng. C.* **2017**, *80*, 771–784. [CrossRef]
39. Chittepu, O.R. Isolation and characterization of biosurfactant producing bacteria from groundnut oil cake dumping site for the control of foodborne pathogens. *Grain Oil Sci. Technol.* **2019**, *2*, 15–20. [CrossRef]
40. Nayarisseri, A.; Singh, P.; Singh, S.K. Screening, isolation and characterization of biosurfactant producing *Bacillus subtilis* strain ANSKLAB03. *Bioinformation* **2018**, *14*, 304–314. [CrossRef]
41. Jahan, R.; Bodratti, A.M.; Tsianou, M.; Alexandridis, P. Biosurfactants, natural alternatives to synthetic surfactants: Physicochemical properties and applications. *Adv. Colloid Interface Sci.* **2020**, *275*, 102061. [CrossRef]
42. Mnif, I.; Segovia, R.; Bouallegue, A.; Ghribi, D.; Rabanal, F. Identifcation of diferent lipopeptides isoforms produced by *Bacillus mojavensis* BI2 and evaluation of their surface activities for potential environmental application. *J. Polym. Environ.* **2023**, *31*, 2668–2685. [CrossRef]
43. Luft, L.; Confortin, T.C.; Todero, I.; Zabot, G.L.; Mazutti, M.A. An overview of fungal biopolymers: Bioemulsifiers and biosurfactants compounds production. *Crit. Rev. Biotechnol.* **2020**, *40*, 1059–1080. [CrossRef]
44. Uzoigwe, C.; Burgess, J.G.; Ennis, C.J.; Rahman, P.K.S.M. Bioemulsifiers are not biosurfactants and require different screening approaches. *Front. Microbiol.* **2015**, *6*, 245. [CrossRef]
45. Al-Sahlany, S.T.G.; Al-Kaabi, W.J.; Al-Manhel, A.J.A.; Niamah, A.K.; Altemimi, A.B.; Al-Wafi, H.; Cacciola, F. Effects of β-glucan extracted from *Saccharomyces cerevisiae* on the quality of bio-yoghurts: In vitro and in vivo evaluation. *J. Food Meas. Charact.* **2022**, *16*, 3607–3617. [CrossRef]
46. Abriata, J.P.; Turatti, R.C.; Luiz, M.T.; Raspantini, G.L.; Tofani, L.B.; do Amaral, R.L.F.; Swiech, K.; Marcato, P.D.; Marchetti, J.M. Development, characterization and biological in vitro assays of paclitaxel-loaded PCL polymeric nanoparticles. *Mater. Sci. Eng. C* **2019**, *96*, 347–355. [CrossRef]
47. Filippov, S.K.; Khusnutdinov, R.; Murmiliuk, A.; Inam, W.; Zakharova, L.Y.; Zhang, H.; Khutoryanskiy, V.V. Dynamic light scattering and transmission electron microscopy in drug delivery: A roadmap for correct characterization of nanoparticles and interpretation of results. *Mater Horiz* **2023**, *10*, 5354–5370. [CrossRef]
48. Khayata, N.; Abdelwahed, W.; Chehna, M.F.; Charcosset, C.; Fessi, H. Preparation of vitamin e loaded nanocapsules by the nanoprecipitation method: From laboratory scale to large scale using a membrane contactor. *Int. J. Pharm.* **2012**, *423*, 419–427. [CrossRef] [PubMed]
49. Alshamsan, A. Nanoprecipitation is more efficient than emulsion solvent evaporation method to encapsulate cucurbitacin I in PLGA nanoparticles. *Saudi Pharm. J.* **2014**, *22*, 219–222. [CrossRef]
50. Bhattacharjee, S. DLS and zeta potential—What they are and what they are not? *J. Control. Release* **2016**, *235*, 337–351. [CrossRef]
51. Bouallegue, A.; Sabbah, M.; Di Pierro, P.; Salamatullah, A.M.; Bourhia, M.; Ellouz-Chaabouni, S. Properties of active levan-bitter vetch protein films for potential use in food packaging applications. *ACS Omega* **2023**, *8*, 42787–42796. [CrossRef]

52. Elakkiya, V.T.; SureshKumar, P.; Alharbi, N.S.; Kadaikunnan, S.; Khaled, J.M.; Govindarajan, M. Swift production of rhamnolipid biosurfactant, biopolymer and synthesis of biosurfactant-wrapped silver nanoparticles and its enhanced oil recovery. *Saudi J. Biol. Sci.* **2020**, *27*, 1892–1899. [CrossRef]
53. Vecino, X.; Rodríguez-López, L.; Rincón-Fontán, M.; Cruz, J.M.; Moldes, A.B. Chapter Six—Nanomaterials synthesized by biosurfactants. In *Comprehensive Analytical Chemistry*; Verma, S.K., Das, A.K., Eds.; Elsevier: Amsterdam, The Netherlands, 2021; pp. 267–301. [CrossRef]
54. Bootz, A.; Vogel, V.; Schubert, D.; Kreuter, J. Comparison of scanning electron microscopy, dynamic light scattering and analytical ultracentrifugation for the sizing of poly(butyl cyanoacrylate) nanoparticles. *Eur. J. Pharm. Biopharm.* **2004**, *57*, 369–375. [CrossRef]
55. Bezza, F.A.; Tichapondwa, S.M.; Chirwa, E.M.N. Synthesis of biosurfactant stabilized silver nanoparticles, characterization and their potential application for bactericidal purposes. *J. Hazard. Mater.* **2020**, *393*, 122319. [CrossRef]
56. Femina, C.C.; Kamalesh, T. Advances in stabilization of metallic nanoparticle with biosurfactants- a review on current trends. *Heliyon* **2024**, *10*, e29773. [CrossRef]
57. Gómez-Graña, S.; Perez-Ameneiro, M.; Vecino, X.; Pastoriza-Santos, I.; Perez-Juste, J.; Cruz, J.M.; Moldes, A.B. Biogenic synthesis of metal nanoparticles using a biosurfactant extracted from corn and their antimicrobial properties. *Nanomaterials* **2017**, *7*, 139. [CrossRef]
58. Belletti, D.; Grabrucker, A.M.; Pederzoli, F.; Menrath, I.; Cappello, V.; Vandelli, M.A.; Forni, F.; Tosi, G.; Ruozi, B. Exploiting the versatility of cholesterol in nanoparticles formulation. *Int. J. Pharm.* **2016**, *511*, 331–340. [CrossRef]
59. Bonaccorso, A.; Musumeci, T.; Carbone, C.; Vicari, L.; Lauro, M.R.; Puglisi, G. Revisiting the role of sucrose in PLGA-PEG nanocarrier for potential intranasal delivery. *Pharm. Dev. Technol.* **2018**, *23*, 265–274. [CrossRef]
60. Khalid, H.F.; Tehseen, B.; Sarwar, Y.; Hussain, S.Z.; Khan, W.S.; Raza, Z.A.; Bajwa, S.Z.; Kanaras, A.G.; Hussain, I.; Rehman, A. biosurfactant coated silver and iron oxide nanoparticles with enhanced anti-biofilm and anti-adhesive properties. *J. Hazard. Mater.* **2019**, *364*, 441–448. [CrossRef]
61. Woodruff, M.A.; Hutmacher, D.W. The return of a forgotten polymer—Polycaprolactone in the 21st Century. *Prog. Polym. Sci.* **2010**, *35*, 1217–1256. [CrossRef]
62. Abamor, E.S.; Tosyali, O.A.; Bagirova, M.; Allahverdiyev, A. *Nigella sativa* oil entrapped polycaprolactone nanoparticles for leishmaniasis treatment. *IET Nanobiotechnol.* **2018**, *12*, 1018–1026. [CrossRef]
63. Morsy, S.M.I. Role of surfactants in nanotechnology and their applications. *Int. J. Curr. Microbiol. App. Sci.* **2014**, *3*, 237–260.
64. Banik, B.L.; Fattahi, P.; Brown, J.L. Polymeric nanoparticles: The future of nanomedicine. *Wiley Interdiscip. Rev. Nanomed. Nanobiotechnol.* **2016**, *8*, 271–299. [CrossRef]
65. El-Say, K.M.; El-Sawy, H.S. Polymeric nanoparticles: Promising platform for drug delivery. *Int. J. Pharm.* **2017**, *528*, 675–691. [CrossRef]
66. Usman, M.; Farooq, M.; Wakeel, A.; Nawaz, A.; Cheema, S.A.; Rehman, H.U.; Ashraf, I.; Sanaullah, M. Nanotechnology in agriculture: Current status, challenges and future opportunities. *Sci. Total Environ.* **2020**, *721*, 137778. [CrossRef] [PubMed]
67. Albuquerque, P.M.; Azevedo, S.G.; de Andrade, C.P.; D'Ambros, N.C.d.S.; Pérez, M.T.M.; Manzato, L. Biotechnological applications of nanoencapsulated essential oils: A review. *Polymers* **2022**, *14*, 5495. [CrossRef]
68. Fierascu, R.C.; Fierascu, I.C.; Dinu-Pirvu, C.E.; Fierascu, I.; Paunescu, A. The application of essential oils as a next-generation of pesticides: Recent developments and future perspectives. *Z. Naturforsch. C J. Biosci.* **2020**, *75*, 183–204. [CrossRef] [PubMed]
69. Maes, C.; Bouquillon, S.; Fauconnier, M.L. Encapsulation of essential oils for the development of biosourced pesticides with controlled release: A review. *Molecules* **2019**, *24*, 2539. [CrossRef] [PubMed]
70. Karam, T.K.; Ortega, S.; Ueda Nakamura, T.; Auzély-Velty, R.; Nakamura, C.V. Development of chitosan nanocapsules containing essential oil of *Matricaria chamomilla* L. for the treatment of cutaneous leishmaniasis. *Int. J. Biol. Macromol.* **2020**, *162*, 199–208. [CrossRef]
71. Bezza, F.A.; Nkhalambayausi Chirwa, E.M. Biosurfactant-enhanced bioremediation of aged polycyclic aromatic hydrocarbons (PAHs) in creosote contaminated soil. *Chemosphere* **2016**, *144*, 635–644. [CrossRef] [PubMed]
72. Gayathiri, E.; Prakash, P.; Karmegam, N.; Varjani, S.; Awasthi, M.K.; Ravindran, B. Biosurfactants: Potential and eco-friendly material for sustainable agriculture and environmental safety—A review. *Agronomy* **2022**, *12*, 662. [CrossRef]
73. Vázquez-Núñez, E.; Molina-Guerrero, C.E.; Peña-Castro, J.M.; Fernández-Luqueño, F.; de la Rosa-Álvarez, M.G. Use of nanotechnology for the bioremediation of contaminants: A review. *Processes* **2020**, *8*, 826. [CrossRef]

processes

MDPI

Article

Integration of Thermal Solar Power in an Existing Combined Cycle for a Reduction in Carbon Emissions and the Maximization of Cycle Efficiency

Adham Mohamed Abdelhalim [1], Andrés Meana-Fernández [2,*] and Ines Suarez-Ramon [2]

[1] Mechanical Engineering Department, College of Engineering and Technology, Arab Academy for Science, Technology and Maritime Transport, Alexandria 21611, Egypt; adhammuhamed90@aast.edu

[2] Thermal Machines and Engines Area, Department of Energy, University of Oviedo, 33204 Gijon, Spain; ines@uniovi.es

* Correspondence: andresmf@uniovi.es

Abstract: The energy transition towards renewable energy sources is vital for handling climate change, air pollution, and health-related problems. However, fossil fuels are still used worldwide as the main source for electricity generation. This work aims to contribute to the energy transition by exploring the best options for integrating a solar field within a combined cycle power plant. Different integration positions at the gas and steam cycles for the solar field were studied and compared under several operating conditions using a thermodynamic model implemented in MATLAB R2024a. Fuel-saving and power-boosting (flowrate and parameter boosting) strategies were studied. The results revealed that, for a maximum fuel savings of 7.97%, the best option was to integrate the field into the steam cycle before the economizer stage. With an integrated solar thermal power of 3 MW, carbon dioxide emissions from fuel combustion were reduced to 8.3 g/kWh. On the other hand, to maximize power plant generation, the best option was to integrate the field before the superheater, increasing power generation by 24.2% for a solar thermal power of 4 MW. To conclude, guidelines to select the best integration option depending on the desired outcome are provided.

Keywords: integrated solar combined cycle; energy efficiency; carbon emissions reduction; power boosting; fuel saving; flowrate boosting; parameter boosting; solar thermal power

1. Introduction

For more than 50 years, global energy consumption has been increasing at rates between 1% and 2% [1], with the only exceptions being the early 1980s (the energy crisis), 2009 (the financial crisis), and 2020 (the COVID crisis). In addition, the average energy consumption annual growth rate of 1.5% from 2010 to 2019 reached a maximum of 2.2% in the year 2023 [2]. Currently, fossil fuels provide more than 80% of the primary energy, with coal representing 27% of this total [3,4]. Between 1965 and 2022, the use of fossil fuels increased globally by 96,796 TWh, becoming around 2.4 times higher. Asia reached a total generation of 775,566 TWh from fossil fuels, and in Europe, fossil fuel generation grew by 21,391 TWh [1]. Iran experienced a growth of 3518%, passing from 92 to 3335 TWh. On the other hand, the United Kingdom reduced fossil fuel generation by 33%, from 2259 to 1519 TWh [1].

As long as fossil fuels lead the energy system, the world will continue to face energy scarcity for millions of people and the worsening of climate change and pollution effects. As the world population increases, so will the energy demand. Therefore, fuel consumption is expected to increase unless the efficiency of power generation systems is improved. In addition, low-carbon energy sources should replace fossil fuels in the energy mix to handle climate change, pollution, and health-related problems.

With the social demand for cleaner energy sources and technologies, most countries are making significant efforts to adopt renewable generation, which increased from 2795 TWh in 1965 to 23,848 TWh in 2022 [1]. Asia had the highest renewable energy consumption in 2022, with 10,879 TWh. South America increased renewable generation by 2270% from 1965 to 2022, passing from 117 TWh to 2773 TWh. As a consequence of those efforts, the global share of renewable energy in electricity generation is now around 30% [5]. The share of solar and wind power increased from 2.8% in 2012 to 12.1% in 2022 [6], with the investment in solar power increasing up to 310 billion dollars, a 36% increase from 2018 to 2022 [5]. The International Renewable Energy Agency (IRENA) expects the share of renewable energy consumption to reach 28% by 2030 and 66% by 2050 [7]. The share of renewables in the electricity sector is expected to increase more, reaching 57% by 2030 and 86% by 2050 [8].

Solar energy is one of the most important renewable energy sources. It is available and affordable, and it requires low maintenance costs [9]. Between 1991 and 2020, solar energy has expanded at an exponential rate and become a common energy source. In fact, it has been claimed that smart solar energy systems could supply the whole world energy demand without additional energy sources [10]. In addition, the carbon footprint of solar panels is 95% lower than coal-based technologies [11]. According to a study by Lawrence Berkeley National Laboratory in USA, the implementation of solar and wind energy between 2019 and 2022 generated USD 249 billion in climate, pollution, and health benefits, avoiding from 1200 to 1600 premature deaths [12]. In addition, the cost of renewable technologies has dropped by around 60%, especially in the case of solar panels [9]. Solar energy is predicted to become extremely cost-competitive by 2030, with prices from 0.02 to 0.08 USD/kWh [12].

Despite the advances in renewable technologies, gas power plants currently generate 22% of global electricity, with natural gas consumption increasing up to 6100 TWh in 2021 [6]. Combined cycles (CC) are the most common power plants, using exhaust gases from a top gas cycle to generate steam in a Heat Recovery Steam Generator (HRSG) and power a bottom steam cycle. A feasible strategy for reducing the environmental impact of combined cycles is the integration of solar energy in the so-called Integrated Solar Combined Cycles (ISCC), especially in tropical regions. These cycles, which combine gas-fired power cycles and Concentrated Solar Power (CSP) technologies, have the advantage of preventing power outer risks that could result from relying only on solar power. The thermal energy obtained from the combustion of natural gas is complemented by the thermal energy produced by solar concentrators, increasing the total efficiency of the system [13]. Although parabolic trough solar power plants were proposed in the 1990s by Luz Solar International [14], economic factors prevented the building of power plants before the 2000s, when the Global Environment Facility financed USD 50 million for the construction of four ISCC power plants in developing countries with intense solar irradiation, most of them in the Middle East. This incentive renewed the interest in Concentrated Solar Power (CSP) technologies, specifically in Parabolic Trough Collectors (PTC) [15]. It has been predicted that CSP power plants will represent 25% of global power generation by 2050 [16]. Due to the lower cost of thermal energy storage with respect to batteries, CSP technologies seem more suitable for baseload power generation than photovoltaic systems. Nevertheless, solar fields are still relatively costly [17].

Research has been conducted on solar thermal power integration at the top (Brayton) and the bottom (Rankine) cycles, with several hybrid setups [18,19]. When integrated into the top gas cycle, solar power is used to preheat compressed air before entering the combustion chamber [14]. When integrated into the bottom steam cycle, it is typically used to generate more steam to power the turbine [20,21]. Barigozzi et al. [22] investigated the performance of an ISCC with solar integration at the top and bottom cycles. A higher solar-to-electricity efficiency was obtained when solar power was integrated at the top cycle, but power generation was higher through integration in the bottom cycle.

According to Behar [23], PTCs with synthetic oils as the heat transfer fluid (HTF) are the most efficient method for solar power integration at the bottom cycle. The results from the work of Manente et al. [24] showed the highest solar-to-electricity efficiency values when synthetic oil was used to evaporate water at the high pressure level of the HRSG. This conclusion matches the results from Elmohlawy et al. [25], who found an increase in the thermal efficiency by 1.2% when injecting the steam at the high pressure level instead of at the intermediate one. El Mohalawy et al. [26] developed a model for two ISCC configurations with PTCs for a plant with an original capacity of 503 MW. In the first configuration, a solar steam generator (SSG) was used to complement the intermediate pressure evaporator and superheater. In the second configuration, the feedwater from the deaerator was superheated using the SSG. They found that the second configuration generated more power than the first one, allowing to reduce CO_2 emissions by around 51,671 ton.

Rovira et al. presented an innovative hybrid configuration [27] with a partially recuperative Brayton cycle for fuel saving with the introduction of solar power, achieving higher solar power shares than standard layouts. The 135 MW Kurymat plant in Egypt, in operation since 2011 [28], works by heating synthetic oil with PTCs and heating a portion of the high-pressure water of the steam cycle before it returns to the HRSG. Abdel Dayem et al. [28] developed a model of this plant, finding that the increase in direct normal irradiance (DNI) could increase the turbine power and the solar share by 10% and 25%, respectively. All these sources, along with the work of Muñoz, Rovira, and Montes [29], show that solar integration into the bottom cycle with PTCs and synthetic oils is the most common configuration in current or developing projects, with solar share values from 3% to 14%. The best thermodynamic performance is obtained when integrating solar energy at the high pressure level of the HRSG for steam evaporation and/or superheating. Javadi et al. [30] examined different possibilities for integrating solar power into a combined cycle with two pressure levels: preheating the fuel or air before the combustion chamber or integrating it at the high pressure level of the HRSG. In line with previous studies, the highest power generation at the lowest cost was found when solar power was integrated into the high-pressure line of the HRSG.

Hosseini et al. [31] compared six thermal power plants, claiming an ISCC with a 67 MW solar field to be the optimal configuration. This plant could avoid the emission of 2.4 Mt of CO_2 and save USD 59 million in fuel consumption over its 30-year operational life. Compared to a combined cycle and a simple gas turbine, its levelized cost of electricity (LCOE) is 10% and 33% less expensive. Aghdam et al. [32] explored the integration of solar power into an operating power plant in Iran, finding an increase in plant capacity and electrical efficiency from 714 to 728 MW and from 45 to 47%, respectively. A similar study was performed by Anwar [33] to assess the performance of solar integration of PTCs into the Al-Abdaliya CC in Kuwait with an Engineering Equation Solver (EES) model. The plant and solar capacities were 280 MW and 60 MW, respectively. The results showed that the ISCC efficiency was 20% higher than the original CC and that carbon emissions fall by around 64 kton/year. Ameri and Mohammadzadeh [34] conducted a thermodynamic, thermo-economic, and Life Cycle Analysis of three hybrid designs for a conventional plant in Iran. They reported an increase in power production of 6 MW and a reduction in carbon emissions of 10 g/kWh when the solar field was integrated into the superheater of the bottom steam cycle. Achour et al. [35] developed a thermodynamic model to calculate the thermal performance of an ISCC in Algeria. The overall plant efficiency reached 60%, while the solar-to-electricity efficiency reached 14.4%. Another model was generated by Manente [36] to evaluate the integration of solar energy into a combined cycle, finding that the solar-to-electricity efficiency was between 24 and 29%, but the drop in the gas turbine efficiency at lower load values decreased the ISCC thermal efficiency. Durán-García et al. [37] examined solar thermal power integration in parallel to the HRSG of a combined cycle with two pressure levels. When they introduced the solar field in parallel to the high-pressure economizer, the cycle efficiency increased by 1.32%, but when the solar field was coupled to the low-pressure superheater, the efficiency increase was higher at 3.22%.

Regarding earlier studies that examined the integration of solar thermal power in a combined cycle power plant, some of them focused on solar integration at the top gas cycle, others focused on the bottom steam cycle, and most of them sought to increase plant output power generation. In this work, a study of solar thermal power integration in an existing combined cycle power plant is presented. A real combined cycle power plant in Egypt was examined with the aim of optimizing cycle efficiency and reducing fuel consumption and carbon emissions. Solar thermal power integration was studied at several positions in the top gas and bottom steam cycles and considering different operating strategies, namely fuel saving (FS) and power boosting (PB), providing a comprehensive study of the different possibilities for solar power integration. Firstly, the development of the thermodynamic model of the original combined cycle is presented. Then, the modifications of the model to be adapted to the different ISCC configurations and operating strategies are explained. Finally, the results from the model are assessed, providing guidelines for solar thermal power integration depending on the benefits sought: increasing cycle efficiency, maximizing power delivery, or reducing fuel consumption and carbon emissions.

2. Thermodynamic Model of the Original Combined Cycle

2.1. Description of the Combined Cycle

The combined cycle studied in this work is a 90.5 MW power plant in Alexandria, Egypt (latitude 31°12′ N, longitude 29°55′ E, altitude 18 m), property of Egyptian Petrochemicals Co. (EPC) [38]. Figure 1 shows the main components of the power plant: the top gas cycle, the bottom steam cycle, and the HRSG. The steam turbine is a DK-M 045 model fabricated by Brown, Boveri, and Cie (Baden, Switzerland), and the gas turbine is a GT8C model fabricated by ASEA Brown Boveri (Zurich, Switzerland).

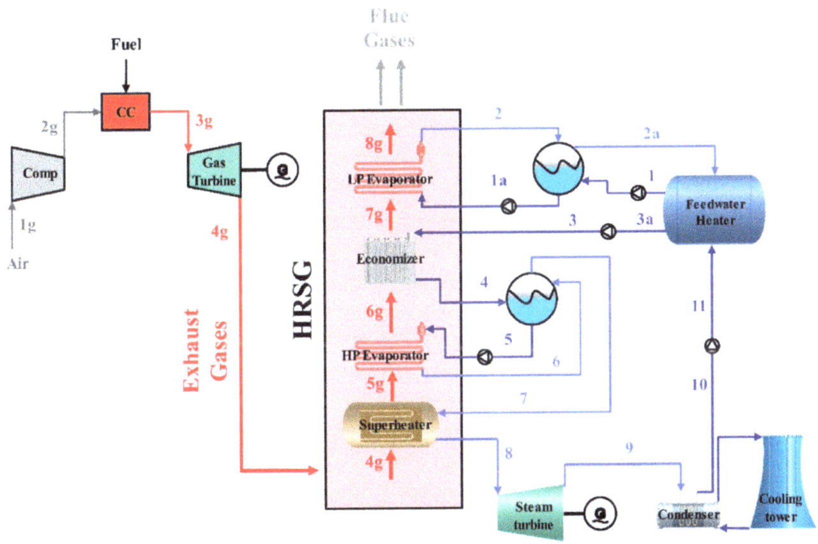

Figure 1. Diagram of the original combined cycle power plant.

Table 1 collects the main characteristics of the cycle, with a cycle efficiency of 56.1%, whereas Figure 2 displays its T-s diagram.

Table 1. Technical data of the combined cycle power plant.

Gas Cycle		Steam Cycle	
Ambient temperature	24 °C	Steam inlet pressure	43 bar
Ambient pressure	1 bar	Steam inlet temperature	457 °C
Combustion chamber inlet temperature	379 °C	LP evaporator pressure	2.4 bar
Turbine pressure	15.7 bar	Condenser pressure	0.08 bar
Turbine inlet temperature	1174 °C	Economizer outlet temperature	228 °C
Turbine exhaust temperature	549 °C	LP evaporator mass flowrate	5 kg/s
Exhaust mass flowrate	174.7 kg/s	HP evaporator mass flowrate	25 kg/s

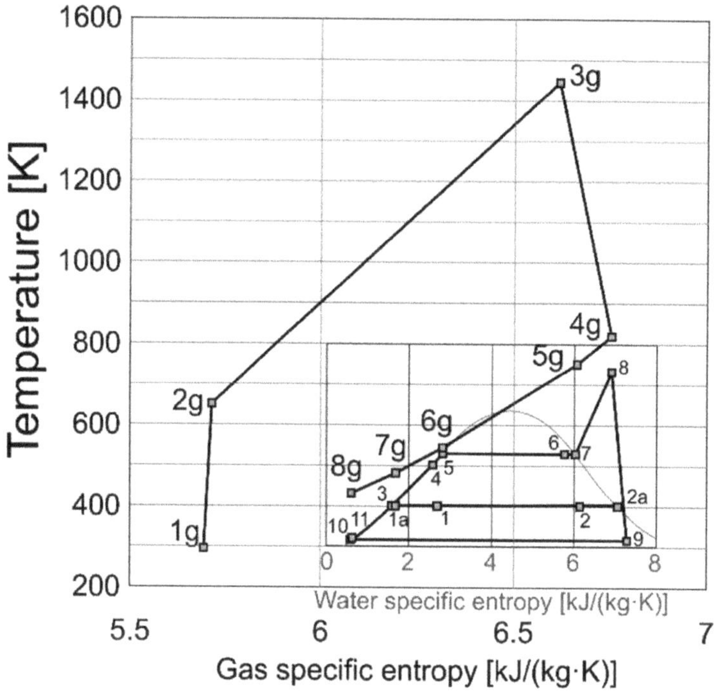

Figure 2. T-s diagram of the original combined cycle.

2.2. Thermodynamic Model

The thermodynamic model of the power plant was developed with MATLAB software [39], using the toolboxes Ideal Air [40] and X-Steam [41] to obtain water and air thermodynamic properties. As depicted on the left side of Figure 1, ambient air enters the compressor (1g), where it increases its temperature and pressure (2g). Then, it is mixed with fuel and burns in the combustion chamber, producing high-temperature gases (3g), which are expanded in the turbine up to ambient pressure (4g), generating power and entering the HRSG afterwards. From the pressure ratio r_p, pressures P_{ig} in bar and temperatures T_{ig} in K may be calculated as follows:

$$r_p = \frac{P_{2g}}{P_{1g}} = \frac{P_{3g}}{P_{4g}} \tag{1}$$

$$r_p^{\frac{k-1}{k}} = \frac{T_{2g}}{T_{1g}} \tag{2}$$

where the heat capacity ratio k is the ratio between the specific heat at constant pressure c_p and at constant volume c_v in kJ/(kg·K). The following equations were used to obtain the power of the gas turbine $\dot{W}_{GT}$ and compressor $\dot{W}_{comp}$, the thermal power supplied in the combustion chamber Q_{cc}, and the net power of the gas cycle $\dot{W}_{G_{net}}$ in kW:

$$\dot{W}_{GT} = \dot{m}_g \cdot (h_{3g} - h_{4g}) \tag{3}$$

$$\dot{W}_{comp} = \dot{m}_a (h_{2g} - h_{1g}) \tag{4}$$

$$\dot{Q}_{cc} = \dot{m}_f \cdot LHV = \dot{m}_g h_{3_g} - \dot{m}_a h_{2g} \tag{5}$$

$$\dot{W}_{G_{net}} = \dot{W}_{GT} - \dot{W}_{comp} \tag{6}$$

The mass flowrates of gases $\dot{m}_g$, air $\dot{m}_a$, and fuel $\dot{m}_f$ are expressed in kg/s, and the enthalpy h is expressed in kJ/kg. The natural gas lower heating value LHV is 47,000 kJ/kg [42]. The thermal efficiency of the top gas cycle is obtained as follows:

$$\eta_T = \frac{\dot{W}_{G_{net}}}{\dot{Q}_{cc}} \tag{7}$$

The main components of the bottom steam cycle, on the right side of Figure 1, are the turbine, condenser, and preheater. The steam turbine power in kW may be obtained:

$$\dot{W}_{ST} = \dot{m}_s \cdot (h_8 - h_9) \tag{8}$$

The power values of the high-pressure pump $\dot{W}_{hp_{pump}}$ and the feedwater pump $\dot{W}_{fw_{pump}}$ are as follows:

$$\dot{W}_{hp_{pump}} = \dot{m}_s \cdot (h_3 - h_{3a}) \tag{9}$$

$$\dot{W}_{fw_{pump}} = \dot{m}_s \cdot (h_{11} - h_{10}) \tag{10}$$

Then, the net power of the steam cycle can be calculated:

$$\dot{W}_{S_{net}} = \dot{W}_{ST} - \dot{W}_{hp_{pump}} - \dot{W}_{fw_{pump}} \tag{11}$$

where $\dot{m}_s$ is the steam flowrate in kg/s, and h_i is the steam enthalpy in kJ/kg. Consequently, the power plant net power and efficiency can be calculated:

$$\dot{W}_{Total} = \dot{W}_{G_{net}} + \dot{W}_{S_{net}} \tag{12}$$

$$\eta_{CC} = \frac{\dot{W}_{G_{net}} + \dot{W}_{S_{net}}}{\dot{Q}_{cc}} \tag{13}$$

The HRSG allows the exchange of thermal energy between the gas turbine exhaust gases and the water from the steam cycle. It consists of four heat exchangers: a superheater, a high-pressure (HP) evaporator, an economizer, and a low-pressure (LP) evaporator. As the UA values and specific configurations of the heat exchangers of the real power plant were not available, it was decided to calculate equivalent UA values using the effectiveness-Number of Transfer Units (ε-NTU) method [43] with a simplified analysis of an equivalent counterflow heat exchanger that operates with the same terminal temperatures and heat transfer rates as the original power plant. The pinch and approach temperatures were obtained from the available power plant data, allowing to adjust the model to match real operating conditions.

Initially, fluid outlet temperatures were guessed to calculate a first value of the Logarithmic Mean Temperature Difference (LMTD). Then, calculations were performed to obtain new values of the outlet temperatures. The LMTD is calculated as follows:

$$LMTD = \frac{\Delta T_1 - \Delta T_2}{\ln(\Delta T_1/\Delta T_2)} \quad (14)$$

where ΔT_1 and ΔT_2 are the temperature differences between the hot and cold fluids at the inlet and outlet in K. The product of the heat transfer area A in m^2 and the heat transfer coefficient U in $W/(m^2{\cdot}K)$ can be determined:

$$UA = \frac{\dot{Q}}{LMTD} \quad (15)$$

where $\dot{Q}$ is the heat transfer rate in kW. Once (UA) is calculated, the Number of Transfer Units (NTU) is obtained:

$$NTU = \frac{UA}{C_{min}} \quad (16)$$

where C_{min} is the smaller of the two heat capacity rates, i.e., C_{cold} and C_{hot}, of the cold and hot fluids in kW/K, determined from the mass flowrates $\dot{m}_i$ in kg/s and the fluid specific heats Cp_i in kJ/(kg·K):

$$C_{hot} = \dot{m}_{hot}.Cp_{hot} \qquad C_{cold} = \dot{m}_{cold}.Cw_{cold} \quad (17)$$

To obtain the relationship between the heat exchanger effectiveness ε and the NTU, the ratio between the smaller and greater heat capacity rates is calculated as follows:

$$C_r = \frac{C_{min}}{C_{max}} \quad (18)$$

The relationship between ε and NTU is obtained from the equation for heat exchangers in counterflow arrangement with a single pass:

$$\varepsilon = \frac{1 - \exp[-NTU\cdot(1 - C_r)]}{1 - C_r\cdot\exp[-NTU\cdot(1 - C_r)]} \quad (19)$$

Which, for a phase change heat exchanger ($C_r \cong 0$), becomes the following:

$$\varepsilon = 1 - \exp[-NTU] \quad (20)$$

The value of ε obtained allows to relate the actual and maximum possible thermal energy transfer rates $\dot{Q}_{actual}$ and $\dot{Q}_{maximum}$ in kW:

$$\varepsilon = \frac{\dot{Q}_{actual}}{\dot{Q}_{maximum}} \quad (21)$$

The maximum possible heat exchanged $\dot{Q}_{maximum}$ can be expressed as given below:

$$\dot{Q}_{maximum} = C_{min}(T_{hot,in} - T_{cold,in}) \quad (22)$$

This equation can be specified for two different cases:

$$C_c < C_h:\ C_{min} = C_c \rightarrow \varepsilon = \frac{(T_{cold,out} - T_{cold,in})}{(T_{hot,in} - T_{cold,in})} \quad (23a)$$

$$C_h < C_c:\ C_{min} = C_h \rightarrow \varepsilon = \frac{(T_{hot,in} - T_{hot,out})}{(T_{hot,in} - T_{cold,in})} \quad (23b)$$

where $T_{i,in}$ and $T_{i,out}$ are the fluid inlet and outlet temperatures and are in K. A new value for the first fluid (with C_{min}) outlet temperature $T_{1,out}$ is then obtained. Assuming no heat losses in the exchanger, the actual heat transfer rate and the outlet temperature of the second fluid (with C_{max}) are calculated from the following equations:

$$\dot{Q}_{actual} = \dot{m}_{hot} \cdot C_{P_{hot}} \cdot (T_{hot,in} - T_{hot,out}) \quad (24a)$$

$$\dot{Q}_{actual} = \dot{m}_{cold} \cdot C_{P_{cold}} \cdot (T_{cold,out} - T_{cold,in}) \quad (24b)$$

Figure 3 shows the temperature–heat transfer rate diagram of the original combined cycle, where the evolution of temperatures across the HRSG may be observed. The pinch and approach temperatures are 17.5 K and 28 K, whereas the UA values that fit the power plant data are 449 kW/K for the feedwater heater, 164.5 kW/K for the low-pressure evaporator, 175.5 kW/K for the economizer, 475 kW/K for the high-pressure evaporator, and 84.5 kW/K for the superheater.

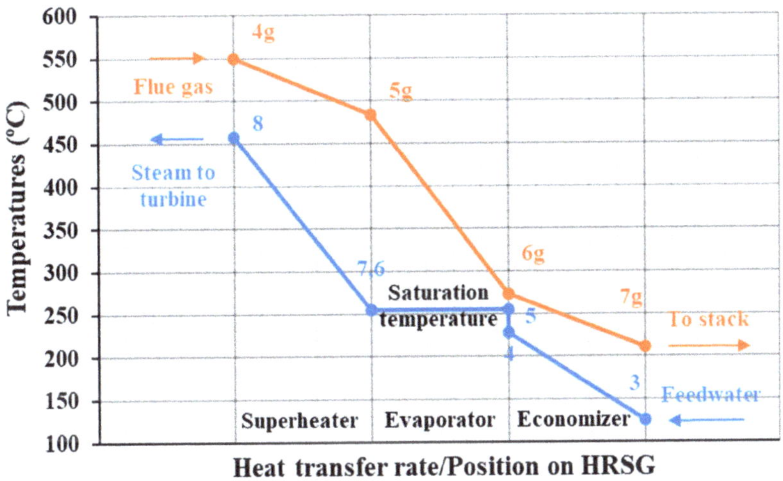

Figure 3. T-Q diagram of the original combined cycle.

2.3. Validation of the Model

As explained in the previous subsection, one part of the data obtained from the EPC power plant was used as input data for the model, whereas the rest (intermediate temperatures, pinch, and approach points) were used to validate the model. A comparison between the EPC power plant real values and the values obtained from the model is presented in Table 2. The results show good agreement, enabling the developed model to be used for the study of solar power integration into the original combined cycle.

Table 2. Results of the thermodynamic model vs. actual values from the EPC power plant.

Operating & Design Conditions	Model	EPC Power Plant
Gas turbine cycle		
Air mass flowrate, kg/s	171.2	171.2
Air to fuel ratio	50	50
Pressure ratio, r_p	15.7	15.7
Turbine inlet temperature, °C	1174	1100
Exhaust temperature, °C	549	540
Power output, MW	90,569	90,569
Top gas cycle efficiency, %	39.84%	39.84%
Steam Turbine cycle		
LP steam mass flowrate, kg/s	5	5
HP steam mass flowrate, kg/s	25	25
Turbine inlet pressure, bar	43	43
Power output, MW	26,292	26,292
Bottom steam cycle efficiency, %	27.1	NA
Heat recovery steam generator (HRSG)		
Pinch point temperature, K	17.5	17.5
Approach temperature, K	28	28
Stack temperature, °C	160	172
(UA) Feedwater heater, kW/K	449	NA
(UA) Low-pressure evaporator, kW/K	164.5	NA
(UA) Economizer, kW/K	175.5	NA
(UA) High-pressure evaporator, kW/K	475	NA
(UA) Superheater, kW/K	84.5	NA
Combined cycle		
Total output power, MW	90,569	90,569
Efficiency, %	56.13	56.13

3. Study of Solar Power Integration (ISCC)

The validated model presented in the previous section was modified to integrate solar thermal power into the combined cycle. Two operating strategies, fuel saving (FS) and power boosting (PB), were analyzed. Figure 4 shows the four possible solar integration positions A, B, C, and D in the gas and steam cycles.

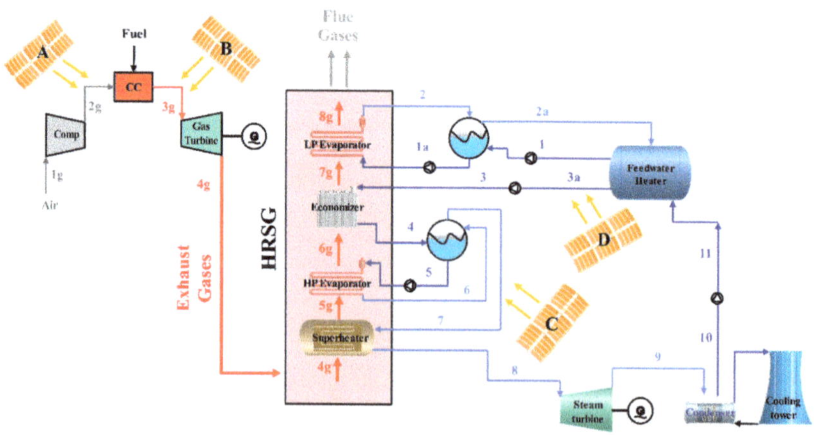

Figure 4. Solar field integration options.

3.1. Fuel-Saving Mode

For fuel-saving operation, the solar field was integrated into the gas or steam cycle to allow a reduction in fuel consumption while keeping the output power of the cycle constant. Once the amount of saved fuel was obtained, the direct reduction in CO_2 emissions was calculated from the natural gas LHV and the natural gas/CO_2 emission ratio $EF_{NG \to CO_2}$ = 0.252 kg/kWh [44]:

$$CO_{2,avoided} = \dot{m}_{f_{saved}} \cdot LHV \cdot EF_{NG \to CO_2} \cdot \Delta t \quad (25)$$

where Δt is the mean solar operation time for Alexandria, i.e., 275 h/month [45], and $\dot{m}_{f_{saved}}$ is the fuel consumption reduction thanks to solar thermal power integration in kg/h. Solar integration at the gas cycle differs from integration at the steam, as explained in the following two subsections.

3.1.1. Gas Cycle Integration

As shown in Figure 4, solar thermal power can be integrated at two positions: after the air compressor in order to heat compressed air before it enters the combustion chamber (case A) and after the combustion chamber in order to heat combustion gases before they enter the turbine (case B). According to the literature, case A is the most typical alternative, but case B is worth investigating. The assumptions considered for gas cycle integration in the FS scheme are as follows:

- Mass flowrates of fuel and air are altered depending on the solar thermal power;
- Compression specific work is constant;
- Gas turbine inlet and outlet conditions are constant;
- The turbine specific work is constant;
- The top gas cycle output power is constant;
- The mass flowrate of fuel is reduced;
- The bottom steam cycle is unaffected;
- The ISCC overall output power remains constant.

(a) Case A: After air compressor

As shown in Figure 5, the solar field is integrated after the compressor, heating the compressed air before it enters the combustion chamber.

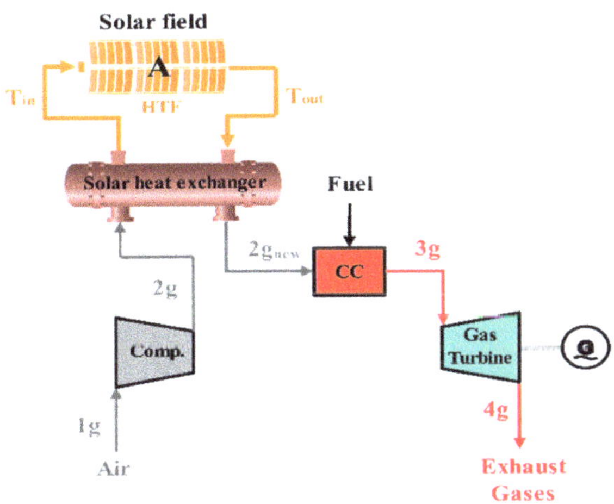

Figure 5. Case A: solar field integration after air compressor.

The original thermodynamic model was adapted by modifying the air and fuel mass flowrates $\dot{m}_{a_{new}}$ and $\dot{m}_{f_{new}}$, so compression power $\dot{W}_{comp}$ becomes the following:

$$\dot{W}_{comp} = \dot{m}_{a_{new}}(h_{2g} - h_{1g}) \tag{26}$$

The energy balance in the combustion chamber is reformulated as given below:

$$\dot{m}_{a_{new}} \cdot h_{2g_{new}} + \dot{Q}_{cc} = \dot{m}_{a_{new}} \cdot h_{2g_{new}} + \dot{m}_{f_{new}} \cdot LHV = \dot{m}_g h_{3g} \tag{27}$$

The solar heat power integrated $\dot{Q}_{Solar}$ in kW, assuming no heat losses, becomes the following:

$$\dot{Q}_{Solar} = \dot{m}_{a_{new}} \cdot \left(h_{2g_{new}} - h_{2g}\right) \tag{28}$$

(b) Case B: After combustion chamber

As depicted in Figure 6, the solar field is integrated after the combustion chamber to heat combustion gases before they enter the gas turbine, resulting in the new thermodynamic state $3g_{new}$. The challenge of heating hot gases from the combustion chamber is significant since they must reach a very high temperature before entering the turbine. The thermodynamic model uses the same assumptions as for case A. As the turbine inlet and outlet conditions are the same as for the original cycle, solar thermal power will allow to reduce fuel consumption in the combustion chamber, reducing the temperature of $3g_{new}$.

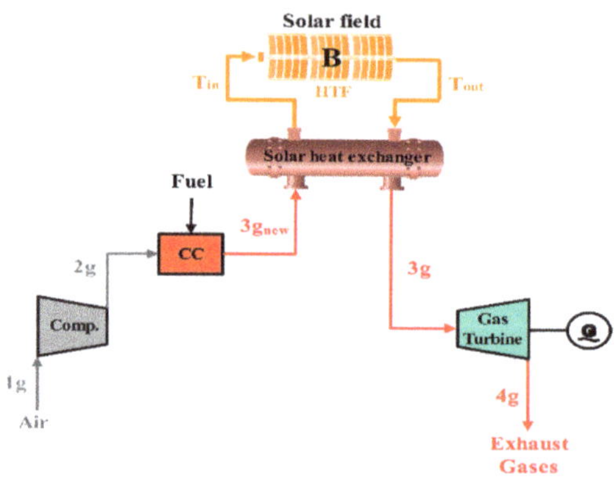

Figure 6. Case B: solar field integration after combustion chamber.

An energy balance in the combustion chamber yields the following:

$$\dot{m}_{a_{new}} \cdot h_{2g} + \dot{Q}_{cc} = \dot{m}_{a_{new}} \cdot h_{2g} + \dot{m}_{f_{new}} \cdot LHV = \dot{m}_g h_{3g_{new}} \tag{29}$$

And the solar thermal power integrated, assuming no heat losses, becomes the following:

$$\dot{Q}_{Solar} = \dot{m}_{a_{new}} \cdot \left(h_{3g} - h_{3g_{new}}\right) \tag{30}$$

3.1.2. Steam Cycle Integration

When working in the fuel-saving operation mode, solar thermal power can be integrated into the bottom steam cycle as well. In this case, the solar integration will compensate for the loss of the gas turbine output power due to the reduction in fuel consumption. Two integration positions were examined: before the superheater, so that saturated steam from the HP drum is heated before entering the actual superheater stage (case C), and before the economizer, with feedwater being preheated before the economizer (case D).

(a) Case C: Integration before superheater

In this configuration, as shown in Figure 7, outlet steam from the HP drum is heated by the solar field before it enters the superheater. The HRSG temperature distribution will change as water and steam temperatures increase. Hence, the steam turbine will generate more power to compensate for the reduction in the top gas cycle power, allowing to reduce fuel consumption.

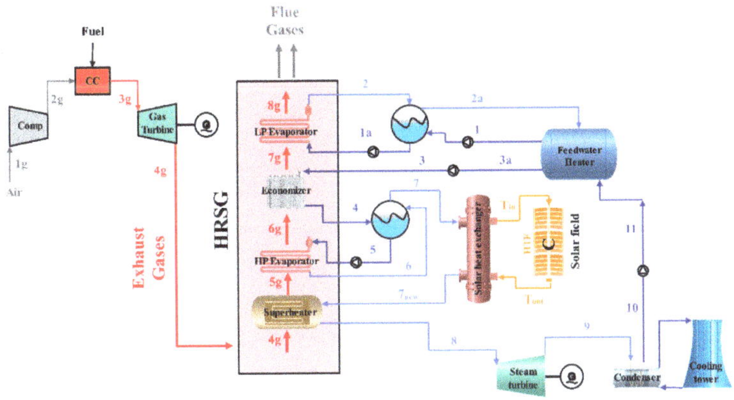

Figure 7. Case C: solar field integration before superheater.

The solar heat power integrated, assuming no heat losses, results in the following:

$$\dot{Q}_{Solar} = \dot{m}_S \cdot (h7_{new} - h7) \quad (31)$$

(b) Case D: Integration at economizer

The solar field can be integrated into the bottom steam cycle after the feedwater outlet to preheat water before it enters the economizer, as depicted in Figure 8. As in case C, the temperature distribution along the HRSG will be shifted upwards, increasing the steam turbine output power and allowing the use of less fuel in the gas cycle.

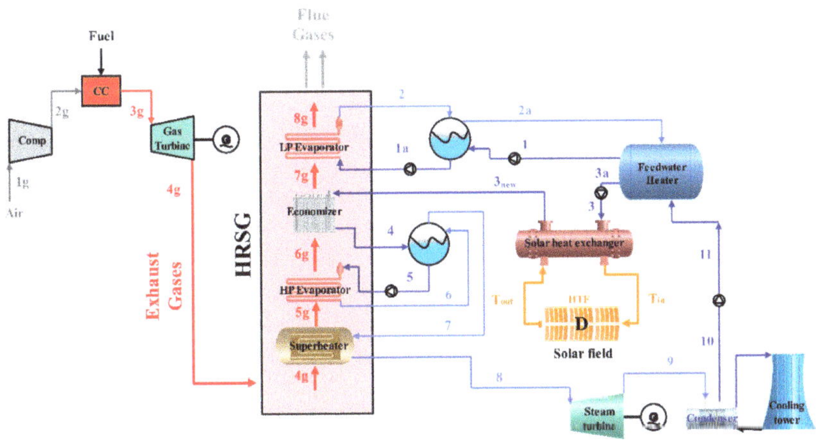

Figure 8. Case D: solar field integration at economizer.

The solar heat power integrated, assuming no heat losses, is as follows:

$$\dot{Q}_{Solar} = \dot{m}_s \cdot (h_{3_{new}} - h_3) \tag{32}$$

3.2. Power-Boosting Mode

In the power-boosting mode, the same fuel consumption as for the original combined cycle is kept constant, so the integration of the solar field increases the output power of the plant. The same four integration positions examined for the fuel-saving mode, indicated in Figure 4, were studied, but the assumptions for the model change.

3.2.1. Gas Cycle Integration

In this case, the added solar heat will result in an increase in the power output of the gas turbine. Solar thermal power integration was studied after the air compressor (case A, Figure 5) and after the combustion chamber (case B, Figure 6). The developed thermodynamic models were modified with the following assumptions:

- Air and gas mass flowrates change depending on the integrated solar thermal power;
- Fuel mass flowrate is steady;
- Compression work increases;
- Gas turbine inlet and outlet conditions are constant;
- The total output power of the upper gas cycle increases;
- The bottom steam cycle is unaffected. The ISCC overall output power increases.

3.2.2. Steam Cycle Integration

In this case, the gas cycle works at the same conditions as in the original cycle, and the integration of solar power increases the power output of the bottom steam cycle. The same two integration positions as for fuel saving, i.e., before the superheater (case C, Figure 7) and before the economizer (case D, Figure 8) of the HRSG, were studied. Two different operating modes, flowrate and parameter boosting, were considered for each integration position. In the flowrate-boosting mode, the integrated power is used to increase the steam flowrate, whereas in the parameter boosting, it modifies the thermodynamic states of the steam cycle, which continues working with the same steam flowrate.

3.3. Solar Field Technology Selection

Before moving on to the results, considerations about the solar field technology to be used are presented, depending on their operating temperatures. Table 3 collects the characteristics of different solar concentration technologies so that, depending on the solar power integration position, the most suitable technology can be selected. According to the literature, the most common technology in ISCCs is the use of PTCs with Therminol VP-1 as HTF. Therminol VP-1 is characterized by a low dynamic viscosity and a high heat capacity over a large operational temperature range [46]. However, its maximum operating temperature is 390 °C. As the temperature of the cycle working fluids could be higher, solar molten salts could be an alternative HTF [47], as they are able to reach much higher temperatures up to 550 °C. Nevertheless, for temperatures too high, PDR or heliostats will be the only option.

Table 3. Concentrating solar collectors [48,49].

Collector Type	Parabolic Trough Collectors (PTC)	Parabolic Dish Reflectors (PDR)	Heliostat Field Collectors (Solar Power Tower)
Description	Parabolic sheet of reflective material.Linear receiver (metal pipe with heat transfer fluid)	Large reflective parabolic dish with stirring high engine receiver at focal point	Large heliostat field with tall tower in its center. Receiver: water/HTF boiler at top
Operating range (°C)	50–400	150–1500	300–2000
Relative cost	Low	Very high	High
Concentration ratio [1]	15–45	100–1000	150–1500
Tracking	One-Axis	Two-Axis	Two-Axis
Efficiency (%)	~18	~30	~25–28

[1] Ratio of the effective area of the aperture to the receiver/absorber area of the collector.

4. Results

Every studied configuration was considered in both fuel-saving and power-boosting operating modes. For fuel saving, maximum reductions in fuel consumption and CO_2 emissions were the target; for power boosting, maximization of the output power was the goal. In addition, the maximum solar thermal power that can be integrated into the cycle was evaluated. To make reading easier, the detailed results of all the studied configurations are collected in Appendix A (Tables A1–A8), leaving only the most relevant data in this section.

4.1. Fuel-Saving Mode

4.1.1. Gas Cycle Integration

The results of the fuel-saving cases alongside the original values of the combined cycle are collected in Table 4. Total net power remains constant and equal to the original cycle value, 90,569 MW, but the cycle efficiency increases slightly to 56.15%. When compared to the original CC, cases A and B show significant benefits, such as the reduction in fuel consumption of 6.23% when 10 MW solar thermal power is integrated into the cycle. Fuel saving as a function of the integrated solar thermal power is represented in Figure 9a, showing linear behavior. With 28.2 MJ/kg specific work per fuel unit mass, both cases A and B result in cutting carbon emissions by 6.4 g CO_2/kWh. In case A, PTC technology could be employed for the solar field placed after the compressor. However, molten salts should be used as HTF, as the maximum output temperature of the solar heat exchanger ($T2g_{new}$) reaches 433 °C at 10 MW of integrated solar power, as shown in Figure 9b.

In case B, although global values are the same as in case A, the temperatures of the different states of the gas cycle change, as collected in Table A1. The outlet temperature of the combustion chamber state $3g_{new}$ becomes lower, requiring less fuel because the solar heat exchanger will provide the additional heat necessary for reaching the temperature of the state 3g just before the turbine inlet. In case B, when solar power is integrated into the cycle, heat must be transferred to gases at temperatures from 1126.5 °C ($3g_{new}$) to 1174 °C (3g), as depicted in Figure 9b. Only heliostat field collectors will be able to provide the required solar thermal power at those temperatures. Comparing options A and B, case A shows a clear advantage, as it allows integrating more solar field technologies.

Table 4. Original CC vs. ISCC (case A and case B) "Fuel saving".

Mass Flowrates	Original CC	ISCC Case A	ISCC Case B
Fuel flowrate (kg/s) Fuel saving (%)	3.42 --	3.21 6.23	
Solar heat integration	Original CC	ISCC Case A	ISCC Case B
Integrated solar heat (MW)	--	10	
Cycle efficiency	Original CC	ISCC Case A	ISCC Case B
Gas turbine cycle (%) Combined cycle (%)	39.84 56.13	39.85 56.15	
Cycle power breakdown	Original CC	ISCC Case A	ISCC Case B
Gas cycle (kW)	64,277	64,277	64,277
Steam cycle (kW)	26,292	26,292	26,292
Total net power (kW)	90,569	90,569	90,569
Specific work per fuel unit mass flow (kJ/kg)	26,439	28,198	28,198
CO_2 emissions (Mt/year)	0.2971	0.2785	0.2785
CO_2 emissions saved (kg CO_2/kWh)	-	0.0064	0.0064

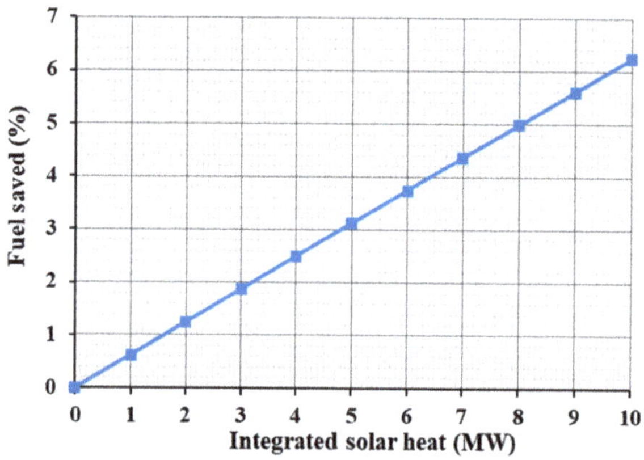

(**a**) Fuel saving (%) as a function of integrated solar heat

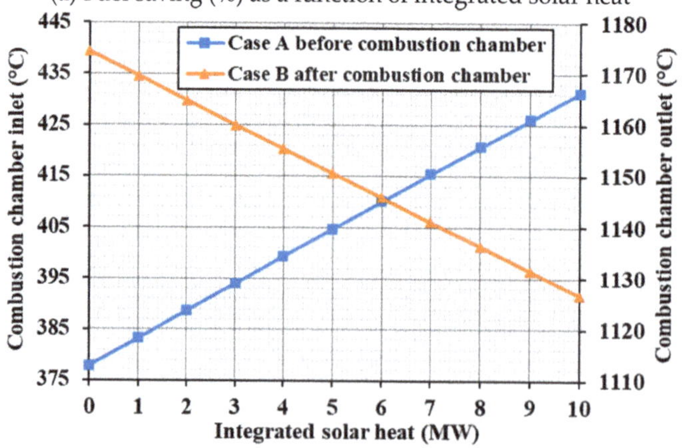

(**b**) Temperature changes as a function of integrated solar heat

Figure 9. Fuel saving (**a**) and temperature changes (**b**) for integration options A and B.

4.1.2. Steam Cycle Integration

When solar thermal power is integrated into the bottom steam cycle, attention must be paid to steam temperatures. If they rise too much, the direction of heat transfer might be reversed inside the HRSG. To prevent this issue, temperature evolutions inside the HRSG were controlled, obtaining the maximum solar thermal power that may be integrated into the cycle. The detailed results from cases C and D are collected in Table A2.

The results from the study of cases C and D are collected in Table 5. In both cases, the top gas cycle was unaffected by solar power integration. The configuration of case C allowed to integrate a maximum of 15 MW solar thermal power before the superheater stage, avoiding the heat transfer reversal inside the HRSG, as depicted in the T-Q diagram shown in Figure 10. This configuration could reduce fuel consumption to 3.3 kg/s, a decrease of 3.49% of the original value. However, the total ISCC efficiency was 53.06%, lower than for the original cycle. On the other hand, the specific work per fuel unit mass increased to 27.4 MJ/kg, leading to a potential reduction in emissions of 3.5 g CO_2/kWh. For the configuration presented in case C, as the maximum temperature reached is 480 °C for 15 MW of integrated solar power, the solar field used could be either PDR, heliostats, or even PTCs with molten salts as HTF.

Table 5. Original CC vs. ISCC (case C and case D) "Fuel saving".

Mass Flowrates	**Original CC**	**ISCC Case C**	**ISCC Case D**
Fuel flowrate (kg/s)	3.42	3.3	3.15
Fuel saving (%)	--	3.49	7.97
Solar heat integration	Original CC	ISCC Case C	ISCC Case D
Integrated solar heat (MW)	--	15	3
Cycle efficiency	Original CC	ISCC Case C	ISCC Case D
Gas turbine cycle (%)	39.84	39.84	39.84
Combined cycle (%)	56.13	53.06	59.79
Cycle power breakdown	Original CC	ISCC Case C	ISCC Case D
Compressor (kW)	62,450	60,266	57,471
Gas turbine (kW)	126,727	122,294	116,622
Gas cycle (kW)	64,277	62,028	59,152
Steam cycle (kW)	26,292	28,542	31,417
Total net power (kW)	90,569	90,569	90,569
Specific work per unit fuel mass flow (kJ/kg)	26,439	27,399	28,730
CO_2 emissions (Mt/year)	0.2971	0.2867	0.2734
CO_2 emissions saved (kg CO_2/kWh)	--	0.0035	0.0083

Regarding the configuration of case D, the maximum solar thermal power that could be integrated before the economizer was limited to 3 MW. However, looking at the T-Q diagram in Figure 10, the temperature evolutions of gas and steam are nearer, hinting at a more effective heat transfer inside the HRSG. Indeed, fuel saving reaches a maximum of 7.97%, more than twice the value obtained with 15 MW solar power in case C with just one-fifth of the solar power integrated, as may be observed in Figure 11. Consequently, overall cycle efficiency increases up to 59.79%, the highest value of the four configurations studied for the fuel-saving operation mode. As collected in Table 5, case D reaches a specific work of 28.7 kJ/kg fuel, leading to potential savings of 8.3 g CO_2/kWh with only 3 MW of integrated solar power. In addition, due to the lower operating temperatures for the solar heat exchanger, PTCs and PDRs could be used, with PTC and synthetic oils becoming a feasible option.

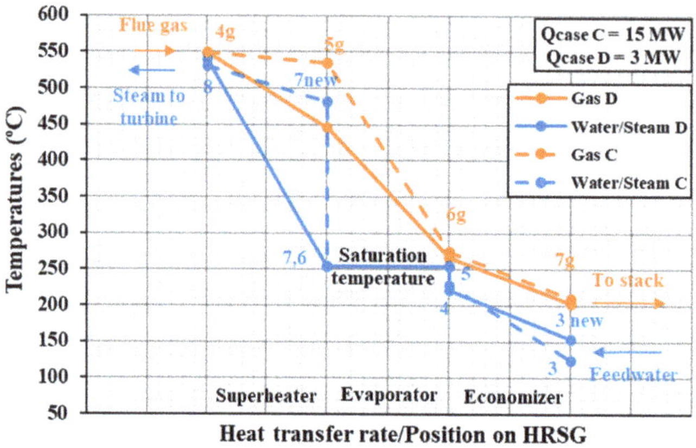

Figure 10. T-Q diagram for cases C and D (fuel saving).

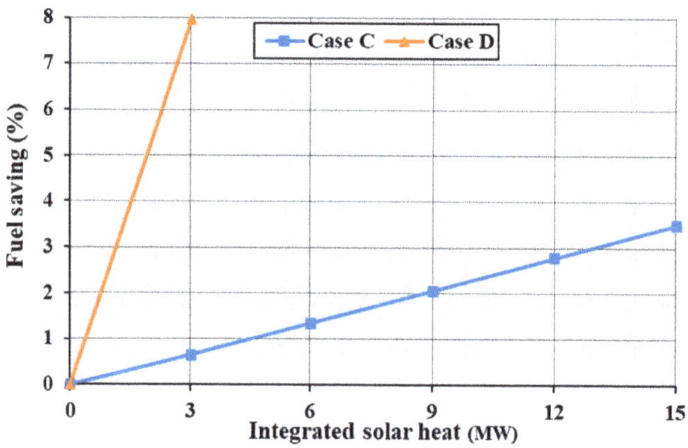

Figure 11. Fuel saving (%) for steam cycle integration options.

4.2. Power-Boosting Mode

4.2.1. Gas Cycle Integration

Table 6 collects the results from power-boosting operation when solar power is integrated into the top gas cycle. For case A, an extra power of 4 MW (4.41%) could be obtained by integrating 10 MW of solar thermal power. Generation capacity increased to 27.6 MJ/kg. However, the back work ratio increases slightly to 49.3% due to the higher air-fuel ratio, and the cycle efficiency drops to 55.19%. Temperatures for this case reaches 379 °C at state 2g and 430 °C at state $2g_{new}$, allowing the use of PTCs with solar molten salts, PDRs, or a heliostat field. Considering case B, global cycle parameters are the same as for case A. The main difference is the temperature of state 3g, which reaches 1129.5 °C for 10 MW of integrated solar thermal power, thus requiring a heliostat as the solar field technology. The evolution of power boosting and cycle efficiency as a function of the solar thermal power is depicted in Figure 12, where the increase in the power output alongside a slight decrease in the cycle efficiency becomes apparent.

Table 6. Original CC vs. ISCC (case A and case B) "Power boosting".

Solar Heat Integration	Original CC	ISCC Case C	ISCC Case D
Integrated solar heat (MW)	--	10	
Cycle efficiency	Original CC	ISCC Case C	ISCC Case D
Gas turbine cycle (%)	39.84	39.83	
Combined cycle (%)	56.13	55.19	
Cycle power breakdown	Original CC	ISCC Case C	ISCC Case D
Compressor (kW)	62,450	66,455	
Gas turbine (kW)	126,727	134,693	
Gas cycle (kW)	64,277	68,239	
Steam cycle (kW)	26,292	26,323	
Total net power (kW)	90,569	94,562	
Power boosted (%)	--	4.41	
Back work ratio (%)	49.279	49.33	
Specific work per unit fuel mass flow (kJ/kg)	26,439	27,605	

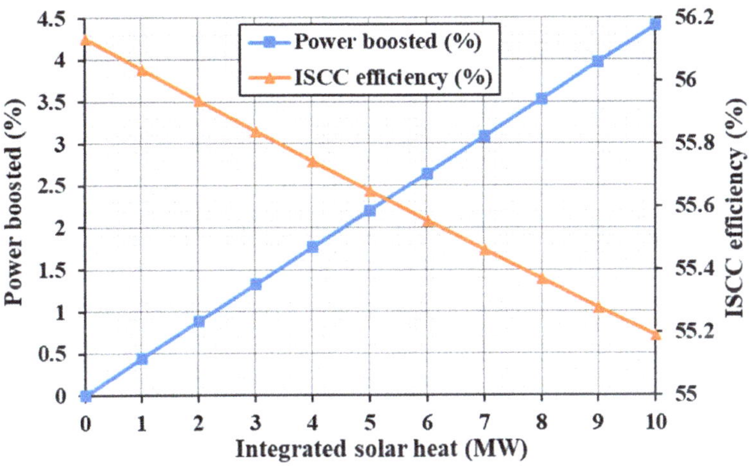

Figure 12. Power boosting (%) and cycle efficiency (%) for integration options A and B.

4.2.2. Steam Cycle Integration: Flowrate Boosting

Firstly, the results from flowrate boosting are discussed. In the configuration proposed in case C, a maximum of 4 MW solar thermal power could be integrated before the superheater, resulting in the T-Q diagram represented in Figure 13. As shown in Table 7, the cycle output power increased to 112.5 MW (24.2% boost) thanks to the increase in the steam flowrate from 25 to 45.84 kg/s. Consequently, overall cycle efficiency increased by 11.9%. Leaving the top gas cycle unaffected, it was possible to generate 32.8 MJ/kg fuel, increasing power production in 6.4 MJ/kg fuel. In case C, the maximum steam temperature at the solar heat exchanger was slightly above 300 °C, so selecting PTC technology with synthetic oil as HTF for the solar field becomes a feasible option.

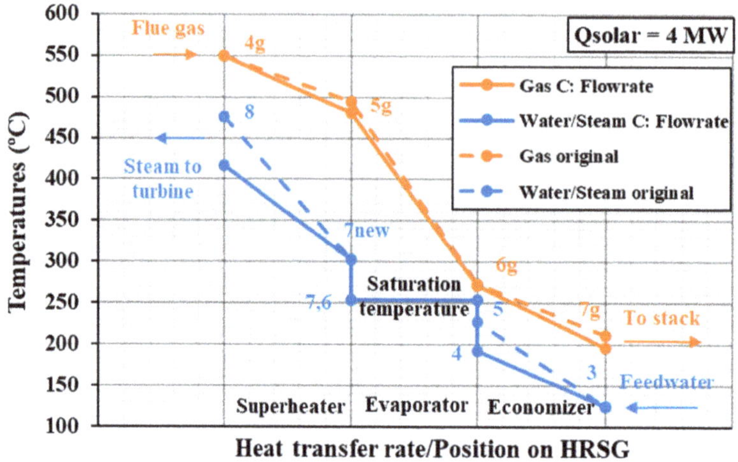

Figure 13. T-Q diagram for case C (flowrate power boosting).

Table 7. Original CC vs. Flowrate boosting (case C and case D).

Mass Flowrates	Original CC	ISCC Case C	ISCC Case D
LP evaporator mass flowrate (kg/s)	5	9.17	6.54
HP evaporator mass flowrate (kg/s)	25	45.84	32.72
Solar heat integration	Original CC	ISCC Case C	ISCC Case D
Integrated solar heat (MW)	--	4	12
Cycle efficiency	Original CC	ISCC Case C	ISCC Case D
Gas turbine cycle (%)	39.84	39.84	39.84
Combined cycle (%)	56.13	68.03	56.93
Cycle power breakdown	Original CC	ISCC Case C	ISCC Case D
Gas cycle (kW)	64,277	64,277	64,277
Steam cycle (kW)	26,292	48,214	34,412
Total net power (kW)	90,569	112,491	98,689
Power boosted (%)	--	24.2	8.96
Specific work per unit fuel mass flow (kJ/kg)	26,439	32,840	28,810

Regarding the configuration of case D, the maximum solar thermal power that could be integrated before the economizer reached 12 MW. In the T-Q diagram of the HRSG shown in Figure 14, it may be appreciated how water and gas temperatures became slightly closer at the economizer stage. As collected in Table 7, the maximum output power was around 98.7 MW (8.96% boost), with overall cycle efficiency increasing up to 56.93%. The work per fuel unit mass increased to 28.8 MJ/kg. In this configuration, solar integration at the economizer allows to use both PDRs and PTCs, with PTC easily matching the low operating temperature ranges for case D.

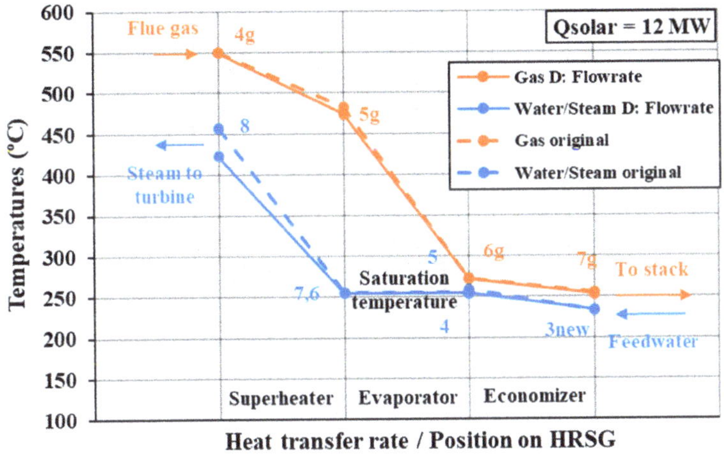

Figure 14. T-Q diagram for case D (flowrate power boosting).

The evolution of the power boosted with respect to solar thermal power is depicted in Figure 15. Despite the limitation in the integrated solar power of 4 MW, the power boosting in case C, i.e., 24.2%, is almost three times the boost in case D for 12 MW of solar power: 8.96%.

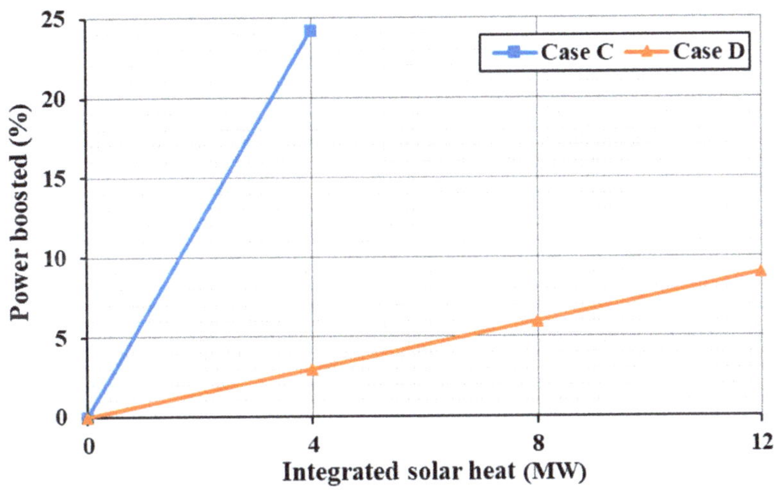

Figure 15. Flowrate power boosting (%) for steam cycle integration configurations.

4.2.3. Steam Cycle Integration: Parameter Boosting

Parameter boosting was the other option studied for power boosting through solar power integration at the bottom steam cycle. For the configuration of case C, several HP evaporator pressure values were studied, from −50% to +50% of the original value in 10% interval steps. (Please refer to Tables A5 and A6 for detailed results.) Operating pressure affected the maximum solar power that could be integrated into the cycle, increasing from 7 MW at −50% pressure to 9 MW at +50% pressure. Therefore, the comparison was performed at 7 MW to select the optimum operating pressure. It was observed that integrating 7 MW of solar power at the original HP evaporator pressure increased power generation by 2.18%, as shown in Figure 16. This figure shows the evolution of power boosting as a function of working pressure for 7 MW of integrated solar power, where it may be appreciated that reducing the pressure increases the power boosted. The minimum and maximum power-boosting values of 1.37 and 2.82% were obtained for the extremes of the studied pressure range: −50% pressure and + 50% pressure. Overall cycle efficiency also varied between 54.54% for the +50% pressure case and 55.32% for the −50% pressure case, as depicted in Figure 17. For case C, PTC can be used as the solar field technology for all the pressure values studied.

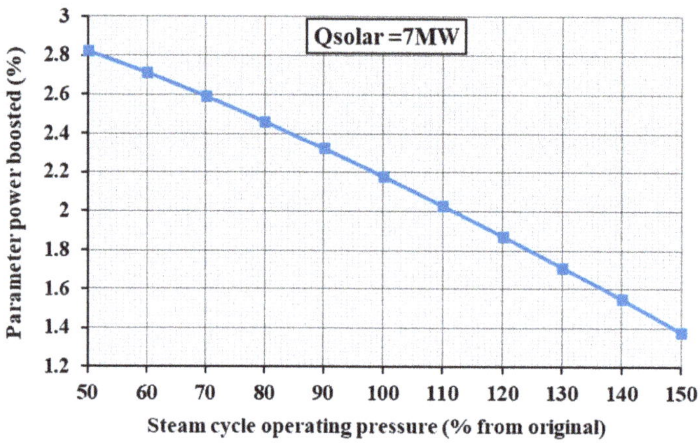

Figure 16. Parameter power boosting (%) at different pressure levels for case C.

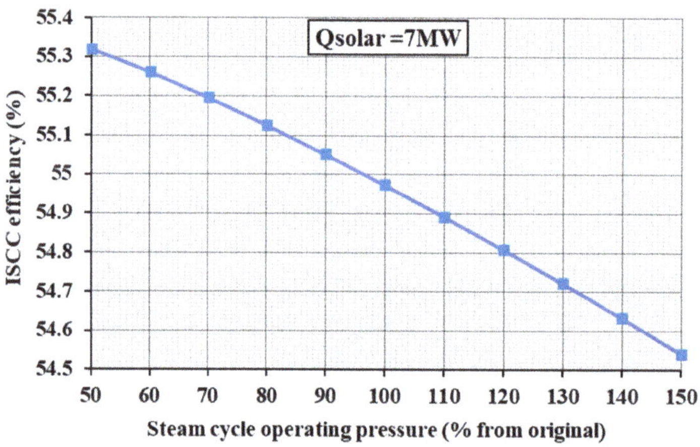

Figure 17. Overall efficiency at different pressure levels for case C.

As with −50% HP evaporator pressure the maximum power boost was obtained, the evolution of power boosting with respect to the integrated solar power is shown in Figure 18. It may be observed that just reducing evaporating pressure increases overall output power by 0.86% (0.77 MW) even without solar power; however, for 7 MW, power is boosted by 2.82% (2.5 MW). Figure 19 shows the temperature distribution inside the HRSG for this last case, where it may be appreciated that exhaust gas temperatures come nearer to steam temperatures.

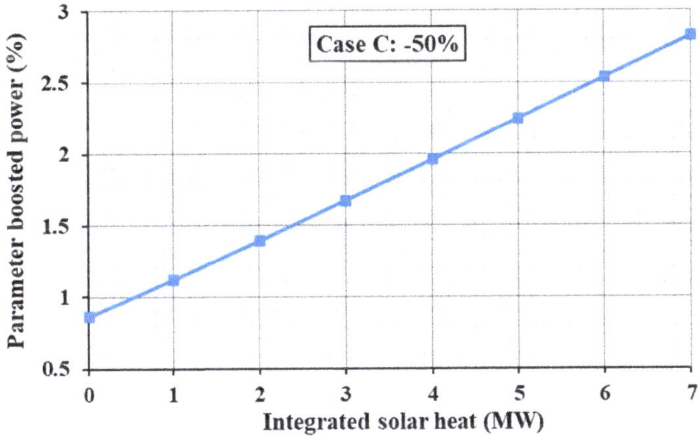

Figure 18. Parameter power boosting as a function of integrated solar power for case C: −50% HP.

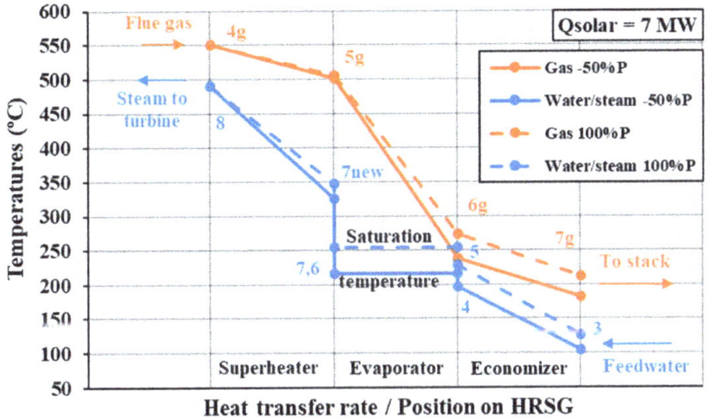

Figure 19. T-Q diagram for case C parameter power boosting (−50% HP evaporator pressure).

Considering solar power integration before the economizer (case D), the evaporator operating pressure was also changed between −50% and +50% of the original pressure at 10% intervals, with the detailed results collected in Tables A7 and A8. Again, the maximum solar thermal power that could be integrated was affected by the operating pressure, varying in the range between 1.5 and 2 MW. Hence, to compare results, a value of 1.5 MW was chosen. Figure 20 shows the power boosting as a function of the HP evaporator pressure. When 1.5 MW solar power was integrated at original operating conditions, the delivered power increased by 4.9%. As in case C, the increase in operating pressure decreased output power, reaching the lowest increase of 4.35% at the +50% pressure case (58.04% cycle efficiency). Nevertheless, for case D, it was possible to find a maximum in power boosting for the −30% pressure case, reaching 5.01% power boosting with respect to the original CC. As with flowrate boosting in case D, integrating the solar field before the economizer makes PTC technology with synthetic oils a suitable option.

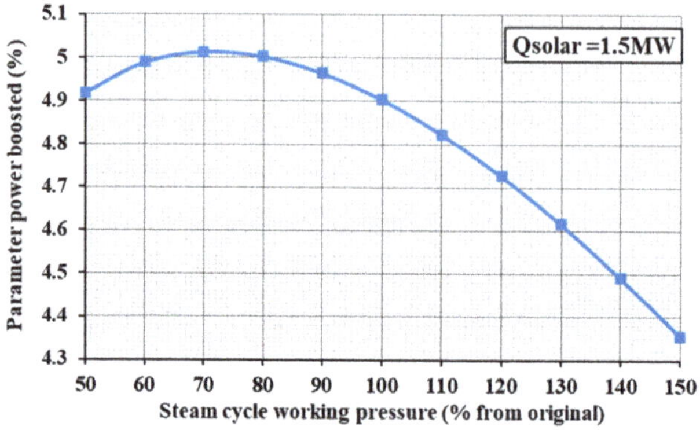

Figure 20. Parameter power boosting (%) at different pressure levels for case D.

Focusing on the −30% HP evaporator pressure, Figure 21 shows power boosting as a function of the integrated solar power, up to the maximum limit of 1.5 MW. It may be observed that the decrease in the evaporator pressure only increases overall output power by 41 kW (0.04%), so the effect of solar power integration becomes more determinant. Even with just 1.5 MW of solar power, power boosting is 5.01% (4.54 MW), with an overall cycle efficiency of 58.4%. Looking at the T-Q diagram of the HRSG under these conditions, shown in Figure 22, it may be appreciated that gas temperatures come much closer to water temperatures in both the economizer and superheater.

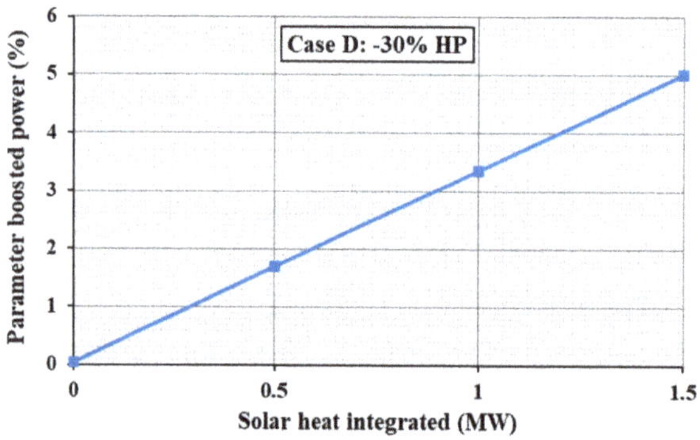

Figure 21. Parameter power boosting (%) as a function of integrated solar power for case D: −30%.

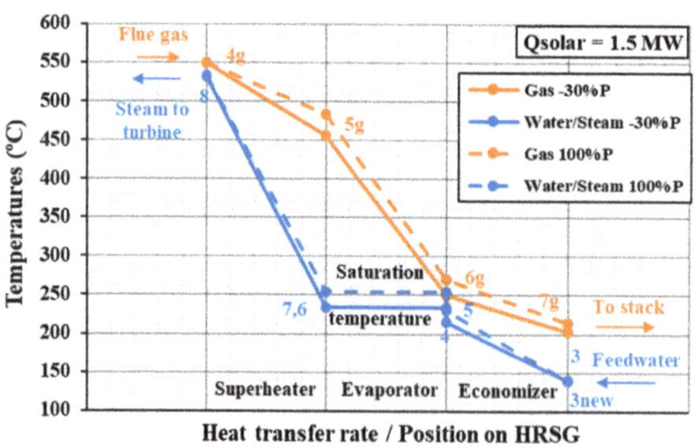

Figure 22. T-Q diagram for case D parameter power boosting (−30% LP evaporator pressure).

5. Discussion

From the analysis of the results, some considerations for solar thermal power integration in existing combined cycles were derived. Table 8 collects the main considerations obtained, while Figure 23 shows graphically the main guidelines to be followed for solar power integration, with the aim of providing the best course of action depending on the desired outcome.

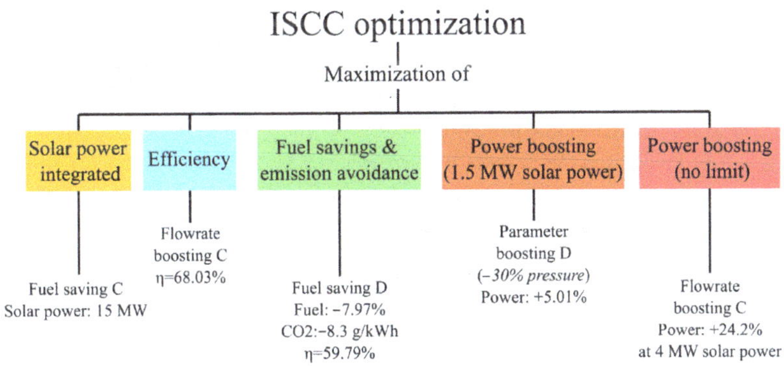

Figure 23. Optimum ISCC strategies depending on the desired outcome.

Regarding fuel-saving operation, cases A and B must adapt to the same gas turbine inlet conditions, so both were able to save the same amount of fuel when 10 MW solar thermal power was integrated: 6.23%. However, case A exhibited better flexibility in terms of the solar field technology to be used (parabolic dish reflectors or heliostat field collectors), as it benefits from lower operating temperatures. For the steam cycle integration options, case C was only able to save 3.49% by requiring 15 MW of integrated solar thermal power, resulting in the lowest fuel savings per MW of solar power. However, it was the configuration that could integrate the highest solar power: 15 MW. The configuration presented in case D, on the contrary, allowed to reduce fuel consumption by 7.97% with just 3 MW of solar power. Due to its lower operating temperatures, parabolic trough collectors are a suitable option for solar power integration in the steam cycle. In addition, for the same integrated solar power of 3 MW, cases A and B were only able to save 1.87% of fuel, whereas case C had the lowest savings of all configurations: 0.65%.

Considering power-boosting operation, cases A and B can boost power by 4.41% with 10 MW of integrated solar power. However, the flowrate-boosting strategy with integration of solar power before the steam cycle superheater was found to have the best impact on the cycle. In this sense, an increase in cycle output power of 24.2% was found for case C when 4 MW of solar power was integrated. With the same solar power, case D was only able to increase cycle output power by 2.98%. Nevertheless, for the parameter-boosting strategy, the opposite behavior was observed. With 7 MW of integrated solar power, case C showed the lowest boosting performance, with only 2.82% when the HP evaporator pressure was reduced to half of that of the original cycle. On the other hand, with only 1.5 MW of integrated solar power, case D was able to boost power by 5.01% when the HP evaporator pressure was reduced to 70% of the original value.

Table 8. Considerations for integration of solar thermal power in existing combined cycles.

	Strategy		Considerations/Recommendations for Solar Thermal Power Integration
Fuel saving	A		• Parabolic dish reflector or heliostat field collector technology must be used. • Parabolic trough collector could be an alternative, but HTF must withstand high temperatures (molten salts). • Recommended if implementation at the top gas cycle is requested.
	B		• Heliostat field collector technology must be used. • Not recommended due to technology restrictions.
	C		• Parabolic dish reflector or heliostat field collector technology must be used. • Parabolic trough collector could be an alternative, but HTF must withstand high temperatures (molten salts). • Lowest fuel saving per MW of solar thermal power. • Can absorb the highest solar thermal power. • Recommended for maximizing solar power integration.
	D		• Can work with all solar field technologies and HTFs. • Highest fuel saving per MW of solar thermal power. • Highest ISCC efficiency achieved among fuel-saving cases. • Recommended for fuel-saving operation.
Power boosting	A		• Parabolic dish reflector or heliostat field collector technology must be used. • Parabolic trough collector could be an alternative, but HTF must withstand high temperatures (molten salts). • Lowest power boosting per MW of solar thermal power. • Recommended if implementation at the top gas cycle is requested.
	B		• Heliostat field collector technology must be used. • Lowest power boosting per MW of solar thermal power. • Not recommended due to technology restrictions and low efficiency.
	C	Flowrate	• Can work with all solar field technologies and HTFs. • Highest power boosting per MW of solar thermal power. • Highest ISCC efficiency achieved. • Recommended for power-boosting operation.
		Parameter	• Can work with all solar field technologies and HTFs. • Low power boosting per MW of solar thermal power. • Not recommended.
	D	Flowrate	• Can work with all solar field technologies and HTFs. • Is clearly outperformed by flowrate option C. • Not recommended.
		Parameter	• Can work with all solar field technologies and HTFs. • Maximizes power boosting for solar power < 1.5 MW. • Recommended for low solar thermal power values.

Finally, the results of this work may be compared with relevant findings from the recent literature. Abdel Dayem et al. [28] found that the increase in DNI, due to changes in climate conditions, could increase steam turbine power by 10%. In the present work, it was found that with only 4 MW of solar power, the steam turbine power could be increased by 24.2% with a flowrate-boosting strategy. The results from Aghdam et al. [32] revealed an increase of 2% in the plant efficiency and from 714 to 728 MW in the plant capacity when the solar field was integrated before the superheater of the bottom steam cycle. In the present work, for the same integration point and with a flowrate-boosting strategy, power was boosted by 24.2%, and the cycle efficiency increased by 11.9%. Comparing the results of the present work with the work of Barigozzi et al. [22], it was also found that power-boosting strategies with solar integration at the bottom steam cycle performed better than those with integration at the top gas cycle. Behar [23] proposed PTCs with synthetic oil as HTF as the most efficient method for solar power integration at the bottom steam cycle. However, it was found that this technology is not suited for all types of solar integration at the bottom steam cycle (see case C for fuel saving). Nevertheless, PTC is the most suitable technology for most of the bottom steam cycle-integration cases. Elmohalawy [25] found an increase in thermal efficiency of 1.2% when steam was injected at the high pressure level. In the present work, the highest efficiency increase, 11%, was found when integrating solar power before the high-pressure superheater to heat saturated steam. Finally, Ameri and Mohammadzadeh [34] found an increase of 6 MW in power generation and a reduction of 10 g/kWh in carbon emissions when the solar field was integrated before the superheater of the bottom steam cycle for a total power output of 300 MW. In the present work, output power was boosted by 22 MW (24.2%) and 2.6 MW (2.82%) for flowrate and parameter boosting, respectively, and carbon emissions could be reduced by 3.5 g/kWh for total power outputs of 112.5 and 93.1 MW.

6. Conclusions

With the focus set on the optimization of the efficiency of combined cycles and a reduction in fuel consumption and carbon emissions, the integration of solar power in a real and existing combined cycle power plant was analyzed in this work. Using a thermodynamic model, it is possible to provide recommendations for solar power integration in combined cycles depending on the desired outcome. In this sense, the results from this work could be valuable for the specific retrofitting of existing combined cycle power plants with different technical or environmental constraints.

The integration of solar power increases the energy content of the cycle streams. Integration at the top gas cycle level may be constrained due to the higher temperatures and technical requirements of the solar field and heat transfer fluid. In this sense, integration should be performed after the compressor and before the combustion chamber to allow for the use of either parabolic dish reflectors or heliostat field collectors. However, high-temperature heat transfer fluids such as molten salts should be used. It is thus advisable to integrate solar power at the bottom steam cycle to also allow for the use of parabolic trough collectors and other heat transfer fluids.

Considering the effects of power integration on the cycle, if the objective is to integrate as much solar power as possible, then the best option is to perform the integration before the superheater of the steam cycle for fuel saving. If the aim is to increase overall cycle efficiency, the best option is integrating solar power before the steam cycle superheater with a flowrate-boosting strategy. If focus is set on reducing fuel consumption and avoiding carbon emissions, then a fuel-saving strategy by solar power integration before the economizer is the best option. Finally, if the objective is to boost power as much as possible, depending on the available solar resource, two different strategies are recommended. For small solar field sizes, a parameter-boosting strategy with solar integration before the economizer is the best choice. If there is no limit on the solar field size, flowrate boosting by integrating solar power before the superheater is the best option.

Future works could focus on the dynamic study of the ISCC configurations proposed in this work, coupling the model to a comprehensive solar database for different locations. Another research interest could be coupling the ISCC with a heat storage system to continue using renewable energy during the night. In addition, combinations of the proposed integrating positions could be studied at the same time and compared with the single-integration cases. Finally, a solar field design based on the maximum solar power to be integrated and an economic study could help to decide the best option for solar power integration for each particular situation.

Author Contributions: Conceptualization, I.S.-R. and A.M.-F.; methodology, A.M.A., A.M.-F. and I.S.-R.; software, A.M.A., A.M.-F. and I.S.-R.; validation, I.S.-R. and A.M.-F.; formal analysis, A.M.A., A.M.-F. and I.S.-R.; investigation, A.M.A., A.M.-F. and I.S.-R.; resources, A.M.-F. and I.S.-R.; data curation, A.M.A., A.M.-F. and I.S.-R.; writing—original draft preparation, A.M.A. and A.M.-F.; writing—review and editing, A.M.-F. and I.S.-R.; visualization, A.M.A., A.M.-F. and I.S.-R.; supervision, A.M.-F. and I.S.-R.; project administration, I.S.-R. All authors have read and agreed to the published version of the manuscript.

Funding: This research received no external funding.

Data Availability Statement: The original contributions presented in the study are included in the article material; further inquiries can be directed to the corresponding author.

Conflicts of Interest: The authors declare no conflicts of interest.

Appendix A. Detailed Results of Each Studied Configuration

Table A1. Original CC vs. ISCC (Case A and Case B) "Fuel saving".

Mass Flowrates	**Original CC**	**ISCC Case A**	**ISCC Case B**
Air to fuel ratio	50	53.39	53.39
Turbine gas flowrate (kg/s)	174.7	174.7	174.7
Air flowrate (kg/s)	171.28	171.49	171.49
Fuel flowrate (kg/s)	3.42	3.21	3.21
Fuel saving (%)	--	6.23	6.23
LP evaporator mass flowrate (kg/s)	5	5	5
HP evaporator mass flowrate (kg/s)	25	25	25
Operating temperatures	Original CC	ISCC Case A	ISCC Case B
Compressor inlet (°C)	24	24	24
Combustion chamber inlet (°C)	378	431	378
Gas turbine inlet (°C)	1174	1174	1174
Gas turbine outlet (°C)	549	549	549
Solar heat integration	Original CC	ISCC Case A	ISCC Case B
Integrated solar heat (MW)	--	10	
Cycle efficiency	Original CC	ISCC Case A	ISCC Case B
Gas turbine cycle (%)	39.84	39.85	
Combined cycle (%)	56.13	56.15	
Cycle power breakdown	Original CC	ISCC Case A	ISCC Case B
Compressor (kW)	62,450	62,450	62,450
Gas turbine (kW)	126,727	126,727	126,727
Gas cycle (kW)	64,277	64,277	64,277
Steam cycle (kW)	26,292	26,292	26,292
Total net power (kW)	90,569	90,569	90,569
Back work ratio (%)	49.279	49.279	49.279
Specific work per unit fuel mass flow (kJ/kg)	26,439	28,198	28,198
CO_2 emissions (Mt/year)	0.2971	0.2785	0.2785
CO_2 emissions saved (kg CO_2/kWh)	--	0.0064	0.0064

Table A2. Original CC vs. ISCC (Case C and Case D) "Fuel saving".

Mass Flowrates	**Original CC**	**ISCC Case C**	**ISCC Case D**
Air to fuel ratio	50	50	50
Turbine gas flowrate (kg/s)	174.7	168.59	160.7
Air flowrate (kg/s)	171.28	165.28	157.61
Fuel flowrate (kg/s)	3.42	3.3	3.15
Fuel saving (%)	--	3.49	7.97
LP evaporator mass flowrate (kg/s)	5	5	5
HP evaporator mass flowrate (kg/s)	25	25	25
Operating temperatures	Original CC	ISCC Case C	ISCC Case D
Compressor inlet (°C)	24	24	24
Combustion chamber inlet (°C)	378	378	378
Gas turbine inlet (°C)	1174	1174	1174
Gas turbine outlet (°C)	549	549	549

Table A2. *Cont.*

Solar heat integration	Original CC	ISCC Case C	ISCC Case D
Integrated solar heat (MW)	--	15	3
Cycle efficiency	Original CC	ISCC Case C	ISCC Case D
Gas turbine cycle (%)	39.84	39.84	39.84
Combined cycle (%)	56.13	53.06	59.79
Cycle power breakdown	Original CC	ISCC Case C	ISCC Case D
Compressor (kW)	62,450	60,266	57,471
Gas turbine (kW)	126,727	122,294	116,622
Gas cycle (kW)	64,277	62,028	59,152
Steam cycle (kW)	26,292	28,542	31,417
Total net power (kW)	90,569	90,569	90,569
Back work ratio (%)	49.279	49.279	49.279
Specific work per unit fuel mass flow (kJ/kg)	26,439	27,399	28,730
CO_2 emissions (Mt/year)	0.2971	0.2867	0.2734
CO_2 emissions saved (kg CO_2/kWh)	--	0.0035	0.0083

Table A3. Original CC vs. ISCC (Case A and Case B) "Power boosting".

Mass Flowrates	**Original CC**	**ISCC Case A**	**ISCC Case B**
Air to fuel ratio	50	53.2	
Turbine gas flowrate (kg/s)	174.7	185.68	
Air flowrate (kg/s)	171.28	182.25	
Fuel flowrate (kg/s)	3.42	3.42	3.42
LP evaporator mass flowrate (kg/s)	5	5	5
HP evaporator mass flowrate (kg/s)	25	25	25
Operating temperatures	Original CC	ISCC Case A	ISCC Case B
Compressor inlet (°C)	24	24	24
Combustion chamber inlet (°C)	378	430	378
Gas turbine inlet (°C)	1174	1174	1174
Gas turbine outlet (°C)	549	549	549
Solar heat integration	Original CC	ISCC Case A	ISCC Case B
Integrated solar heat (MW)	--	10	
Cycle efficiency	Original CC	ISCC Case A	ISCC Case B
Gas turbine cycle (%)	39.84	39.83	
Combined cycle (%)	56.13	55.19	
Cycle power breakdown	Original CC	ISCC Case A	ISCC Case B
Compressor (kW)	62,450	66,455	
Gas turbine (kW)	126,727	134,693	
Gas cycle (kW)	64,277	68,239	
Steam cycle (kW)	26,292	26,323	
Total net power (kW)	90,569	94,562	
Power boosted (%)	--	4.41	
Back work ratio (%)	49.279	49.33	
Specific work per unit fuel mass flow (kJ/kg)	26,439	27,605	

Table A4. Original CC vs. ISCC (Case C and Case D) "Flowrate boosting".

Mass Flowrates	**Original CC**	**ISCC Case C**	**ISCC Case D**
Air to fuel ratio	50	50	50
Turbine gas flowrate (kg/s)	174.7	174.7	174.7
Air flowrate (kg/s)	171.28	171.28	171.28
Fuel flowrate (kg/s)	3.42	3.42	3.42
LP evaporator mass flowrate (kg/s)	5	9.17	6.54
HP evaporator mass flowrate (kg/s)	25	45.84	32.72
Operating temperatures	Original CC	ISCC Case C	ISCC Case D
Compressor inlet (°C)	24	24	24
Combustion chamber inlet (°C)	378	378	378
Gas turbine inlet (°C)	1174	1174	1174
Gas turbine outlet (°C)	549	549	549
Inlet steam temperature (°C)	457	416.5	423
Pinch temperature (°C)	17.5	17.3	17
Economizer outlet temperature (°C)	228	192.5	254.5
Approach temperature (°C)	28	62	0.5
Operating pressures	Original CC	ISCC Case C	ISCC Case D
Inlet steam pressure (bar)	43	43	43
LP evaporator pressure (bar)	2.4	2.4	2.4
Condenser pressure (bar)	0.08	0.08	0.08
Solar heat integration	Original CC	ISCC Case C	ISCC Case D
Integrated solar heat (MW)	--	4	12
Cycle efficiency	Original CC	ISCC Case C	ISCC Case D
Gas turbine cycle (%)	39.84	39.84	39.84
Combined cycle (%)	56.13	68.03	56.93
Cycle power breakdown	Original CC	ISCC Case C	ISCC Case D
Compressor (kW)	62,450	62,450	62,450
Gas turbine (kW)	126,727	126,727	126,727
Gas cycle (kW)	64,277	64,277	64,277
Steam cycle (kW)	26,292	48,214	34,412
Total net power (kW)	90,569	112,491	98,689
Power boosted (%)	--	24.2	8.96
Back work ratio (%)	49.279	49.279	49.279
Specific work per unit fuel mass flow (kJ/kg)	26,439	32,840	28,810

Table A5. Original CC vs. Parameter boosting "Case C" (+10%, +20%, +30%, +40%, and +50%).

Mass Flowrates	**Original ISCC**	**ISCC "Case C" (Superheater)**				
		+10%	**+20%**	**+30%**	**+40%**	**+50%**
Turbine gas flowrate (kg/s)	174.7					
Air flowrate (kg/s)	171.27					
Fuel flowrate (kg/s)	3.42					
LP evaporator mass flowrate (kg/s)	5					
HP evaporator mass flowrate (kg/s)	25					
Operating temperatures	Original ISCC	+10%	+20%	+30%	+40%	+50%
Compressor inlet (°C)	24					
Combustion chamber inlet (°C)	379					
Gas turbine inlet (°C)	1174					

Table A5. *Cont.*

Mass Flowrates	Original ISCC	ISCC "Case C" (Superheater)				
		+10%	+20%	+30%	+40%	+50%
Gas turbine outlet (°C)			549			
Inlet steam temperature (°C)	491	491	490.5	490.5	490	489.5
Pinch temperature (°C)	19.3	19	18.5	18.2	17.9	17.5
Economizer outlet temperature (°C)	228	232.5	237	241	244.5	48
Approach temperature (°C)	26.5	27.5	29	30	31	32
Operating pressures	Original ISCC	+10%	+20%	+30%	+40%	+50%
Inlet steam pressure (bar)	2.4	2.64	2.88	3.12	3.36	3.6
LP evaporator pressure (bar)	43	47.3	51.6	55.9	60.2	64.5
Condenser pressure (bar)			0.08			
Solar heat integration	Original ISCC	+10%	+20%	+30%	+40%	+50%
Integrated solar heat (MW)			7			
Cycle efficiency	Original ISCC	+10%	+20%	+30%	+40%	+50%
Gas turbine cycle (%)			39.84			
Combined cycle (%)	54.97	54.89	54.81	54.72	54.63	54.54
Cycle power breakdown	Original ISCC	+10%	+20%	+30%	+40%	+50%
Compressor (kW)			62,450			
Gas turbine (kW)			126,727			
Gas cycle (kW)			64,277			
Steam cycle (kW)	28,265	28,128	27,987	27,843	27,694	27,539
Total net power (kW)	92,542	92,405	92,264	92,120	91,971	91,816
Power boosted (%)	2.18	2.02	1.87	1.71	1.55	1.37
Back work ratio (%)			49.279			
Specific work per unit fuel mass flow (kJ/kg)	27,016	26,976	26,935	26,892	26,849	26,804

Table A6. Original CC vs. Parameter boosting "Case C" (−10%, −20%, −30%, −40%, and −50%).

Mass Flowrates	Original ISCC	ISCC "Case C" (Superheater)				
		−10%	−20%	−30%	−40%	−50%
Turbine gas flowrate (kg/s)			174.7			
Air flowrate (kg/s)			171.27			
Fuel flowrate (kg/s)			3.42			
LP evaporator mass flowrate (kg/s)			5			
HP evaporator mass flowrate (kg/s)			25			
Operating temperatures	Original ISCC	−10%	−20%	−30%	−40%	−50%
Compressor inlet (°C)			24			
Combustion chamber inlet (°C)			379			
Gas turbine inlet (°C)			1174			

Table A6. *Cont.*

Mass Flowrates	Original ISCC	ISCC "Case C" (Superheater)				
		−10%	−20%	−30%	−40%	−50%
Gas turbine outlet (°C)			549			
Inlet steam temperature (°C)	491	491	491	491	491	490.5
Pinch temperature (°C)	19.3	19.7	20	20.5	21.	21.5
Economizer outlet temperature (°C)	228	223	218	212	205	197.5
Approach temperature (°C)	26.5	25	23.5	22	20.5	18.5
Operating pressures	Original ISCC	−10%	−20%	−30%	−40%	−50%
Inlet steam pressure (bar)	43	38.7	34.4	30.1	25.8	21.5
LP evaporator pressure (bar)	2.4	2.16	1.92	1.68	1.44	1.2
Condenser pressure (bar)			0.08			
Solar heat integration	Original ISCC	−10%	−20%	−30%	−40%	−50%
Integrated solar heat (MW)			7			
Cycle efficiency	Original ISCC	−10%	−20%	−30%	−40%	−50%
Gas turbine cycle (%)			39.84			
Combined cycle (%)	54.97	55.05	55.12	55.19	55.26	55.32
Cycle power breakdown	Original ISCC	−10%	−20%	−30%	−40%	−50%
Compressor (kW)			62,450			
Gas turbine (kW)			126,727			
Gas cycle (kW)			64,277			
Steam cycle (kW)	28,265	28,396	28,521	28,640	28,750	28,849
Total net power (kW)	92,542	92,673	92,798	92,917	93,027	93,126
Power boosted (%)	2.18	2.32	2.46	2.59	2.71	2.82
Back work ratio (%)			49.279			
Specific work per unit fuel mass flow (kJ/kg)	27,016	27,054	27,091	27,125	27,157	27,186

Table A7. Original CC vs. Parameter boosting "Case D" (+10%, +20%, +30%, +40%, and +50%).

Mass Flowrates	Original ISCC	ISCC "Case D" (Economizer)				
		+10%	+20%	+30%	+40%	+50%
Turbine gas flowrate (kg/s)			174.7			
Air flowrate (kg/s)			171.27			
Fuel flowrate (kg/s)			3.42			
LP evaporator (kg/s)			5			
HP evaporator kg/s)			25			
Operating temperatures	Original ISCC	+10%	+20%	+30%	+40%	+50%
Compressor inlet (°C)			24			
Combustion chamber inlet (°C)			379			
Gas turbine inlet (°C)			1174			
Gas turbine outlet (°C)			549			
Inlet steam temperature (°C)	534	534.5	535	535	535	534.5
Pinch temperature (°C)	15	15	14.5	14	13.5	13.5

Table A7. *Cont.*

Mass Flowrates	Original ISCC	ISCC "Case D" (Economizer)				
		+10%	**+20%**	**+30%**	**+40%**	**+50%**
Economizer outlet temperature (°C)	229	233	236	239.5	242	245
Approach temperature (°C)	25.5	27.5	29.5	31.5	33.5	35
Operating pressures	Original ISCC	+10%	+20%	+30%	+40%	+50%
Inlet steam (bar)	43	47.3	51.6	55.9	60.2	64.5
LP evaporator (bar)	2.4	2.64	2.88	3.12	3.36	3.6
Condenser (bar)			0.08			
Solar heat integration	Original ISCC	+10%	+20%	+30%	+40%	+50%
Integrated solar heat (MW)			1.5			
Cycle efficiency	Original ISCC	+10%	+20%	+30%	+40%	+50%
Gas turbine cycle (%)			39.84			
Combined cycle (%)	58.34	58.3	58.24	58.18	58.65	58.04
Cycle power breakdown	Original ISCC	+10%	+20%	+30%	+40%	+50%
Compressor (kW) Gas turbine (kW) Gas cycle (kW)			62,450 126,727 64,277			
Steam cycle (kW)	30,733	30,660	30,573	30,472	30,360	30,237
Total net power (kW)	95,010	94,937	94,850	94,749	94,637	94,514
Power boosted (%)	4.9	4.82	4.72	4.61	4.49	4.35
Back work ratio (%)			49.279			
Specific work per unit fuel mass flow (kJ/kg)	27,736	27,715	27,689	27,660	27,627	27,591

Table A8. Original CC vs. Parameter boosting "Case D" (−10%, −20%, −30%, −40%, −50%).

Mass Flowrates	Original ISCC	ISCC "Case D" (Economizer)				
		−10%	**−20%**	**−30%**	**−40%**	**−50%**
Turbine gas flowrate (kg/s) Air flowrate (kg/s) Fuel flowrate (kg/s) LP evaporator (kg/s) HP evaporator kg/s)			174.7 171.27 3.42 5 25			
Operating temperatures	Original ISCC	−10%	−20%	−30%	−40%	−50%
Compressor inlet (°C) Combustion chamber inlet (°C) Gas turbine inlet (°C) Gas turbine outlet (°C)			24 379 1174 549			
Inlet steam temperature (°C)	534	533	532	530	527.5	524.5
Pinch temperature (°C)	15	15.5	16	16.5	17.5	18
Economizer outlet temperature (°C)	229	225	221	216	211	205
Approach temperature (°C)	25.5	23	20.5	18	14.5	11
Operating pressures	Original ISCC	−10%	−20%	−30%	−40%	−50%
Inlet steam (bar)	43	38.7	34.4	30.1	25.8	21.5
LP evaporator (bar)	2.4	2.16	1.92	1.68	1.44	1.2
Condenser (bar)			0.08			

Table A8. *Cont.*

Mass Flowrates	Original ISCC	ISCC "Case D" (Economizer)				
		−10%	**−20%**	**−30%**	**−40%**	**−50%**
Solar heat integration	Original ISCC	−10%	−20%	−30%	−40%	−50%
Solar heat (MW)			1.5			
Cycle efficiency	Original ISCC	−10%	−20%	−30%	−40%	−50%
Gas turbine cycle (%)			39.84			
Combined cycle (%)	58.34	58.38	58.4	58.4	58.39	58.35
Cycle power breakdown	Original ISCC	−10%	−20%	−30%	−40%	−50%
Compressor (kW) Gas turbine (kW) Gas cycle (kW)			62,450 126,727 64,277			
Steam cycle (kW)	30,733	30,788	30,823	30,833	30,811	30,746
Total net power (kW)	95,010	95,065	95,100	95,110	95,088	95,023
Power boosted (%)	4.9	4.96	5	5.01	4.98	4.92
Back work ratio (%)			49.279			
Specific work per unit fuel mass flow (kJ/kg)	27,736	27,752	27,762	27,765	27,759	27,740

References

1. U.S Energy Information Administration "EIA". Energy Institute Statistical Review of World Energy. 2012. Available online: https://ourworldindata.org/ (accessed on 13 November 2024).
2. Enerdata. World Energy & Climate Statistics—Yearbook 2024. Available online: https://yearbook.enerdata.net/total-energy/world-consumption-statistics.html (accessed on 1 November 2024).
3. Shahabuddin, M.; Bhattacharya, S. Effect of reactant types (steam, CO_2 and steam + CO_2) on the gasification performance of coal using entrained flow gasifier. *Int. J. Energy Res.* **2021**, *45*, 9492–9501. [CrossRef]
4. Alam, M.T.; Dai, B.; Wu, X.; Hoadley, A.; Zhang, L. A critical review of ash slagging mechanisms and viscosity measurement for low-rank coal and bio-slags. *Front. Energy* **2021**, *15*, 46–67. [CrossRef]
5. REN21. Renewables 2023 Global Status Report: Energy Supply Module. 2023. Available online: https://www.ren21.net/wp-content/uploads/2019/05/GSR-2023_Energy-Supply-Module.pdf (accessed on 13 November 2024).
6. Statista. Global Data and Business Intelligence Platform with an Extensive Collection of Statistics. 2023. Available online: https://www.statista.com/ (accessed on 5 August 2024).
7. Imteaz, M.A.; Shanableh, A.; Rahman, A.; Ahsan, A. Optimisation of rainwater tank design from large roofs: A case study in Melbourne, Australia. *Resour. Conserv. Recycl.* **2011**, *55*, 1022–1029. [CrossRef]
8. Gielen, D.; Boshell, F.; Saygin, D.; Bazilian, M.D.; Wagner, N.; Gorini, R. The role of renewable energy in the global energy transformation. *Energy Strateg. Rev.* **2019**, *24*, 38–50. [CrossRef]
9. Zhu, L.; Fang, W.; Rahman, S.U.; Khan, A.I. How solar-based renewable energy contributes to CO_2 emissions abatement? Sustainable environment policy implications for solar industry. *Energy Environ.* **2023**, *34*, 359–378. [CrossRef]
10. Weldekidan, H.; Strezov, V.; Town, G. Review of solar energy for biofuel extraction. Renew. Sustain. *Energy Rev.* **2018**, *88*, 184–192. [CrossRef]
11. Tsoutsos, T.; Frantzeskaki, N.; Gekas, V. Environmental impacts from the solar energy technologies. *Energy Policy* **2005**, *33*, 289–296. [CrossRef]
12. International Renewable Energy Agency "IRENA". Future of Solar Photovoltaic. 2019. Available online: https://www.irena.org/-/media/Files/IRENA/Agency/Publication/2019/Nov/IRENA_Future_of_Solar_PV_2019.pdf (accessed on 25 October 2024).
13. U.S. Department of Energy. Solar Parabolic Trough. 2009. Available online: https://www1.eere.energy.gov/ba/pba/pdfs/solar_trough.pdf (accessed on 31 October 2024).
14. Rovira, A.; Montes, M.J.; Varela, F.; Gil, M. Comparison of Heat Transfer Fluid and Direct Steam Generation technologies for Integrated Solar Combined Cycles. *Appl. Therm. Eng.* **2013**, *52*, 264–274. [CrossRef]
15. The World Bank. Implementation Completion and Results Report (TF-91289) on A Grand in The Amount of US $49.80 Million to the Arab Republic of Egypt for the Kuraymat Solar Thermal Hybrid Project. 2012. Available online: http://documents.worldbank.org/curated/en/168831468332487486/Main-report (accessed on 13 November 2024).
16. Islam, M.T.; Huda, N.; Abdullah, A.B.; Saidur, R. A comprehensive review of state-ofthe-art concentrating solar power (CSP) technologies: Current status and research trends. *Renew. Sustain. Energy Rev.* **2018**, *91*, 987–1018. [CrossRef]

17. Sumayli, H.; El-Leathy, A.; Danish, S.N.; Al-Ansary, H.; Almutairi, Z.; Al-Suhaibani, Z.; Saleh, N.S.; Saeed, R.S.; Alswaiyd, A.; Djajadiwinata, E.; et al. Integrated CSP-PV hybrid solar power plant for two cities in Saudi Arabia. *Case Stud. Therm. Eng.* **2023**, *44*, 102835. [CrossRef]
18. Powell, K.M.; Rashid, K.; Ellingwood, K.; Tuttle, J.; Iverson, B.D. Hybrid concentrated solar thermal power systems: A review. *Renew. Sustain. Energy Rev.* **2017**, *80*, 215–237. [CrossRef]
19. Pramanik, S.; Ravikrishna, R.V. A review of concentrated solar power hybrid technologies. *Appl. Therm. Eng.* **2017**, *127*, 602–637. [CrossRef]
20. Wang, S.; Zhang, G.; Fu, Z. Performance analysis of a novel integrated solar combined cycle with inlet air heating system. *Appl. Therm. Eng.* **2019**, *161*, 114010. [CrossRef]
21. Barakat, S.; Ramzy, A.; Hamed, A.M.; El Emam, S.H. Enhancement of gas turbine power output using earth to air heat exchanger (EAHE) cooling system. *Energy Convers. Manag.* **2016**, *111*, 137–146. [CrossRef]
22. Barigozzi, R.; Franchini, G.; Perdichizzi, A.; Ravelli, S. Simulation of Solarized Combined Cycles: Comparison Between Hybrid GT and ISCC Plants. In Proceedings of the ASME Turbo Expo 2013: Turbine Technical Conference and Exposition, San Antonio, TX, USA, 3–7 June 2013; Volume 4. [CrossRef]
23. Behar, O. Solar thermal power plants—A review of configurations and performance comparison. *Renew. Sustain. Energy Rev.* **2018**, *92*, 608–627. [CrossRef]
24. Manente, G.; Rech, S.; Lazzaretto, A. Optimum choice and placement of concentrating solar power technologies in integrated solar combined cycle systems. *Renew. Energy* **2016**, *96*, 172–189. [CrossRef]
25. Elmohlawy, A.E.; Ochkov, V.F.; Kazandzhan, B.I. Thermal performance analysis of a concentrated solar power system (CSP) integrated with natural gas combined cycle (NGCC) power plant. *Case Stud. Therm. Eng.* **2019**, *14*, 100458. [CrossRef]
26. Elmohlawy, A.E.; Ochkov, V.F.; Kazandzhan, B.I. Study and prediction the performance of an integrated solar combined cycle power plant. *Energy Procedia* **2019**, *156*, 72–78. [CrossRef]
27. Rovira, A.; Abbas, R.; Sánchez, C.; Muñoz, M. Proposal and analysis of an integrated solar combined cycle with partial recuperation. *Energy* **2020**, *198*, 117379. [CrossRef]
28. Dayem, A.M.A.; Metwally, M.N.; Alghamdi, A.S.; Marzouk, E.M. Numerical Simulation and Experimental Validation of Integrated Solar Combined Power Plant. *Energy Procedia* **2014**, *50*, 290–305. [CrossRef]
29. Muñoz, M.; Rovira, A.; Montes, M.J. Thermodynamic cycles for solar thermal power plants: A review. *WIREs Energy Environ.* **2022**, *11*, e420. [CrossRef]
30. Javadi, M.; Jafari Najafi, N.; Khalili Abhari, M.; Jabery, R.; Pourtaba, H. 4E analysis of three different configurations of a combined cycle power plant integrated with a solar power tower system. *Sustain. Energy Technol. Assess.* **2021**, *48*, 101599. [CrossRef]
31. Hosseini, R.; Soltani, M.; Valizadeh, G. Technical and economic assessment of the integrated solar combined cycle power plants in Iran. *Renew Energy* **2005**, *30*, 1541–1555. [CrossRef]
32. Hajizadeh Aghdam, M.; Khoshgoftar Manesh, M.H.; Khani, N.; Yazdi, M. Energy, Exergy-Based and Emergy-Based Analysis of Integrated Solar PTC with a Combined Cycle Power Plant. *Int. J. Thermodyn.* **2021**, *24*, 17–30. [CrossRef]
33. Binamer, A.O. Al-Abdaliya integrated solar combined cycle power plant: Case study of Kuwait, part I. *Renew. Energy* **2019**, *131*, 923–937. [CrossRef]
34. Ameri, M.; Mohammadzadeh, M. Thermodynamic, thermoeconomic and life cycle assessment of a novel integrated solar combined cycle (ISCC) power plant. *Sustain. Energy Technol. Assess.* **2018**, *27*, 192–205. [CrossRef]
35. Achour, L.; Bouharkat, M.; Behar, O. Performance assessment of an integrated solar combined cycle in the southern of Algeria. *Energy Rep.* **2018**, *4*, 207–217. [CrossRef]
36. Manente, G. High performance integrated solar combined cycles with minimum modifications to the combined cycle power plant design. *Energy Covers. Manag.* **2016**, *111*, 186–197. [CrossRef]
37. Dolores, D.G.; Rafael, A.S.; Galileo, M.C. Estudio del acoplamiento de diferentes configuraciones de ciclo combinado con planta solar de canal parabólico. *Ing. Investig. Tecnol.* **2015**, *16*, 253–264. [CrossRef]
38. Egyptian Petrochemicals Company. Available online: www.egy-petrochem.com (accessed on 26 November 2023).
39. Math Works. MATLAB Software. Available online: https://www.mathworks.com/products.html?s_tid=nav_products (accessed on 13 November 2024).
40. Math Works. Ideal Air Toolbox. Available online: https://www.mathworks.com/matlabcentral/fileexchange/71269-ideal-air-properties-at-constant-pressure-1-atm (accessed on 19 April 2019).
41. Math Works. XSteam Toolbox. Available online: https://www.mathworks.com/matlabcentral/fileexchange/9817-x-steam-thermodynamic-properties-of-water-and-steam (accessed on 19 April 2019).
42. World Nuclear Association. Heat Values of Various Fuels. Available online: https://world-nuclear.org/information-library/facts-and-Figures/heat-values-of-various-fuels.aspx (accessed on 22 December 2023).
43. Bergman, T.L.; Lavine, A.S.; Incropera, F.P.; Dewitt, D.P. Heat Exchangers. In *Fundamentals of Heat and Mass Transfer*, 7th ed.; John Wiley & Sons, Inc.: Hoboken, NJ, USA, 2011; pp. 706–747.
44. "Recognized Document of the Regulation of Thermal Installations in Buildings (RITE)" Joint Resolution of the Ministries of Industry, Energy and Tourism, and the Ministry of Public Works. CO2 Emission Factors and Passage Coefficients to Primary Energy. Available online: https://energia.gob.es/desarrollo/EficienciaEnergetica/RITE/Reconocidos/Reconocidos/Otrosdocumentos/Factores_emision_CO2.pdf (accessed on 15 October 2023).

45. World Weather & Climate Information. 2023. Available online: https://weather-and-climate.com/average-monthly-hours-Sunshine,Alexandria,Egypt (accessed on 20 July 2023).
46. Solutia. Therminol VP-1: Vapor Phase/Liquid Phase Heat Transfer Fluid. Available online: http://twt.mpei.ac.ru/tthb/hedh/htf-vp1.pdf (accessed on 18 July 2021).
47. Ruegamer, T.; Kamp, H.; Kuckelkorn, T.; Schiel, W.; Weinrebe, G.; Nava, P.; Riffelmann, K.; Richert, T. Molten Salt for Parabolic Trough Applications: System Simulation and Scale Effects. *Energy Procedia* **2014**, *49*, 1523–1532. [CrossRef]
48. Barlev, D.; Vidu, R.; Stroeve, P. Innovation in concentrated solar power. *Sol. Energy Mater. Sol. Cells.* **2011**, *95*, 2703–2725. [CrossRef]
49. Kalogirou, S.A. Solar thermal collectors and applications. *Prog. Energy Combust. Sci.* **2004**, *30*, 231–295. [CrossRef]

processes

MDPI

Article

Design and Technical-Economic-Environmental Evaluation of a Biorefinery Using Non-Marketable Edible Mushroom Waste

Brenda Lazaro-Molina [1] and Teresa Lopez-Arenas [2,*]

[1] Posgrado en Ciencias Naturales e Ingeniería, Universidad Autónoma Metropolitana—Cuajimalpa, Av. Vasco de Quiroga 4871, Mexico City 05348, Mexico
[2] Departamento de Procesos y Tecnología, Universidad Autónoma Metropolitana—Cuajimalpa, Av. Vasco de Quiroga 4871, Mexico City 05348, Mexico
* Correspondence: mtlopez@cua.uam.mx

Abstract: Edible mushrooms are gaining popularity as functional foods, not only for their distinctive taste and subtle flavor but also for their potential health benefits. They are rich in essential nutrients, including carbohydrates, proteins, fiber, minerals, and vitamins. However, it is estimated that up to 30% of total mushroom production generates non-marketable waste, which is currently used as animal feed, fertilizer, or compost. From a circular economy perspective, the objective of this work is to propose a conceptual design for a biorefinery to produce high-value-added products from non-marketable edible mushroom waste and to conduct a comprehensive assessment using modeling and simulation tools for process engineering. The general approach first involves identifying high-potential products, then determining the best processing routes, followed by developing a process flowsheet diagram for a case study (*A. bisporus*), and ultimately conducting a comprehensive assessment of the biorefinery to evaluate its sustainability. As a result, the proposed biorefinery may produce chitin, citric acid, and fertilizer, demonstrating the technical feasibility of waste valorization in terms of product yields, with positive profitability in terms of the rate of return on investment and payback period, and low environmental impact in terms of water and energy consumption as well as CO_2 emissions.

Keywords: biorefinery; technical-economic-environmental evaluation; process modeling; process simulation; circular economy

1. Introduction

It is estimated that there are around 2.3 to 3.8 million species of fungi in the world. In particular, there are around 140,000 species of macromycetes (such as edible, medicinal, hallucinogenic, and poisonous mushrooms), of which only between 14,000 and 21,000 have been taxonomically characterized, and around 10 species have reached an industrial scale of production [1]. A dramatic acceleration of the total production of cultivated mushrooms worldwide has occurred in the last decades; for example, annual production was 0.90 million tons in 1975, 2.18 million tons in 1986, 6.16 million tons in 1997, 7 million tons in 1999 [2], reaching a global production of 48 million tons in 2022 [3]. The most widely cultivated and consumed edible mushroom worldwide is *Agaricus bisporus* (with an estimated annual production of 2 and 4 million tons in 1997 and 2009, respectively), followed by *Lentinus edodes*, *Pleurotus* spp. and *Flammulina velutipes*. China is the largest producer of champignon or button mushrooms (*A. bisporus*) and oyster mushrooms (*Pleurotus* spp.) in the world, while Mexico is the main producer in Latin America [1,4].

Non-marketable edible mushrooms (NEM) primarily include waste from (a) mushroom cultivation that cannot be sold, such as damaged, undersized, or diseased mushrooms, trimmings like stems, and spoiled mushrooms (between 5% and 20% of farm production [5]), and (b) spoiled mushrooms that have deteriorated due to improper storage, transport, or extended shelf life. Therefore, the amount of NEM generated could be up to 30% of total mushroom production. Currently, this waste material is repurposed for animal feed, fertilizer, or compost. Despite the negative physical characteristics of NEM, the basic composition of mushrooms remains intact. Thus, NEM could be valorized due to its bioactive components, as edible mushrooms are quite rich in carbohydrates (such as glucans, hemicelluloses, chitin, among others), proteins, minerals, vitamins, and fiber, while being low in fat and containing a significant amount of essential fatty acids. It is important to note that spent mushroom substrate (SMS), which is the lignocellulosic material remaining after mushroom harvesting, is another important form of mushroom waste; however, it is not considered part of NEM waste, as it has a different composition and characteristics.

From a circular economy perspective, NEM could be transformed into several bioproducts (such as biofuels, bioenergy, biopolymers, organic and amino acids, etc.), reusing, recycling, and valorizing waste, thereby bringing economic, social, and environmental benefits. This is possible through the implementation of facilities such as biorefineries that allow for the separation of bioactive compounds present in mushrooms and their transformation into bioproducts using chemical and biotechnological processes.

There are currently numerous reports of the reuse of SMS [3], the development of biorefineries that use SMS for valorization, mainly in biofuels such as bioethanol [6], and the conceptualization of the recovery of bioactive compounds from NEM [5]. However, to our knowledge, the design and evaluation of biorefineries that use NEM waste as feedstock have not been reported. For this reason, the purpose of this work is to promote research for the development and evaluation of biorefineries based on the use of NEM waste through bioprocess modeling and simulation. In particular, non-marketable button mushrooms (*A. bisporus*) are considered as a case study, determining the synthesis and design of a proposed biorefinery for the recovery of chitin and the additional production of citric acid and animal feed, as well as performing parametric sensitivity analyses to study the effects on profitability and sustainability. The results of the technical-economic-environmental evaluation are relevant for decision-making at an early stage of biorefinery design.

2. Methodology

The general methodology followed for the development of a biorefinery based on NEM waste is summarized in Figure 1. In the following sections, details of each of the steps involved will be provided.

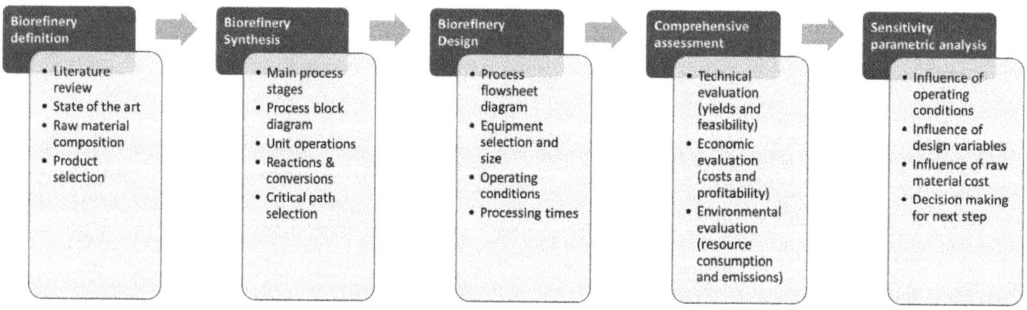

Figure 1. Methodology implemented for the modeling and simulation of a biorefinery.

2.1. *Raw Material: NEM Waste (A. bisporus)*

Mushrooms contain a high percentage of moisture, depending on the harvest, growth, and storage conditions. For the case study of this work, *A. bisporus* (button mushroom) is considered because it is the most cultivated and consumed mushroom, for which a composition has been reported [4] as follows: moisture 91.27%, carbohydrates 6.46% (including polysaccharides, glucans, chitin, hemicelluloses, and pectic substances), proteins 1.23%, fatty acids 0.19% (mainly linoleic, stearic, palmitic, and oleic), tocopherols (0.005%), and ash 0.845% (including minerals such as potassium, sodium, iron, copper, zinc, magnesium, and selenium). The chitin content in *A. bisporus* was reported as 4.69% on dry basis, which is significantly higher than that of other mushrooms [7]. While the glucan content was reported as 10.05% on a dry basis (with 1.54% α-glucan and 8.51% β-glucan, of which 54–82% is insoluble and 16–46% is soluble) [8]. For biorefinery simulation purposes, the composition of the NEM waste is adjusted to a moisture content of 90.0%, such that the remainder is assumed to be 1.00% glucan, 0.47% chitin, 5.93% other carbohydrates, 1.41% proteins, 0.22% fat, and 0.97% other solids.

An important aspect is the acquisition cost of NEM waste; however, to date, no value has been found reported commercially or in the literature. In Mexico, NEM waste is usually free, as it is often considered waste. In some cases, producers may even pay to dispose of this waste or offer incentives to those who collect it for other uses. However, if it were used for biorefineries, its acquisition cost could be estimated based on the costs of collection, transportation, and treatment. These, in turn, can vary considerably depending on several factors, such as geographic location, waste quality, demand, and availability [9]. Based on reported cases of agro-industrial waste used in biorefineries and taking into account all the aspects mentioned, the cost of NEM waste could range from 0.1 to 0.6 USD/kg.

2.2. Product Selection

2.2.1. Chitin

Mushrooms contain chitin in their cell walls, which is a polysaccharide and a precursor for obtaining chitosan, widely used in various industries (agriculture, food, environmental, pharmaceutical, and health) due to its biocompatibility, biodegradability, and non-toxicity. The global chitosan market will reach a value of around USD 12 billion in 2023 and is estimated to grow by 21% annually over the next decade [10]. One of the key trends driving market growth is the technological advancement in chitosan production, mainly in chitin extraction processes. It is important to mention that the traditional method of obtaining chitin is through its extraction from crustacean shells (such as shrimp and crabs). Although the fungal chitin content is lower than that of crustacean chitin, it is not limited by seasonal and regional variation, and its extraction does not require the aggressive acid treatment that crustacean chitin requires for purification and demineralization. Therefore, fungal chitin extraction is a less aggressive process and has lower energy consumption [11].

2.2.2. Bioproducts

Bioproducts are the result of the application of industrial biotechnology through physical, chemical, and biological processes, including biofuels (such as bioethanol, biodiesel or biogas), biopolymers (such as polyhydroxybutyrate—PHB—or polylactic acid—PLA—), amino acids (such as L-lysine or L-threonine), enzymes (such as xylanase or alpha-amylase), organic acids (such as citric acid or succinic acid), food precursors (such as baker's yeast or sorbitol), bioenergy (thermal or electrical energy), etc. Thus, part of the carbohydrates contained in NEM waste can be transformed into glucose, and this can be fermented by microorganisms to generate many of the bioproducts mentioned.

In particular, in this work, citric acid is selected as one of the bioproducts with high potential to valorize NEM waste. Citric acid is one of the most widely used organic acids due to its flavor, low toxicity, antioxidant, and buffering properties. Global citric acid production reached 2.70 million tons in 2024, and its demand is expected to grow at a rate of approximately 4% per year in the following decade [12]. The highest demand for citric acid is in the food industry (approximately 70%), but it also has wide applications in the pharmaceutical, cosmetic, and cleaning industries [13].

Although citric acid can be obtained through chemical synthesis, it represents higher costs and lower yields compared to those obtained by microbial fermentation. Citric acid can be produced by different fermentation methods (surface, submerged, or solid state) and different microorganisms. However, this work only considers mature processing technologies and industrially tested microorganisms. Therefore, the production of citric acid by submerged fermentation using the fungus *Aspergillus niger* in glucose-rich media will be considered since it has been reported that around 80% of citric acid is produced industrially in the world with this method [13].

2.2.3. Animal Feed

Animal feed consists of a mixture of raw materials that can come from plant, animal, and mineral sources, with the purpose of obtaining a nutritious diet for animals. There are two types of feed: complete and complementary. Complete animal feed provides all the nutrients required in its diet, while complementary animal feed is formulated to be combined with other raw materials such as forage. One of the most important nutritional parameters in animal feed formulations is the protein content, whose recommendation is in the range of 3–6%. Furthermore, if the animal feed comes from vegetable waste, it is suggested that the water content should be less than 12% or as necessary to maintain its quality during its shelf life [14].

In particular, the main source of vegetable protein for livestock feed is soy, so the search for other protein sources is of great interest. Both mushrooms and NEM constitute an important source of protein, which makes them suitable to be considered directly as raw materials in the preparation or formulation of animal feed. However, another protein source is the biomass generated at the end of a fermentation culture, which is also rich in protein and consists mainly of microbial growth. Since this work proposes the production of citric acid by fermentation of glucose (recovered from NEM waste) using *Aspergillus niger*, the residual biomass after fermentation could also be considered as a by-product for sale as complementary animal feed. The yield and productivity of animal feed will depend on the operating conditions of the citric acid fermentation process and the drying techniques.

2.2.4. Bioenergy

Industrial processes are energy-intensive, which underlines the importance of exploring alternative ways of obtaining renewable energy from biomass. From an energy perspective, biomass is assumed to be any renewable resource derived from organic matter, whether of animal or plant origin, generated through photosynthesis and that can be used in the production of value-added materials and bioenergy. In this context, NEM waste can be considered as biomass suitable for bioenergy production, either in the form of thermal and electrical energy.

NEM waste can be subjected to various processes, such as anaerobic digestion, fermentation, combustion, or gasification to be transformed into biofuels (biogas, bioethanol, biodiesel, among others) or steam, which can drive generators for the production of electricity. This could have a positive impact on the industry, as it provides a renewable energy source that would cover energy needs and contribute to reducing associated costs. It would also represent a sustainable alternative to the limited availability of fossil fuels, contributing to the reduction of greenhouse gas emissions such as CO_2 [15].

2.3. *Biorefinery Synthesis*

Once the raw material and products have been defined, alternatives are proposed with different reaction routes, technologies, and process configurations that can carry out the chemical and biological conversion of NEM waste efficiently. Under this vision, a process block diagram was built for the conceptual representation of the biorefinery (Figure 2), where the general overview of the processes that can be carried out for the valorization of NEM waste can be seen.

As can be seen in Figure 2, the conceptual design of the biorefinery proposes the generation of new products with high added value that can enter other marketing and/or production chains. Among these products are the following:

- Biogas, obtained from the anaerobic digestion of NEM waste;
- Chitin, precursor of chitosan, through extraction treatments;
- Bioproducts, generated through the fermentation process of converted sugars;

- Biofertilizer, organic waste from enzymatic or fermentation processes;
- Animal feed, produced by drying the residual biomass from the fermentation process;
- Bioenergy (steam and electricity) through the cogeneration of organic waste, and
- Treated water, through recycling in a wastewater treatment plant (WWTP), with the aim of achieving a sustainable process with zero waste.

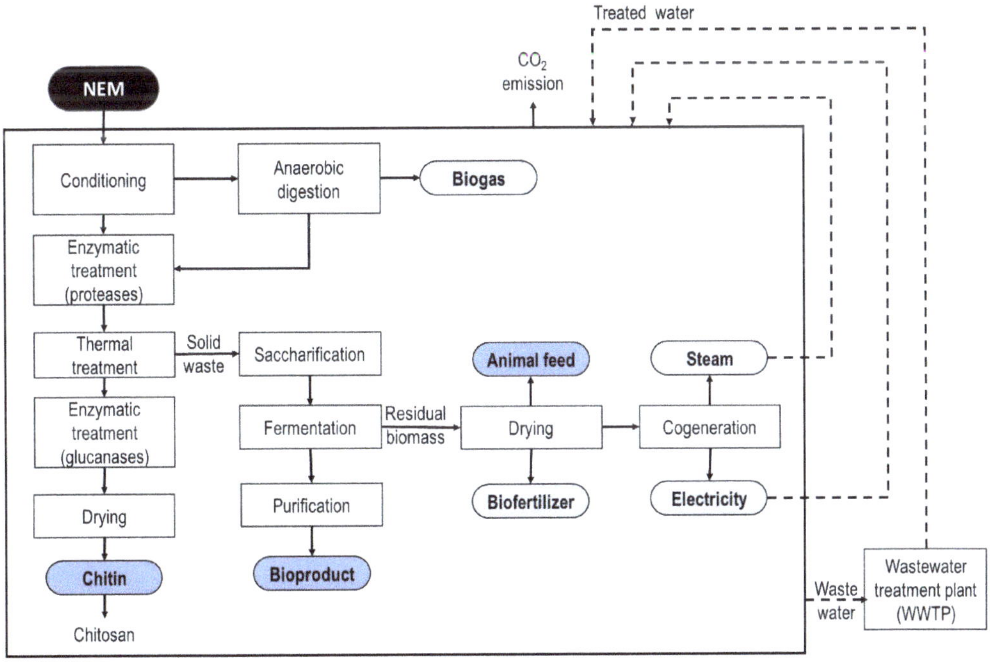

Figure 2. Conceptual biorefinery using NEM as the main raw material (the rectangles indicate the processes, and the ovals represent the raw material and the possible products).

To delimit the scope of this contribution, from the general diagram presented in Figure 2, a selection of the critical path of the processes to be implemented was made, considering as the potential products: chitin, citric acid, and animal feed. For the extraction of chitin, stages of conditioning of the raw material and enzymatic (using proteases and glucanases) treatments will be considered. Subsequently, a thermal treatment is carried out that will favor the separation of soluble glucans, with the aim of obtaining fermentable sugars (mainly glucose). Then, the bioproduct can be produced through fermentation with selected microorganisms, followed by a purification stage. Finally, the residual biomass generated after fermentation will undergo a drying process for sale as animal feed.

2.4. Biorefinery Design

The biorefinery design focuses on the detail of the selection of unit operations, the specification of each of the pieces of equipment, the operating conditions, and the control parameters (such as processing times) that are needed to carry out the proposed process. Figure 3 shows the flowsheet diagram of the biorefinery implemented in SuperPro Designer (modular process simulator), which is divided into four sections: 01 Conditioning, 02 Chitin extraction, 03 Saccharification and fermentation, 04 Animal feed purification, and 05 Citric acid purification.

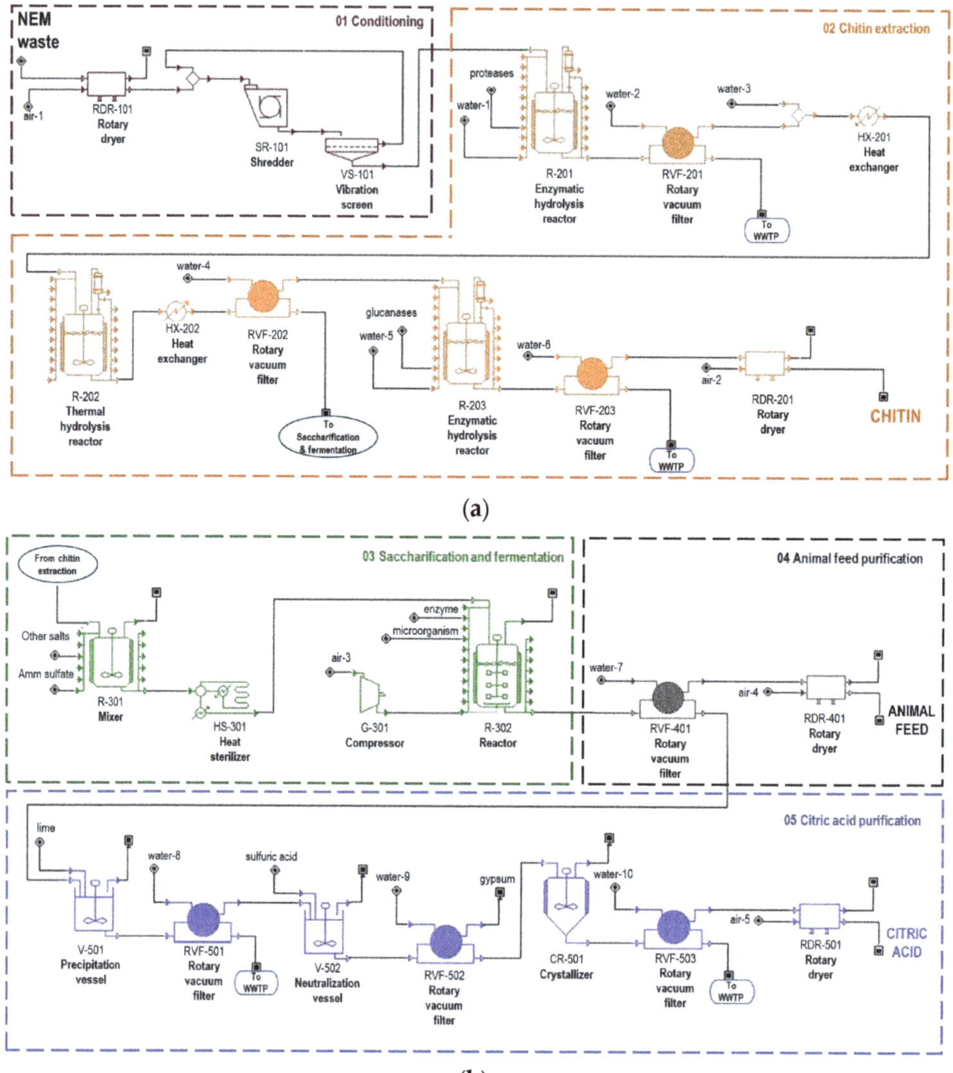

Figure 3. Process flowsheet diagram for: (**a**) chitin production; (**b**) animal feed and citric acid production.

2.4.1. Conditioning Area

In order to stabilize the raw material and prevent its deterioration, NEM waste is subjected to a drying process. The objective of the conditioning section is to obtain a fine powder (flour) from the NEM waste that enters a rotary dryer (RDR-101), then a shredder (SR-101), and subsequently a vibrating screen (VS-101) that has a recirculation system to return the raw material that does not meet the appropriate particle size to the beginning of the section.

2.4.2. Chitin Extraction Section

The unit operations for chitin recovery were adapted based on previously reported operating conditions [11]. First, an enzymatic treatment is performed on the NEM flour in a reactor (R-201), adding enzymes (proteases) for deproteinization. The hydrolysate obtained is passed through a filter (RVF-201) obtaining supernatant 1 (soluble or hydrolyzed material that is sent to the WWTP) and precipitate 1 (insoluble material, or fraction enriched in chitin and glucans). Precipitate 1 is mixed with a stream of water and enters a heater (HX-201), to be incorporated into the reactor (R-202), where thermal hydrolysis is performed to extract compounds such as lipids, minerals, vitamins, and remaining proteins. The output stream from this reactor passes through a cooler and is transferred to a filter to be separated into two streams: supernatant 2 (which will be transferred to the saccharification and fermentation stage) and precipitate 2. The latter contains the chitin-glucan complex and other unreacted insoluble solids, which enter the next reactor (R-203) to be subjected to enzymatic hydrolysis by glucanases, in order to separate this complex. The fraction enriched with chitin is separated by a filter (RVF-203), which will be subjected to a drying process (RDR-201) to reach a final humidity percentage of 0.10% and a chitin purity of approximately 80%.

2.4.3. Saccharification and Fermentation Section

The supernatant stream 2 from the chitin extraction section enters a tank (R-301) to be mixed with the nutrients. The mixture is sterilized (HS-301) and transferred to the fermentation reactor (R-302), where the saccharification process is carried out (addition of beta-glucanases) to achieve the conversion to glucose, and later in the same reactor, the fermentation process is carried out (addition of *A. niger* and oxygen) to obtain citric acid in the liquid phase. The operating conditions were taken from the work reported by [16].

2.4.4. Animal Feed Purification Section

Once the fermentation process is complete, the generated biomass (rich in proteins) is removed by filtration (RVF-401). Once separated, it is subjected to a drying stage (RDR-401) to obtain dry animal feed in order to prevent the growth of microbiological contamination in the final product before it is packaged and distributed.

2.4.5. Citric Acid Purification Section

For this section, the operating conditions were taken from a previous work [17]. The clarified liquid from the fermentation reactor (R-302) is taken to a neutralizing tank (V-501), where $Ca(OH)_2$ is added to precipitate calcium citrate. The latter is separated by means of a rotary filter (RVF-501), and the filter cake is acidified with dilute sulfuric acid to form a calcium sulfate precipitate (gypsum). Citric acid is separated from the gypsum by filtration (RVF-502) to be concentrated and crystallized (CR-501). The crystals are separated again by filtration (RVF-502) and subsequently passed through a dryer (RDR-501). Finally, a product of citric acid crystals with a humidity of 0.5% is obtained. The aqueous waste from the entire process must be sent to a WWTP for recirculation (although the process is not included in this simulation study, the operating costs are considered for its evaluation).

2.5. *Comprehensive Assessment*

Conducting technical-economic and environmental analyses is essential to assess the viability, profitability, and sustainability of the proposed biorefinery. These studies usually integrate process modeling, engineering design, and comprehensive evaluation through process simulation tools, which allow identifying critical points and financial risks at an early stage of development for decision making. For this purpose, evaluation parameters are established that allow us to compare design configurations with different plant scenarios at the industrial level.

2.5.1. Technical Evaluation

To analyze the design and operation of the proposed biorefinery on an industrial scale, the following aspects are taken into account: mass and energy balances; the stoichiometry and conversions of the reactive processes, or their reaction kinetics; the sizing and occupancy times of the equipment, as well as the processing cycles; and the installed capacity of the plant. That is, all operational aspects that are necessary for its correct operation are evaluated. Thus, the following technical parameters are established in this study:

(a) The annual consumption of raw materials, to propose scenarios that allow verifying the input of raw material required and their availability to establish the logistics of collection and transfer.
(b) The production cycle time, as a measure of the efficiency of the production process, allows identifying downtime and bottlenecks to improve the process flow and increase productivity.
(c) Product yield per kg of raw material, as a measure to evaluate the efficiency of resource use, since it allows determining how much raw material is actually converted into the desired product and how much is converted into by-products or lost in waste.

2.5.2. Economic Evaluation

To determine profitability, an economic method without discounted cash flow is used, since it provides a quick evaluation of the economics of the process and is usually applied to make initial estimates when comparing alternative flowsheet diagrams in the synthesis phase of the process design [18]. Thus, in this work, to determine whether it is profitable or not, the following economic parameters are considered:

(a) The unit production cost (UPC), which includes the direct and indirect costs associated with the manufacture of the selected products. Direct costs include materials, labor and services (such as heat transfer agents and energy), and indirect costs include construction and installation of equipment, depreciation, maintenance, and general administration expenses. The lower the UPC value, the greater the economic benefit.
(b) The rate of return on investment (ROI), which provides a measure of the effectiveness of management and the ability of a company to generate a satisfactory return on investment. It is a criterion for forecasting profits and its acceptance value is between 15 and 20% [18].
(c) The payback period (PBP), which determines the time needed to recover the capital invested in starting up an industrial plant. The desired PBP must be less than 4 years; otherwise, the investment is considered unprofitable [18].

2.5.3. Environmental Evaluation

A successful industrial design depends not only on its profitability, but also on the rational use of resources and the reduction of waste, from a circular economy perspective. This type of assessment seeks to ensure that environmental implications are considered during the planning phase of projects, and that measures are taken to mitigate negative impacts. Environmental impact studies are applied at different stages of the design process, both in early development phases and in construction and implementation, as well as the evaluation of plans, programs, or public policies. For the purposes of this project, the parameters focus on general aspects of environmental sustainability that would affect climate change:

(a) Water consumption, as a measure of resource use and avoiding damage to surrounding ecosystems;
(b) Energy consumption, as a factor affecting global warming, and to identify the most energy-consuming processes and improve them in later design stages;
(c) CO_2 emissions, as a measure of the contribution of greenhouse gas (GHG) emissions.

It is important to note that water consumption is calculated in terms of process water demand (i.e., for dilution, washing, filtration, etc.); however, it is not a permanent demand (only initial) as the waste water is sent to the PWWT and recycled. While the water required for the heat transfer agent demand (i.e., steam and cooling water) remains in a closed loop, it affects global warming and contributes to CO_2 emissions due to the generation of steam in boilers.

2.6. Some Social Considerations

Increased mushroom cultivation could contribute to the development of new agriculture and meet consumer demand for healthy products. This can meet the three interrelated dimensions of sustainable development proposed by the United Nations Environment Program (UNEP): environmental, economic, and social. Therefore, the biorefineries for NEM valorization should be located, as much as possible, as an extension of the cultivation process in order to take advantage of the NEM waste on site, and thus not generate additional costs for its collection and transportation.

Aspects such as the climate of the geographical area must also be considered, since mushrooms grow at temperate temperatures (approximately 18 °C), so climates with large fluctuations will require the use of energy (for heating or cooling), which makes mushroom production more expensive. Another benefit of having the industrial biorefinery on-site would be to generate bioenergy from NEM waste that would allow mushrooms to be produced continuously under a controlled environment in greenhouses.

3. Results and Discussion

3.1. Base Case Assumptions and Evaluation

Technical, economic, and environmental assessments were performed using a commercial modular process simulator (SuperPro Designer). The industrial biorefinery was implemented in batch operation mode, with an annual operation time of 336 days. The implementation considers material loading, process operation, material unloading, and equipment cleaning times, as applicable.

To define the availability of NEM waste that will be fed to the biorefinery, the case of *A. bisporus* production in Mexico was considered, whose reported annual value was between 87,000–109,000 T [19], concentrated in six states of the country: Puebla with 30,000–36,000 T, Querétaro with 25,000–30,000 T, the State of Mexico with 15,000–20,000 T, Tlaxcala with 7000–10,000 T, Guanajuato with 5000–7000 T, and Jalisco with 5000–6000 T. Considering the state of Puebla with the highest production, and assuming 20% as NEM waste [5], then there would be approximately 7200 T/y of NEM. Thus, the technical evaluation was carried out using this reference value, obtaining the results for this *Base Case*:

(a) The batch size is 150 T/batch, giving an installed capacity of the plant of 7350 T/y of NEM waste.
(b) The recipe batch time is 437.4 h (18.2 days), processing 49 batches/year, and with a production cycle time of 156.2 h.
(c) Achieving a production of 44,333 T/y of chitin, 1109 T/y of citric acid and 3035 T/y of animal feed, equivalent to product yields of 6.03 kg chitin/kg NEM, 0.41 kg citric acid/kg NEM, and 3.57 kg animal feed/kg NEM. Chitin is the product with the greatest contribution, followed by animal feed and finally citric acid.

Additional assumptions for the economic evaluation included: all costs in US dollars, a 30% income tax, a 12-year depreciation period, a product selling price of 220 USD/kg for chitin [20], 2.0 USD/kg for citric acid [16], and 0.2 USD/kg for animal feed [17]. Costs for equipment, utilities, and other materials were estimated directly from the simulator database. As indicated in Section 2.1, the acquisition cost of NEM waste could vary in the range of 0.1–0.6 USD/kg. For cost-effectiveness purposes, the value of 0.60 USD/kg will be taken for the main case studies; at the end of this study, the influence of raw material cost in the range of 0.1–0.6 USD/kg will be analyzed. The economic parameters calculated for the *Base Case* were as follows:

(1) UPC = 295.49 USD/kg of product, which will be a reference value to compare subsequent configurations or scenarios.
(2) ROI = 3.0%, which is much lower than the recommended 20%, so it is not a satisfactory value.
(3) PBP = 33.3 years, which is much greater than 4 years, so it is not within the acceptable limit for the investment to be recovered.

Summarizing, the *Base Case* is not profitable according to the values established in Section 2.5.2. This aspect will be analyzed and improved with the profitability and parametric sensitivity analyses below.

As for the environmental parameters, the following were calculated for the *Base Case*:

(a) Process water consumption = 264.1 kg/kg of chitin, steam consumption = 0.35 T/kg of chitin, and cooling water consumption = 17.1 T/kg of chitin.
(b) Electricity consumption = 28.5 kW-h/kg chitin.
(c) CO_2 emissions = 0.13 kg/kg chitin.

These values are reported based on the installed capacity for chitin production (as it is the main product with the highest added value) and will be compared with other scenarios later on.

3.2. Equipment Occupancy Analysis

By analyzing the flow of materials and movements within the process (i.e., equipment occupancy), it is possible to identify downtimes, bottlenecks, and areas for improvement. This helps optimize movement paths, reduce delays, and streamline material handling. Figure 4a shows the equipment operation time schedule for the *Base Case* (each color corresponds to a batch operation), where long equipment downtimes are observed. The longest processing times are given by the saccharification and fermentation reactor R-302 (153 h), which is the main bottleneck, followed by the mixer R-203 for the preparation of the culture medium (98 h), and then by the enzymatic hydrolysis reactor R-301 (85 h). Therefore, to increase the occupancy times and reduce the downtimes, the number of reactors installed was increased in a staggered manner for the R-203, 301, and 302 equipment. The optimal equipment occupancy was achieved using a set of five staggered reactors, R-203, R-301, and R-302, as shown in Figure 4b. This modification, of course, impacts the amount of NEM waste processed as well as the profitability of the process, as will be discussed in the next section.

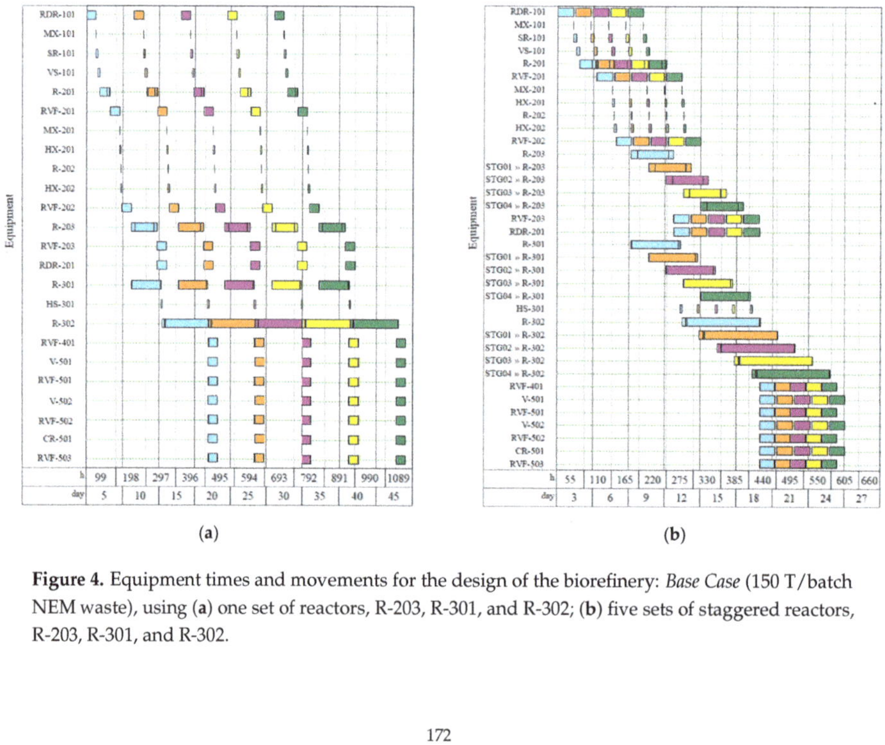

(a) (b)

Figure 4. Equipment times and movements for the design of the biorefinery: *Base Case* (150 T/batch NEM waste), using (**a**) one set of reactors, R-203, R-301, and R-302; (**b**) five sets of staggered reactors, R-203, R-301, and R-302.

3.3. Profitability Analysis

Once the process flowsheet diagram was implemented and the technical feasibility of the biorefinery was verified, a profitability analysis was carried out based on the amount of NEM waste processed and the set of staggered reactors implemented. The results are presented in Table 1, which shows the values of the economic parameters.

Table 1. Profitability analysis for the *Base Case* (chitin, citric acid, and animal feed production), varying the raw material input and the set number of staggered reactors, R-203, R-301, and R-302 (The grey highlights indicate the best case and NA means not available).

Set of Staggered Reactors	UPC (USD/kg)/ROI(%)/PBP (y)/C_{NEM} (T/y) * Batch Size (T/Batch NEM Waste) 50	100	150	200
1	390.1/−3.0/NA/2500	317.9/1.9/51.4/5000	307.3/3.0/33.3/7350	284.2/5.7/17.5/9800
2	305.1/2.7/37.8/4950	262.5/8.6/11.7/9900	243.8/11.8/8.5/14,700	228.6/15.5/6.4/19,600
3	278.2/6.7/15.0/7450	236.1/14.5/6.9/14,800	222.4/18.6/5.4/22,050	215.1/21.5/4.7/29,200
4	261.4/9.6/10.4/9900	227.6/17.8/5.6/19,700	215.6/22.7/4.4/29,400	211.8/23.2/4.3/33,200
5	252.3/11.9/8.4/12,400	219.1/22.1/4.5/24,600	212.2/24.6/4.1/32,700	215.1/21.3/4.7/33,200
6	256.8/10.7/9.4/12,450	222.5/20.2/5.0/24,800	217.1/21.3/4.7/32,700	218.4/19.5/5.1/33,200

* C_{NEM} is the annual consumption of NEW waste.

As can be seen, by fixing the feed quantity, as the number of reactors increases, the UPC decreases, reaching a minimum UPC value using five sets of reactors for feeds ≤ 150 T/batch, while for a NEM waste feed of 200 T/batch, the minimum UPC value is achieved with four sets of reactors. Likewise, the ROI and PBP reach satisfactory values (ROI greater than 20% and PBP around 4 years) with five sets of reactors. The optimum profitability value was achieved for 150 T/batch and five sets of reactors: UPC = 212.2 USD/kg, ROI = 24.6%, and PBP = 4.1 years.

3.4. Reduced Case Assumptions and Evaluation

From the technical-economic evaluation, two relevant results were detected: (1) the highest contribution in yield was chitin, followed by animal feed. The citric acid yield was very low, due to the low amount of fermentable sugars recovered, which in future work could be improved by optimizing the operating conditions or implementing a fed-batch mode. (2) Although the best scenario involves a batch size of 150 T of NEM waste, the annual consumption of NEM waste increased up to 32,700 T/y (see Table 1) by increasing to five sets of staggered reactors, which would be unfeasible for the *Base Case* studied, as all the NEM waste from Mexico would not be sufficient.

Therefore, a second *Reduced Case* is proposed for the design of the biorefinery, considering exclusively the chitin recovery section and omitting the rest of the products. Table 2 shows the results generated by different scenarios for this *Reduced Case*.

Table 2. Profitability analysis for the *Reduced Case* (chitin production), varying the raw material input and the set number of staggered reactors R-203 (The grey highlights indicate the best case).

Set of Staggered Reactors	UPC (USD/kg)/ROI (%)/ PBP (y)/C_{NEM} (T/y) Batch Size (T/Batch of NEW Waste) 10	50
1	242.3/14.4/6.9/2500	181.3/50.0/2.0/11,150
2	244.0/13.8/7.3/2500	179.6/54.2/1.9/12,700
3	245.8/13.2/7.6/2500	180.5/51.9/1.9/12,700
5	249.4/12.1/8.3/2500	182.4/47.8/2.1/12,700
1	242.3/14.4/6.9/2500	181.3/50.0/2.0/12,700

The evaluation indicates an improvement in terms of profitability parameters, with the best scenario being the process with 50 T/batch and implementing two sets of R-203 staggered reactors. For this scenario, the annual consumption of NEM waste required is 12,700 T/y, which is a more reasonable and feasible amount, as there would be several alternatives: (a) collecting NEM waste from two states (regions) of Mexico; (b) including not only the waste from the button mushroom (*A. bisporus*) but also the waste from other mushrooms, such as the oyster mushroom (*Pleurotus* spp.), as both of them are the most cultivated in Mexico; or (c) this proposal could be applicable to other countries with a higher production of mushrooms.

3.5. Technical-Economic-Environmental Assessment

The technical-economic-environmental report is presented in Table 3 for the most relevant scenarios studied. The first section of this table shows the technical report with the annual quantities of NEM waste consumption and generation of each product, as well as the product yields, as a measure of the valorization of NEM waste. As can be seen, the highest yield is achieved in the recovery of chitin, followed by the production of animal feed, and finally, citric acid. The production cycle time is also reported as a measure of the process downtime, which is sometimes optimized by increasing the number of staggered reactors (for example, Scenario 4 could not be improved by increasing the number of reactors).

Table 3. Technical-economic-environmental report for selected scenarios.

Concept	Scenario 1	Scenario 2	Scenario 3	Scenario 4
Biorefinery case	*Base Case*	*Base Case*	*Reduced Case*	*Reduced Case*
Batch size (T/batch NEW waste)	150	50	50	10
Set of staggered reactors	5	5	2	1
Technical report				
Annual consumption of raw material (T/y)	32,700	12,400	2550	12,700
Annual production of chitin (kg/y)	197,236	74,793	15,381	76,603
Annual production of animal feed (kg/y)	13,502	5286	-	-
Annual production of citric acid (kg/y)	116,772	44,284	-	-
Production cycle time (h)	35	31.2	31	31
Chitin yield (kg/kg NEM waste)	6.03	6.03	6.03	
Animal feed yield (kg/kg NEM waste)	3.57	3.57	-	-
Citric acid yield (kg/kg NEM waste)	0.41	0.41	-	-
Economic report				
Total investment (USD)	41,146,000	21,392,000	3,916,000	8,851,000
Annual operating cost (USD/y)	32,539,000	14,673,000	2,897,000	10,696,000
Annual revenues (USD/y)	43,628,252	16,544,086	3,383,780	16,852,553
Unit revenue cost (USD/kg)	284.5	284.5	282.9	282.9
UPC, unit production cost (USD/kg)	212.2	252.3	242.3	179.6
ROI, return on investment (%)	24.6	11.9	14.4	54.2
PBP payback period (y)	4.1	8.4	6.9	1.9
Environmental report				
Process water consumption (kg/kg chitin)	264.1	271.2	257.7	256.0
Steam requirement (T/kg chitin)	0.35	0.35	0.28	0.28
Cooling water requirement (T/kg chitin)	17.1	17.3	7.2	7.2
Electricity consumption (kW-h/kg chitin)	28.5	46.4	138.8	33.5
CO_2 emissions (kg CO_2/kg chitin)	0.13	0.13	0.0	0.0

Regarding the economic report, the second section of Table 3 summarizes some of the costs involved, such as total investment (calculated as the sum of direct fixed capital, working capital, and start-up cost), operating cost (calculated as the sum of raw material costs, labor, transfer agent services, electricity consumption, quality control, and waste disposal), and total revenues (sum of annual revenues from the sale of each product). These costs are used to calculate the unit revenue cost, as well as the previously defined economic parameters (UPC, ROI, and PBP). This report shows that Scenario 4 is the most profitable, requiring 12,700 T/y of NEM waste followed by Scenario 1, which requires a higher feed of 32,700 T/y of NEM waste. Depending on the available NEM waste, the alternatives would be the Scenarios 2 and 3, requiring a moderate feed (12,400/y) or low feed (7350 T/y) of NEM waste, respectively. Although these last two scenarios do not meet the recommended profitability parameters [18], they have positive values and could be considered acceptable, taking into account that waste is being valued.

Regarding the environmental report, the third section of Table 3 shows the values obtained for the environmental parameters for each scenario. According to the process water requirements, for all scenarios, there is a record of more than 250 kg of water per kg of chitin, which indicates that it is a process that uses a high amount of water. Therefore, it is essential to implement a WWTP within the industrial biorefinery to achieve a sustainable process with which the treated water could be reintroduced into the process, thus reducing the impact on the environment, in addition to representing an economic benefit by not having an additional charge for the disposal of aqueous waste. Concerning the use of heat transfer agents (steam and cooling water), the requirement is high in terms of thermal energy consumption and generation costs. Although these heat transfer agents are in a closed circuit, it would be highly advisable to perform a pinch analysis of the process to implement heat integration strategies that allow the optimization of these energy resources. Regarding electrical consumption, it is observed that it is one of the services with the highest demand in the process, detecting that the raw material conditioning section is the one that requires the highest consumption of the biorefinery, followed by the operation of the reactors. Some possible alternatives to reduce the electric demand include trying to reduce reaction times through research on more efficient enzymes or microorganisms, as well as research related to heat integration, or exploring other process conditions, i.e., using other extraction methods with shorter times to reduce negative effects on the environment. Finally, carbon dioxide emissions are very low for the *Base Case*, as they come only from the fermentation process of sugars to form citric acid. In the *Reduced Case*, as there are no fermentation processes, there are thus no CO_2 emissions. Although the use of energy resources involves the combustion of fossil fuels, which in turn involves the generation of CO_2, it must be considered that the CO_2 generated in this biorefinery would be absorbed in the growth cycle of edible mushrooms [21]. Therefore, in future works, it is recommended to evaluate the life cycle analysis (LCA) of CO_2 to determine carbon footprint fixation.

3.6. Profitability Analysis: Variation in the NEM Waste Cost

In Section 3.1, it was mentioned that the evaluation of the main case studies would be conducted with the maximum value of 0.6 USD/kg for the cost of acquiring NEM waste. However, this cost could vary between 0.1 and 0.6 USD/kg, so in this section as a final study, a parametric sensitivity analysis is carried out by varying this cost for the same scenarios already analyzed in Table 3. The corresponding results are shown in Table 4, where it can be seen that this sensitivity analysis has significant effects on the profitability parameters for each of the scenarios. As expected, better profitability values are achieved by decreasing the cost of acquiring NEM waste.

Table 4. Profitability analysis varying NEM waste costs for main scenarios.

Scenario	UPC (USD/kg)/ROI (%)/PBP (y)		
	NEM Cost (USD/kg)		
	0.1	0.3	0.6
1	105.6/54.3/1.8	148.2/42.2/2.4	212.2/24.6/4.1
2	146.9/32.4/3.1	189.6/24.0/4.2	252.3/11.9/8.4
3	73.0/111.6/0.9	115.6/87.7/1.1	242.3/14.4/6.9
4	135.6/38.3/2.6	178.3/28.6/3.5	179.6/54.2/1.9

It is relevant to mention that not all scenarios are profitable at a cost of 0.6 USD/kg NEM (noting that profitability is mainly achieved with ROI values > 20% and PBP < 4 years). All scenarios become moderately and highly profitable when the cost is 0.3 and 0.1 USD/kg NEM, respectively. These results highlight the importance of the acquisition cost of NEM waste, which will depend on the geographic location of the waste and the installation of the biorefinery (due to the effects of collection and transportation costs), the quantity and quality of the waste generated on agricultural farms associated with the biorefinery, the characteristics of the waste (for example, whether it has undergone drying, grinding, or other preparations), and, of course, on supply and demand.

4. Conclusions

The creation of alternatives for the synthesis, design, and operation of biorefineries that produce high added-value products from non-marketable edible mushrooms (NEM) waste represents a promising, profitable and sustainable option. In this work, a generalized conceptual design of a biorefinery was proposed, showing the processing routes and alternatives of added-value products that could be generated from NEM waste. Additionally, a comprehensive evaluation methodology and technical-economic-environmental parameters were presented that support decision-making to select a design or configuration, improve process efficiency, or even determine research points of greater interest. According to the analysis and the results obtained, the decision-making to select the best scenario for the biorefinery will depend on the availability of NEM waste. Scenario 4 was the best, with ROI = 54.2%, PBP = 1.9 y, requiring 12,700 T/y of NEM waste to produce only chitin, followed by Scenario 1, with ROI = 24.6%, PBP = 4.1 y, requiring 32,700 T/y of NEM waste to produce chitin, citric acid, and animal feed.

This work has been an initial investigation into the comprehensive evaluation of a biorefinery to valorize NEM waste. However, from a circular economy perspective, several aspects of improvement were identified to increase feasibility and profitability, as well as to reduce environmental impact, such as the following:

(1) Including secondary reactions and changing stoichiometries for reaction rates (such as Monod kinetics for fermentations, Michaelis–Menten for enzymatic reactions, etc.);
(2) Optimizing the operating conditions for each of the unit operations involved, which allows for improving product yields, reducing time and consumption of services (i.e., implementing new drying techniques);
(3) Improving product yields in reactors by optimizing operating conditions (i.e., pH, temperature, feed concentrations) and reducing reaction time by designing a fed-batch operation;
(4) Carrying out the synthesis of the biorefinery to analyze other bioproducts (for example, lactic acid or a biopolymer through sugar fermentation) or producing biofuels (such as biogas through anaerobic digestion or bioethanol through sugar fermentation);
(5) Studying the use of mixtures of various types of edible mushroom waste, which will allow for processing more raw material and achieving higher productions;
(6) Studying alternatives to reduce the consumption of services (such as the integration of heat to reduce steam and cooling water consumption);
(7) Reducing process water consumption by optimizing water resource use in rotary vacuum filters, or looking for filtering alternatives with lower consumption;
(8) Incorporating rigorous environmental impact studies, such as life cycle analysis, among others.

Supplementary Materials: The following supporting information can be downloaded at: https://www.mdpi.com/article/10.3390/pr12112450/s1, Table S1: Technical Report for Scenario 1; Table S2: Economic Report for Scenario 1.

Author Contributions: Conceptualization, B.L.-M. and T.L.-A.; methodology, T.L.-A.; software, T.L.-A.; validation, B.L.-M.; formal analysis, B.L.-M.; investigation, B.L.-M.; resources, T.L.-A.; data curation, B.L.-M. and T.L.-A.; writing—original draft preparation, B.L.-M. and T.L.-A.; writing—review and editing, T.L.-A.; visualization, T.L.-A.; supervision, T.L.-A.; project administration, T.L.-A.; funding acquisition, T.L.-A. All authors have read and agreed to the published version of the manuscript.

Funding: This research was funded by Conahcyt in 2024, grant number CBF2023-2024-3615.

Data Availability Statement: Data is contained within the article or Supplementary Material.

Conflicts of Interest: The authors declare no conflicts of interest.

References

1. Sande, D.; Pereira de Oliveira, G.; Aparecida Fidelis e Moura, M.; de Almeida Martins, B.; Nogueira Silva Lima, M.T.; Aparecida Takahashi, J. Edible mushrooms as a ubiquitous source of essential fatty acids. *Food Res. Int.* **2019**, *125*, 108524. [CrossRef]
2. Chang, S.T.; Miles, P.G. *Mushrooms: Cultivation, Nutritional Value, Medicinal Effect, Environmental Impact*, 2nd ed.; CRC Press: Boca Raton, FL, USA, 2004.
3. Viriato, V.; Carvalho, S.A.D.d.; Santoro, B.d.L.; Bonfim, F.P.G. A Business Model for Circular Bioeconomy: Edible Mushroom Production and Its Alignment with the Sustainable Development Goals (SDGs). *Recycling* **2024**, *9*, 68. [CrossRef]
4. Reis, F.S.; Barros, L.; Martins, A.; Ferreira, I.C. Chemical composition and nutritional value of the most widely appreciated cultivated mushrooms: An inter-species comparative study. *Food Chem. Toxicol.* **2012**, *50*, 191–197. [CrossRef] [PubMed]
5. Ramos, M.; Burgos, N.; Barnard, A.; Evans, G.; Preece, J.; Graz, M.; Preece, J.; Jiménez, A. *Agaricus bisporus* and its by-products as a source of valuable extracts and bioactive compounds. *Food Chem.* **2019**, *292*, 176–187. [CrossRef] [PubMed]
6. Leong, Y.K.; Ma, T.W.; Chang, J.S.; Yang, F.C. Recent advances and future directions on the valorization of spent mushroom substrate (SMS): A review. *Bioresour. Technol.* **2022**, *344 Pt A*, 126157. [CrossRef] [PubMed]
7. Nitschke, J.; Altenbach, H.J.; Malolepszy, T.; Mölleken, H. A new method for the quantification of chitin and chitosan in edible mushrooms. *Carbohydr. Res.* **2011**, *346*, 1307–1310. [CrossRef] [PubMed]
8. Khan, A.A.; Gani, A.; Masoodi, F.A.; Mushtaq, U.; Naik, A.S. Structural, rheological, antioxidant, and functional properties of β–glucan extracted from edible mushrooms *Agaricus bisporus*, *Pleurotus ostreatus* and *Coprinus attrimentarius*. *Bioact. Carbohydr. Diet. Fibre* **2017**, *11*, 67–74. [CrossRef]
9. Awasthi, M.K.; Sindhu, R.; Sirohi, R.; Kumar, V.; Ahluwalia, V.; Binod, P.; Juneja, A.; Kumar, D.; Yan, B.; Sarsaiya, S.; et al. Agricultural waste biorefinery development towards circular bioeconomy. *Renew. Sustain. Energy Rev.* **2022**, *158*, 112122. [CrossRef]
10. Expert Market Research. Global Chitosan Market Report and Forecast 2024–2032. Available online: https://www.expertmarketresearch.com/reports/chitosan-market (accessed on 1 October 2024).
11. Urbina-Salazar, A.; Inca-Torres, A.R.; Aguilar, M.D.P.C.; Palomas, J.B. Preparación de quitina fúngica a partir de subproductos de hongos comestibles (*Agaricus bisporus*). *Polo Del Conoc. Rev. Científico-Prof.* **2020**, *5*, 115–140.
12. Expert Market Research. Global Citric Acid Market Report and Forecast 2024–2032. Available online: https://www.expertmarketresearch.com/reports/citric-acid-market (accessed on 1 October 2024).
13. Wang, J.; Cui, Z.; Li, Y.; Cao, L.; Lu, Z. Techno-economic analysis and environmental impact assessment of citric acid production through different recovery methods. *J. Clean. Prod.* **2020**, *249*, 119315. [CrossRef]
14. San Martin, D.; Ramos, S.; Zufía, J. Valorisation of food waste to produce new raw materials for animal feed. *Food Chem.* **2016**, *198*, 68–74. [CrossRef] [PubMed]
15. Mignogna, D.; Szabó, M.; Ceci, P.; Avino, P. Biomass Energy and Biofuels: Perspective, Potentials, and Challenges in the Energy Transition. *Sustainability* **2024**, *16*, 7036. [CrossRef]
16. Heinzle, E.; Biwer, A.P.; Cooney, C.L. *Development of Sustainable Bioprocesses: Modeling and Assessment*; John Wiley & Sons: Chichester, UK, 2007.
17. Anaya-Reza, O.; Lopez-Arenas, T. Design of a sustainable biorefinery for the production of lactic acid from sugarcane molasses. *Rev. Mex. Ing. Química* **2018**, *17*, 243–259. [CrossRef]
18. Seider, D.W.; Seader, J.D.; Lewis, D.R.; Widagd, S. *Product and Process Design Principles: Synthesis Analysis and Desing*; John Wiley & Sons: New York, NY, USA, 2009.
19. SIAP (Servicio de Información Agroalimentaria y Pesquera). Estadísticas de Producción Agrícola. Champiñón Blanco (Agaricus bisporus). Secretaría de Agricultura y Desarrollo Rural (SADER), Gobierno de México. 2020. Available online: https://www.gob.mx/siap (accessed on 1 October 2024).
20. Pighinelli, L. Methods of Chitin Production a Short Review. *Am. J. Biomed. Sci. Res.* **2019**, *3*, 307–314. [CrossRef]
21. Robinson, B.; Winans, K.; Kendall, A.; Dlott, J.; Dlott, F. A life cycle assessment of *Agaricus bisporus* mushroom production in the USA. *Int. J. Life Cycle Assess.* **2019**, *24*, 456–467. [CrossRef]

processes

MDPI

Article

Preparation of Polyvinyl Alcohol–Chitosan Nanocellulose–Biochar Nanosilver Composite Hydrogel and Its Antibacterial Property and Dye Removal Capacity

Licheng Xie [1], Zhichao Zhang [1,2,3], Yucai He [2,*] and Yan Jiang [4,*]

[1] Changzhou University Huaide College, Jingjiang 214500, China; lichengxie@smail.cczu.edu.cn (L.X.); zhangzhichao9088@163.com (Z.Z.)
[2] School of Pharmacy & Biological and Food Engineering, Changzhou University, Changzhou 213164, China
[3] School of Chemistry and Chemical Engineering, Guangxi University, Nanning 530004, China
[4] School of Petrochemical Engineering, Changzhou University, Changzhou 213164, China
* Correspondence: yucaihe@cczu.edu.cn (Y.H.); jy@cczu.edu.cn (Y.J.)

Abstract: In this research, silver-loaded biochar (C-Ag) was acquired from a waste fish scale, and nanocellulose (CNF) was prepared from the waste wheat stalk. Then C-Ag was loaded into chitosan-polyvinyl alcohol hydrogel (CTS-PVA) with CNC as a reinforcement agent, and a novel nanocomposite material was acquired, which could be efficiently applied for antibacterial and dye removal. By plate diffusion analysis, the inhibition areas of C-Ag-CTS-PVA-CNF (C/CTS/PVA/CNF) hydrogel against *E. coli* ATCC25922, *S. aureus* ATCC6538, and *P. aeruginosa* ATCC9027 could reach 22.5 mm, 22.0 mm, and 24.0 mm, respectively. It was found that the antibacterial rate was 100% in the water antibacterial experiment for 2 h, and the antibacterial activity was more than 90% within 35 days after preparation, and the antibacterial rate was more than 90% after repeated antibacterial tests for five times. Through swelling, water adsorption, water loss rate, and water content tests, the hydrogel manifested good moisturizing properties and could effectually block the loss of water and improve the stability of the C/CTS/PVA/CNF hydrogel. The pseudo-first-order and pseudo-second-order models were built, and the adsorption capacity of hydrogel to dye was analyzed, and the dye removal was more consistent with the pseudo-first-order kinetic model. The best removal effect for Congo red was 96.3 mg/g. The C/CTS/PVA/CNF hydrogel had a remarkable removal efficacy on Malachite green, Methyl orange, Congo red, and Methylene blue. As a result, the C/CTS/PVA/CNF hydrogels had robust antibacterial properties and reusability. In addition, the present research developed a facile strategy for effectual dyes removal from the aqueous medium.

Keywords: antibacterial composite; antibacterial ability; composite hydrogel; dye removal; silver-loaded biochar

1. Introduction

To date, the rapid modern industrial development and the complexity of human life activities have accelerated the pollution of water resources, resulting in a series of problems such as bacteria, heavy metal ions, and dye pollution [1,2]. Polluted wastewater has become a carrier for the spread of diseases and cause harm to human health [3]. Accordingly, bacteriostatic materials have attracted the attention of researchers. Considering the tolerance of different bacteria and the safety of antibacterial materials, it is urgent to acquire a biocompatible and effectual antibacterial material with a wide application [4,5]. As a renewable resource, biochar is cheap and easy to acquire. The porous structure of biochar is extensively utilized as a carrier of nano-metal ions, which is often utilized in the field of adsorption [6,7]. Aquaculture and fish slaughter produce a large amount of fish scale waste [8,9]. They are commonly dumped into the sea or shipped to landfills because they have little commercial value. It is known that fish scale biochar (FSB) has a dense and porous structure [10], so making full use of the porous characteristics of FSB and reusing fish scale waste has become a hot topic.

Silver nanomaterials are extensively used in life because of their broad antibacterial properties and durability [11]. Silver nanoparticles (AgNPs) have a small particle size, which can be attached to the surface of materials and have the merits of a wide application range and low biological toxicity [12]. AgNPs may promote bacterial resistance because nanoparticles can contact directly with bacterial cell walls, altering charges around the cell membrane, resulting in cell membrane damage, leading to the leakage of intracellular compounds and bacterial death [13]. Although the antibacterial properties of silver-carrying biochar (C-Ag) are effectual and durable [14,15], the small particle size of C-Ag is not easy to recover and recycle, resulting in material loss [16]. Consequently, environment-friendly AgNP antibacterial materials with fast recovery and easy preparation have been extensively considered.

Chitosan (CTS) and its derivatives are natural polysaccharides extracted from chitin [17]. They have excellent antibacterial, biocompatible, biodegradable, and adsorption properties [18]. Polyvinyl alcohol (PVA) is a biocompatible and hydrophilic biomaterial [19,20]. PVA-based materials find extensive applications in drug delivery, fruit packaging, pollutant removal, etc. [21]. PVA evidences excellent hydrophilicity and is often utilized as a support for immobilizing antimicrobial agents [22], whereas the water-soluble degradation of PVA-based composite materials limits their applications. Wheat straw is a plentiful and renewable material with potential value and can be utilized for preparing biodegradable composite materials [23]. A large amount of wheat straw is acquired from agricultural production [24]. However, this renewable agricultural residue is often wasted through disposal or incineration [25]. Nanocellulose (CNF) can be extracted from wheat straw [26]. Cellulose is a plentiful and renewable carbohydrate. The good mechanical properties and biodegradability of CNF make it an ideal material for preparing polymer nanocomposites [27]. CNF is compatible with both PVA and CTS, and it substantially enhances the mechanical strength of PVA materials [28,29]. Research has showcased that CTS/PVA hydrogels exhibit a relatively low internal porosity [30]. The introduction of C-Ag and CNF into the hydrogel alters its pore structure and improves hydrophobicity.

In this research, CTS-PVA hydrogel was used as the matrix, C-Ag as the filler, and CNF as the enhancer to acquire C/CTS/PVA/CNF hydrogels. The incorporation of CNF enhanced the mechanical strength of hydrogel, while the loading of carbon biochar contributed to recycling and environmental pollution issues. The antibacterial properties of hydrogel were testified, along with the antibacterial mechanisms of hydrogel. The experimental data on dye removal were analyzed using pseudo-first-order and pseudo-second-order kinetic equations. Additionally, the stability and antibacterial efficacy of the hydrogel were examined after regular preparation. Milk-simulation experiments and cytotoxicity tests were conducted to assess the antibacterial capability of the hydrogel. The influence of CTS on the swelling ratio, water-loss rate, water content, water-absorption rate, and degradation performance of the hydrogel were testified. By establishing kinetic models, the removal capacity of C/CTS/PVA/CNF hydrogel was assessed. The hydrogel material manifested excellent antibacterial efficiency, outstanding physical properties, and removal ability, holding significant promising prospects for applications in antimicrobial and dye removal.

2. Materials and Methods

2.1. Materials

Silver nitrate, dimethyl sulfoxide (DMSO), chitosan (CTS) (molecular weight 1526.45), polyvinyl alcohol (PVA > 98.5%), glutaraldehyde ($C_5H_8O_2$: 50% in water), and other chemicals were from Shanghai Lingfeng Reagents Co., (Shanghai, China). Wheat straw and discarded fish scales are both sourced from the agricultural market in Changzhou (China).

2.2. Fish Scale Carbon Composite Material (C-Ag) Preparation

C-Ag was prepared as described previously [6]. Fish scales were soaked and rinsed in water, followed by boiling in water to further eliminate impurities. After drying, the fish scales were placed in a muffle furnace and calcined for 120 min at 300 °C. After cooling, the calcined fish scales were retrieved and ground into powder. Afterwards, 10 g powders were supplemented with a stirring solution of 200 mL of $AgNO_3$ (500 mg/L) and mixed for 120 min. A certain amount of sodium citrate (400 mg) was supplemented to the mixture to reduce Ag^+. The solution was then stirred magnetically for 1 day. After rinsing, filtering, and drying the solution, the biochar was loaded into a crucible and placed in a muffle furnace, heated to a predetermined temperature of 250 °C, and calcined for 120 min. Eventually, the fish scale carbon composite material (C-Ag) was ground into powder for further use.

2.3. Nanocellulose Extraction

Wheat straw was subjected to multiple washing cycles with water to remove soil or dust particles. The washed wheat straw was oven-dried (60 °C) for 12 h and further pulverized into 60-mesh of powders. Afterwards, dewaxing treatment was performed by soaking the pulverized wheat straw in ethanol liquid-to-solid mass ratio 10:1 for 6 h. The treated wheat straw fibers were rinsed several times with DI water and then dried to eliminate moisture from the fibers. A 3.0 g sample of dewaxed fibers was soaked with 90 mL of DI water, and a suspension was prepared by adding acetic acid (0.75 m) and sodium chlorite (4.5 g) buffer solution. The suspension was then subjected to leaching at 80 °C for 240 min, with additional replenishment of the acetic acid (0.75 mL) and sodium chlorite (0.75 g) buffer solution every hour. This step was repeated three times. The fibers turned whiter with longer bleaching time and were washed multiple times with DI water, maintaining a pH value of 7.0, followed by another round of drying. The dried fibers were soaked with 17.5 wt% of sodium hydroxide solution for 1 h, rinsed several times with DI water until neutral, and then dried entirely. After the alkali treatment, the fibers were milled to acquire uniformly sized cellulose nanofibers (CNF) (Figure S1, see Supplementary File).

2.4. Preparation of C/CTS/PVA/CNF Hydrogel

At room temperature, 1 g of chitosan (CTS) powder was dissolved in a 2 wt% solution of 50 mL ice acetic acid. Simultaneously, 1 g of polyvinyl alcohol (PVA) was added to DI water and mixed, followed by stirring in a water bath (90 °C) until entirely dissolved. Afterwards, 1.0 g/L of C-Ag and 0.05 g of cellulose nanofiber (CNF) were uniformly mixed in the CTS-PVA solution for 1 h. Then, 1 mL of glutaraldehyde solution was supplemented for gelation, and the mixture was stirred until hydrogel formation occurred. Eventually, the C/CTS/PVA/CNF hydrogel was acquired by allowing it to stand overnight in a refrigerator at 4 °C and stored for later use.

2.5. C/CTS/PVA/CNF Hydrogel Characteristics

The C/CTS/PVA/CNF hydrogel was dried in an oven (60 °C) to constant weight. FT-IR (Thermo Fisher Scientific, Waltham, MA, USA) was employed for qualitative and quantitative analysis of the dried C/CTS/PVA/CNF hydrogel within the range of 500–4000 cm^{-1}. SEM (SUPRA-55, Zeiss, Oberkochen, Germany) was applied to observe the surface morphology and structural features of the dried hydrogel composite material.

2.6. Antibacterial Testing

The antibacterial performance of the antimicrobial material was tested against *P. aeruginosa* ATCC9027, *S. aureus* ATCC6538, and *E. coli* ATCC25922. The antibacterial activity of the material was determined through the plate-counting analysis, and the antibacterial efficacy was assessed through the agar-diffusion method. A suspension of the bacteria (0.10 mL) was evenly spread on solid agar LB culture medium, forming holes with a diameter of 9 mm [31]. The C/CTS/PVA/CNF hydrogel (wet weight) at a quantity of 0.3 g was supplemented to the holes. The plates were then incubated at 37 °C for 1 day. Experimental data were recorded, and the antibacterial rate was given as below:

$$\text{Antibacterial rate } (\%) = \frac{N0 - N1}{N0} \times 100 \tag{1}$$

where $N0$ represents the colony number without inhibition $N1$ represents the colony number after inhibition.

2.7. Optimization C/CTS/PVA/CNF Hydrogel Composite and Its Antibacterial Ability

The hydrogel prepared by incorporating cellulose nanofiber (CNF) into the chitosan-polyvinyl alcohol (CTS-PVA) matrix was named C/P/F. The hydrogel prepared by combining CTS-PVA with C-Ag was named C/P/A. The hydrogel synthesized using CTS, C-Ag, and CNF was denoted as C/A/F. The hydrogel composed of PVA, C-Ag, CNF, and CTS was named C/P/A/F. The effects of C-Ag content and CTS solution concentration on the antibacterial efficacy of the hydrogels and the influencing factors were testified. The impact of different hydrogel combinations on the antimicrobial activity was observed using the agar-diffusion method. The optimal material combination was assayed by varying the C-Ag content (A content: 0.01, 0.05, 0.1, 0.2, 0.3, 0.4, 0.5, 0.6 wt%) and CTS concentration (C content: 1.0, 1.25, 1.5, 1.75, 2.0, 2.5 wt%).

The optimization of hydrogel dosage and incubation duration was conducted using *P. aeruginosa* ATCC9027, *S. aureus* ATCC6538, and *E. coli* ATCC25922 as test strains. The initial concentration of bacterial suspension for the plate-counting method was 10^8 CFU/mL [32]. The hydrogel (wet weight) was supplemented to the bacterial suspension at dosages of 0.5, 1.0, 1.5, 2.0, and 2.5 g/L. The antimicrobial hydrogel was entirely mixed with the bacterial suspension at 37 °C. Antimicrobial efficacy was assessed through the plate counting analysis.

Reusability is one of the important factors for assessing the practical application of antimicrobial materials [33]. The antimicrobial activity of the C/CTS/PVA/CNF hydrogel against *P. aeruginosa* ATCC9027, *S. aureus* ATCC6538, and *E. coli* ATCC25922 in water was assayed. Wet weight of 0.3 g of the C/CTS/PVA/CNF hydrogel was supplemented with a bacterial suspension (10^8 CFU/mL, 50 mL), and the bacterial count in the suspension was determined every 0.5 h after incubation. After each antimicrobial test, the hydrogel was washed and used for the next test. The antimicrobial efficacy of the hydrogel was assayed after eight cycles of antimicrobial experiments. The stability of antimicrobial materials is another important characteristic of their wide application [34]. C/CTS/PVA/CNF hydrogel was stored indoors, and its antimicrobial performance was tested at different storage durations (5–35 days). Antimicrobial effectiveness was recorded and analyzed for each test, evaluating the stability of the antimicrobial material.

2.8. Swelling Ratio, Moisture Content, Moisture Adsorption, and Water Loss of C/CTS/PVA/CNF Hydrogel

One of the important indicators for evaluating the performance of antibacterial gel materials is the swelling ratio in water. Different CTS contents (1.0–2.5 wt%) of C/CTS/PVA/CNF hydrogels were separately weighed at 100.0 mg. The hydrogels were immersed in DI water and retrieved every 60 min. The surface moisture was blotted dry with filter paper, and the mass was determined. The expansion rate was calculated as below:

$$\text{Expansion rate } (\%) = \frac{W2 - W1}{W1} \times 100 \tag{2}$$

where $W2$ represents the pellet weight after treatment, and $W1$ represents pellet weight before treatment.

Water content is a key indicator for evaluating their hydrogel moisturizing performance. The hydrogel water content with different CTS concentrations (1.0–2.5 wt%) was measured to assess their moisturizing performance.

The water uptake capacity is one of the important indicators for evaluating the daily storage performance of hydrogels [35]. Hydrogels with different CTS concentrations (1.0–2.5 wt%) were prepared and dried for subsequent use. Each sample (0.1 g) was placed in a light-protected corner. The samples were weighed every 24 h, and the morphological changes of hydrogels with different CTS concentrations were observed, along with the measurement of their water content. Data were then processed to analyze the impact of CTS concentration on the water absorption performance of hydrogels.

Hydrogels with different CTS concentrations (1.0–2.5 wt%) were prepared and left undisturbed. Water was allowed to evaporate in a 60 °C oven, and samples were withdrawn at 1–60 min after placement. The samples were weighed to record the mass loss, investigating the effect of CTS on the water loss rate of the hydrogels as below equation:

$$\text{Water loss rate }(\%) = \frac{M1 - M2}{M1} \times 100 \quad (3)$$

where $M2$ indicates the gel bead weight after treatment, and $M1$ represents the gel bead weight before treatment.

2.9. Dye Removal by C/CTS/PVA/CNF Hydrogel

Methyl orange (0.5 g/L), Methylene blue (1 g/L), Congo red (2.5 g/L), and Malachite green (2.5 g/L) solutions were individually prepared. The prepared dye solution (5 mL) was added into 25 mL conical flasks, and 0.3 g of C/CTS/PVA/CNF hydrogel (wet weight) was added to this dye solution. This mixture was withdrawn once an hour for 9 h of oscillating with a thermostatic oscillator (150 rpm, 30 °C). The extracted samples were diluted and separated in a centrifuge at a speed of 8000 rpm for 2 min. The supernatant was determined by a UV-visible spectrophotometer.

The removal kinetics were modeled using pseudo-first- and pseudo-second-order model [36]. The adsorption (mg/g) of C/CTS/PVA/CNF hydrogel under balance was defined as below:

$$q_e = \frac{(C_0 - C_e)V}{M} \quad (4)$$

where C_0 (mg/L) is the initial dye concentration. C_e (mg/L) is the equilibrium dye content. V (L) represents the dye solution volume. M (g) represents the mass of carbon aerogel. q_e (mg/g) represents the capacity of equilibrium adsorption.

The equations representing the pseudo-first-order kinetic model and pseudo-second-order kinetic model were denoted below [36]:

$$q_t = q_e[1 - \exp(-k_1 t)] \quad (5)$$

$$q_t = \frac{k_2 q_e^2 t}{1 + k_2 q_e t} \quad (6)$$

where q_t (mg/g) is the adsorption amount when the removal time is t (h). q_e (mg/g) is the adsorption amount when the adsorption equilibrium is reached. k_1 and k_2 are the rates of the pseudo-first-order and pseudo-second-order dynamics model, respectively.

3. Results and Discussion

3.1. Characterization of C/CTS/PVA/CNF Hydrogel Composite

Fourier Transform Infrared Spectroscopy (FTIR) is often implemented to measure specific chemical functional groups in materials and analyze molecular-level interactions between CTS, PVA, C-Ag, and CNF (Figure 1). The enhanced peak in the vicinity of 3448 cm^{-1} was associated with the hydrogen bonding formed between CTS, C-Ag, and PVA moieties [37]. The peaks near 2927 cm^{-1} and 1383 cm^{-1} were ascribed to the stretching and bending vibrations of C-H [38]. C/P/A/F, C/P/A, and C/A/F manifested clear adsorption near 1575 cm^{-1}, which was ascribed to the stretching vibration of C=C in PVA. The significant adsorption around 1263 cm^{-1} was found in C/P/A/F and C/A/F, which was attributed to the C-O stretching vibration produced by C-Ag and CNF [39]. The range from 1078 cm^{-1} to 1024 cm^{-1} indicated the interaction between C-O and Ag [14]. The weak absorption peaks near 841 cm^{-1} and 642 cm^{-1} were ascribed to C-H bending vibrations and hydroxyl group rotations [10].

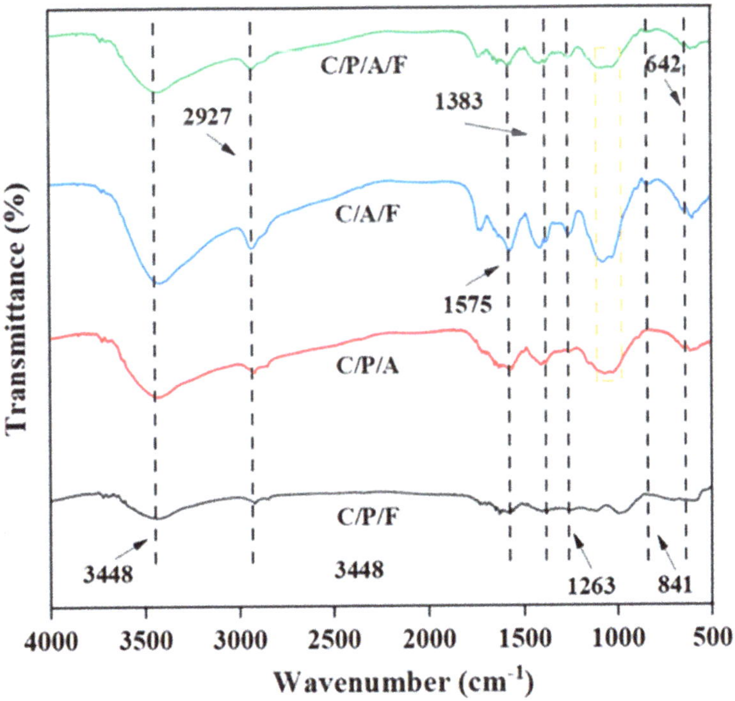

Figure 1. FT-IR spectra of C/P/F hydrogels, C/P/A hydrogels, C/A/F hydrogels, and C/P/A/F hydrogels.

The C/CTS/PVA/CNF hydrogel was characterized by SEM (Figure 2). Its surface exhibited a porous structure with embedded cellulose nanofibers within the network structure constructed by CST and PVA. At a magnification of 200 times, the dried hydrogel surface revealed the presence of a certain number of pores. As the magnification increased to 1000 times and 5000 times, the hydrogel exhibited a complex porous structure, which was advantageous for water transport and the release of antibacterial agents. At a magnification of 30,000 times, some AgNPs were found to be embedded in C/CTS/PVA/CNF hydrogel.

3.2. *Antimicrobial Property*

3.2.1. Effect of CST and C-Ag

The composition of materials and the dosage of antimicrobial substances in the preparation of hydrogels can affect their antimicrobial efficacy [40]. Figure 3a showcased that hydrogel without the supplementary of C-Ag acquired weak antibacterial performance. Hydrogels without the addition of PVA and CNF demonstrated similar antibacterial performance. The C/CTS/PVA/CNF hydrogel exhibited a significant inhibitory effect on bacteria. The positively charged amino groups on CTS interacted with the negatively charged components of microbial cell membranes, leading to the leakage of bacterial proteins and other cell components [41]. AgNPs could also affect the charge difference inside and outside of cells, causing cell leakage and inducing microbial oxidative stress (ROS) [42].

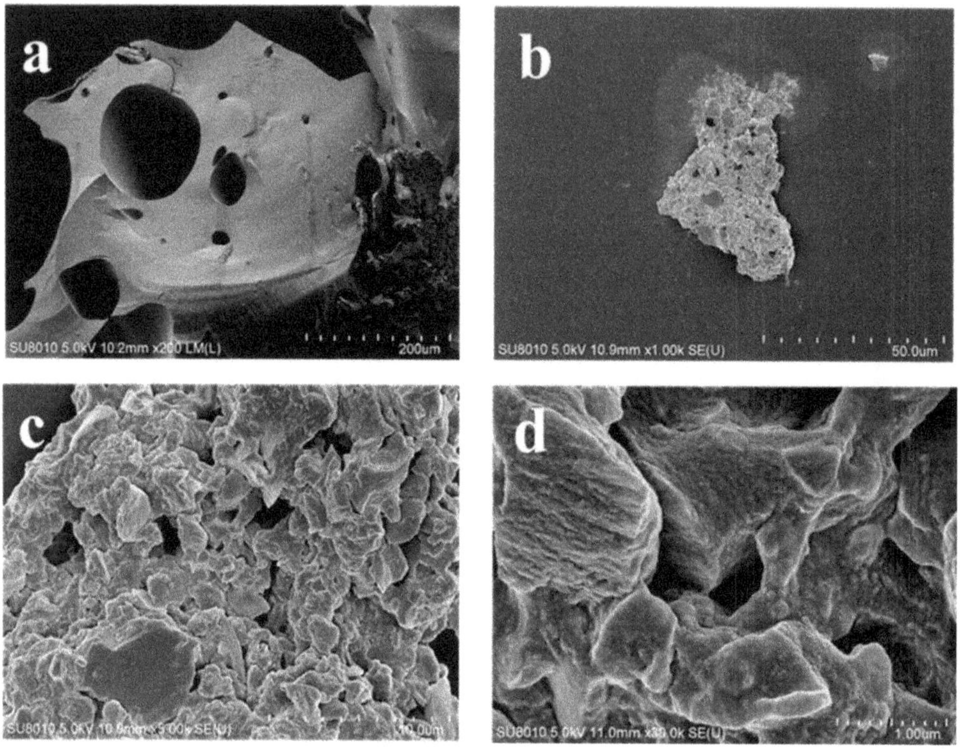

Figure 2. SEM images C/CTS/PVA/CNF hydrogels ×200 (**a**), ×1000 (**b**), ×5000 (**c**), ×30,000 (**d**).

Figure 3b revealed that the inhibitory capacity of bacteria by C-Ag increased with the increase in dosage at low loading concentrations (1 g/L). However, when the loading amount was too high, AgNPs aggregated within the gel, which hindered the liberation of silver ions and weakened the antibacterial effect [43]. Figure 3c showcased that the gel exhibited maximum antibacterial activity when the CTS content was 15 g/L. The inhibition areas of hydrogel against *E. coli*, *S. aureus*, and *P. aeruginosa* could reach 22.5 mm, 22.0 mm, and 24.0 mm, respectively. When the CTS content was excessively high, the tightly cross-linked structure formed by PVC and CTS could affect the release of AgNPs and amino groups, substantially impacting the antibacterial efficacy [44]. PVA/starch hydrogel containing turmeric and glutaraldehyde could inhibit *E. coli* and *S. aureus*, with an inhibition zone of 9.9–11.3 mm [19]. The royal jelly/chitosan/polyvinyl alcohol gel could inhibit *P. aeruginosa* with an inhibition zone of 13.0 mm [20]. The inhibition zones against *P. aeruginosa* ATCC9027, *S. aureus* ATCC6538, and *E. coli* ATCC25922 were over 20 mm when CST dosage was 15 g/L. Mesoporous Zn^{2+}/Ag^{+} doped hydroxyapatite nanoparticles were utilized to inhibit *P. aeruginosa* with an inhibition zone of 7–14 mm [5]. Incorporating silver nanoparticles into solvent-free synthesized PEG-based hydrogels was used for antibacterial, acquiring the maximum antibacterial zone of inhibition against *E. coli* and *S. aureus* were 17.4 and 15.9 mm [4], respectively. In our work, the prepared C/CTS/PVA/CNF hydrogel had high antibacterial activity.

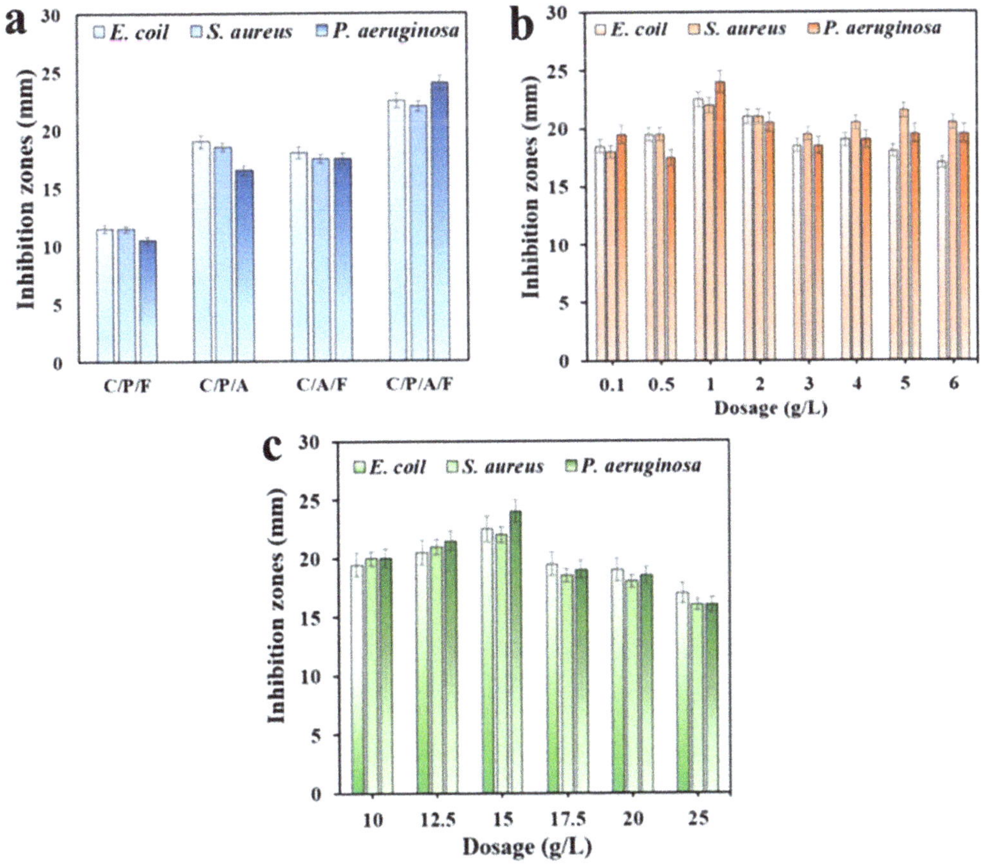

Figure 3. Antibacterial effect of gels prepared from different materials (C/P/F, C/P/A, C/P/F, and C/P/A/F) (**a**), C–Ag dosage (0.1, 0.5, 1, 2, 3, 4, 5, and 6 g/L) (**b**), chitosan dosage (10, 12.5, 15, 17.5, 20, and 25 g/L) (**c**).

3.2.2. Effect of C/CTS/PVA/CNF Hydrogel Dosage and Incubation Time

By increasing the material dosage and incubation time, the antibacterial efficiency of C/CTS/PVA/CNF hydrogel could be elevated (Figure 4). Figure 4a indicated that increasing the dosage of the C/CTS/PVA/CNF hydrogel led to a noticeable enhancement in the antibacterial effect on *E. coli* within 1 h. The difference in antibacterial effect decreased by 1.5 h, and the antibacterial rate was 100% by 2 h. However, increasing the gel dosage did not substantially improve the antibacterial efficiency. In the previous research, a concentration of 0.6 g/L of the antibacterial material acquired a 90% antibacterial effect within 5 h [14]. In our work, a C/CTS/PVA/CNF hydrogel dosage of 0.50 g/L acquired a 100% antibacterial rate within 2 h.

Inhibitors of *S. aureus* have been extensively studied, with some studies reporting inhibition rates as high as 95% for antibacterial materials [15]. In our research, the C/CTS/PVA/CNF hydrogel load was 0.50 g/L. After an incubation period of 1.5 h, the antibacterial rate approached 90% (Figure 4b), manifesting that the C/CTS/PVA/CNF hydrogel exhibited a good antibacterial effect against *S. aureus*. *P. aeruginosa* is a naturally occurring strain with strong drug resistance and good adaptability [45]. After 1 h of antibacterial treatment with the gel (1.5 g/L), the inhibition rate against *P. aeruginosa* could exceed 90%. By increasing the dosage of C/CTS/PVA/CNF hydrogel, the antibacterial rate also elevated (Figure 4c). For antibacterial time exceeding 90 min, the minimum C/CTS/PVA/CNF hydrogel dosage acquired a 100% inhibition rate. However, as the antibacterial duration increased, the inhibitory effect on bacteria no longer manifested significant enhancement. The antibacterial tests testified that the C/CTS/PVA/CNF hydrogel exhibited substantial and rapid bactericidal effects against both Gram-positive and Gram-negative bacteria. Even at low dosages, the hydrogel manifested excellent antibacterial activity during prolonged antibacterial processes.

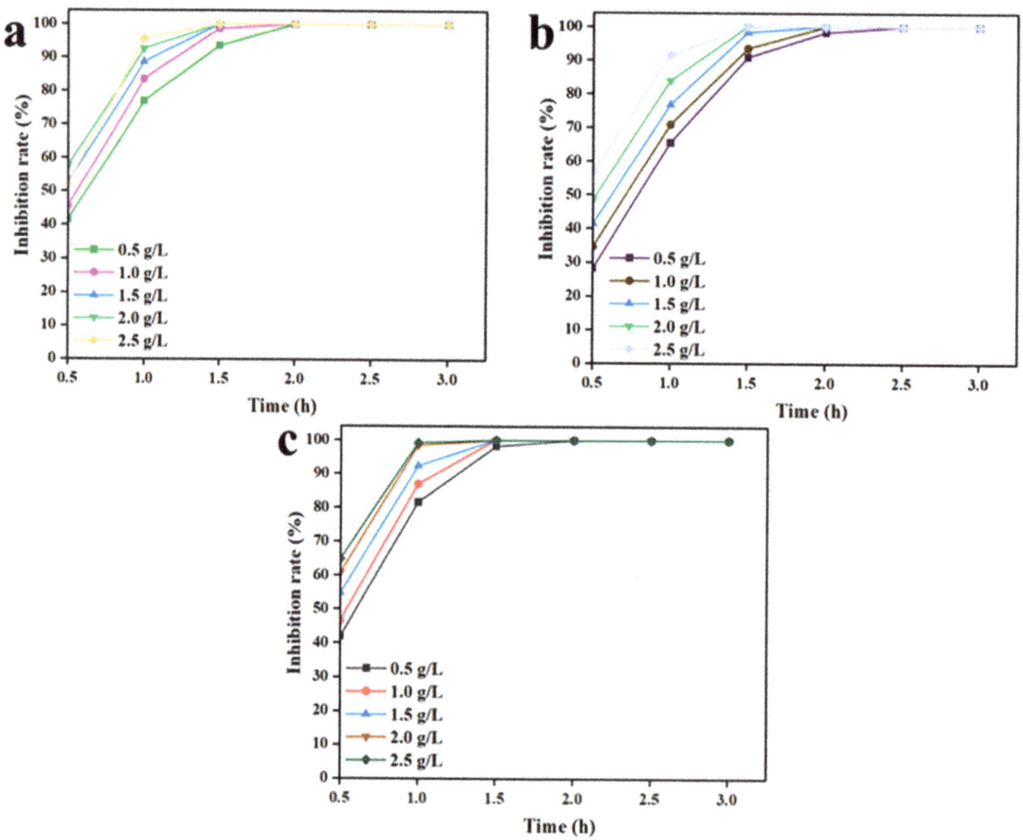

Figure 4. Antibacterial activity against *E. coli* (**a**), *S. aureus* (**b**), and *P. aeruginosa* (**c**) was observed in C/CTS/PVA/CNF hydrogel composite gel at different dosages (0.5, 1.0, 1.5, 2.0, and 2.5 g/L) and time (0.5, 1.0, 1.5, 2.0, 2.5, and 3.0 h).

3.3. *Stability and Reusability of C/CTS/PVA/CNF Hydrogels*

C/CTS/PVA/CNF hydrogel manifested strong stability and high inhibition rates, which might decrease performance costs and minimize potential pollution. Figure 5a shows that the C/CTS/PVA/CNF hydrogel maintained long-term stability in its antibacterial performance. In addition, it could be repeatedly used. The antibacterial rate of C/CTS/PVA/CNF hydrogel was 100% within 10 days and remained above 90% within 30 days after storage. In some stability studies of antibacterial gels, the inhibition rate declined to 90% after 15 days of preparation [46]. As showcased in Figure 5b, when the fifth batch of reuse experiment was over, the antibacterial rate was over 85%. Meanwhile, the antibacterial rate began to weaken apparently after the sixth run, which resulted from the loss of antibacterial compounds. The antibacterial durability of natural antibacterial materials might be relatively weak, and the antibacterial effect of biofiber material was less than 30% after the fifth test [47]. These results implied that the C/CTS/PVA/CNF hydrogel possessed good stability and reusability.

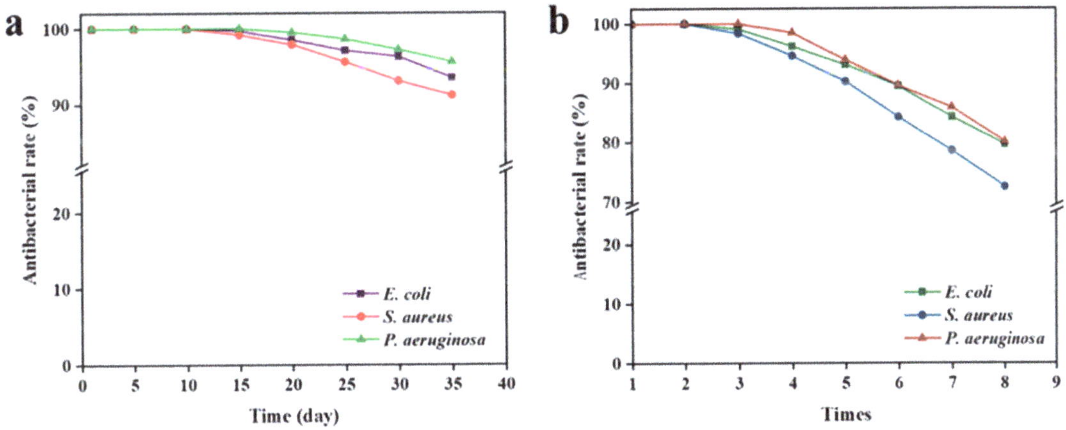

Figure 5. Antibacterial effect images of C/CTS/PVA/CNF hydrogels prepared on different days (5, 10, 15, 20, 25, 30, and 35 days) (**a**), repetitive antibacterial properties (1, 2, 3, 4, 5, 6, 7, and 8 times) (**b**).

3.4. Synergistic Antibacterial Mechanism of C/CTS/PVA/CNF Hydrogels

Biochar was combined with silver nanoparticles to form C-Ag, which exhibited high bactericidal activity. CTS is a natural antibacterial material capable of inhibiting the proliferation of many bacteria. PVA is a cross-network structure of polymer, which might be used as a carrier for dispersing C-Ag and CTS in C/CTS/PVA/CNF hydrogels. CTS, PVA, C-Ag, and CNF can cross-link to build a gel network structure for antibacterial assistance. In addition, CTS and PVA are hydrophilic biomaterials, and the prepared C/CTS/PVA/CNF hydrogels might absorb water and further expand. C-Ag will be released through its dispersion in C/CTS/PVA/CNF hydrogels, which have bacteriostatic action. The positively charged amino group ($-NH_2$) in CTS and C-Ag contained in the C/CTS/PVA/CNF hydrogels can combine with the negatively charged cell membrane, resulting in the cell membrane structural alteration and damage [48–50]. Afterwards, bacteriostatic chemicals and materials will inhibit the formation of a cell wall, block the synthesis of protein, destroy ion transport channel, affect the function of the membrane, inhibit the biosynthesis of nucleic acid, and influence specific metabolic pathways [51–53], causing the death of the bacteria (Figure 6). The utilization of bio-based waste and natural antibacterial agents reduced the antibacterial cost. Improving the eco-friendly and sustainable aspects of antibacterial agents or materials holds great promising prospects for their application in antimicrobial and dye removal. For the antibacterial mechanism, in-depth exploration needs to be implemented in the future.

3.5. Swelling Ratio, Moisture Adsorption, Water Loss, and Moisture Content of C/CTS/PVA/CNF Hydrogels

Swelling rate is one of the most important properties of hydrogels [53]. Within a certain period of time, the swelling ratio of hydrogel materials increased with the prolongation of immersion time in water (Figure 7a). When the CTS content was 1.0, 1.25, 2.0, and 2.25 wt%, the gel reached equilibrium swelling within 200 min. For CTS contents of 1.5 and 1.75 wt%, the gel reached equilibrium swelling around 240 min. Within a certain CTS concentration range, the swelling capacity of the hydrogel increased with increasing concentration. This was ascribed to the sufficient cross-linking of CTS and PVA, which enlarged the pore structure of the hydrogel, promoting swelling [54]. The highest swelling ratio was observed at approximately 400% when the CTS concentration was 1.75 wt%.

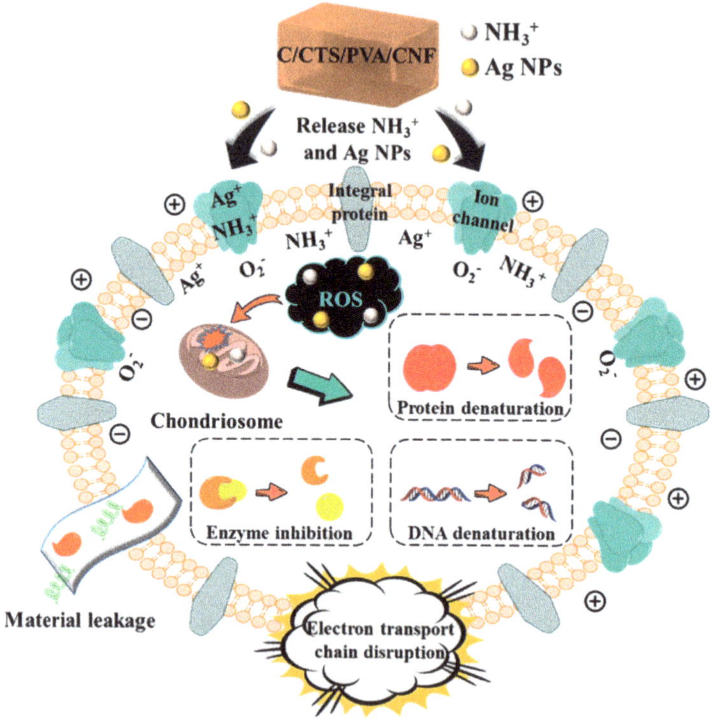

Figure 6. Synergistic antibacterial mechanism of C/CTS/PVA/CNF hydrogels.

In the dehydration test experiment, as the hydrogel is subjected to increasing time in the oven, the water content within the hydrogel starts to diminish. The intermolecular interactions between CTS and PVA affected the water loss in the gel [55]. Figure 7b shows the influence of CTS dosage on the dehydration rate of the hydrogel. Within a certain CTS concentration range, the water loss rate of the gel gradually declined with increasing CTS dosage. However, when the CTS concentration exceeded 1.5 wt%, the dehydration rate of hydrogel started to increase. When the CTS concentration was 1.5 wt%, the water loss rate reached 63.4% after drying for 60 min. As CTS concentration reached 1.0 wt% and 2.25 wt%, the water loss rate approached ~80%. These results manifested that an appropriate CTS dosage substantially promoted the water retention capability of the hydrogel.

Moisture absorption is represented by the water ratio, which is the ratio of the weight of water contained in the material over the weight of the material in the absolute dry state [56]. It was manifested that the CTS content affected the moisture absorption rate and moisture content of C/CTS/PVA/CNF hydrogel (Figure 7c,d). As CTS was 1.5 wt%, this prepared gel continued to exhibit an increasing trend in moisture absorption even after 168 h, surpassing the gels with lower CTS content. This implied that the hydrogel manifested superior moisture absorption performance within a certain CTS concentration range. In the moisture content test, C/CTS/PVA/CNF hydrogel displayed strong water-holding capacity, with a moisture content of 2563.7% when the CTS concentration was 1.5 wt%. For CTS concentrations below 1.5 wt%, both the MA and MC of the hydrogel increased with increasing CTS dosage. This was attributed to the influence of CTS concentration on the gel's structural morphology, which facilitated the diffusion of water within the network-like adhesive structure, a typical scenario of water diffusion within a reticular adhesive structure [57]. The incorporation of C-Ag effectually enhanced the frictional force within the hydrogel, possibly because -OH and -NH_2 groups might interact with AgNPs, as well as the cross-linking of polymer chains, which would weaken the water permeability of the prepared material [58]. The addition of CNF also strengthened the internal network structure of this prepared hydrogel to some extent.

Overall, C/CTS/PVA/CNF hydrogel exhibited excellent physical properties, and its complex and diverse internal network structure effectually controlled water permeation.

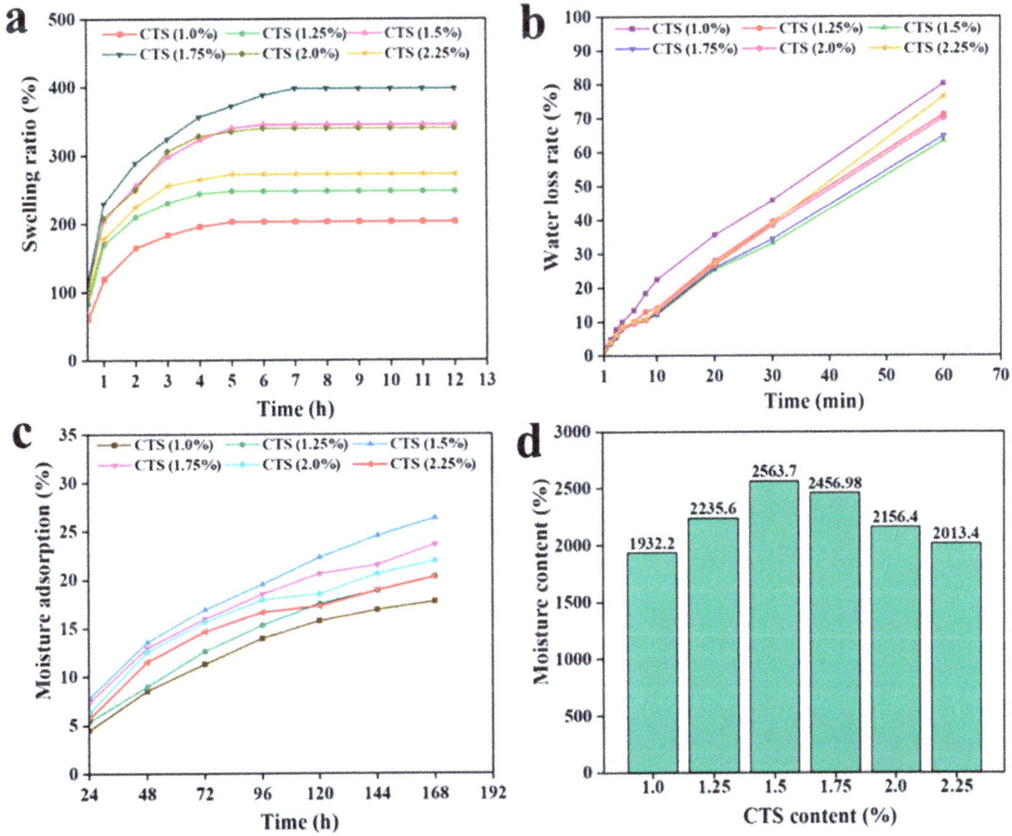

Figure 7. Swelling effect (**a**), water loss (**b**), moisture adsorption (**c**), and moisture content (**d**) images of different CTS dosage (1.0, 1.25, 1.5, 1.75, 2.0, and 2.25 wt%).

3.6. C/CTS/PVA/CNF Hydrogel Dye-Removal Properties

In order to test the ability and property of dye removal by the C/CTS/PVA/CNF hydrogel, the dye-removal kinetics were studied (Figure 8). The removal results of dyes indicated that the removal rate of MB, MG, and MO reached equilibrium at around 5 h, while the removal rate of CR reached equilibrium at around 6 h. High adsorption rate of MB and MO occurred within 1/2 h, while high adsorption rate of MG and CR happened within 2 h. This result implied that a large amount of dye was eliminated around these time points. Through data fitting, it was found that the hydrogel manifested outstanding affinity for CR removal, with a maximum removal capacity of 96.32 mg/g. This was comparable to the removal capacity of some nanomaterial [59]. Table 1 illustrated that the removal kinetics of C/CTS/PVA/CNF hydrogel well fitted the pseudo-first-order kinetics, with a correlation coefficient ($R^2 \geq 0.99$) for MB, MO and CR, while the correlation coefficient (R^2)

for the pseudo-second-order kinetic equation was less than 0.99 for three sets (MB, MG and CR).

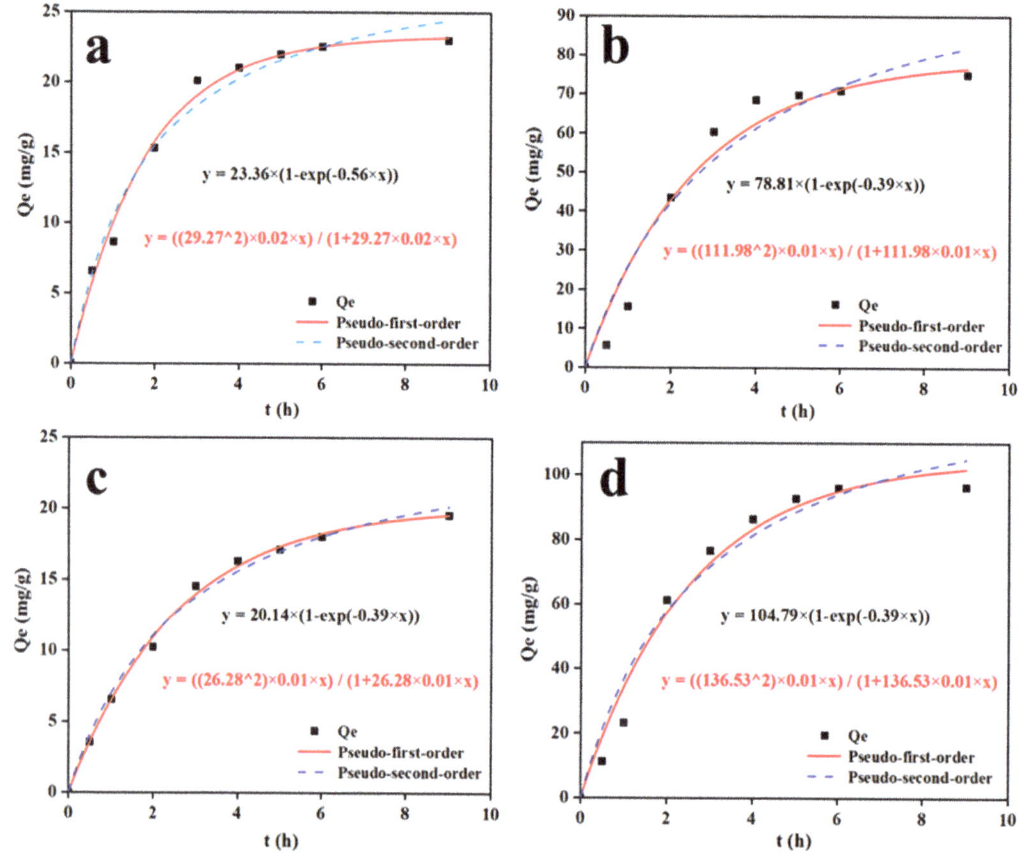

Figure 8. Kinetic fitting results for methylene blue (MB: 1 g/L) (**a**), Malachite green (MG: 2.5 g/L) (**b**), Methyl orange (MO: 1 g/L) (**c**), and Congo red (CR: 2.5 g/L) (**d**) adsorption onto C/CTS/PVA/CNF hydrogels.

Table 1. Kinetic parameters for the adsorption of dyes on C/CTS/PVA gel.

		Pseudo-First-Order Model			Pseudo-Second-Order Model		
	$q_{e\ exp}$ (mg/g)	$q_{e\ cal}$ (mg/g)	k_1 (min^{-1})	R^2	$q_{e\ cal}$ (mg/g)	k_2 (g/mg·min)	R^2
MB	23.01	23.21	0.56	0.99	24.38	0.02	0.98
MG	75.01	76.54	0.39	0.97	81.31	0.01	0.95
MO	19.56	19.55	0.16	0.99	20.14	0.01	0.99
CR	96.32	101.81	0.39	0.99	104.91	0.01	0.98

By fitting the pseudo-first-order kinetic equation, the equilibrium-removal capacities of MB, MG, MO, and CR were calculated to be 23.21, 76.54, 19.55, and 101.81 mg/g. According to the pseudo-second-order kinetic equation, the capacities of equilibrium adsorption ($q_{e\ cal}$) were 24.38, 81.31, 20.14, and 104.91 mg/g for MB, MG, MO, and CR, respectively. The experimental maximum values ($q_{e\ exp}$) were observed to be 23.01, 75.01, 19.56, and 96.32 mg/g for MB, MG, MO, and CR, respectively. Accordingly, the fitting curves better matched the pseudo-first-order kinetic equation: R^2, with a value close to 1 [60]. Consequently, the pseudo-first-order kinetic equation might effectually describe the entire adsorption process. The adsorption experimental results showcased the excellent dye adsorption capacity of the C/CTS/PVA/CNF hydrogel. The acid-promoted UiO-66 had the adsorption capacities of MO (84.8 mg/g) and MB (13.2 mg/g) [61]. The maximum adsorption capacity of ZnTPA-O/Tea with MB dye was 31.81 mg/g [62]. The C/CTS/PVA/CNF hydrogels, with good antibacterial and adsorption properties, have a certain application value in dye adsorption.

Biochar, C-Ag, CTS, and PVA had good adsorption properties [63–68]. The electrostatic interaction between the hydroxyl group (-OH) and the amino group (-NH_2) in CTS molecules caused the dye adsorption on the surface of gels [63]. PVA has a cross-network structure [66], rendering it as a support for dispersive C-Ag and CTS in C/CTS/PVA/CNF hydrogels. The formed network adhesive structure fabricated by CTS, C-Ag, and PVA enhanced swelling properties, improved water retention capability, and improved moisture content of C/CTS/PVA/CNF hydrogels, which would favor expanding the adsorption area of dyes.

Hydrogels have shown potential in antibacterial and waste adsorption [69]. In this research, the C/CTS/PVA/CNF hydrogel has a high potential for antibacterial and dye-removal control. However, the involved mechanism is not clear yet. In-depth exploration of this subject needs to be well implemented through the characterization of prepared C/CTS/PVA/CNF hydrogel (e.g., Brunner−Emmet−Teller (BET), X-ray Diffractometer (XRD), Atomic Force Microscope (AFM), Differential Scanning Calorimeter (DSC), Thermal Gravimetric Analyzer (TGA), Transmission Electron Microscope (TEM), Energy Dispersive Spectroscopy (EDS), Elemental Mapping (EM), etc.). In addition, optimal antibacterial and dye removal control processes need to be well developed in the future.

4. Conclusions

This study adhered to the principle of waste utilization by employing discarded fish scales to prepare C-Ag and utilizing waste wheat straw to extract CNF for the preparation of a C/CTS/PVA/CNF hydrogel with antibacterial properties and dye-removal capacity. The hydrogel's porous hydrophobic structure enhanced stability and degradation ability, while also strengthening the antibacterial effect by facilitating the liberation of silver ions and amino groups to promote synergistic antibacterial activity. Additionally, the hydrogel manifested a maximum removal capacity of 96.3 mg of Congo red dye/g. In summary, the C/CTS/PVA/CNF hydrogel was an environmentally sustainable antibacterial material with significant potential in sewage treatment.

Supplementary Materials: The following supporting information can be downloaded at: https://www.mdpi.com/article/10.3390/pr12102277/s1, Figure S1. SEM image of CNF.

Author Contributions: Conceptualization, methodology, formal analysis, investigation, resources, data curation, writing—original draft: L.X.; Conceptualization, methodology, software, formal analysis, investigation, data curation, writing—original draft: Z.Z.; Supervision, writing—review and editing: Y.H. and Y.J. All authors have read and agreed to the published version of the manuscript.

Funding: This research received no external funding.

Data Availability Statement: Data are contained within the article.

Acknowledgments: The authors thank the Analysis and Testing Center (Changzhou University) for the analysis of samples with FT-IR and SEM. All individuals included in this section have consented to the acknowledgment.

Conflicts of Interest: The authors declare no conflict of interest to this research, and the paper has not been submitted to any other journal simultaneously.

References

1. He, Q.; Zhang, H.; Ma, M.; He, Y.; Jia, J.; Hu, Q.; Gong, Y. Critical assessment of protozoa contamination and control measures in mass culture of the diatom *Phaeodactylum tricornutum*. *Bioresour. Technol.* **2022**, *359*, 127460. [CrossRef] [PubMed]
2. Jiang, S.; Meng, L.; Lou, Y.; Yan, Z.; Xi, J.; Bian, H.; Wu, W.; Xiao, H. Fabrication of multifunctional air filter paper with flame retardant, antibacterial and hydrophobic properties. *J. Environ. Chem. Eng.* **2023**, *11*, 111540. [CrossRef]
3. Hezma, A.M.; Shaltout, W.A.; Kabary, H.A.; El-Bahy, G.S.; Abdelrazzak, A.B. Fabrication, characterization and adsorption investigation of nano zinc oxide–sodium alginate beads for effective removal of chromium (VI) from aqueous solution. *J. Inorg. Organomet. Polym. Mater.* **2023**, *33*, 1400–1408. [CrossRef]
4. Kazeminava, F.; Arsalani, N.; Ahmadi, R.; Kafil, H.S.; Geckeler, K.E. A facile approach to incorporate silver nanoparticles into solvent-free synthesized PEG-based hydrogels for antibacterial and catalytical applications. *Polym. Test.* **2021**, *101*, 106906. [CrossRef]
5. Phatai, P.; Prachumrak, N.; Kamonwannasit, S.; Kamcharoen, A.; Roschat, W.; Phewphong, S.; Futalan, C.M.; Khemthong, P.; Butburee, T.; Youngjan, S.; et al. Zinc-Silver doped mesoporous hydroxyapatite synthesized via ultrasonic in combination with sol-gel method for increased antibacterial activity. *Sustainability* **2022**, *14*, 11756. [CrossRef]
6. Zhang, Z.; He, Y. Synthesis and characteristics of a fish scale-based biochar–nanosilver antibacterial material. *Processes* **2023**, *11*, 1992. [CrossRef]
7. Jiang, W.; Cai, Y.; Liu, D.; Yu, X.; Wang, Q. Enhanced adsorption performance of oxytetracycline in aqueous solutions by Mg-Fe modified suaeda-based magnetic biochar. *Environ. Res.* **2024**, *241*, 117662. [CrossRef]
8. Cai, Q.; Bai, X.; Pu, J. Author Correction: Adaptive VAlCN-Ag composite and VAlCN/VN-Ag multilayer coatings intended for applications at elevated temperature. *J. Mater. Sci.* **2022**, *57*, 15674–15675. [CrossRef]
9. Oliveira, Í.M.; de Jesus, R.A.; Nascimento, V.R.S.; Bilal, M.; Iqbal, H.M.N.; Ferreira, L.F.R.; Cestari, A.R. Bioremediation potential of Dicentrarchus labrax fish scales for dye-based emerging contaminants by ANN–GA hybrid modeling. *Bioprocess Biosyst. Eng.* **2022**, *45*, 1189–1200. [CrossRef]
10. Xia, D.; Liu, Y.; Cheng, X.; Gu, P.; Chen, Q.; Zhang, Z. Temperature-tuned fish-scale biochar with two-dimensional homogeneous porous structure: A promising uranium extractant. *Appl. Surf. Sci.* **2022**, *591*, 153136. [CrossRef]
11. Kesarwani, V.; Rai, V.K. Impact of AgNPs on the optical thermometry and stability of bismuth modified tellurium-tungstate upconverting glass. *J. Non-Cryst. Solids* **2023**, *603*, 122129. [CrossRef]
12. Yang, D.; Fan, B.; Sun, G.; He, Y.-C.; Ma, C. Ultraviolet blocking ability, antioxidant and antibacterial properties of newly prepared polyvinyl alcohol-nanocellulose-silver nanoparticles-ChunJian peel extract composite film. *Int. J. Biol. Macromol.* **2023**, *252*, 126427. [CrossRef] [PubMed]
13. Hariram, M.; Vivekanandhan, S.; Ganesan, V.; Muthuramkumar, S.; Rodriguez-uribe, A.; Mohanty, A.K.; Misra, M. *Tecoma stans* flower extract assisted biogenic synthesis of functional Ag-Talc nanostructures for antimicrobial applications. *Bioresour. Technol. Rep.* **2019**, *7*, 100298. [CrossRef]
14. Hu, Z.; Zhang, L.; Zhong, L.; Zhou, Y.; Xue, J.; Li, Y. Preparation of an antibacterial chitosan-coated biochar-nanosilver composite for drinking water purification. *Carbohydr. Polym.* **2019**, *219*, 290–297. [CrossRef]
15. Cui, J.; Liang, Y.; Yang, D.; Liu, Y. Facile fabrication of rice husk based silicon dioxide nanospheres loaded with silver nanoparticles as a rice antibacterial agent. *Sci. Rep.* **2016**, *6*, 21423. [CrossRef]
16. Zhou, X.; Fu, Y.; Chen, L.; Wang, R.; Wang, X.; Miao, Y.; Ji, X.; Bian, H.; Dai, H. Diisocyanate modifiable commercial filter paper with tunable hydrophobicity, enhanced wet tensile strength and antibacterial activity. *Carbohydr. Polym.* **2020**, *248*, 116791. [CrossRef]
17. Potaś, J.; Szymańska, E.; Winnicka, K. Challenges in developing of chitosan—Based polyelectrolyte complexes as a platform for mucosal and skin drug delivery. *Eur. Polym. J.* **2020**, *140*, 110020. [CrossRef]
18. Singh, S.; Arputharaj, E.; Dahms, H.U.; Patel, A.K.; Huang, Y.L. Chitosan-based nanocomposites for removal of Cr(VI) and synthetic food colorants from wastewater. *Bioresour. Technol.* **2022**, *351*, 127018. [CrossRef]
19. Sekhavat Pour, Z.; Ghaemy, M. Removal of dyes and heavy metal ions from water by magnetic hydrogel beads based on poly(vinyl alcohol)/carboxymethyl starch-g-poly(vinyl imidazole). *RSC Adv.* **2015**, *5*, 64106–64118. [CrossRef]
20. Su, J.F.; Li, G.Q.; Wen, Q.; Xue, L.; Chen, C.L.; Huang, T.L. Highly efficient nitrate and phosphorus removal and adsorption of tetracycline by precipitation in a chitosan/polyvinyl alcohol immobilized bioreactor. *Bioprocess Biosyst. Eng.* **2020**, *43*, 1761–1771. [CrossRef]
21. Bandyopadhyay, S.; Saha, N.; Brodnjak, U.V.; Sáha, P. Bacterial cellulose and guar gum based modified PVP-CMC hydrogel films: Characterized for packaging fresh berries. *Food Packag. Shelf Life* **2019**, *22*, 100402. [CrossRef]
22. Ma, S.; Shi, W.; Li, H.; Zhang, Y. Biomimetic mineralization of nacre-inspired multiple crosslinked PVA/CaAlg/SiO_2 membrane with simultaneously enhanced mechanical and separation properties. *Int. J. Biol. Macromol.* **2023**, *234*, 123650. [CrossRef] [PubMed]
23. Alemdar, A.; Sain, M. Isolation and characterization of nanofibers from agricultural residues—Wheat straw and soy hulls. *Bioresour. Technol.* **2008**, *99*, 1664–1671. [CrossRef] [PubMed]
24. Froese, A.G.; Sparling, R. Cross-feeding and wheat straw extractives enhance growth of *Clostridium thermocellum*-containing co-cultures for consolidated bioprocessing. *Bioprocess Biosyst. Eng.* **2021**, *44*, 819–830. [CrossRef] [PubMed]

25. Zhang, C.-W.; Li, F.-Y.; Li, J.-F.; Li, Y.-L.; Xu, J.; Xie, Q.; Chen, S.; Guo, A.-F. Novel treatments for compatibility of plant fiber and starch by forming new hydrogen bonds. *J. Clean. Prod.* **2018**, *185*, 357–365. [CrossRef]
26. Kumar Trivedi, A.; Kumar, A.; Gupta, M.K. Extraction of nanocellulose from wheat straw and its characterization. *Mater. Today Proc.* **2023**, *78*, 48–54. [CrossRef]
27. Wang, Y.; Xu, T.; Liu, K.; Zhang, M.; Zhao, Q.; Liang, Q.; Si, C. Nanocellulose-based advanced materials for flexible supercapacitor electrodes. *Ind. Crops Prod.* **2023**, *204*, 117378. [CrossRef]
28. Srivastava, K.R.; Dixit, S.; Pal, D.B.; Mishra, P.K.; Srivastava, P.; Srivastava, N.; Hashem, A.; Alqarawi, A.A.; Abd_Allah, E.F. Effect of nanocellulose on mechanical and barrier properties of PVA–banana pseudostem fiber composite films. *Environ. Technol. Innov.* **2021**, *21*, 101312. [CrossRef]
29. Bai, H.; Liang, Z.; Wang, D.; Guo, J.; Zhang, S.; Ma, P.; Dong, W. Biopolymer nanocomposites with customized mechanical property and exceptionally antibacterial performance. *Compos. Sci. Technol.* **2020**, *199*, 108338. [CrossRef]
30. Luo, C.; Guo, A.; Zhao, Y.; Sun, X. A high strength, low friction, and biocompatible hydrogel from PVA, chitosan and sodium alginate for articular cartilage. *Carbohydr. Polym.* **2022**, *286*, 119268. [CrossRef]
31. Balouiri, M.; Sadiki, M.; Ibnsouda, S.K. Methods for in vitro evaluating antimicrobial activity: A review. *J. Pharm. Anal.* **2016**, *6*, 71–79. [CrossRef] [PubMed]
32. Parmar, A.; Kapil, S.; Sachar, S.; Sharma, S. Design of experiment based methodical optimization and green syntheses of hybrid patchouli oil coated silver nanoparticles for enhanced antibacterial activity. *Curr. Res. Green Sustain. Chem.* **2020**, *3*, 100016. [CrossRef]
33. Kumar, A.; Negi, Y.S.; Bhardwaj, N.K.; Choudhary, V. Synthesis and characterization of methylcellulose/PVA based porous composite. *Carbohydr. Polym.* **2012**, *88*, 1364–1372. [CrossRef]
34. Lin, D.; Kelly, A.L.; Maidannyk, V.; Miao, S. Effect of concentrations of alginate, soy protein isolate and sunflower oil on water loss, shrinkage, elastic and structural properties of alginate-based emulsion gel beads during gelation. *Food Hydrocoll.* **2020**, *108*, 105998. [CrossRef]
35. Xie, L.; Zhang, Z.; He, Y. Antibacterial effect of polyvinyl alcohol/biochar–nano silver/sodium alginate gel beads. *Processes* **2023**, *11*, 2330. [CrossRef]
36. Feng, Q.; Fan, B.; He, Y. Antibacterial, antioxidant, Cr (VI) adsorption and dye adsorption effects of biochar-based silver nanoparticles-sodium alginate-tannic acid composite gel beads. *Int. J. Biol. Macromol.* **2024**, *271*, 132453. [CrossRef]
37. Xiang, X.; Yi, X.; Zheng, W.; Li, Y.; Zhang, C.; Wang, X.; Chen, Z.; Huang, M.; Ying, G.G. Enhanced biodegradation of thiamethoxam with a novel polyvinyl alcohol (PVA)/sodium alginate (SA)/biochar immobilized *Chryseobacterium* sp. H5. *J. Hazard. Mater.* **2023**, *443*, 130247. [CrossRef]
38. Salunke, A.S.; Salunke, S.T.; Deokate, R.J.; Kale, B.B. Tuning of photoluminescence behavior of gold coated chitosan-polyvinyl alcohol binding with graphene quantum dots. *Mater. Today Proc.* **2022**, *62*, 1752–1757. [CrossRef]
39. Bian, H.; Chen, L.; Dong, M.; Wang, L.; Wang, R.; Zhou, X.; Wu, C.; Wang, X.; Ji, X.; Dai, H. Natural lignocellulosic nanofibril film with excellent ultraviolet blocking performance and robust environment resistance. *Int. J. Biol. Macromol.* **2021**, *166*, 1578–1585. [CrossRef]
40. Abbaszadegan, A.; Ghahramani, Y.; Gholami, A.; Hemmateenejad, B.; Dorostkar, S.; Nabavizadeh, M.; Sharghi, H. The effect of charge at the surface of silver nanoparticles on antimicrobial activity against Gram-positive and Gram-negative bacteria: A preliminary study. *J. Nanomater.* **2015**, *2015*, 720654. [CrossRef]
41. Dhandapani, P.; Santhoshkumar, M.; Narenkumar, J.; AlSalhi, M.S.; Kumar, P.A.; Devanesan, S.; Kokilaramani, S.; Rajasekar, A. Bio-approach: Preparation of RGO-AgNPs on cotton fabric and interface with sweat environment for antibacterial activity. *Bioprocess Biosyst. Eng.* **2022**, *45*, 1825–1837. [CrossRef] [PubMed]
42. Wang, D.; Zhao, L.; Ma, H.; Zhang, H.; Guo, L.H. Quantitative analysis of reactive oxygen species photogenerated on metal oxide nanoparticles and their bacteria toxicity: The role of superoxide radicals. *Environ. Sci. Technol.* **2017**, *51*, 10137–10145. [CrossRef] [PubMed]
43. Yang, D.; Fan, B.; He, Y.C. UV-blocking, antibacterial, corrosion resistance, antioxidant, and fruit packaging ability of lignin-rich alkaline black liquor composite film. *Int. J. Biol. Macromol.* **2024**, *275*, 133344. [CrossRef] [PubMed]
44. Janani, B.; Okla, M.K.; Abdel-Maksoud, M.A.; AbdElgawad, H.; Thomas, A.M.; Raju, L.L.; Al-Qahtani, W.H.; Khan, S.S. CuO loaded ZnS nanoflower entrapped on PVA-chitosan matrix for boosted visible light photocatalysis for tetracycline degradation and anti-bacterial application. *J. Environ. Manag.* **2022**, *306*, 114396. [CrossRef] [PubMed]
45. Masilan, K.; Neethiselvan, N.; Shakila, R.J.; Muralidharan, N.; Karthy, A.; Ravikumar, T.; Parthiban, F. Investigation on the coacervation of fish scale gelatin hydrogel with seafood waste hydrolysates for the development of artificial fish bait: Physico-chemical, thermodynamic, and morpho-structural properties. *J. Indian Chem. Soc.* **2022**, *99*, 100783. [CrossRef]
46. Zhao, H.; Li, X.; Zhang, L.; Hu, Z.; Zhong, L.; Xue, J. Preparation and bacteriostatic research of porous polyvinyl alcohol/biochar/nanosilver polymer gel for drinking water treatment. *Sci. Rep.* **2021**, *11*, 12205. [CrossRef]
47. Thakur, K.; Kalia, S.; Kaith, B.S.; Pathania, D.; Kumar, A.; Thakur, P.; Knittel, C.E.; Schauer, C.L.; Totaro, G. The development of antibacterial and hydrophobic functionalities in natural fibers for fiber-reinforced composite materials. *J. Environ. Chem. Eng.* **2016**, *4*, 1743–1752. [CrossRef]

48. Qi, D.; Zhao, S.; Zhang, H.; Liu, B.; She, P.; Yue, X. Development of high-strength porous polyetheretherketone foam/nanosilver antibacterial composites for the prevention of postoperative infections in bone repair. *Compos. Commun.* **2022**, *31*, 101127. [CrossRef]
49. Velidandi, A.; Pabbathi NP, P.; Dahariya, S.; Baadhe, R.R. Green synthesis of novel Ag–Cu and Ag–Znbimetallic nanoparticles and their in vitro biological, eco-toxicity and catalytic studies. *Nano-Struct. Nano-Objects* **2021**, *26*, 100687. [CrossRef]
50. Ahmed, B.; Hashmi, A.; Khan, M.S.; Musarrat, J. ROS mediated destruction of cell membrane, growth and biofilms of human bacterial pathogens by stable metallic AgNPs functionalized from bell pepper extract and quercetin. *Adv. Powder Technol.* **2018**, *29*, 1601–1616. [CrossRef]
51. Jiang, B.; Tian, C.; Song, G.; Pan, Q.; Wang, Z.; Shi, L.; Qiao, Y.; Fu, H. A green route to synthesize novel Ag/C antibacterial agent. *Mater. Res. Bull.* **2012**, *47*, 458–463. [CrossRef]
52. Aryan, N.; Behpour, M.; Benvidi, A.; Jookar Kashi, F.; Azimzadeh, M.; Zare, H.R. Evaluation of sodium alendronate drug released from TiO_2 nanoparticle doped with hydroxyapatite and silver–strontium for enhancing antibacterial effect and osteoinductivity. *Mater. Chem. Phys.* **2023**, *295*, 126934. [CrossRef]
53. Vityazev, F.V.; Khramova, D.S.; Saveliev, N.Y.; Ipatova, E.A.; Burkov, A.A.; Beloserov, V.S.; Belyi, V.A.; Kononov, L.O.; Martinson, E.A.; Litvinets, S.G.; et al. Pectin-glycerol gel beads: Preparation, characterization and swelling behaviour. *Carbohydr. Polym.* **2020**, *238*, 116166. [CrossRef] [PubMed]
54. Sethi, V.; Kaur, M.; Thakur, A.; Rishi, P.; Kaushik, A. Unravelling the role of hemp straw derived cellulose in CMC/PVA hydrogel for sustained release of fluoroquinolone antibiotic. *Int. J. Biol. Macromol.* **2022**, *222*, 844–855. [CrossRef] [PubMed]
55. Rezagholizade-shirvan, A.; Fathi Najafi, M.; Behmadi, H.; Masrournia, M. Preparation of nano-composites based on curcumin/chitosan-PVA-alginate to improve stability, antioxidant, antibacterial and anticancer activity of curcumin. *Inorg. Chem. Commun.* **2022**, *145*, 110022. [CrossRef]
56. Bhat, V.G.; Masti, S.P.; Narasagoudr, S.S.; Chougale, R.B.; Kumar, P.; Vantamuri, A.B. Development and characterization of Chitosan/Guar gum/Gum ghatti bionanocomposites with in situ silver nanoparticles. *Chem. Data Collect.* **2023**, *44*, 101009. [CrossRef]
57. Mathew, S.; Jayakumar, A.; Kumar, V.P.; Mathew, J.; Radhakrishnan, E.K. One-step synthesis of eco-friendly boiled rice starch blended polyvinyl alcohol bionanocomposite films decorated with in situ generated silver nanoparticles for food packaging purpose. *Int. J. Biol. Macromol.* **2019**, *139*, 475–485. [CrossRef]
58. Li, Q.; Lu, F.; Zhou, G.; Yu, K.; Lu, B.; Xiao, Y.; Dai, F.; Wu, D.; Lan, G. Silver inlaid with gold nanoparticle/chitosan wound dressing enhances antibacterial activity and porosity, and promotes wound healing. *Biomacromolecules* **2017**, *18*, 3766–3775. [CrossRef]
59. Aghaei, F.; Tangestaninejad, S.; Bahadori, M.; Moghadam, M.; Mirkhani, V.; Mohammadpoor-Baltork, I.; Khalaji, M.; Asadi, V. Green synthesize of nano-MOF-ethylcellulose composite fibers for efficient adsorption of Congo red from water. *J. Colloid Interface Sci.* **2023**, *648*, 78–89. [CrossRef]
60. Chen, L.; Mi, B.; He, J.; Li, Y.; Zhou, Z.; Wu, F. Functionalized biochars with highly-efficient malachite green adsorption property produced from banana peels via microwave-assisted pyrolysis. *Bioresour. Technol.* **2023**, *376*, 128840. [CrossRef]
61. Qiu, J.; Feng, Y.; Zhang, X.; Jia, M.; Yao, J. Acid-promoted synthesis of UiO-66 for highly selective adsorption of anionic dyes: Adsorption performance and mechanisms. *J. Colloid Interface Sci.* **2017**, *499*, 151–158. [CrossRef] [PubMed]
62. Arunkumar, G.; Pannipara, M.; Deviga, G.; Mariappan, M.; Al-Sehemi, A.G.; Anthony, S.P. Natural tea extract coated porous MOF nano/microparticles for highly enhanced and selective adsorption of cationic dyes from aqueous medium. *J. Mol. Liq.* **2024**, *394*, 123747. [CrossRef]
63. Liu, W.; Lou, T.; Wang, X. Enhanced dye adsorption with conductive polyaniline doped chitosan nanofibrous membranes. *Int. J. Biol. Macromol.* **2023**, *242*, 124711. [CrossRef] [PubMed]
64. Liu, Y.; Wu, Y.; He, Y.C.; Ma, C. Synthesis of furoic acid from biomasses by sequential catalysis with fish scale-rice husk-based heterogeneous chemocatalyst and dehydrogenase biocatalyst. *Ind. Crops Prod.* **2023**, *202*, 117033. [CrossRef]
65. Zhang, H.; Li, R.; Zhang, Z. A versatile EDTA and chitosan bi-functionalized magnetic bamboo biochar for simultaneous removal of methyl orange and heavy metals from complex wastewater. *Environ. Pollut.* **2022**, *293*, 118517. [CrossRef]
66. Wang, J.; Liang, J.; Sun, L.; Li, G.; Temmink, H.; Rijnaarts, H.H.M. Granule-based immobilization and activity enhancement of anammox biomass via PVA/CS and PVA/CS/Fe gel beads. *Bioresour. Technol.* **2020**, *309*, 123448. [CrossRef]
67. Rodwihok, C.; Suwannakeaw, M.; Charoensri, K.; Wongratanaphisan, D.; Woon Woo, S.; Kim, H.S. Alkali/zinc-activated fly ash nanocomposites for dye removal and antibacterial applications. *Bioresour. Technol.* **2021**, *331*, 125060. [CrossRef]
68. Tomczyk, A.; Sokołowska, Z.; Boguta, P. Biomass type effect on biochar surface characteristic and adsorption capacity relative to silver and copper. *Fuel* **2020**, *278*, 118168. [CrossRef]
69. Bhuyan, M.M.; Jophous, M.; Jeong, J.H. Preparation of pectin–acrylamide–(vinyl phosphonic acid) hydrogel and its selective adsorption of metal ions. *Polym. Bull.* **2023**, *80*, 4625–4641. [CrossRef]

processes

MDPI

Article

Production and Application of a New Biosurfactant for Solubilisation and Mobilisation of Residual Oil from Sand and Seawater

Ivison Amaro Silva [1,2], José Gabriel Lima Alcântara Fortunato [2,3], Fabíola Carolina Gomes Almeida [2], Romulo Nepomuceno Alves [2], Maristela Casé Costa Cunha [2], Raquel Diniz Rufino [3], Mucio Luiz Banja Fernandes [2,4] and Leonie Asfora Sarubbo [2,3,*]

1 Rede Nordeste de Biotecnologia (RENORBIO), Universidade Federal Rural de Pernambuco (UFRPE), Rua Dom Manuel de Medeiros, s/n—Dois Irmãos, Recife 52171-900, PE, Brazil; ivison.silva@iati.org.br

2 Instituto Avançado de Tecnologia e Inovação (IATI), Rua Potyra, n. 31, Prado, Recife 50070-280, PE, Brazil; j.gabrielfortunato99@gmail.com (J.G.L.A.F.); fabiola.almeida@iati.org.br (F.C.G.A.); romulo.dirmam@gmail.com (R.N.A.); maristela.case@iati.org.br (M.C.C.C.); mucio.banja@iati.org.br (M.L.B.F.)

3 Escola UNICAP Icam Tech, Universidade Católica de Pernambuco (UNICAP), Rua do Príncipe, n. 526, Boa Vista, Recife 50050-900, PE, Brazil; raquel.rufino@unicap.br

4 Departamento de Ciências Biológias, Universidade de Pernambuco (UPE), Av. Gov. Agamenon Magalhães, Santo Amaro, Recife 50100-010, PE, Brazil

* Correspondence: leonie.sarubbo@unicap.br

Abstract: Significant research has been conducted to minimise environmental impacts and promote the sustainable use of resources and raw materials. Microbial surfactants are an example of advanced materials obtained from sustainable production processes. In the present study, a biosurfactant was produced by the yeast *Starmerella bombicola* ATCC 22214 grown in a previously selected low-cost mineral medium containing 10% sucrose, 1.2% canola oil, and 0.5% corn steep liquor. The biosurfactant reduced surface tension from 72 $\pm$ 0.1 to 32.76 $\pm$ 0.3 mN/m. The yield was 23 g/L, and the critical micelle concentration was 0.6 g/L. The biosurfactant emulsified 96.25 $\pm$ 0.08% of used motor oil, was characterised as a sophorolipid, and exhibited stability under extreme conditions with no significant loss of its properties. Toxicity was assessed by exposing the microcrustacean *Artemia salina* and the zebrafish (*Danio rerio*) to the biosurfactant. The biosurfactant proved efficient for use in remediation processes, removing 97.8% and 69.2% of the petroleum derivative from sand in kinetic and static tests, respectively, and removed 91.5% of the contaminant from seawater. The results indicate the potential of this new biosurfactant for the mobilisation and solubilisation of hydrocarbons in the marine environment. This green biomolecule is a promising technology for the replacement of chemical dispersants in the remediation of aquatic and soil systems.

Keywords: *Starmerella bombicola*; biosurfactant; bioemulsifier; toxicity; oil derivative; bioremediation

1. Introduction

Oil and its derivatives have played a central role in driving the economy for more than a century [1]. The primary sources of water and soil contamination by petroleum hydrocarbons are oil spills and the improper disposal of oily waste generated from leaks during the production, drilling, extraction, transportation, and storage of oil. This includes damage to pipelines and leaks from underground storage tanks [2]. When released into the environment, oil hydrocarbons spread horizontally, affecting a large area, and are decanted due to the action of gravity, resulting in the blockage of pores in the soil [3]. These durable, stable contaminants remain in the environment for long periods of time and do not easily undergo degradation [4].

Separation from the soil is difficult for two main reasons: (1) contaminants can be strongly absorbed by organic matter and encapsulated in minerals in the soil, which hampers the remediation process; and (2) soil is a complex, heterogeneous system and mass transfer processes play an important role in separation. Organic and inorganic colloids, flora, fauna, and microorganisms in the soil can also interfere with remediation [3,5].

Different methods are used to treat oily wastewater, such as flotation, sedimentation, coagulation, filtration, ultrafiltration, and reverse osmosis. As water and oil are practically immiscible, they are easy to separate. Water containing suspended, emulsified, or solubilised residual oil is treated and sent to an appropriate destination [6].

As environmental contamination with oil hydrocarbons constitutes a considerable threat to human health, different technologies are employed to remediate contaminated sites. Environmental remediation constitutes a set of methods used to mitigate the harmful effects of these pollutants. However, such methods involve the use of synthetic surfactants [7], which are highly toxic [8]. Thus, replacing synthetic compounds with natural products has attracted growing interest.

Concerns related to the depletion of fossil fuels have shifted the focus toward sustainable alternatives to conventional chemical processes that rely on petroleum [9]. The advancement of biorefinery practices has facilitated the obtainment of fuels, polymers, and chemicals produced from microbial sources [10]. Fermentation techniques that employ microbial strains enable the obtainment of high-value products, such as vitamins, carboxylic acids, biofuels, enzymes, etc. Natural products derived from microbial cells offer ecological compatibility and also require less land and water [11]. An environmental biodiversity analysis revealed that 99% of microbes exist in the form of consortia and have applications as functional ingredients in different industries [9,12].

There are approximately one million types of products of a natural origin. One-quarter of these are biologically active compounds. More than half are derived from plants, and the remainder are obtained from microorganisms, which produce about 23,000 secondary metabolites, with fungi accounting for 42% and filamentous bacteria accounting for 32% [13]. These statistics demonstrate the considerable biodiversity and utility of microorganisms for industrial purposes. Natural products constituted approximately 52% of all novel chemical products that received approval from the US Food and Drug Administration between the years 1981 and 2006 [14]. Numerous strategies have been developed and put into practice to obtain byproducts from microorganisms. However, a small number of microbial-based natural products are employed in the industrial sector [15], which underscores the need to establish a commercial market for bioproducts derived from microbes.

Biosurfactants constitute a valuable by-product obtained from microbial cells and have become increasingly competitive with synthetic surfactants derived from petroleum [16]. The increasing interest in microbial surfactants is due to the fact that such compounds are expected to replace synthetic petroleum surfactants, such as sodium dodecylbenzenesulfonate (SDBS), which have a slow degradation process. For instance, sulfonate surfactants are produced from alkyl aryl hydrocarbons, such as dodecylbenzene, which have a linear hydrocarbon structure without an aromatic component, and degradation takes three to eight days, compared to the 24 days that synthetic petroleum surfactants require [17].

Biosurfactants are biomolecules with hydrophobic and hydrophilic portions. The hydrophobic portion has long-chain fatty acids, whereas the hydrophilic portion may be an amino acid, carbohydrate, phosphate carboxyl acid, cyclic peptide, or alcohol [18]. This amphipathic nature gives biosurfactants surface-active properties that enable the reduction of surface tension and interfacial tension in aqueous solutions and mixtures with hydrocarbons. These metabolites are synthesised by yeasts, bacteria, and filamentous fungi of the genera *Candida, Pseudomonas, Bacillus, Starmerella, Rhodococcus*, and others [19–21].

The advantages of biosurfactants over synthetic surfactants include lower toxicity, greater biodegradability, and high stability over a broad range of pH, salinity, and temperature values. Thus, these biomolecules have applications in a variety of fields, including the food, biomedical, and environmental industries [22]. Moreover, the critical micelle concentration (CMC) of biosurfactants is lower. The CMC is the lowest amount of a surfactant needed to achieve the greatest reduction in surface tension, improving economic efficiency in different applications.

The properties of biosurfactants include humectation, emulsification, foaming, phase solubilisation, and dispersion. Depending on the combination of molar mass, mode of action, and physicochemical properties, biosurfactants can have low or high molecular weight. Those with low molecular weight reduce surface tension and interfacial tension, whereas those with high molecular weight are denominated bioemulsifiers and are more effective at ensuring the stabilisation of emulsions [18,23]. Biosurfactants generally have a molar mass ranging from 500 to 1500 Da [24]. With regards to the chemical composition, these biomolecules can be glycolipids (rhamnolipids, mannosylerythritol lipids, trehalose lipids), lipopeptides (surfactins, fengycins, lichenysines), glycolipopeptides, glycoproteins, phospholipids, neutral lipids, polymeric biosurfactants (emulsan, alasan, biodispersan), and particular biosurfactants (protein–sugar–lipid complex molecules) [25].

Biosurfactants can be used to enhance the washing and removal of lyophilic contaminants through displacement and solubilisation. Displacement occurs when the concentration of biosurfactant is below the CMC, whereas solubilisation occurs at higher concentrations. With the displacement mechanism, biosurfactant molecules accumulate at the interface between the soil and pollutant or between water and soil, causing the soil to roll and changing the affinity of the system for water. The adsorption of biosurfactant molecules to the surface of the contaminant results in repulsion forces between the main chemical groups of the contaminant and the soil particles, enhancing the separation of the contaminant. With the solubilisation mechanism, the contaminant is incorporated into the micelles formed by the presence of the biosurfactant, favouring partitioning towards the water phase. Pollutants that partition towards micelles can be recovered and demulsified, electrochemically destroyed, or adsorbed to activated carbon. The washing solution (biosurfactant) can be discarded or recycled to reduce remediation costs. Biosurfactants also increase the bioavailability of organic pollutants in the soil to microbial cells by lowering the surface tension of the aqueous phase, thereby facilitating biodegradation [26].

The compound annual growth rate of the global biosurfactant market is expected to be 0.8%, increasing from USD 1.3754 billion in 2020 to USD 1.4427 billion in 2026, although the cost of producing a biosurfactant is not yet compatible with the market demand. Foaming during processing, limited yields, expensive raw materials, and costs related to purification and downstream processing constitute some of the challenges to face when producing biosurfactants on an industrial scale. To solve this problem, industrial and agricultural byproducts have been used as substrates. Moreover, the use of waste products minimises pollution and reduces waste treatment costs. Statistical approaches and engineering methods have also been successfully used to reduce costs and optimise biosurfactant production operations [18,27].

The viability of industrial biosurfactant production depends on the target market. Production can only be performed on a small scale for food, medicinal, and cosmetic products due to the purification steps required. The use of crude fermentation broths, on the other hand, could be a viable solution for environmental applications, which do not require a purification step. Moreover, biosurfactants for such applications can be produced from microorganisms grown in media containing a combination of low-cost carbon sources, ensuring economic and environmental sustainability [28]. Thus, crude biosurfactants are promising for environmental remediation and wastewater treatment, taking advantage of the hydrophobicity of the microbial cell surface, which is an essential aspect of biodegradation [29].

The main challenges for biosurfactants are related to technical and economic issues. Technical problems include low production yields, low product concentration, high mass intensity, and high specific energy demands [30,31]. Economic issues arise from biosurfactant separation and purification processes, which involve technologies such as foam fractionation, membranes, gravity separation (e.g., acid precipitation, crystallization), and ultrafiltration, all of which have high capital and operating costs [32]. These challenges have hindered the widespread replacement of chemical surfactants with biosurfactants. Various process improvements have been proposed, including metabolic engineering, bioprocess engineering, chemical engineering, and process engineering. For example, genetically modified microorganisms (GMOs) have been developed to increase the yield of biosurfactants [33]. Hybrid production schemes, which integrate product formation and separation, have also been studied to reduce processing steps and production costs, but these methods are still in the research stage [34]. Few studies have focused on the conceptual design of biosurfactant production processes from a techno-economic and environmental perspective to explore potential technologies for upscaling. However, it is important for the development of biosurfactants to expand beyond the academic sector, as the industrial development of biosurfactants is linked to establishing a circular bioeconomy by using renewable sources for production [35]. The increasing development of biosurfactants is driven by current laws and policies regulating the use of environmentally harmful chemicals. Such laws and policies have been announced and implemented throughout the world, further promoting the shift towards the use of sustainable eco-friendly products [22]. For example, BASF SE (Ludwigshafen, Germany) has entered partnership agreements with Allied Carbon Solutions Co. Ltd. (Numazu, Japan) and Holiferm Ltd. (Manchester, United Kingdom) to advance sustainable biosurfactant production for the personal and home care sector. These actions set an example to encourage the production of bio-based products in line with policies, laws, and financial incentives [36].

The research addressed in this paper focuses on technical and environmental information regarding the production of a new biosurfactant. The aim was to produce a biosurfactant from the yeast *Starmerella bombicola* ATCC 22214 and evaluate its properties, toxicity, and safety for use in remediating soil and water contaminated with an oil derivative. In the following sections, we will explain how we were able to achieve high yields in the production of this novel biosurfactant using low-cost substrates. This biomolecule is highly efficient, non-toxic, and environmentally friendly, and can be used without requiring multiple purification steps.

2. Materials and Methods

2.1. Microorganism, Maintenance Medium, and Growth Medium

The yeast *S. bombicola* ATCC 22214 purchased from the American Type Culture Collection was used for biosurfactant production and was maintained in yeast mould agar (YMA) medium at 5 °C. The medium was composed of distilled water (100 mL) with peptone (0.5%), agar (2%), D-glucose (1%), and yeast extract (0.3%), pH 7.0. To maintain viability, transfers to fresh agar slants were performed every month. The growth medium was yeast mould broth (YMB), with the same composition as the YMA medium, but without the agar.

2.2. Growth of Inoculum

To standardise the inoculum, the culture was transferred to a tube containing the YMA medium at 28 °C, obtaining a young culture, and the sample was placed in a 250 mL Erlenmeyer flask with YMB medium (50 mL). Incubation was performed under aerobic conditions, with constant agitation (150 rpm) for 48 h at 28 °C. The mixture was diluted until reaching 10^4 cells/mL. A Neubauer chamber was used for the cell count. The inoculum was used at a concentration of 5% (v/v).

2.3. Production Media and Culture Conditions

Different media (500 mL) were used for biosurfactant production based on descriptions in the literature (Table 1). Erlenmeyer flasks with a capacity of 1000 mL were used for fermentation to produce biosurfactants. The pH was adjusted to 6.0. An autoclave operating at 121 °C was used to sterilise the media (15 min), which were then incubated under aerobic conditions with 5% of the pre-inoculum and kept under orbital agitation at 200 rpm for

192 h at a temperature of 28 °C. The pH of the media was not adjusted during cultivation. All analyses were performed in triplicate and did not vary more than 5%.

Table 1. Composition of biosurfactant production media.

Medium	Components of Production Medium (g/L)
Medium 1	Sunflower oil: 50; Glucose: 25; Yeast extract: 1; KH_2PO_4: 0.5; $MgSO_4{\cdot}7H_2O$: 0.5; $NaNO_3$: 3
Medium 2	Sunflower oil: 50; Sucrose: 25; Yeast extract: 1; KH_2PO_4: 0.5; $MgSO_4{\cdot}7H_2O$: 0.5; $NaNO_3$: 3
Medium 3	Canola oil: 12; Glucose: 100; Corn steep liquor: 5; K_2HPO_4: 1; $(NH_4)_2SO_4$: 4; $MgSO_4{\cdot}7H_2O$: 0.5
Medium 4	Canola oil: 12; Sucrose: 100; Corn steep liquor: 5; K_2HPO_4: 1; $(NH_4)_2SO_4$: 4; $MgSO_4{\cdot}7H_2O$: 0.5
Medium 5	Canola oil: 12; Glucose: 100; Corn steep liquor: 5
Medium 6	Canola oil: 12; Sucrose: 100; Corn steep liquor: 5
Medium 7	Crude cotton seed oil: 100; Glucose: 100; Urea: 1.5; K_2HPO_4: 1; Corn steep liquor: 4; NaCl: 0.1
Medium 8	Refined cotton seed oil: 100; Glucose: 100; Urea: 1.5; K_2HPO_4: 1; Corn steep liquor: 4; NaCl: 0.1
Medium 9	Crude cotton seed oil: 100; Sucrose: 100; Urea: 1.5; K_2HPO_4: 1; Corn steep liquor: 4; NaCl: 0.1
Medium 10	Refined cotton seed oil: 100; Sucrose: 100; Urea: 1.5; K_2HPO_4: 1; Corn steep liquor: 4; NaCl: 0.1

2.4. Isolation of Biosurfactant

Liquid–liquid extraction was used to isolate the biosurfactant. For such, ethyl acetate (proportion of 1:4 (v/v) with the non-centrifuged medium) was used twice. After centrifugation of the organic phase at 2600× g for 20 min, filtration was performed, and the filtrate was placed in a separatory funnel with a solution of saturated sodium chloride (NaCl) for separation of the remaining aqueous phase. Next, the organic phase was placed into an Erlenmeyer flask, followed by the addition of anhydrous magnesium sulphate ($MgSO_4$) until the formation of granules. Filtration was then performed using a qualitative paper filter (Whatman No. 1), followed by drying at a temperature of 50 °C [37].

2.5. Biosurfactant Characterisation

The ionic charge of the biosurfactant was determined using the agar double diffusion method [38]. Two rows of wells were prepared in 1% agar. The wells of one row received the isolated biosurfactant solution, and the wells of the other row received a pure compound, the ionic charge of which was known. The anionic substance was sodium dodecyl sulphate (SDS) (20 mM), and the cationic substance was barium chloride (50 mM). The ionic nature of the biosurfactant was indicated by precipitation lines between the wells after monitoring for 48 h at room temperature.

^{1}H and ^{13}C nuclear magnetic resonance (NMR) analyses were performed in a 500 MHz spectrometer (Bruker INOVA, Varian, Palo Alto, CA, USA). For such, 20 mg of the isolated biosurfactant was dissolved in deuterated chloroform (CDCl3; Sigma-Aldrich, Taufkirchen, Germany) (500 μL) at 300 MHz and 298.1 K. The ppm scale relative to normal tetramethylsilane (TMS) was considered for the analysis of chemical shifts (δ). Fourier transform infrared (FTIR) spectroscopy (400 Perkin Elmer) was also used to characterise the isolated biosurfactant in the wavenumber range of 4000 to 400 (resolution: 4 cm^{-1}).

2.6. Surface Tension

A Sigma 700 Tensiometer (KSV Instruments Ltd., Helsinki, Finland) with a du Noüy ring was used at room temperature for the automatic measurement of surface tension in samples of the cell-free broth (crude biosurfactant) centrifuged at 10,000× g for 15 min.

2.7. Emulsification Index (E_{24})

Two mL of the crude biosurfactant solution (cell-free broth) were placed in a screw-top tube (100 mm × 13 mm) to which 2 mL of used motor oil was added for the determination of emulsification activity following the method proposed by Cooper and Goldenberg [39]. Motor oil used as a contaminant was obtained from a local automotive manufacturer in the city of Recife, Brazil. This oil is commercially available for use in flex engines (gasoline, CNG, and alcohol) and is labelled SAE 20W-50 with synthetic blend (PETROBRAS, Rio de Janeiro, Brazil). It is composed of a paraffinic base lubricating oil (a complex mixture of hydrocarbons) and includes performance-enhancing additives. The viscosity of the oil is 98.0 cSt (at 40 °C) and its density is 0.9420 g/mL (at 20 °C). The contents of the tube were mixed in a vortex at 50 Hz for two minutes. The emulsification index (E_{24}) was determined after 24 h using Equation:

$$E_{24} = (he/ht) \times 100$$

in which: he = height of emulsion layer; ht = total height of mixture measured with a ruler in mm. The samples were stored at 27 °C [40].

2.8. Effect of Environmental Factors

The effects of environmental factors on surface tension and emulsification activity in solutions of the crude biosurfactant (cell-free broth) were investigated as described in Sections 2.6 and 2.7, considering different temperatures (0, 5, 28, 70, 100, and 120 °C) for 60 min, pH (2.0, 4.0, 6.0, 8.0, 10.0, and 12.0) after adjustments with HCl or NaOH 6.0 M, and concentrations of NaCl (2, 4, 6, 8, 10, and 12%) at 28 °C [41].

2.9. Determination of Critical Micelle Concentration

The critical micelle concentration (CMC) was determined by diluting sodium hydroxide (NaOH) in a small fraction of distilled water, to which the crude extract of the biosurfactant was added at a proportion of 1:7 (v/v) ratio. The product was washed in acetone, followed by filtration through a sintered glass filter and drying for evaporation of the solvent. The product (0.1 g) was successively diluted with distilled water, followed by the quantification of surface tension with the aid of the KSV Sigma 700 tensiometer and du Noüy ring up to a constant value (standard deviation less than 0.4 mN/m during 10 successive measurements) to obtain the CMC, which was expressed as g/L of biosurfactant. The ring method involves raising the liquid until it touches the surface. The sample is then lowered again to stretch the film formed beneath the liquid to determine maximum force, which is then used to calculate surface tension. The instrument was calibrated using Mill-Q-4 ultrapure distilled water from Millipore (Burlington, MA, USA). Before use, the platinum plate and all glassware were washed with chromic acid, deionized water, and acetone in sequence and then flamed with a Bunsen burner. Samples were read three times for accuracy [37].

2.10. Toxicity Test with Artemia salina as Indicator

Brine shrimp (*Artemia salina*) larvae were used as the bioindicator in the toxicity test of the biosurfactant. Eggs of the microcrustacean were purchased from a local store, and larvae were obtained after 24 h of incubation. Ten larvae were placed in 10 mL flasks with seawater (5.0 mL), together with 5.0 mL of the crude biosurfactant (cell-free broth) or different concentrations of the isolated biosurfactant (½ CMC, CMC, 2 × CMC, 3 × CMC, and 5 × CMC). The control treatment was seawater alone (without biosurfactant). Mortality was determined after 24 h [42].

2.11. Ecotoxicity Tests with Danio rerio as Indicator

Adult zebrafish (*Danio rerio*) were fed nauplii of *Artemia* sp. four times per day. A 50 L aquarium was used, into which eight females and four males were placed for reproduction. Fertilised eggs were examined using an inverted microscope at a magnification of 40 times. Fertilisation was greater than 90%. Eggs with opacity or coagulation were discarded. The environmental variables of interest were pH (7.5 to 7.9), temperature (27 ± 0.5 °C), and dissolved oxygen (5 to 6.5 mg/L).

The fish embryo test (FET) was used, in which fertilised eggs were exposed to the biosurfactant [43]. The signs of embryo death were egg coagulation, absence of somites after 24 h, as well as the absence of a heartbeat or movement. The number of deaths after 96 h of exposure was compared to the total exposed to each sample (20 individuals) for the calculation of the mortality rate [44].

The general morphology score (sum partial scores for each embryo during morphological development in 96 h of exposure) was used to determine sublethal effects. Developmental markers were investigated at 24 h intervals, with the determination of abnormalities indicating sublethal effects. The effect of the different concentrations of the biosurfactant on the embryos was determined by comparisons with the control. The following characteristics and respective time intervals were considered: detachment of the tail during the initial development of the embryo (24 h); formation of somites (24 and 48 h); development and pigmentation of eyes (24 to 96 h); movement of the embryo (24 to 96 h); the presence of blood circulation (24 to 96 h); the presence of heartbeats (48 to 96 h); pigmentation of head and body (48 to 96 h); pigmentation of the tail (48 to 96 h); the presence of an extension of a nearly empty vitelline sac related to a nearly completely resorbed vitelline sac (96 h), enabling a space where the swim bladder will be; presence of pectoral fins (72 to 96 h); presence of a salient mouth (72 to 96 h); hatching (72 to 96 h). The maximum GMS is 18 at the end of 96 h, indicating a perfectly developed larva [44–46].

Statistical analysis: A logistic curve was used to calculate the lethal effects of $LC_{50/96h}$ with the aid of R software 4.0.2 (R Development Core Team, 2020, Auckland, New Zealand) [47]. One-way analysis of variance (ANOVA) was used to determine mean GMSs obtained from embryos exposed to different concentrations of the biosurfactant, considering a 5% significance level. Dunnett's post hoc test was used to detect significant differences from the control. Statistical analysis was performed with the aid of the SigmaPlot software, version 12 (Jandel Scientific, Erkrath, Germany).

2.12. Remediation Experiment with Oil Derivative Adsorbed to Sand—Kinetic Test

Sand (10 g) contaminated with a 10% motor oil solution was placed in 100 mL of drinking water, to which 1 mL of sugarcane molasses donated by a local processing plant was added. The mixture was sterilised under fluent vapor and constituted the control condition. Next, 2% solutions of different concentrations of the isolated biosurfactant (CMC and 2 × CMC) were added, followed by 15% of the inoculum containing 10^7 colony-forming units/mL cultivated in the YMB medium. The mixtures were incubated at 150 rpm and 28 °C for 75 days. The experiments were performed in triplicate using 250 mL Erlenmeyer flasks. The following conditions were analysed: Control—contaminated sand + molasses; Condition 1: contaminated sand + molasses + *S. bombicola*; Condition 2: contaminated sand + molasses + biosurfactant (CMC) + *S. bombicola*; Condition 3: contaminated sand + molasses + *S. bombicola* + biosurfactant (2 × CMC). Molasses (1%) was added at regular intervals (Days 15, 30, 45, and 60). Aliquots (5 mL) were withdrawn every 15 days for analysis, totalling five samplings (Days 15, 30, 45, 60, and 75) [48]. The oil removal rate was determined by gravimetry, as described in Section 2.14.

2.13. Removal of Oil Derivative Adsorbed to Sand in Packed Columns—Static Test

Sand (10 g) contaminated with a 10% motor oil solution (*w*/*w*) was placed in glass columns (55 × 6 cm). The surface was then inundated with 200 mL of the biosurfactant solution at the CMC (Condition 1) and 2 × CMC (Condition 2) under the action of gravity.

The crude biosurfactant (cell-free broth) was tested with the same quantity (Condition 3). A column containing the sand and water (200 mL) was the control. After 24 h, no further percolation of the biosurfactant solutions was observed [48,49]. The oil removal rate was determined by gravimetry, as described in Section 2.14.

2.14. Analysis of Oil Derivative Removed from Sand

One hundred mL of n-hexane was added to the liquid phase in a decantation funnel and agitated for 10 min. The mixture was either placed into a rotary evaporator to evaporate the hexane or hexane was evaporated in a laboratory oven at 68–70 °C. The beaker with the residual oil was weighed.

The role of the aging factor in pollution phenomena of soil and sand particles, which is an important element in the effective dynamics of contaminant removal, was considered using motor oil samples that were previously exposed to room temperature (30–35 °C) for a period of one year prior to use.

2.15. Remediation Experiment of Oil Derivative in Seawater

Bioremediation tests were performed based on the methods described in the Standard Methods for the Examination of Water and Wastewater [50]. Motor oil removal experiments were conducted in 250 mL Erlenmeyer flasks with 50 mL of seawater collected from Port Suape and 1% motor oil. The medium was sterilised, followed by inoculation with 5% of the inoculum of the biosurfactant-producing microorganism (10^7 colony-forming units/mL with an O.D. of 0.7 to 600 nm). The flasks were agitated at 150 rpm in a rotary shaker for 30 days, with samples withdrawn for analysis every 10 days (totalling three samples). The experiments involved the following different conditions: Control − seawater + motor oil; Condition 1: seawater + motor oil + *S. bombicola;* Condition 2: seawater + motor oil + *S. bombicola* + biosurfactant (CMC); Condition 3: seawater + motor oil + *S. bombicola* + biosurfactant (2 × CMC). The oil degradation efficiency was determined as described in Section 2.16.

2.16. Calculation of Degradation Efficiency of Oil Derivative from Seawater

The oil degraded from the samples and control medium was quantified following extraction with n-hexane. The residual oil was separated using a separatory funnel with the same volume of hexane in a beaker that had previously been weighed.

2.17. Statistical Analysis

Statistical analysis was performed with the aid of Statistica® (version 7.0) using the one-way procedure, followed by linear one-way analysis of variance (ANOVA). The results of triplicate experiments were expressed as mean and standard deviation. Tukey's post hoc test was used with a 95% significance level for the determination of significant differences.

3. Results and Discussion

3.1. Biosurfactant Production, Isolation, and Emulsifying Capacity

Biosurfactants were produced by *S. bombicola* ATCC 22214 using different media, followed by the determination of the surface tension of the crude biosurfactants, yield (through the isolation of the organic solvent), and emulsifying capacity. The results are displayed in Table 2.

Surface tension is one of the most important properties for the determination of the effectiveness of a biosurfactant [51]. According to Akbari et al. [52], biosurfactants with the capacity to reduce the surface tension of water from 72 to 35 mN/m are effective. Thus, all biosurfactants produced in the present study achieved satisfactory results (Table 2). The similar surface tension of the different biosurfactants demonstrates that *S. bombicola* ATCC 22214 can produce biosurfactants using a variety of substrates. Previous studies have also reported the versatility of this yeast in producing biosurfactants in different media [53–55]. Jiménez-Peñalver et al. [56] produced a biosurfactant from *S. bombicola*

ATCC 22214 in a low-cost medium that lowered surface tension to 33.8 mN/m. Jadhav et al. [57] cultivated *S. bombicola* MTCC 1910 in a medium in which the carbon source was 10% residue from a sunflower oil refinery and obtained a biosurfactant that lowered the surface tension to 35.50 mN/m. Shah et al. [58] cultivated *S. bombicola* ATCC 22214 in a medium with 10% palm oil and produced a biosurfactant that lowered the surface tension to 35.35 mN/m. Gaur et al. [59] produced a biosurfactant from the yeast *Candida albicans* SC5314 that reduced the surface tension to 42 mN/m. These results are similar to those found in the present investigation.

Table 2. Surface tension results, yield, and motor oil emulsification index of biosurfactants produced by *S. bombicola* ATCC 22214 in different production media (data expressed as mean ± SD of triplicate determinations).

Biosurfactant	Surface Tension (mN/m)	Yield (g/L)	Emulsification Index (%)
Medium 1	32.4 ± 0.2	8.1	83.3 ± 0.1
Medium 2	32.8 ± 0.1	7.3	84.4 ± 0.4
Medium 3	38.0 ± 0.1	11.4	77.0 ± 0.1
Medium 4	32.7 ± 0.3	23.0	96.2 ± 0.1
Medium 5	32.8 ± 0.5	7.7	90.2 ± 0.1
Medium 6	32.9 ± 0.2	5.3	90.5 ± 0.1
Medium 7	33.6 ± 0.6	5.4	72.9 ± 0.1
Medium 8	33.1 ± 0.1	8.7	91.0 ± 0.1
Medium 9	33.4 ± 0.4	10.1	89.7 ± 0.1
Medium 10	31.3 ± 0.1	19.5	92.4 ± 0.5

The simplified isolation method carried out in the laboratory was used to determine biosurfactant yields. The advantage of this method is the elimination of the initial centrifugation and filtration steps involved with other methods and the use of a smaller quantity of solvent. The present results are in agreement with data described in previous studies involving the isolation of biosurfactants produced by microorganisms of the genus *Candida*. Marcelino et al. [60] cultivated *S. bombicola* in a mineral medium supplemented with soybean oil and corn industry residue, obtaining a biosurfactant yield of 15.6 g/L. Dierickx et al. [61] cultivated *S. bombicola* in a 7.5 L bioreactor and obtained a biosurfactant yield of 87.12 g/L, indicating that it is possible to scale up the production of the biosurfactant produced by this species.

The emulsification index was calculated to determine the capacity of the biosurfactants produced in the different media to emulsify residual motor oil. The results were above 90% for all tests, indicating the high emulsifying activity of the biomolecules. Using a biosurfactant produced by *C. albicans* IMRU 3669, El-Sheshtawy et al. [62] obtained 65% emulsification of a petroleum derivative. Lira et al. [63] produced a biosurfactant from *C. guilliermondii* UCP 0992 in a medium supplemented with 5% corn steep liquor, 5% soybean waste frying oil, and 5% sugarcane molasses and obtained 71.4% emulsification of motor oil. Santos et al. [64] produced a biosurfactant from *C. lipolytica* UCP 0988 in a medium supplemented with industrial waste products and achieved 60% emulsification of motor oil.

Emulsion systems containing hydrocarbons and water have low stability. Therefore, surfactants are used to stabilise these systems. The stability provided by surfactants demonstrates the surface activity of the compound. However, it is important to note that surfactants and emulsifiers serve different purposes. Surfactants primarily function to reduce interfacial tension, while emulsifiers adsorb more slowly to the droplet surface, providing long-term stability [65]. The biosurfactant produced by *S. bombicola* in medium 4 (1.2% canola oil, 10% sucrose, 0.5% corn steep liquor, 0.1% K_2HPO_4, 0.4% $(NH_4)_2SO_4$, and 0.05% $MgSO_4{\cdot}7H_2O$) was selected for further experiments, as the best yield and the highest emulsification index were achieved with this medium. The replacement of glucose with sucrose is an important point, as it reduces the final production cost.

3.2. Biosurfactant Characterisation

The double diffusion method in agar showed that the biosurfactant is anionic. Using the same method, other biosurfactants produced by yeasts were also described as anionic [66,67].

A ^{1}H NMR spectrum was obtained from the purified biosurfactant (Figure 1). The peaks between 0 and 3 ppm suggest aliphatic groups, with the presence of hydrogens of methyl groups (0–1.2 ppm), aliphatic carbons (1.3–1.8 ppm, 1.8–2.0 ppm), and the carbonyl group (2.2–2.8 ppm). The peaks between 4 and 4.4 ppm suggest the presence of hydroxyl (-OH). Moreover, a double bond was found at 5.3 ppm. Gaur et al. [59] found similar peaks in the characterisation of a sophorolipid. Similar peaks were also found in the analysis of the biosurfactant produced by *S. bombicola* NRRL Y-17069 [68].

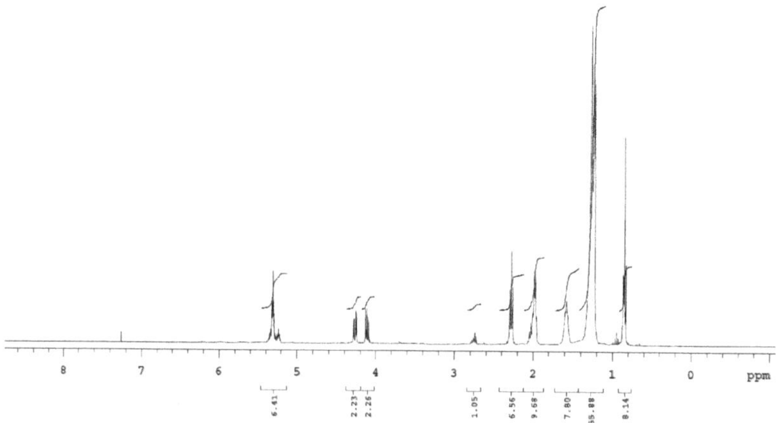

Figure 1. ^{1}H NMR spectrum (CD3OH, 300 MHz) of biosurfactant isolated from *S. bombicola* ATCC 22214 cultivated in 10% sucrose, 0.5% corn steep liquor, 1.2% canola oil, 0.1% K_2HPO_4, 0.4% $(NH_4)_2SO_4$, and 0.05% $MgSO_4{\cdot}7H_2O$.

In the ^{13}C NMR spectrum, the peak at 173 ppm was attributed to the C=O of carboxyl acid or ester. Double-bond peaks were found between 120 and 140 ppm. Hydroxyl (-OH) was detected between 60 and 70 ppm. Signals were also detected between 10 and 40 ppm, which are characteristic of aliphatic carbons (Figure 2).

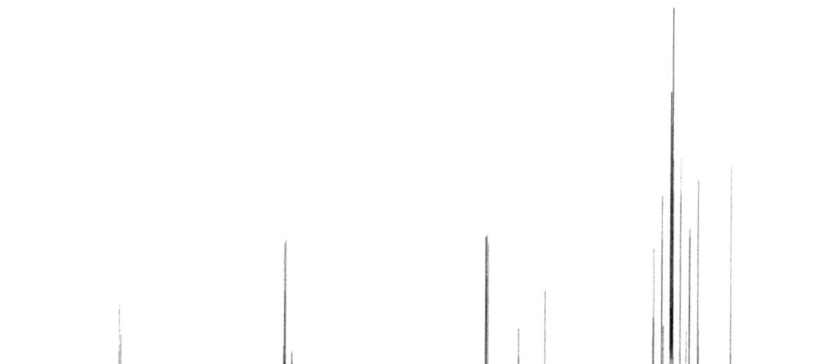

Figure 2. ^{13}C NMR spectrum (CD3OD, 300 MHz) of biosurfactant isolated from *S. bombicola* ATCC 22214 cultivated in 10% sucrose, 0.5% corn steep liquor, 1.2% canola oil, 0.1% K_2HPO_4, 0.4% $(NH_4)_2SO_4$, and 0.05% $MgSO_4{\cdot}7H_2O$.

FTIR spectra (Figure 3) revealed a characteristic stretching of O–H near 3500 cm^{-1} in the structure of the biosurfactant. The peak at 3006 cm^{-1} was attributed to =C–H stretching. The peaks at 2924 cm^{-1} and 2854 cm^{-1} were attributed to –C–H stretching. An absorbance band was found at 1747 cm^{-1} and attributed to the vibration of the stretching of –C=O. The bands at approximately 1463 cm^{-1} and 1377 cm^{-1} are associated with the asymmetrical and symmetrical bending of CH_3, respectively. Stretching characteristic of C (=O)–O–C was found at 1163 cm^{-1}. C–O–C stretches were obtained at 1120 cm^{-1} and 1096 cm^{-1}, suggesting a glycosidic bond. The structural details of the biosurfactant produced by *S. bombicola* ATCC 22214 were similar to those described for sophorolipid biosurfactants characterised in previous studies [58,59,69,70].

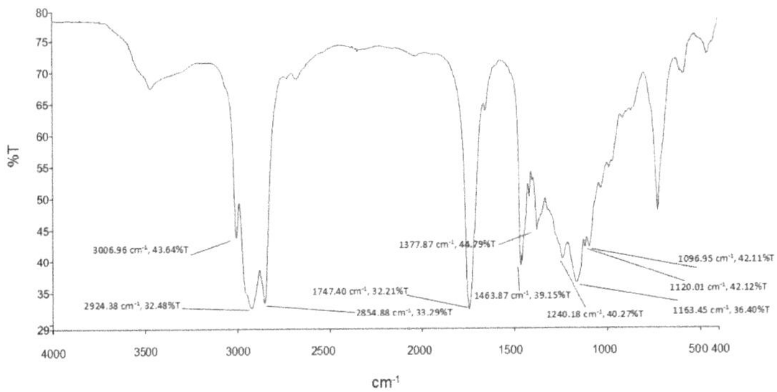

Figure 3. FTIR absorption spectra of biosurfactant produced by *S. bombicola* ATCC 22214 cultivated in 10% sucrose, 0.5% corn steep liquor, 1.2% canola oil, 0.1% K_2HPO_4, 0.4% $(NH_4)_2SO_4$, and 0.05% $MgSO_4{\cdot}7H_2O$.

3.3. Critical Micelle Concentration

The effectiveness of a biosurfactant in reducing surface tension is determined by its critical micelle concentration (CMC), which is the concentration at which the surfactant starts forming micelles. Therefore, a lower CMC indicates a more effective surfactant, making it more desirable for the industries by improving its cost–performance profile, which determines its commercial viability [71,72]. Figure 4 shows the change in surface tension as a function of the concentration of the biosurfactant produced in medium 4. The CMC of the biosurfactant produced by *S. bombicola* ATCC 22214 was reached at a concentration of 0.6 g/L, indicating satisfactory efficiency. Studying a biosurfactant produced by *C. bombicola* URM 3718, Silva et al. [37] determined a CMC of 0.5 g/L. Ashish and Debnath [73] produced a biosurfactant from *C. tropicalis* MTCC230 and determined a CMC of 0.0325 g/L.

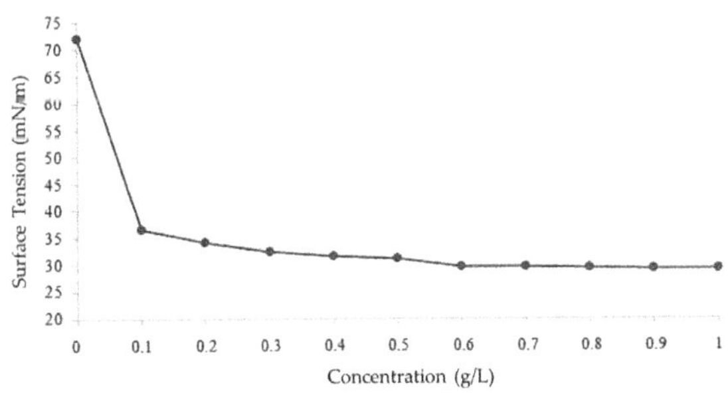

Figure 4. CMC of biosurfactant produced by *S. bombicola* ATCC 22214 in medium composed of 10% sucrose, 0.5% corn steep liquor, 1.2% canola oil, 0.1% K_2HPO_4, 0.4% $(NH_4)_2SO_4$, and 0.05% $MgSO_4{\cdot}7H_2O$.

3.4. Stability of Biosurfactant

The stability study of a biosurfactant is required to determine its applicability, as applications in specific environments can pose a challenge. For a biosurfactant to have industrial use, it must maintain its surface-active characteristics irrespective of the environmental conditions to which it is subjected [74].

Biosurfactant yields obtained in the fermentation process are essential for their use in the bioremediation of large areas contaminated with hydrocarbons. Thus, using crude biosurfactants (cell-free broth) is recommended in view of economic considerations. Therefore, the stability of the biosurfactant produced in medium 4 was investigated in its crude form considering the effect on surface tension and emulsification capacity in the presence of residual motor oil (Table 3).

Table 3. Influence of saline (NaCl) concentration, temperature, and pH on reduction in surface tension and emulsifying activity of residual motor oil in cell-free broth containing biosurfactant produced by *S. bombicola* ATCC 22214 cultivated in 10% sucrose, 0.5% corn steep liquor, 1.2% canola oil, 0.1% K_2HPO_4, 0.4% $(NH_4)_2SO_4$, and 0.05% $MgSO_4 \cdot 7H_2O$ (data expressed as mean ± SD of triplicate determinations).

NaCl (v/v)	Surface Tension (%)	Emulsification Index (%)
2	33.3 ± 0.02	95.5 ± 0.3
4	33.7 ± 0.03	95.4 ± 0.3
6	32.2 ± 0.01	96.2 ± 0.2
8	33.5 ± 0.02	96.2 ± 0.1
10	31.8 ± 0.02	96.2 ± 0.2
12	32.4 ± 0.01	96.9 ± 0.1
Temperature (°C)	**Surface Tension (mN/m)**	**Emulsification Index (%)**
0	33.7 ± 0.02	96.3 ± 0.2
5	33.9 ± 0.01	96.4 ± 0.2
28	32.7 ± 0.01	96.3 ± 0.4
70	32.8 ± 0.00	92.7 ± 0.2
100	32.8 ± 0.00	92.6 ± 0.4
120	33.5 ± 0.18	90.4 ± 0.3
pH	**Surface Tension (mN/m)**	**Emulsification Index (%)**
2	35.0 ± 0.02	94.4 ± 0.1
4	34.9 ± 0.03	94.5 ± 0.3
6	32.7 ± 0.01	95.5 ± 0.2
8	31.8 ± 0.01	95.5 ± 0.2
10	34.2 ± 0.01	96.4 ± 0.2
12	33.9 ± 0.01	97.6 ± 0.1

The biosurfactant maintained the ability to reduce surface tension in the presence of all concentrations of NaCl added to the cell-free broth (2–12%), indicating good tolerance to salinity. The concentrations of NaCl also did not exert a substantial influence on the emulsification index. As the salinity of the ocean is around 3%, the biosurfactant produced by *S. bombicola* ATCC 22214 can be applied in environments with a high saline concentration.

Surface tension remained around 33 mN/m, with little variation in the cell-free broth at temperatures ranging from 0 to 120 °C. This indicates that the biosurfactant can be applied in environments that undergo a significant change in temperature, such as industries in which sterility is achieved by heat. The emulsification indices of motor oil also demonstrated thermal stability.

The surface tension of the cell-free broth fluctuated somewhat with the change in pH, remaining relatively stable (around 35 mN/m) at more acidic pH (2 and 4) and more basic pH (around 34 mN/m) and dropping to 32 mN/m at pH 6 and 8. The emulsification of the motor oil increased with the increase in pH. Ashish and Debnath [74] found similar behaviour.

Based on the results, the crude biosurfactant can be applied in environments with extreme salinity, temperature, and pH, as in oil recovery activities and the bioremediation of polluted marine environments, with no significant change in its properties. This factor is important, as the purification step can correspond to as much as 60% of the total production cost of a biosurfactant. The elimination of this step lowers the application cost of the biosurfactant produced by *S. bombicola* ATCC 22214, constituting another advantage of this novel biomolecule in the petroleum market.

3.5. Toxicity of Biosurfactants to Artemia salina

The literature suggests that biosurfactants are less harmful than synthetic surfactants and dispersants. However, the impact of these biomolecules on the environment has not been studied enough [75]. Indeed, recent research emphasises the importance of conducting thorough investigations to understand the properties of new biosurfactants before release into the environment. According to Silva et al. [76], biosurfactants are commonly non-toxic to microorganisms at concentrations close to the CMC.

A bioassay was conducted involving larvae of the microcrustacean *Artemia salina* to determine the toxicity of the biosurfactant produced by *S. bombicola* ATCC 22214 (Table 4). No mortality occurred after exposure to the crude biosurfactant and different concentrations of the isolated biosurfactant (½ CMC, CMC, and 2 × CMC) for 24 h, indicating the absence of toxicity. In contrast, mortality was 10 and 20% at concentrations of 3 × CMC and 5 × CMC, respectively. Acute toxicity tests of a biosurfactant produced by *C. bombicola* to *A. salina* larvae also demonstrated low toxicity in a previous study [77].

Table 4. Toxicity of biosurfactant produced by *S. bombicola* ATCC 22214 cultivated in 10% sucrose, 0.5% corn steep liquor, 1.2% canola oil, 0.1% K_2HPO_4, 0.4% $(NH_4)_2SO_4$, and 0.05% $MgSO_4 \cdot 7H_2O$.

Biosurfactant Concentration in Saline Water	Mortality of Brine Shrimp Larvae (%)
Cell-free broth	no mortality
½ × CMC	no mortality
CMC	no mortality
2 × CMC	no mortality
3 × CMC	10.000 ± 0.000
5 × CMC	20.000 ± 0.000

3.6. Ecotoxicity of Biosurfactant to Danio rerio (Zebrafish)

Surfactants stand out among synthetic materials due to their unique properties, which enable their application in diverse fields compared to conventional solvents. However, approximately 60% of chemical surfactants enter aquatic environments [78], and the continual emissions negatively alter the health of such environments. Thus, biosurfactants constitute a viable option to diminish the harmful effects on natural ecosystems due to their low toxicity while maintaining the same functions as synthetic products [79]. To assess the toxicity level of these compounds, it is necessary to carry out controlled, standardised ecotoxicology tests that use established organisms as adequate biological models for such analyses. Among the test organisms used for this purpose, the teleost fish *D. rerio* (zebrafish) is currently one of the main biological models of vertebrates used in ecotoxicological tests for environmental monitoring and the laboratory assessment of toxicity at lethal and sublethal levels of isolated substances or mixtures, including morphological and behavioural biomarkers [44,80]. Toxicity tests were performed on samples of the biosurfactant produced by *S. bombicola* ATCC 22214, with the analysis of lethal and sublethal effects [43,45].

One hundred ninety-two embryos were used in the tests performed in culture plates: 24 in the culture water (control) and 7 in plates with different concentrations of the biosurfactant. The mortality of the embryos is displayed in Table 5.

Table 5. Quantity of dead individuals exposed to different concentrations of biosurfactant with percentage of deaths 96 h post-exposure (hpe). Twenty individuals used in each treatment.

Concentration (mg/L)	Deaths 24 hpe	Deaths 48 hpe	Deaths 96 hpe	Mortality Rate (%) at End of Test (96 h)
600	20	-	-	100
300	20	-	-	100
150	9	8	3	100
75	0	4	16	100
37.50	0	4	16	100
18.750	0	3	14	85
9.375	0	0	5	25

The data showed the absence of toxicity with less than 24 h of exposure for all concentrations less than 75 mg/L, unlike what was found for exposure to three synthetic surfactants (dodecyl dimethyl benzyl ammonium chloride, sodium dodecyl sulphate, and fatty alcohol polyoxyethylene ether), for which the mortality rate was 53% at concentrations of 1 mg/L in the first 10 h of exposure, demonstrating high toxicity [81]. A study using a biosurfactant for the control of aquatic pathogens (SPH6) reported 10% toxicity at a concentration of 20 mg/L in 24 h, by which the surfactant was considered a product with low toxicity [82]. In the present study, 15% mortality was found beginning with 48 h of exposure at a concentration of 18.75 mg/L, which demonstrates lower toxicity of the biosurfactant produced by *S. bombicola* ATCC 22214.

The lethal concentration that kills fifty percent of the organisms (LC_{50}) was 134.4, 100.8, and 15 mg/L after 24, 48, and 96 h of exposure, respectively, which, based on data from the U.S. Fish and Wildlife Service, denotes low toxicity [83]. Previous studies using commercial surfactants reported lower LC_{50} than the values found in the present investigation, such as the 18.3 μg/L described by Al-asmakh et al. [84] using AEO-7. Yi et al. [79] performed tests involving sodium dodecylbenzenesulfonate, nonylphenol exthoxylate (NPE), and stearyl trimethylammonium bromide and found LC_{50} values of 5.77 mg/L, 17.24 mg/L, and 0.73 mg/L, respectively, which are in agreement with the low toxicity found in the present study. In a study involving a biosurfactant produced by *Pseudomonas putida*, the LC_{50} was 60 mg/L when zebrafish embryos were exposed for 48 h, which is considered low toxicity. Johann et al. [85] reported an LC_{50} of 100.8 mg/L in the same period used in the present investigation.

With regards to sublethal effects, embryo–larval development was only analysed at the lowest concentrations (9.37 and 18.75 mg/L) due to the low mortality found after exposure for 96 h. No significant differences were found when these concentrations were compared to the control (Figure 5).

Despite the absence of toxicity in the GMS analysis at the lowest concentrations, some embryos exhibited pericardial oedema and haemorrhage when exposed to other concentrations of the biosurfactant (Figure 6), with a frequency of 63% at 150 mg/L, 18.75% at 75 mg/L, and 12.5% at 37.5 mg/L. Such pathologies were not found at the other concentrations. In previous studies, pericardial oedema was also found in zebrafish embryos and larvae exposed to 12.8 μg/L of AEO-7 [84], 10 mg/L of NPE, and 0.5 mg/L of STAB [79], which are much lower concentrations than the lowest concentration at which this effect was found in the present study (37.5 mg/L).

The tests carried out with the biosurfactant produced by *S. bombicola* ATCC 22214 demonstrated low toxicity to zebrafish embryos and larvae at environmentally relevant concentrations and the absence of toxicity at the lowest concentrations. Thus, the biosurfactant is a safe product for use in natural aquatic environments, offering low toxicity to non-target organisms.

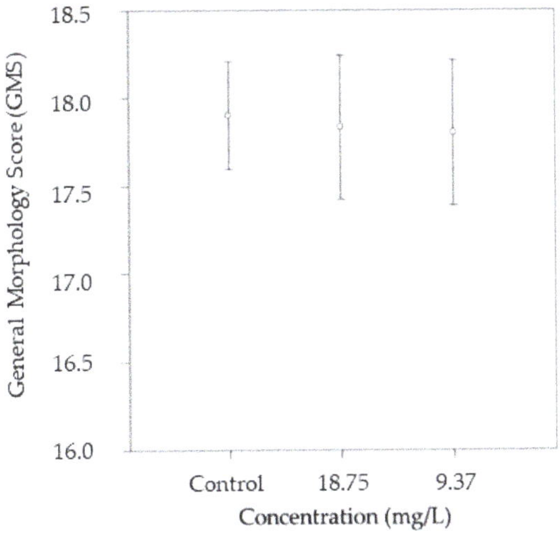

Figure 5. General morphology score for *D. rerio* embryos and larvae following exposure to different concentrations of biosurfactant produced by *S. bombicola* ATCC 22214.

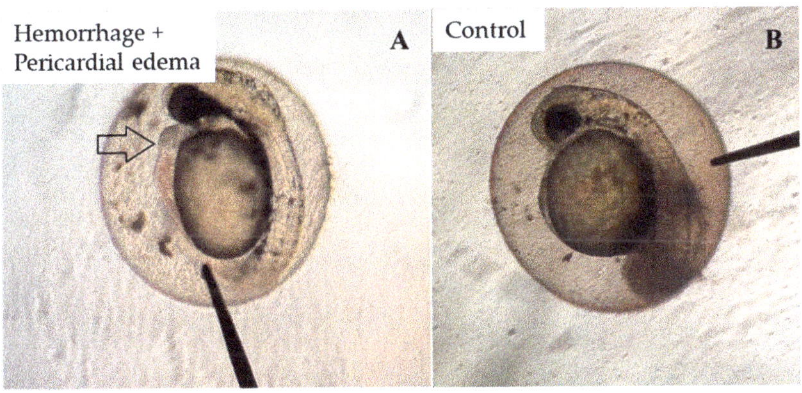

Figure 6. Larva with haemorrhage and pericardial oedema (**A**) exposed to 75 mg/L of biosurfactant produced by *S. bombicola* and control larva without pathologies (**B**).

In the context of environmental impact and regulations on the use of biosurfactants, it is important to emphasize that chemical dispersants have been used in the USA since 1969. During the oil spill from Deepwater Horizon in 2010, an unprecedented amount of Corexit dispersants, which contain the anionic surfactant sodium dioctyl sulfosuccinate (DOSS), was used. This raised concerns with regards to the potential toxicity to organisms in the water column. Corexit 9527 and 9500 were extensively on the oil spill. The use of Corexit 9580 was discontinued due to its toxic surfactants and a component that was found to be carcinogenic (2-butoxyethanol) [76,86]. In Brazil, only two chemical dispersants (Corexit EC9500—Nalco Holding Company, Watchung, NJ, USA, and Ultrasperse II®—Ingredion, Westchester, IL, USA) are authorized by the National Environment Council [87] for the treatment of oil spills in the marine environment. Ultrasperse II® is a blend of alcohol, alcohol sulphate, and fatty ester ethoxylate, and few studies have reported its effects on marine life. Although it is allowed in some countries and used by some oil companies with intellectual property protection, its toxicity to marine fish has been demonstrated [86].

Current dispersants are less toxic and more effective than the products used in past decades. However, several challenges to understanding toxicity have been pointed out, such as the limitations of lab tests and differences in exposure conditions in the field [87]. Laboratory experiments are good for maintaining consistent test material concentrations during exposure, which is necessary for the accurate measurement of toxicological responses. However, these methods fail to fully replicate real exposure scenarios and can affect the availability of the compounds being tested. Despite these challenges, chemical toxicity distribution (CTD) is a risk assessment method that assists in assessing the environmental risks of dispersants. A study by Berninger et al. [88] suggested that dispersants are less toxic than oil alone but more toxic than oil when mixed with this hydrocarbon. Assessing the toxicity of untreated and dispersant-treated oil is complex due to the various toxic compounds to which aquatic organisms are exposed. The presence of polycyclic aromatic hydrocarbons (PAHs) in chemically dispersed oils is also linked to their toxicity. The toxicity of dispersants can be measured using LC_{50} values, which range from 200 to 500 mg/L, with higher concentrations indicating lower toxicity. The US Environmental Protection Agency uses a five-step scale to classify pesticides based on their acute toxicity to aquatic organisms. Microbial biosurfactants are considered eco-friendly alternatives for dispersant formulations due to their low toxicity. Despite the availability of different toxicity assessment methods, the low toxicity of eco-friendly dispersants is likely attributed to the absence of organic solvents and other toxic chemicals, which also enhances the biodegradability of these products [76].

3.7. Remediation of Oil Derivative Adsorbed to Sand by Biosurfactant—Kinetic Test

Oil and its derivatives are among the main environmental problems throughout the world. Bioremediation is considered a promising ecological option for cleaning up oil-contaminated environments with the use of microorganisms or microbial processes to diminish the concentration and/or toxicity of these pollutants. However, the response time can be long, which makes the addition of agents that accelerate this process necessary, such as biosurfactants. The addition of biosurfactants increases the solubility of hydrophobic organic compounds, enhancing their desorption from soil [29,89,90].

Figure 7 displays the results of the bioremediation of soil contaminated with motor oil in the presence of the yeast *S. bombicola* and the biosurfactant produced by the *S. bombicola* ATCC 22214 strain in a kinetic test.

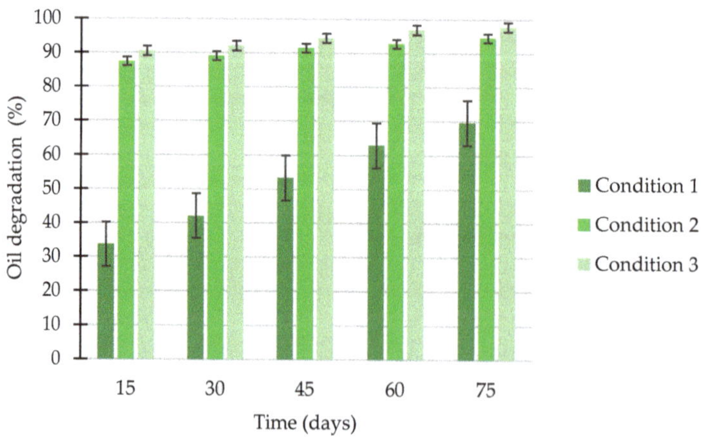

Figure 7. Degradation of oil adsorbed to sand by bioremediation process using biosurfactant produced by *S. bombicola* ATCC 22214. Condition 1: contaminated sand + molasses + *S. bombicola;* Condition 2: contaminated sand + molasses + biosurfactant (CMC) + *S. bombicola;* Condition 3: contaminated sand + molasses + *S. bombicola* + biosurfactant (2 × CMC). Error bars illustrate standard deviations calculated from three independent experiments.

The motor oil degradation rate was increased by the addition of the biosurfactant compared to the control condition (without biosurfactant). The highest removal rate (97.8%) was achieved with the biosurfactant at the 75-day assessment, demonstrating the advantage of this new biosurfactant in remediation processes. The concentration of the isolated biosurfactant exerted an influence on the degradation rate due to the enhancement of solubilisation of the oil in the aqueous phase. According to Oluwaseun et al. [91] and Zhao et al. [92], mobilisation and solubilisation are the main mechanisms of oil removal from soil, which are related to the CMC. Mobilisation occurs when the biosurfactant is used at a concentration lower than the CMC, and solubilisation occurs when the biosurfactant is used at a concentration above the CMC, as stated in Section 1. The reduction in surface and interfacial tensions is associated with the mobilisation mechanism. Surfactants increase the interaction angle between the hydrophobic contaminant and soil, facilitating separation from soil particles. With the mobilisation mechanism, the contaminant is divided in the centre of the micelles of the surfactant.

In this research, the biosurfactant was used at and above its CMC. This means that at higher concentrations, the surfactant molecules replaced water molecules, reducing the polarity of the water phase and surface tension. Consequently, the process of solubilisation of pollutants was accelerated. Micelles were formed, which significantly increased the solubility of the hydrophobic contaminant in the aqueous phase, thus helping to detach it from the soil. Mobilisation is more efficient when pollutants are solubilised in the water phase, enabling removal by either plants and microorganisms (biotic removal) or washing and recovery (abiotic removal) [93].

In a previous study, a biosurfactant produced by *Candida antarctica* was able to remove about half of the oil adsorbed to sand [94]. In a study carried out by Santos et al. [95], a biosurfactant produced from *C. sphaerica* UCP 0995 achieved a 90% motor oil removal rate at a concentration of 2 × the CMC in 90 days.

3.8. Removal of Oil Derivative Adsorbed to Sand by Biosurfactant in Packed Columns—Static Test

Biosurfactants decrease interfacial tension between oil and soil or oil and water, reducing capillary forces that resist the movement of oil through soil. Packed columns were used instead of agitation processes to test the effectiveness of the biosurfactant produced by *S. bombicola* ATCC 22214 under static conditions. Figure 8 displays the results of the static test. The cell-free broth (crude biosurfactant) achieved the best removal rate (69.2%) after 24 h of percolation.

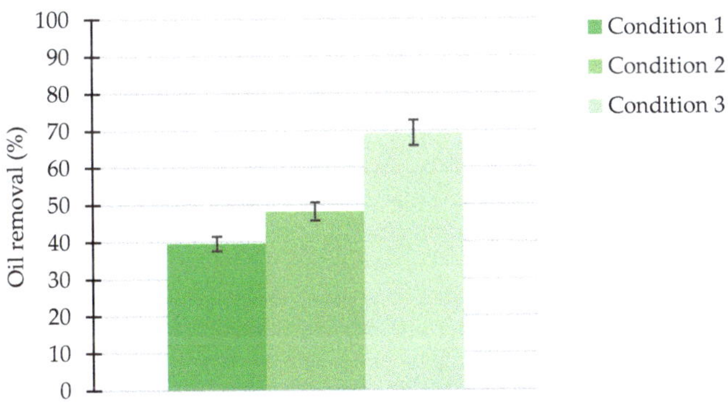

Figure 8. Removal of oil adsorbed to sand by bioremediation process using biosurfactant produced by *S. bombicola* ATCC 22214 in packed columns through static test. Condition 1: biosurfactant at CMC; Condition 2: biosurfactant at 2 × CMC; Condition 3: cell-free broth (crude biosurfactant); Control: distilled water. Error bars illustrate standard deviations calculated from three independent experiments.

This removal capacity is promising, as the biosurfactant did not undergo the extraction process and removed more than half of the oil adsorbed to the sand. The isolated biosurfactant achieved removal rates of 39.5% and 48.1% under Condition 1 (CMC) and Condition 2 (2 × CMC), respectively, whereas water alone (control) was able to remove 19.2% of the contaminant. It is noteworthy that isolation constitutes a large part of the production costs, and high removal rates with the crude biosurfactant are of extreme industrial interest.

Several biosurfactants have shown potential for cleaning soil contaminated with hydrophobic substances in glass columns. Ibrahim et al. [96] reported a 76% oil recovery rate using a biosurfactant in a column in a period of only two hours. Fernandes et al. [97] produced a biosurfactant from *Bacillus subtilis* RI 4114 and reported a 69% recovery rate of residual oil using 600 mg/L in a column. Kavitha et al. [98] produced a biosurfactant from *Bacillus* sp. MTCC 5514 and found a greater than 70% oil removal rate from standard sand and sandy soil. Jain et al. [99] investigated oil removal in glass columns comparing two biosurfactants to synthetic surfactants, reporting greater than 90% recovery rates with the biosurfactants, whereas the synthetic surfactants did not achieve a 70% rate of contaminant removal.

3.9. Remediation of Seawater Contaminated with Spilled Oil Derivative

The bioremediation of seawater requires a surfactant with dispersant capacity. As a phenomenon associated with both interfacial tension and surfactant concentration, dispersion facilitates the access of autochthonous microorganisms to the contaminant, thus promoting bioremediation.

The reduction in surface and interfacial tensions promoted by biosurfactants increases the solubility, mobility, and bioavailability of petroleum hydrocarbons. This facilitates biodegradation by microorganisms, which can break down large oil slicks and make the contaminants more easily accessible for natural processes. As a result, microorganisms can metabolise and reduce or eliminate the contaminants to safe levels [100]. There are two mechanisms by which biosurfactants facilitate hydrocarbon biodegradation: (1) The reduction in surface and interfacial tensions increases the bioavailability of the contaminant to the microorganism; (2) The interaction between the cell surface of the microorganism and biosurfactant alter the cell membrane, facilitating adhesion to the hydrocarbon through the increase in hydrophobicity without causing harm to the membrane. Due to the blocking of hydrogen bonds, biosurfactants enable hydrophobic–hydrophilic interactions that rearrange molecules and reduce the surface tension of the medium, leading to an increase in surface area. This favours bioavailability and consequent biodegradability of the contaminant [101,102].

Time (in days) and the increase in biosurfactant concentration enhanced the degradation rate of the motor oil by the yeast, as shown in Figure 9. The best result was found at 30 days, with the degradation of 91.5% of the oil when the biosurfactant was used at twice its CMC. Good results were also achieved under Conditions 1 and 2 (lower biosurfactant concentrations), with an increase in the degradation rate over time.

Saeki et al. [103] produced a biosurfactant from *Gordonia* sp. JE-1058 that enhanced the degradation polycyclic aromatic hydrocarbons and total saturated hydrocarbons in seawater.

The viscosity of liquid oil plays a crucial role in the performance of cleaning agents [104]. High viscosity slows the dispersion of oil and delays leaching after the collection of the contaminant and the thickness of floating oil exerts a negative impact on the effectiveness and efficiency of treatment [105]. As the residual engine lubricating oil used in the experiments of this work had already undergone physical and chemical changes caused by prolonged storage, the results obtained demonstrate the potential of the biosurfactant in removing very viscous hydrocarbons.

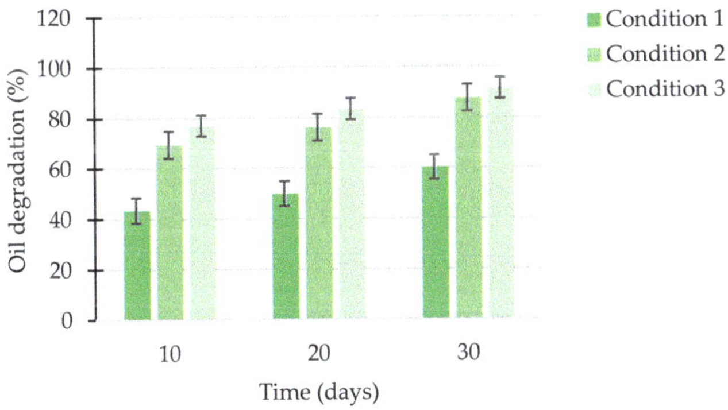

Figure 9. Degradation of oil from seawater by bioremediation process using biosurfactant produced by *S. bombicola* ATCC 22214. Condition 1: seawater + motor oil + *S. bombicola*; Condition 2: seawater + motor oil + *S. bombicola* + biosurfactant (CMC); Condition 3: seawater + motor oil + *S. bombicola* + biosurfactant (2 × CMC).

Several studies have compared biosurfactants with chemical surfactants/dispersants. Couto et al. [106] examined the effects of the chemical surfactant Ultrasperse II® and the biosurfactant surfactin produced by *Bacillus* sp. H2O-1 on marine bacterial communities. The authors found that surfactin stimulated the growth of oil-degrading bacteria more effectively than the chemical surfactant, although the biodegradation of the hydrocarbon was not affected. Additionally, rhamnolipids stimulated hydrocarbon biodegradation in the marine environment more effectively than the chemical surfactants DOSS and GM-2 [107]. Binary systems combining biosurfactants and chemical surfactants have been developed to combat oil spills with less toxicity. For instance, a binary system consisting of the cationic surfactant ethanediyl-1,3-bis(dodecyl dimethyl ammonium bromide) and surfactin produced by *Bacillus subtilis* was successful at reducing the interfacial tension of crude oil [108]. Shah et al. [109] also developed a dispersant based on a binary mixture of an ionic surfactant, choline laurate, and a lactonic sophorolipid produced by *S. bombicola*, which exhibited no toxicity in experiments with fish and had dispersion rates higher than 80%.

4. Conclusions

Despite the advances in biotechnology, few microbial products have reached the industrial scale to replace petroleum-based materials. While biotechnology is important to many industries, the production of microbial surfactants remains too costly to compete with chemical surfactants. Therefore, strategies are needed to improve the affordability of the production of these natural compounds on the industrial level. The microbial strain must be able to use substrates efficiently, and careful selection of the microorganism is required when creating a particular product. The existence of a market for microbial products is another concern, which requires both efficiency and a competitive price. The present study fulfilled some of these requirements. The new biosurfactant produced by *S. bombicola* ATCC 22214 in a low-cost medium demonstrated efficiency and effectiveness and was characterised as a sophorolipid. Moreover, the biosurfactant exhibited stability in the presence of extreme environmental conditions, low toxicity, and the capacity to perform satisfactorily in the removal and degradation of a petroleum derivative in soil and seawater. Thus, the production of this biosurfactant on a large scale for applications in industries as an agent for the mitigation of environmental pollution related to hydrophobic compounds is promising and can significantly contribute to the reduction of environmental impacts on ecosystems. Although the production of surfactants has been a widely explored process for decades, the combination of substrates and cultivation conditions associated with different microorganisms remains a valid strategy for obtaining optimal yields and efficient biomolecules. After the initial establishment of satisfactory conditions to produce this new biomolecule, as described in this study, the next steps will be scale-up in bioreactors and the optimisation of the extraction steps to use crude or semi-purified formulations of the new agent to meet the demands of the oil industry. Joining efforts to improve the entire process of obtaining each biomolecule is essential for these green surfactants to reach the market.

Author Contributions: Conceptualisation, L.A.S.; methodology, L.A.S., I.A.S., R.N.A., R.D.R., M.C.C.C. and F.C.G.A.; validation, L.A.S., I.A.S. and F.C.G.A.; formal analysis, L.A.S. and M.L.B.F.; investigation, I.A.S., R.N.A., R.D.R., J.G.L.A.F. and F.C.G.A.; resources, L.A.S.; data curation, L.A.S. and I.A.S.; writing—original draft preparation, I.A.S., R.N.A., J.G.L.A.F. and F.C.G.A.; writing—review and editing, L.A.S. and M.L.B.F.; visualisation, L.A.S.; supervision, L.A.S.; project administration, L.A.S.; funding acquisition, L.A.S. All authors have read and agreed to the published version of the manuscript.

Funding: This study was funded by the Programa de Pesquisa e Desenvolvimento da Agência Nacional de Energia Elétrica (ANEEL) and by the Brazilian fostering agencies Fundação de Apoio à Ciência e Tecnologia do Estado de Pernambuco (FACEPE), the Conselho Nacional de Desenvolvimento Científico e Tecnológico (CNPq), and the Coordenação de Aperfeicoamento de Pessoal de Nível Superior (CAPES) (Finance Code 001).

Data Availability Statement: The original contributions presented in the study are included in the article; further inquiries can be directed to the corresponding author.

Acknowledgments: The authors are grateful to the Laboratories of Universidade Católica de Pernambuco (UNICAP) and to the Instituto Avancado de Tecnologia e Inovação (IATI), Brazil.

Conflicts of Interest: The authors declare no conflicts of interest.

References

1. Thorat, B.N.; Sonwani, R.K. Current technologies and future perspectives for the treatment of complex petroleum refinery wastewater: A review. *Bioresour. Technol.* **2022**, *355*, 127263. [CrossRef]
2. Wei, Z.; Wei, Y.; Liu, Y.; Niu, S.; Xu, Y.; Park, J.-H.; Wang, J.J. Biochar-based materials as remediation strategy in petroleum hydrocarbon-contaminated soil and water: Performances, mechanisms, and environmental impact. *J. Environ. Sci.* **2024**, *138*, 350–372. [CrossRef] [PubMed]
3. Zhang, T.; Liu, Y.; Zhong, S.; Zhang, L. AOPs-based remediation of petroleum hydrocarbons contaminated soils: Efficiency, influencing factors and environmental impacts. *Chemosphere* **2020**, *246*, 125726. [CrossRef] [PubMed]
4. Ossai, I.C.; Ahmed, A.; Hassan, A.; Hamid, F.S. Remediation of soil and water contaminated with petroleum hydrocarbon: A review. *Environ. Technol. Innov.* **2020**, *17*, 100526. [CrossRef]
5. Rajabi, H.; Sharifipour, M. Geotechnical properties of hydrocarbon-contaminated soils: A comprehensive review. *Bull. Eng. Geol. Environ.* **2019**, *78*, 3685–3717. [CrossRef]
6. Yu, L.; Han, M.; He, F. A review of treating oily wastewater. *Arab. J. Chem.* **2017**, *10*, 1913–1922. [CrossRef]
7. Jabbar, N.M.; Alardhi, S.M.; Mohammed, A.K.; Salih, I.K.; Albayati, T.M. Challenges in the implementation of bioremediation processes in petroleum-contaminated soils: A review. *Environ. Nanotechnol. Monit. Manag.* **2022**, *18*, 100694. [CrossRef]
8. Johnson, P.; Trybala, A.; Starov, V.; Pinfield, V.J. Effect of synthetic surfactants on the environment and the potential for substitution by biosurfactants. *Adv. Colloid Interface Sci.* **2021**, *288*, 102340. [CrossRef]
9. Chaudhary, R.; Nawaz, A.; Fouillaud, M.; Dufossé, L.; Haq, I.u.; Mukhtar, H. Microbial Cell Factories: Biodiversity, Pathway Construction, Robustness, and Industrial Applicability. *Microbiol. Res.* **2024**, *15*, 247–272. [CrossRef]
10. Shi, T.Q.; Darvishi, F.; Cao, M.; Ji, B.; Ji, X.J. Design and construction of microbial cell factories for the production of fuels and chemicals. *Front. Bioeng. Biotechnol.* **2023**, *11*, 1198317. [CrossRef]
11. Gomes, D.; Rodrigues, L.R.; Rodrigues, J.L. Perspectives on the design of microbial cell factories to produce prenylflavonoids. *Int. J. Food Microbiol.* **2022**, *367*, 109588. [CrossRef] [PubMed]
12. Jiang, L.L.; Zhou, J.J.; Quan, C.S.; Xiu, Z.L. Advances in industrial microbiome based on microbial consortium for biorefinery. *Bioresour. Biproc.* **2017**, *4*, 11. [CrossRef] [PubMed]
13. Demain, A.L. Importance of microbial natural products and the need to revitalize their discovery. *J. Ind. Microbiol. Biotechnol.* **2014**, *41*, 185–201. [CrossRef] [PubMed]
14. Thomford, N.E.; Senthebane, D.A.; Rowe, A.; Munro, D.; Seele, P.; Maroyi, A.; Dzobo, K. Natural products for drug discovery in the 21st century: Innovations for novel drug discovery. *Int. J. Mol. Sci.* **2018**, *19*, 1578. [CrossRef] [PubMed]
15. Shrivastava, A.; Pal, M.; Sharma, R.K. Pichia as yeast cell factory for production of industrially important bio-products: Current trends, challenges, and future prospects. *J. Bioresour. Bioprod.* **2023**, *8*, 108–124. [CrossRef]

16. Bi, H.; Mulligan, C.N.; Zhang, B.; Biagi, M.; An, C.; Yang, X.; Lyu, L.; Chen, X. A review on recent development in the use of surface washing agents for shoreline cleanup after oil spills. *Ocean Coast. Manag.* **2023**, *245*, 106877. [CrossRef]
17. Charoentanaworakun, C.; Assabumrungrat, S.; Soottitantawat, A. Techno-economic environmental analysis of sustainable anionic biosurfactant production from palm fatty acid distillate. *ACS Omega* **2023**, *8*, 45045–45055. [CrossRef]
18. Mohanty, S.S.; Koul, Y.; Varjani, S.; Pandey, A.; Ngo, H.H.; Chang, J.-S.; Wong, J.W.C.; Bui, X.-T. A critical review on various feedstocks as sustainable substrates for biosurfactants production: A way towards cleaner production. *Microb. Cell Fact.* **2021**, *20*, 120. [CrossRef]
19. Kurtzman, C.P.; Price, N.P.J.; Ray, K.J.; Kuo, T.-M. Production of sophorolipid biosurfactants by multiple species of the *Starmerella (Candida) bombicola* yeast clade. *FEMS Microbiol. Lett.* **2010**, *311*, 140–146. [CrossRef]
20. Jadav, S.; Sakthipriya, N.; Doble, M.; Sangwai, J.S. Effect of biosurfactants produced by *Bacillus subtilis* and *Pseudomonas aeruginosa* on the formation kinetics of methane hydrates. *J. Nat. Gas Sci. Eng.* **2017**, *43*, 156–166. [CrossRef]
21. Negrete, P.S.; Ghilardi, C.; Pineda, L.R.; Pérez, E.; Herrera, M.L.; Borroni, V. Biosurfactant production by *Rhodococcus* ALDO1 isolated from olive mill wastes. *Biocatal. Agric. Biotechnol.* **2024**, *57*, 103106. [CrossRef]
22. Nagtode, V.S.; Cardoza, C.; Yasin, H.K.; Mali, S.N.; Tambe, S.M.; Roy, P.; Singh, K.; Goel, A.; Amin, P.D.; Thorat, B.R.; et al. Green surfactants (biosurfactants): A petroleum-free substitute for sustainability-comparison, applications, market, and future prospects. *ACS Omega* **2023**, *8*, 11674–11699. [CrossRef] [PubMed]
23. Kashif, A.; Rehman, R.; Fuwad, A.; Shahid, M.K.; Dayarathne, H.N.P.; Jamal, A.; Aftab, M.N.; Mainali, B.; Choi, Y. Current advances in the classification, production, properties and applications of microbial biosurfactants—A critical review. *Adv. Colloid Interface Sci.* **2022**, *306*, 102718. [CrossRef]
24. Thapliyal, U.; Negi, S. Biosurfactants: Recent trends in healthcare applications. *Mater. Today Proc.* 2023; *in press*. [CrossRef]
25. Mouafo, H.T.; Pahane, M.M.; Mbarga, A.J.M.; Sokamte, A.T.; Somashekar, D.; Mbawala, A. Methods of purification and characterization of biosurfactants: An overview. *J. Adv. Biol. Biotechnol.* **2023**, *26*, 35–53. [CrossRef]
26. Sales da Silva, I.G.; Almeida, F.C.G.; Rocha e Silva, N.M.P.; Casazza, A.A.; Converti, A.; Sarubbo, L.A. Soil bioremediation: Overview of technologies and trends. *Energies* **2020**, *13*, 4664. [CrossRef]
27. Singh, P.; Patil, Y.; Rale, V. Biosurfactant production: Emerging trends and promising strategies. *J. Appl. Microbiol.* **2019**, *126*, 2–13. [CrossRef] [PubMed]
28. Santos, D.K.F.; Rufino, R.D.; Luna, J.M.; Santos, V.A.; Sarubbo, L.A. Biosurfactants: Multifunctional biomolecules of the 21st century. *Int. J. Mol. Sci.* **2016**, *17*, 401. [CrossRef] [PubMed]
29. Ambaye, T.G.; Vaccari, M.; Prasad, S.; Rtimi, S. Preparation, characterization and application of biosurfactant in various industries: A critical review on progress, challenges and perspectives. *Environ. Technol. Innov.* **2021**, *24*, 102090. [CrossRef]
30. Kanawal, H.H.; Khan, K.; Abdullah, M. Mass production and factors affecting biosurfactant productivity using bioreactors. In *Green Sustainable Process for Chemical and Environmental Engineering and Science Microbially-Derived Biosurfactants for Improving Sustainability in Industry*; Inamuddin, A.C.O., Asiri, A.M., Eds.; Elsevier Inc.: Amsterdam, The Netherlands, 2021; pp. 379–398.
31. Gaur, V.K.; Sharma, P.; Gupta, S.; Varjani, S.; Srivastava, J.K.; Wong, J.W.C.; Ngo, H.H. Opportunities and challenges in omics approaches for biosurfactant production and feasibility of site remediation: Strategies and advancements. *Environ. Technol. Innov.* **2022**, *25*, 102132. [CrossRef]
32. Aslam, A.; Ishtaiq, M.; Badar, R.; Nazir, M.S.; Tahir, Z. Applications of biosurfactants in the production of industrially relevant bioproducts. In *Green Sustainable Process for Chemical and Environmental Engineering and Science: Microbially Derived Biosurfactants for Improving Sustainability in Industry*; Inamuddin, A.C.O., Asiri, A.M., Eds.; Elsevier Inc.: Amsterdam, The Netherlands, 2021; pp. 173–201.
33. Markande, A.R.; Patel, D.; Varjani, S. A review on biosurfactants: Properties, applications and current developments. *Bioresour. Technol.* **2021**, *330*, 124963. [CrossRef] [PubMed]
34. Dolman, B.; Fuju, W.; Winterburn, J.B.; Ben, M. Integrated production and separation of biosurfactants. *Process Biochem.* **2019**, *83*, 1–8. [CrossRef]
35. Koul, B.; Yakoob, M.; Shah, M.P. Agricultural waste management strategies for environmental sustainability. *Environ. Res.* **2022**, *206*, 112285. [CrossRef] [PubMed]
36. Poveda-Giraldo, J.A.; Solarte-Toro, J.C.; Treinen, C.; Noll, P.; Henkel, M.; Hausmann, R.; Alzate, C.A.C. Assessing the feasibility and sustainability of a surfactin production process: A techno-economic and environmental analysis. *Environ. Sci. Pollut. Res.* **2024**. [CrossRef] [PubMed]
37. Silva, I.A.; Veras, B.O.; Ribeiro, B.G.; Aguiar, J.S.; Guerra, J.M.C.; Luna, J.M.; Sarubbo, L.A. Production of cupcake-like dessert containing microbial biosurfactant as an emulsifier. *PeerJ* **2020**, *8*, e9064. [CrossRef] [PubMed]
38. Meylheuc, T.; Van Oss, C.J.; Bellon-Fontaine, M.N. Adsorption of biosurfactants on solid surfaces and consequences regarding the bioahesion of *Listeria monocytogenes* LO28. *J. Appl. Microbiol.* **2001**, *91*, 822–832. [CrossRef] [PubMed]
39. Cooper, D.G.; Goldenberg, B.G. Surface active agents from two *Bacillus* species. *Appl. Environ. Microbiol.* **1987**, *53*, 224–229. [CrossRef]
40. Han, Y.; Liu, E.; Liu, L.; Zhang, B.; Wang, Y.; Gui, M.; Wu, R.; Li, P. Rheological, emulsifying and thermostability properties of two exopolysaccharides produced by *Bacillus amyloliquefaciens* LPL061. *Carbohydr. Polym.* **2015**, *115*, 230–237. [CrossRef]
41. Das, A.J.; Kumar, R. Production of biosurfactant from agro-industrial waste by Bacillus safensis J2 and exploring its oil recovery efficiency and role in restoration of diesel contaminated soil. *Environ. Technol. Innov.* **2019**, *16*, 100450. [CrossRef]

42. Meyer, B.N.; Ferrigni, N.R.; Putnam, J.E.; Jacobsen, L.B.; Nichols, D.E.; McLaughlin, J.L. Brine shrimp: A convenient general bioassay for active plant constituents. *Planta Med.* **1982**, *45*, 31–34. [CrossRef]
43. OECD. *Test No. 236: Fish Embryo Acute Toxicity (FET) Test*; OECD: Paris, French, 2013.
44. Alves, R.N.; Mariz, C.F., Jr.; Melo, A.M.K.; Cavalcanti, M.G.N.; Melo, T.J.B.; Arruda-Santos, R.H.; Zanardi-Lamardo, E.; Carvalho, P.S.M. Contamination and toxicity of surface Waters along rural and urban regions of the Capibaribe river in tropical Northeastern Brazil. *Environ. Toxicol. Chem.* **2021**, *40*, 3063–3077. [CrossRef] [PubMed]
45. Beekhuijzen, M.; De Koning, C.; Flores-Guillén, M.E.; De Vries-Buitenweg, S.; Tobor-Kaplon, M.; Van De Waart, B.; Emmen, H. From cutting edge to guideline: A first step in harmonization of the zebrafish embryotoxicity test (ZET) by describing the most optimal test conditions and morphology scoring system. *Reprod. Toxicol.* **2015**, *56*, 64–76. [CrossRef] [PubMed]
46. Alves, R.N.; Mariz, C.F.; Paulo, D.V.; Carvalho, P.S.M. Toxicity of effluents from gasoline stations oil-water separators to early life stages of zebrafish *Danio rerio*. *Chemosphere* **2017**, *178*, 224–230. [CrossRef] [PubMed]
47. Ritz, C.; Baty, F.; Streibig, J.C.; Gerhard, D. Dose-response analysis using R. *PLoS ONE* **2015**, *10*, 0146021. [CrossRef] [PubMed]
48. Joo, H.-S.; Ndegwa, P.M.; Shoda, M.; Phae, C.-G. Bioremediation of oil-contaminated soil using *Candida catenulate* and food waste. *Environ. Pollut.* **2008**, *156*, 891–896. [CrossRef] [PubMed]
49. Robert, M.; Mercadé, M.E.; Bosch, M.P.; Parra, J.L.; Espuny, M.J.; Manresa, M.A.; Guinea, J. Effect of the carbon source on biosurfactant production byPseudomonas aeruginosa 44T1. *Biotechnol. Lett.* **1989**, *11*, 871–874. [CrossRef]
50. Eaton, A.D. *Standard Methods for the Examination of Water and Wastewater*, 21st ed.; American Public Health Association: Washington, DC, USA, 2005.
51. Bose, S.; Kumar, P.S.; Rangasamy, G. Exploring the role of biosurfactants in the remediation of organic contaminants with a focus on the mechanism- a review. *J. Mol. Liq.* **2024**, *393*, 123585. [CrossRef]
52. Akbari, S.; Abdurahman, N.H.; Yunus, R.M.; Fayaz, F.; Alara, O.R. Biosurfactants—A new frontier for social and environmental safety: A mini review. *Biotechnol. Res. Innov.* **2018**, *2*, 81–90. [CrossRef]
53. Kaur, G.; Wang, H.; To, M.H.; Roelants, S.L.K.W.; Soetaert, W.; Lin, C.S.K. Efficient sophorolipids production using food waste. *J. Clean. Prod.* **2019**, *232*, 1–11. [CrossRef]
54. Bacille, N.; Babonneau, F.; Banat, I.M.; Ciesielska, K.; Cuvier, A.; Devreese, B.; Everaert, B.; Lydon, H.; Marchant, R.; Mitchell, C.A.; et al. Development of a Cradle-to-Grave Approach for Acetylated Acidic Sophorolipid Biosurfactants. *ACS Sustain. Chem. Eng.* **2017**, *5*, 1186–1198. [CrossRef]
55. Konishi, M.; Yoshida, Y.; Horiuchi, J. Efficient production of sophorolipids by *Starmerella bombicola* using a corncob hydrolysate medium. *J. Biosci. Bioeng.* **2014**, *119*, 317–322. [CrossRef]
56. Jiménez-Peñalver, P.; Castillejos, M.; Koh, A.; Gross, R.; Sánchez, A.; Font, X.; Gea, T. Production and characterization of sophorolipids from stearic acid by solid-state fermentation, a cleaner alternative to chemical surfactants. *J. Clean. Prod.* **2018**, *172*, 2735–2747. [CrossRef]
57. Jadhav, J.V.; Pratap, A.P.; Kale, S.B. Evaluation of sunflower oil refinery waste as feedstock for production of sophorolipid. *Process Biochem.* **2019**, *78*, 15–24. [CrossRef]
58. Shah, M.U.H.; Sivapragasam, M.; Moniruzzaman, M.; Talukder, M.M.R.; Yusup, S.B.; Goto, M. Production of sophorolipids by *Starmerella bombicola* yeast using new hydrophobic substrates. *Biochem. Eng. J.* **2017**, *127*, 60–67. [CrossRef]
59. Gaur, V.K.; Regar, R.K.; Dhiman, N.; Gautam, K.; Srivastava, J.K.; Patnaik, S.; Kamthan, M.; Manickam, N. Biosynthesis and characterization of sophorolipid biosurfactant by *Candida* spp.: Application as food emulsifier and antibacterial agent. *Bioresour. Technol.* **2019**, *285*, 121314. [CrossRef]
60. Marcelino, P.R.F.; Peres, G.F.D.; Terán-Hilares, R.; Pagnocca, F.C.; Rosa, C.A.; Lacerda, T.M.; Dos Santos, J.C.; Da Silva, S.S. Biosurfactants production by yeasts using sugarcane bagasse hemicellulosic hydrolysate as new sustainable alternative for lignocellulosic biorefineries. *Ind. Crop. Prod.* **2019**, *129*, 212–223. [CrossRef]
61. Dierickx, S.; Maes, K.; Roelants, S.L.K.W.; Pomian, B.; Meulebroek, L.V.; De Maeseneire, S.L.; Vanhaecke, L.; Soetaert, W.K. A multi-omics study to boost continuous bolaform sophorolipid production. *New Biotechnol.* **2022**, *66*, 107–115. [CrossRef]
62. El-Sheshtawy, H.S.; Aiad, I.; Osman, M.E.; Abo-ELnasr, A.A.; Kobisy, A.S. Production of biosurfactants by *Bacillus licheniformis* and *Candida albicans* for application in microbial enhanced oil recovery. *Egypt. J. Pet.* **2016**, *25*, 293–298. [CrossRef]
63. Lira, I.R.A.S.; Santos, E.M.S.; Santos, J.C.V.; Silva, R.R.; Silva, Y.A.; Durval, I.J.B.; Guerra, J.C.M.; Sarubbo, L.A.; Luna, J.M. Production of biossurfactant by *Candida guilliermondii* and application in a mayonnaise emulsion. *Chem. Eng. Trans.* **2021**, *87*, 259–264. [CrossRef]
64. Santos, J.C.V.; Santos, E.M.S.; Silva, Y.A.; Lira, I.R.A.S.; Silva, R.R.; Durval, I.J.B.; Sarubbo, L.A.; Luna, J.M. Application of *Candida lipolytica* biosurfactant for bioremediation of motor oil from contaminated environment. *Chem. Eng. Trans.* **2021**, *86*, 649–654. [CrossRef]
65. Sałek, K.; Euston, S.R. Sustainable microbial biosurfactants and bioemulsifiers for commercial exploitation. *Process Biochem.* **2019**, *85*, 143–155. [CrossRef]
66. Rubio-Ribeaux, D.; Andrade, R.F.S.; Silva, G.S.; Holanda, R.S.; Pele, M.A.; Nunes, P.; Junior, J.C.V.; Resende-Stoianoff, M.A.; Campos-Takaki, G.M. Promising biosurfactant produced by a new *Candida tropicalis* UCP 1613 strain using substrates from renewable-resources. *Afr. J. Microbiol. Res.* **2017**, *11*, 981–991. [CrossRef]

67. Camargo, F.P.; Menezes, A.J.; Tonello, P.S.; Santos, A.C.A.; Duarte, I.C.S. Characterization of biosurfactant from yeast using residual soybean oil under acidic conditions and their use in metal removal processes. *FEMS Microbiol. Lett.* **2018**, *365*, fny098. [CrossRef]
68. Price, N.P.J.; Ray, K.J.; Vermillion, K.E.; Dunlap, C.A.; Kurtzman, C.P. Structural characterization of novel sophorolipid biosurfactants from a newly identified species of *Candida* yeast. *Carbohydr. Res.* **2012**, *348*, 33–41. [CrossRef]
69. Daverey, A.; Pakshirajan, K. Sophorolipids from *Candida bombicola* using mixed hydrophilic substrates: Production, purification and characterization. *Colloids Surf. B* **2010**, *79*, 246–253. [CrossRef]
70. Silveira, V.A.I.; Marim, B.M.; Hipólito, A.; Gonçalvez, M.C.; Mali, S.; Kobayashi, R.K.T.; Celligoi, M.A.P.C. Characterization and antimicrobial properties of bioactive packaging films based on polylactic acid-sophorolipid for the control of foodborne pathogens. *Food Packag. Shelf Life* **2020**, *26*, 100591. [CrossRef]
71. Bacille, N.; Poirier, A.; Griel, P.L.; Pernot, P.; Pala, M.; Roelants, S.; Soetaert, W.; Stevens, C.V. Aqueous self-assembly of a wide range of sophorolipid and glucolipid microbial bioamphiphiles (biosurfactants): Considerations on the structure-properties relationship. *Colloids Surf. A Physicochem. Eng. Asp.* **2023**, *679*, 132518. [CrossRef]
72. Roy, A.; Khan, M.R.; Mukherjee, A.K. Recent advances in the application of microbial biosurfactants in food industries: Opportunities and challenges. *Food Control* **2024**, *163*, 110465. [CrossRef]
73. Ashish; Debnath, M. Application of biosurfactant produced by an adaptive strain of *C. tropicalis* MTCC230 in microbial enhanced oil recovery (MEOR) and removal of motor oil from contaminated sand and water. *J. Petrol. Sci. Eng.* **2018**, *170*, 40–48. [CrossRef]
74. Velmurugan, M.; Baskaran, A.; Kumar, S.D.; Sureka, I.; Raj, E.A.; Emelda, J.; Sathiyamurthy, K. Screening, stability and antibacterial potential of rhamnolipids from *Pseudomonas* sp., isolated from hydrocarbon contaminated soil. *J. Appl. Pharm. Sci.* **2015**, *5*, 26–33. [CrossRef]
75. Murawski, S.A.; Ainsworth, C.H.; Gilbert, S.; Hollander, D.J.; Paris, C.B.; Schlüter, M.; Wetzel, D.L. Modernizing protocols for aquatic toxicity testing of oil and dispersant. In *Scenarios and Responses to Future Deep Oil Spills*, 1st ed.; Mitchelmore, C.L., Griffitt, R.J., Coelho, G.M., Wetzel, D.L., Eds.; Springer: Berlin/Heidelberg, Germany, 2020; pp. 239–252.
76. Silva, I.A.; Almeida, F.C.G.; Souza, T.C.; Bezerra, K.G.O.; Durval, I.J.B.; Converti, A.; Sarubbo, L.A. Oil spills: Impacts and perspectives of treatment technologies with focus on the use of green surfactants. *Environ. Monit. Assess.* **2022**, *194*, 143. [CrossRef] [PubMed]
77. Pinto, M.I.; Campos, J.M.; Meira, H.M.; Sarubbo, L.A.; Luna, J.M. A Biosurfactant from *Candida bombicola*: Its synthesis, characterization, and its application as a food emulsions. *Foods* **2022**, *11*, 561. [CrossRef] [PubMed]
78. Pradhan, A.; Bhattacharyya, A. Quest for an eco-friendly alternative surfactant: Surface and foam characteristics of natural surfactants. *J. Clean. Prod.* **2017**, *150*, 127–134. [CrossRef]
79. Yi, X.; Wei, Y.; Zhai, W.; Wang, P.; Liu, D.; Zhou, Z. Effects of three surfactants on the degradation and environmental risk of metolachlor in aquatic environment. *Chemosphere* **2022**, *300*, 134295. [CrossRef] [PubMed]
80. Embry, M.R.; Belanger, S.E.; Braunbeck, T.A.; Galay-Burgos, M.; Halder, M.; Hinton, D.E.; Léonard, M.A.; Lillicrap, A.; Norbeg-King, T.; Whale, G. The fish embryo toxicity test as an animal alternative method in hazard and risk assessment and scientific research. *Aquat. Toxicol.* **2010**, *97*, 79–87. [CrossRef] [PubMed]
81. Wang, Y.; Zhang, Y.; Li, X.; Sun, M.; Wei, Z.; Wang, Y.; Gao, A.; Chen, D.; Zhao, X.; Feng, X. Exploring the effects of different types of surfactants on zebrafish embryos and larvae. *Sci. Rep.* **2015**, *5*, 10107. [CrossRef] [PubMed]
82. Korbut, R.; Skjolding, L.M.; Mathiessen, H.; Jaafar, R.; Li, X.; Jørgensen, L.V.G.; Kania, P.W.; Wu, B.; Buchmann, K. Toxicity of the antiparasitic lipopeptide biosurfactant SPH6 to green algae, cyanobacteria, crustaceans and zebrafish. *Aquat. Toxicol.* **2022**, *243*, 106072. [CrossRef]
83. El-Harbawi, M. Toxicity Measurement of Imidazolium Ionic Liquids Using Acute Toxicity Test. *Procedia Chem.* **2014**, *9*, 40–52. [CrossRef]
84. Al-Asmakh, M.; Majdalawieh, A.F.; Abdullah, A.M.; Younes, N.; Da'as, S.I.; Radwan, A.B.; Sliem, M.H.; Ech-Cherif, H.; Pintus, G.; Nasrallah, G.K. AEO-7 surfactant is "super toxic" and induces severe cardiac, liver, and locomotion damage in zebrafish embryos. *Environ. Sci. Eur.* **2020**, *32*, 149. [CrossRef]
85. Johann, S.; Seiler, T.-B.; Tiso, T.; Bluhm, K.; Blank, L.M.; Hollert, H. Mechanism-specific and whole-organism ecotoxicity of mono-rhamnolipids. *Sci. Total Environ.* **2016**, *548–549*, 155–163. [CrossRef]
86. Bejarano, A.C. Critical review and analysis of aquatic toxicity data on oil spill dispersants. *Environ. Toxicol. Chem.* **2018**, *37*, 2989–3001. [CrossRef]
87. CONAMA. Conselho Nacional de Meio Ambiente, Brasil. 2021. Available online: http://www.mma.gov.br/port/conama/estr.cfm/ (accessed on 3 March 2024).
88. Berninger, J.P.; Williams, E.S.; Brooks, B.W. An initial probabilistic hazard assessment of oil dispersants approved by the United States National Contingency Plan. *Environ. Toxicol. Chem.* **2011**, *30*, 1704–1708. [CrossRef]
89. Nitschke, M.; Pastore, G.M. Biossurfactantes: Propriedades e aplicações. *Quim. Nova* **2002**, *25*, 772–776. [CrossRef]
90. Parus, A.; Ciesielski, T.; Woźniak-Karczewska, M.; Ślachciński, M.; Owsianiak, M.; Ławniczak, Ł.; Loibner, A.P.; Heipieper, H.J.; Chrzanowski, Ł. Basic principles for biosurfactant-assisted (bio)remediation of soils contaminated by heavy metals and petroleum hydrocarbons—A critical evaluation of the performance of rhamnolipids. *J. Hazard. Mater.* **2023**, *443*, 130171. [CrossRef]

91. Oluwaseun, A.C.; Kola, O.J.; Mishra, P.; Singh, J.R.; Singh, A.K.; Cameotra, S.S.; Micheal, B.O. Characterization and optimization of a rhamnolipid from *Pseudomonas aeruginosa* C1501 with novel biosurfactant activities. *Sustain. Chem. Pharm.* **2017**, *6*, 26–36. [CrossRef]
92. Zhao, F.; Li, P.; Guo, C.; Shi, R.-J.; Zhang, Y. Bioaugmentation of oil reservoir indigenous *Pseudomonas aeruginosa* to enhance oil recovery through in-situ biosurfactant production without air injection. *Bioresour. Technol.* **2018**, *251*, 295–302. [CrossRef]
93. Kim, B.K.; Baek, K.; Ko, S.H.; Yang, J.W. Research and field experiences on electrokinetic remediation in South Korea. *Sep. Purif. Technol.* **2011**, *79*, 116–123. [CrossRef]
94. Adamczak, M.; Bednarski, W. Influence of medium composition and aeration on the synthesis of biosurfactants produced by *Candida antarctica*. *Biotechnol. Lett.* **2000**, *22*, 313–316. [CrossRef]
95. Santos, E.M.S.; Lira, I.R.A.S.; Filho, A.A.P.S.; Meira, H.M.; Farias, C.B.B.; Rufino, R.D.; Sarubbo, L.A.; Luna, J.M. Application of the biosurfactant produced by *Candida sphaerica* as a bioremediation agent. *Chem. Eng. Trans.* **2020**, *79*, 451–456. [CrossRef]
96. Ibrahim, M.L.; Ijah, U.J.J.; Manga, S.B.; Bilbis, L.S.; Umar, S. Production and partial characterization of biosurfactant produced by crude oil degrading bacteria. *Int. Biodeterior. Biodegrad.* **2013**, *81*, 28–34. [CrossRef]
97. Fernandes, P.L.; Rodrigues, E.M.; Paiva, F.R.; Ayupe, B.A.L.; McInerney, M.J.; Tótola, M.R. Biosurfactant, solvents and polymer production by *Bacillus subtilis* RI4914 and their application for enhanced oil recovery. *Fuel* **2016**, *180*, 551–557. [CrossRef]
98. Kavitha, V.; Mandal, A.B.; Gnanamani, A. Microbial biosurfactant mediated removal and/or solubilization of crude oil contamination from soil and aqueous phase: An approach with *Bacillus licheniformis* MTCC 5514. *Int. Biodeterior. Biodegrad.* **2014**, *94*, 24–30. [CrossRef]
99. Jain, R.M.; Mody, K.; Mishra, A.; Jha, B. Physicochemical characterization of biosurfactant and its potential to remove oil from soil and cotton cloth. *Carbohydr. Polym.* **2012**, *89*, 1110–1116. [CrossRef]
100. Wang, X.; Cai, T.; Wen, W.; Zhang, Z. Effect of biosurfactant on biodegradation of heteroatom compounds in heavy oil. *Fuel* **2018**, *230*, 418–429. [CrossRef]
101. Aparna, A.; Srinikethan, G.; Hedge, S. Effect of addition of biosurfactant produced by *Pseudomonas* ssp. on biodegradation of crude oil. In *International Proceedings of Chemical, Biological & Environmental Engineering*, 2nd ed.; World Scientific: Singapore, 2011; Volume 6, pp. 71–75.
102. Karlapudi, A.P.; Venkateswarulu, T.C.; Tammineedi, J.; Kanumuri, L.; Ravuru, B.K.; Dirisala, V.; Kodali, V.P. Role of biosurfactants in bioremediation of oil pollution-a review. *Petroleum* **2018**, *4*, 241–249. [CrossRef]
103. Saeki, H.; Sasaki, K.M.; Komatsu, O.; Miura, A.; Matsuda, H. Oil spill remediation by using the remediation agent JE1058BS that contains a biosurfactant produced by *Gordonia* sp. strain JE-1058. *Bioresour. Technol.* **2009**, *100*, 572–577. [CrossRef]
104. Nikolova, C.; Gutierrez, T. Biosurfactants and their applications in the oil and gas industry: Current state of knowledge and future perspectives. *Front. Bioeng. Biotechnol.* **2021**, *9*, 626639. [CrossRef]
105. Hubbe, M.A.; Rojas, O.J.; Fingas, M.; Gupta, B.S. Cellulosic substrates for removal of pollutants from aqueous systems: A review. 3. Spilled oil and emulsified organic liquids. *BioResources* **2013**, *8*, 3038–3097. [CrossRef]
106. Couto, C.R.A.; Jurelevicius, D.A.; Alvarez, V.M.; Elsas, J.D.; Seldin, L. Response of the bacterial community in oil-contaminated marine water to the addition of chemical and biological dispersants. *J. Environ. Manag.* **2016**, *184*, 473–479. [CrossRef]
107. Pi, Y.; Bao, M.; Liu, Y.; Lu, T.; He, R. The contribution of chemical dispersants and biosurfactants on crude oil biodegradation by *Pseudomonas* sp. LSH-7′. *J. Clean. Prod.* **2017**, *153*, 74–82. [CrossRef]
108. Jin, L.; Garamus, V.M.; Liu, F.; Xiao, J.; Eckerlebe, H.; Willumeit-Römer, R.; Mu, B.; Zou, A. Interaction of a biosurfactant, surfactin with a cationic gemini surfactant in aqueous solution. *J. Colloid Interface Sci.* **2016**, *481*, 201–209. [CrossRef] [PubMed]
109. Shah, M.U.H.; Moniruzzaman, M.; Sivapragasam, M.; Talukder, M.M.R.; Yusup, S.B.; Goto, M. A binary mixture of a biosurfactant and an ionic liquid surfactant as a green dispersant for oil spill remediation. *J. Mol. Liq.* **2019**, *280*, 111–119. [CrossRef]

processes

MDPI

Communication

Study on Removal of Nitrogen-Containing Heterocyclic Compounds Contained in Crude Methylnaphthalene Oil by Formamide Extraction

Su Jin Kim

Department of Chemical & Biological Engineering, Chungwoon University, Incheon 22100, Republic of Korea; sujkim@chungwoon.ac.kr

Abstract: This study examined the effect of experimental factors and conditions on the removal of nitrogen-containing heterocyclic compounds (NCHCs) by performing equilibrium extraction using formamide or formamide aqueous solution as a solvent to remove NCHCs contained in crude methylnaphthalene oil (CMNO). The CMNO used as a raw material in this study contained three types of NCHCs (quinoline, isoquinoline, and indole) classified as group A, and six kinds of non-NCHCs (naphthalene, 1-methylnaphthalene, 2-methylnaphthalene, biphenyl, dibenzofuran, and fluorene) classified as group B. Increasing the volume fraction of water to the solvent before the extraction run increased the raffinate residual rate but conversely decreased the removal rate of group A. The increase in the volume fraction of solvent to feed before the extraction run and operating temperature decreased the residual rate of raffinate but conversely increased the removal rate of group A. Over the entire range of extraction conditions performed in this study, the removal rate of group A ranged from 10.8% to 70.7%. Considering that these experimental results were obtained using only a single stage of batch equilibrium extraction, the formamide extraction method applied in this study showed excellent performance in terms of the residual rate of raffinate and the removal rate of group A. Therefore, it was expected to be an alternative to the reaction extraction method using acids and bases applied so far to separate NCHCs in the distillation residue of coal tar.

Keywords: coal tar; crude methylnaphthalene oil; nitrogen-containing heterocyclic compounds; formamide extraction; removal; quality improvement

1. Introduction

Crude methylnaphthalene oil (CMNO; approximately 10,000 tons/year in Korea) is produced as a distillation residue of naphthalene oil (bp 483–533 K) from coal tar after the recovery of crude naphthalene [1]. The CMNO used as a raw material in this study contains a total of 15.23 wt% of nitrogen-containing heterocyclic compounds (NCHCs): quinoline (QNL, 6.72 wt%), iso-quinoline (IQNL, 4.15 wt%), and indole (ID, 4.36 wt%). These NCHCs contained in CMNO, which are hazardous, flammable, and carcinogenic chemicals, are considered undesirable impurities of CMNO because they cause air pollution by NOx generated from combustion, produce a very unpleasant odor, and deteriorate catalyst performance [1–3]; there are also many restrictions on the transportation and handling due to the harmfulness of CMNO. For the above reasons, improving the quality of CMNO by removing NCHCs contained in CMNO would be very significant. Meanwhile, the by-product discharged in the process of improving the quality of CMNO contains a large amount of very useful NCHCs, such as QNL, IQNL, and ID, which are used in the manufacture of drugs, perfumes, pesticides, dyes, and pigments [2–7]. Therefore, we believe that the study on improving the quality of CMNO by removing NCHCs contained in CMNO is very important in improving the quality of CMNO and utilizing the very useful resources contained in the by-products discharged from the process.

So far, the separation of NCHCs contained in the distillation residue of coal tar has been mainly achieved by reactive extraction using acids and bases; however, this method, which uses both strong alkaline (e.g., NaOH) solutions and acidic (e.g., H_2SO_4) solutions, has the disadvantages of high cost, corrosion of the metal separation apparatus, environmental pollution, and complicating the separation process because the separating agent cannot be regenerated [8,9]. Therefore, finding new alternative separation methods that are simpler and more efficient than reactive extraction is significant. Currently, to find an alternative to the reaction extraction method for removing NCHCs containing in distillation residues of coal tar, studies such as adsorption [10–12], supercritical extraction [1,4,8], extraction using ionic liquids [13–16], inclusion complexation [17,18], and organic solvent extraction [3,7,19–25] with a variety of organic solvents, including methanol, ethanol, and formamide, are in progress. Among organic solvent extractions, methanol extraction using CMNO, one of coal tar's distillation residues directly produced in the coal tar distillation industry, showed very high solubility of NCHCs and compounds other than NCHCs. As a result, the methanol extraction method was not satisfactory the separation between NCHCs and compounds other than NCHCs due to the low selectivity of NCHCs to non-NCHCs below 10 [7,21,25].

In a previous study [3], we investigated the recovery of NCHCs contained in wash oil, one of the distillation residues for recovering naphthalene oil in coal tar, using a mixture of formamide and water (MFW) as a solvent. The recovery results reported that MFW is an excellent solvent in terms of balance between solubility and selectivity of NCHCs. Therefore, this study examined the reduction of NCHCs contained in CMNO using MFW as a solvent. For this review, we performed equilibrium extraction using formamide or MFW as a solvent to examine the effect of experimental factors and conditions on the removal of NCHCs.

2. Experimental Section

2.1. Material

The raw material for this study, CMNO, was supplied by OCI Company Ltd. in Seoul, Republic of Korea. For the identification and quantitative analysis of each compound present in CMNO through gas chromatography (GC), we purchased standard reagents Naphthalene (NTL, 99% purity), QNL (98% purity), IQNL (97% purity), ID (≥99% purity), 2-methylnaphthalene (2MNTL, 97% purity), 1-methylnaphthalene (1MNTL, ≥95% purity), biphenyl (BP, ≥99.5% purity), dibenzofuran (DBF, 98% purity), and fluorene (FR, 98% purity) from Sigma-Aldrich Korea (Seoul, Republic of Korea). Formamide (≥99.5% purity), used as a solvent, was also purchased from the same place.

2.2. Method

First, formamide and tap water were mixed to make a solvent of a certain experimental concentration. Next, a 500 mL Erlenmeyer flask containing a certain amount of feed (F_0: CMNO) and solvent (formamide or MFW, S_0) was placed in a shaking water bath maintained at the experimental temperature, and shaking was started. After a certain period, the shaking was stopped and allowed to settle; the mass of each phase was measured after the extract phase, and the raffinate phase was separated using a 500 mL separatory funnel. The concentration of each compound contained in each phase was measured by GC analysis of each sample, to which a small amount of acetone (a diluting solvent for concentration measurement) was added to the extraction and raffinate phases. Analysis of two phases was performed using GC equipped with a flame ionization detector. Details of the analysis apparatus and conditions are presented in Table 1.

Table 1. Analysis apparatus and conditions.

Gas Chromatograph	HP 6890 (Hewlett Packard Co., Houston, TX, USA)
Column (19091Z-416)	Capillary column HP-1
length (m)	60
inner diameter (mm)	0.32
film (μm)	0.25
Carrier gas	N_2
split ratio (-)	0.025
the flow rate in column (mL/min)	1
Sample volume (μL)	1
Injection temperature (K)	523
Column temperature (K)	383–593
increasing rate (K/min)	0 (0–3 min) 5 (383–523 K) 14 (523–593 K)
Detector temperature (K)	593

2.3. Material Systems and Conditions

Table 2 shows the material systems and experimental conditions used in this study. As described above, CMNO and formamide or MFW were used as feed and solvent, respectively. The distribution equilibrium experiment was performed by changing the liquid-liquid contacting time (t), the operating temperature (T), the volume fraction of water to solvent before the extraction run ($y_{w,0}$), and the volume fraction of solvent to feed before extraction run (S_0/F_0).

Table 2. Experimental system and conditions.

System	
Feed crude methylnaphthalene oil (CMNO)	
Solvent formamide, the mixture of formamide and water (MFW)	
Experimental conditions	
Liquid-liquid contacting time, t (h)	24–96
Operating temperature, T (K)	277–343
Volume of total liquid (ml)	400
Volume fraction of water to solvent before extraction run, $y_{w,0}$ (-)	0–0.3
Volume fraction of solvent to feed before extraction run, S_0/F_0 (-)	1–9

3. Results and Discussions

3.1. Gas Chromatogram of CMNO

Figure 1a shows the gas chromatogram of CMNO and the names of each compound identified using standard reagents. The peak numbers 2, 3, and 4, respectively, represent three kinds of NCHCs (QNL, IQNL, and ID) classified as group A, and the peak numbers 1 and 5 to 9, respectively, represent six kinds of non-NCHCs (NTL, 2MNTL, 1MNTL, BP, DBF, and FR) classified as group B. The gas chromatogram showed that the CMNO used in this study contained a relatively small amount of group A compared to group B. The composition of each compound contained in CMNO is presented in Table 3. The compositions of QNL, IQNL, and ID, the target compounds to be removed in this study, in CMNO were 6.72, 4.15, and 4.36 wt%, respectively, and group A, which summed these three kinds of NCHCs, was 15.23 wt%.

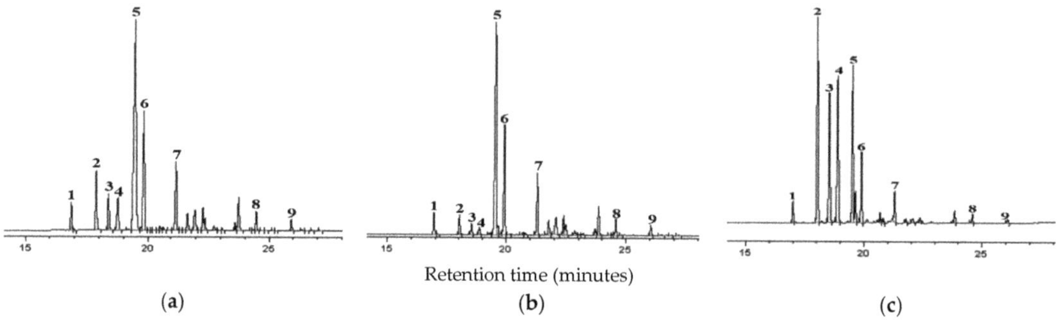

Figure 1. Gas chromatograms of (**a**) feed (CMNO), (**b**) raffinate phase, and (**c**) extract phase. Peak numbers; 1: naphthalene (NTL), 2: quinoline (QNL), 3: iso-quinoline (IQNL), 4: indole (ID), 5: 2-methylnaphthalene (2MNTL), 6: 1-methylnaphthalene (1MNTL), 7: biphenyl (BP), 8: dibenzofuran (DBF), and 9: Fluorene (FR). Extraction conditions: $y_{w,0} = 0.1$, $S_0/F_0 = 9$, T = 303 K, and t = 72 h.

Table 3. Compositions of compounds Contained in CMNO.

		Compound	Composition (wt%)
Group A	Heterocyclic Nitrogen Compounds (NCHCs)	Quinoline (QNL, C_9H_7N)	6.72
		Iso-quinoline (IQNL, C_9H_7N)	4.15
		Indole (ID, C_8H_7N)	4.36
Group B	Non-Heterocyclic Nitrogen Compounds (Non-NCHCs)	Naphthalene (NTL, $C_{10}H_8$)	2.88
		2-Methylnaphthalene (2MNTL, $C_{11}H_{10}$)	38.93
		1-Methylnaphthalene (1MNTL, $C_{11}H_{10}$)	15.11
		Biphenyl (BP, $C_{12}H_{10}$)	8.03
		Dibenzofuran (DBF, $C_{12}H_8O$)	1.92
		Fluorene (FR, $C_{13}H_{10}$)	1.13
Others			16.77

3.2. Checking of Time to Reach Equilibrium

To confirm the time to reach equilibrium, we analyzed the raffinate and extract phases recovered by liquid-liquid contacting between CMNO and MFW (t = 24, 48, 72, 96 h) under a constant experimental condition. We found that the composition of the two phases recovered at t = 72 and 96 h was almost identical. Therefore, the equilibrium reaching time of the system used in this study is within 72 h, so the entire distribution equilibrium experiment was performed in liquid-liquid contact for t = 72 h.

3.3. Definition of Equations

The residual rate of raffinate (RRR), the removal rate of group A (RRGA), the distribution coefficient (m_i) indicating the degree of solvency of component (or group) i, and the selectivity ($\beta_{i,j}$) suggesting the degree of separation efficacy between component (or group) i and a reference component (or group) j were calculated using the following definition equations.

$$\mathrm{RRR} = \frac{\text{mass of raffinate phase}}{\text{mass of feed}} \times 100\%$$

$$\mathrm{RRGA} = \frac{\text{mass of group in feed} - \text{mass of group A in raffinate phase}}{\text{mass of group A in feed}} \times 100\%$$

$$m_i = \frac{\text{mass fraction of component (or group) i in extract phase}}{\text{mass fraction of component (or group) i in raffinate phase}}$$

$$\beta_{i,j} = \frac{\text{distribution coefficient of component (or group) i}}{\text{distribution coefficient of a reference component (or group) j}}$$

3.4. Removal Performance of Group A

Figure 2a–c, respectively, shows the effect of the volume fraction of water to solvent before extraction run ($y_{w,0}$) on (a) residual rate of raffinate (RRR) and removal rate of group A (RRGA), (b) m_{GA} and m_{GB}, which are distribution coefficient of group A (GA) and group B (GB), and selectivity of group A in reference to group B ($\beta_{GA,GB}$), (c) selectivity of compound i in reference to 2MNTL ($\beta_{i,2MNTL}$). From (a), as $y_{w,0}$ increases, RRR increases while RRGA decreases. This is thought to be a tendency caused by an increase in the polarity of the extract phase as $y_{w,0}$ increases. In the range of $y_{w,0}$, RRR and RRGA, respectively, were 95.9% to 99.1% and 10.8% to 19.1%. From (b), we can see that the increase in $y_{w,0}$ increases the polarity of the extract phase, which decreases m_{GA} and m_{GB} but conversely increases $\beta_{GA,GB}$. Additionally, the fact that m_{GA} is much larger than that of group B shows that the polarity of group A is greater than that of group B. According to $y_{w,0}$, $\beta_{i,2MNTL}$ was reviewed to confirm the degree of separation between all the compounds identified using GC in this study. As predicted from the tendency of m_{GA}, m_{GB}, and $\beta_{GA,GB}$, according to $y_{w,0}$, of (b), we can see that the $\beta_{i,2MNTL}$ of each NCHC of group A increased with increasing $y_{w,0}$, but that of each non-NCHCs of group B showed almost constant values regardless of $y_{w,0}$. The $\beta_{i,2MNTL}$ of each NCHC obtained in the $y_{w,0}$ range of this study was approximately 3–5 times greater than that obtained from methanol extraction using wash oil [7,21,25]. In all compounds identified, $\beta_{i,2MNTL}$ showed the following order: ID > QNL = IQNL > NTL > BP > DBF > 2MNTL = 1MNTL > FR. Given the balance between RRR and RRGA, according to $y_{w,0}$, we thought an extraction that maintained $y_{w,0}$ = 0.1 would be favorable for removing group A from CMNO using MFW as a solvent.

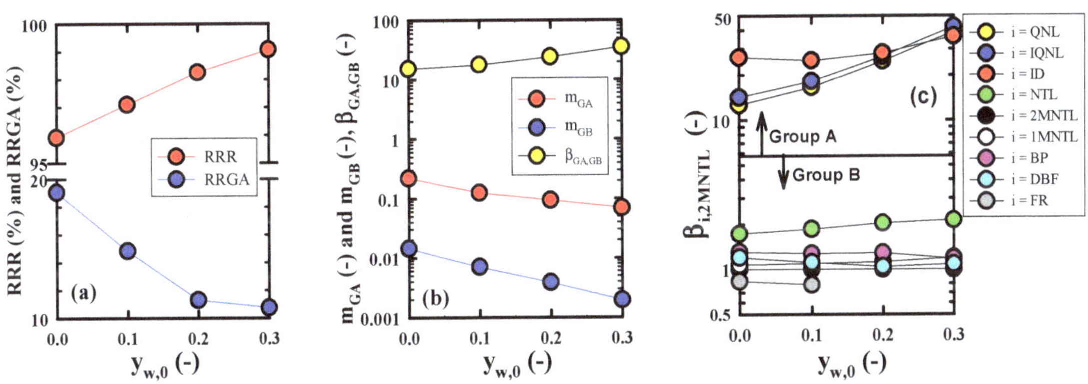

Figure 2. Effect of volume fraction of water to solvent before extraction run ($y_{w,0}$) on (**a**) residual rate of raffinate (RRR) and removal rate of group A (RRGA), (**b**) distribution coefficient of group A (GA) and group B (GB) (m_{GA} and m_{GB}), and selectivity of GA in reference to GB ($\beta_{GA,GB}$), (**c**) selectivity of compound i in reference to 2MNTL ($\beta_{i,2MNTL}$). 2MNTL: 2-Methylnaphthalene. Extraction conditions: S_0/F_0 = 1, T = 303 K, and t = 72 h.

Figure 3a–c, respectively, shows the effect of the volume fraction of solvent to feed before extraction run (S_0/F_0) on (a) residual rate of raffinate (RRR) and removal rate of group A (RRGA), (b) m_{GA} and m_{GB}, which are distribution coefficient of group A (GA) and group B (GB), and selectivity of group A in reference to group B ($\beta_{GA,GB}$), (c) selectivity of compound i in reference to 2MNTL ($\beta_{i,2MNTL}$). An increase in S_0/F_0 resulted in a decrease in RRR and an increase in RRGA. This tendency is caused by a chemical change, such as salvation between the NCHCs and a solvent by S_0/F_0 change [22,25]. When S_0/F_0 = 1 and 9, RRR decreased from 97.1% to 81.3%, but RRGA increased sharply from 14.8% to

70.7%. Through this, it is expected that if the raffinate phase recovered by $S_0/F_0 = 9$ is washed with water (to remove formamide contained in a small amount in the raffinate phase), it can be used as a CMNO with improved quality. It can be seen from (b) that as S_0/F_0 increased, m_{GA} and m_{GB} showed a weak increase trend and then decreased, but $\beta_{GA,GB}$ showed a slight increase trend as S_0/F_0 increased. The $\beta_{i,2MNTL}$ of each NCHC in group A increased with increasing S_0/F_0, while that of each non-NCHC in group B was almost constant regardless of S_0/F_0. Considering the balance of RRR and RRGA per the unit volume of solvent, according to S_0/F_0, it was considered that extraction in $S_0/F_0 = 1$ using MFW as a solvent would be advantageous for removing group A in CMNO.

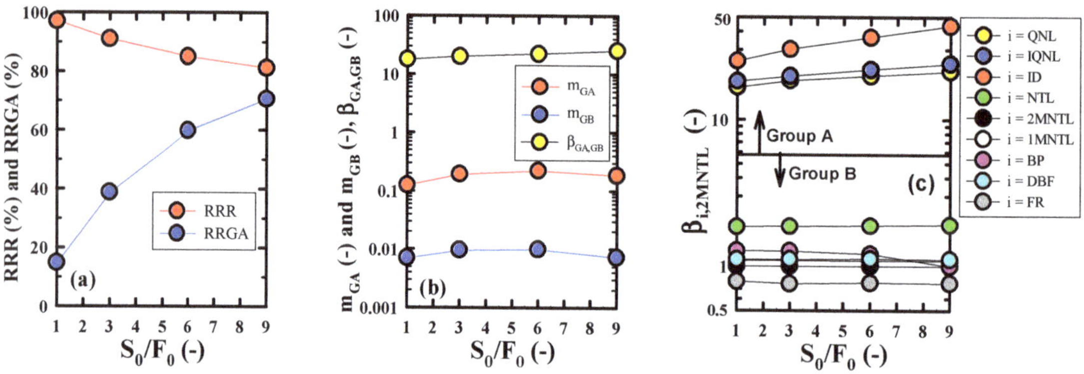

Figure 3. Effect of volume fraction of solvent to feed before extraction run (S_0/F_0) on (**a**) residual rate of raffinate (RRR) and removal rate of group A (RRGA), (**b**) distribution coefficient of GA and GB (m_{GA} and m_{GB}), and selectivity of GA in reference to GB ($\beta_{GA,GB}$), (**c**) selectivity of compound i in reference to 2MNTL ($\beta_{i,2MNTL}$). 2MNTL: 2-Methylnaphthalene. Extraction conditions: $y_{w,0} = 0.1$, T = 303 K, and t = 72 h.

Figure 4a–c, respectively, shows the effect of the operating temperature (T) on (a) residual rate of raffinate (RRR) and removal rate of group A (RRGA), (b) m_{GA} and m_{GB}, which are distribution coefficient of group A (GA) and group B (GB), and GA in reference to GB ($\beta_{GA,GB}$), (c) selectivity of compound i in reference to 2MNTL ($\beta_{i,2MNTL}$). As the operating temperature increased, RRR decreased, but conversely, RRGA increased. The operating temperature increased, the molecular movement of all compounds in CMNO became active, and the movement to the extraction phase through the liquid-liquid interface increased, reducing RRR; on the contrary, it showed a general extraction tendency to increase RRGA. From the results of examining the effect of operating temperature on m_{GA}, m_{GB}, $\beta_{GA,GB}$, and $\beta_{i,2MNTL}$ shown in (b) and (C), it was determined that room temperature operation could be used to remove NCHCs from CMNO.

Figure 1b,c show the gas chromatograms of the raffinate phase and the extract phase recovered through equilibrium extraction under constant conditions ($y_{w,0} = 0.1$, $S_0/F_0 = 9$, T = 303 K, t = 72 h), respectively. The gas chromatogram of the raffinate phase in (b) differed significantly from that of CMNO in Figure 1a, as the peak height of each NCHC of the raffinate phase was greatly reduced as many NCHCs were extracted. From differences in these gas chromatograms, it was possible to reconfirm the effect of removing NCHCs in CMNO by formamide extraction in this study. On the contrary, comparing the gas chromatogram of the extract phase with that of CMNO revealed a significant increase in the peak height of each NCHC compound of group A due to formamide extraction; still, the peak height of the six types of non-NCHCs of group B was greatly decreased. Compared to CMNO, the extract phase recovered from formamide extraction contained many useful NCHCs used to manufacture drugs, perfumes, pesticides, dyes, and pigments, as mentioned in the introduction. If NCHCs (especially ID) can be purified to high purity by recovering the formamide extract phase and adopting an appropriate post-treatment process, this is thought to be very meaningful in terms of recycling resources.

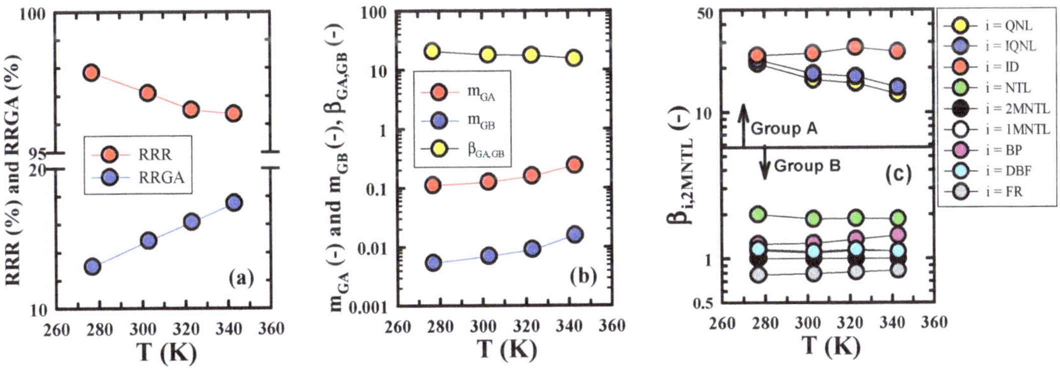

Figure 4. Effect of operating temperature (T) on (**a**) residual rate of raffinate (RRR) and removal rate of group A (RRGA), (**b**) distribution coefficient of GA and GB (m_{GA} and m_{GB}), and selectivity of GA in reference to GB ($\beta_{GA,GB}$), (**c**) selectivity of compound i in reference to 2MNTL ($\beta_{i,2MNTL}$). 2MNTL: 2-Methylnaphthalene. Extraction conditions: $y_{w,0}$ = 0.1, S_0/F_0 = 1, and t = 72 h.

From the results of this study, which comprehensively examined the effects of experimental factors and conditions on the removal of group A contained in CMNO, we considered $y_{w,0}$ = 0.1, S_0/F_0 = 1, and T = room temperature to be the optimal experimental conditions. In addition, considering that these experimental results obtained through this study were obtained using only a single stage of batch equilibrium extraction, it is expected that very high removal efficiency of group A can be obtained from CMNO if formamide extraction is performed using the multi-stage continuous extraction apparatus of the tower type with large liquid-liquid contact area under an optimal extraction condition.

4. Conclusions

To improve the quality of CMNO, this study performed distribution equilibrium between CMNO and formamide, or a mixture of formamide and water, to investigate the effects of experimental parameters and conditions on the removal of NCHCs in CMNO. When extraction operation was performed under the experimental conditions of $y_{w,0}$ = 0.1, S_0/F_0 = 1, and T = 303 K, the very excellent removal efficiency of NCHCs in CMNO was achieved. The formamide extraction method applied in this study showed excellent performance in terms of the residual rate of raffinate and the removal rate of group A (NCHCs), so it was expected to be an alternative to the reaction extraction method using acids and bases applied so far to the separation of NCHCs in the distillation residue of coal tar.

Funding: This research was supported by the Basic Science Research Program through the National Research Foundation of Korea (NRF), funded by the Ministry of Education (No. 2020R1I1A3061492).

Data Availability Statement: The data presented in this study are available within the article (tables and figures).

Conflicts of Interest: The author declares no conflict of interest.

References

1. Sakanishi, K.; Obata, H.; Mochida, I.; Sakaki, T. Removal and recovery of quinoline bases from methylnaphthalene oil in a semicontinuous supercritical CO_2 separation apparatus with a fixed bed of supported aluminum sulfate. *Ind. Eng. Chem. Res.* **1995**, *34*, 4118–4124. [CrossRef]

2. Lobovich, D.V.; Zinov'eva, I.V.; Milevskii, N.A.; Kostanyan, A.E.; Zakhodyaeva, Y.A.; Voshkin, A.A. Extraction kinetics of pyridine, quinoline, and indole from the organic phase with natural deep eutectic solvents and separation study using a centrifugal extractor. *Processes* **2024**, *12*, 488. [CrossRef]
3. Kim, S.J. Upgrading of wash oil through reduction of nitrogen-containing compounds. *Processes* **2021**, *9*, 1869. [CrossRef]
4. Sakanishi, K.; Obata, H.; Mochida, I.; Sakaki, T. Capture and recovery of indole from methylnaphthalene oil in a continuous supercritical CO_2 extraction apparatus over a fixed bed of anion-exchange resin. *Ind. Eng. Chem. Res.* **1996**, *35*, 335–337. [CrossRef]
5. Mindt, M.; Beyraghdar Kashkooli, A.; Suarez-Diez, M.; Ferrer, L.; Jilg, T.; Bosch, D.; Martins dos Santos, V.; Wendisch, V.F.; Cankar, K. Production of indole by corynebacterium glutamicum microbial cell factories for flavor and fragrance applications. *Microb. Cell Factories* **2022**, *21*, 45. [CrossRef] [PubMed]
6. Rogošić, M.; Kučan, K.Z. Deep eutectic solvents based on choline chloride and ethylene glycol as media for extractive denitrification/desulfurization/dearomatization of motor fuels. *J. Ind. Eng. Chem.* **2019**, *72*, 87–99. [CrossRef]
7. Kim, S.J. Comparison of methanol with formamide on separation of mitrogen heterocyclic compounds from medel coal tar fraction by batch concurrent multistage equilibrium extraction. *Polycycl. Aromat. Compd.* **2016**, *36*, 745–757.
8. Mamoru, Y.; Tomonori, K. Separation and purification of indole from coal tar by supercritical fluid extraction. *J. Chem. Eng. Jpn.* **1993**, *26*, 153–158.
9. Xiao, R.H.; Gao, W.H. Study on the recovery of indole from coal tar wash oil. *Coal Convers.* **1998**, *21*, 59–61.
10. Mochida, I.; Fei, Y.Q.; Sakanishi, K. Capture and recovery of basic nitrogen species in coal tar pitch, using nickel sulfate as adsorbent. *Chem. Lett.* **1990**, *19*, 515–518. [CrossRef]
11. Feng, X.; Ma, X.; Li, N.; Shang, C.; Yang, X.; Chen, X.D. Adsorption of quinoline from liquid hydrocarbons on graphite oxide and activated carbons. *RSC Adv.* **2015**, *5*, 74684–74691. [CrossRef]
12. Koriakin, A.; Ponvel, K.M.; Lee, C.H. Denitrogenation of raw diesel fuel by lithium-modified mesoporous silica. *Chem. Eng. J.* **2010**, *162*, 649–655. [CrossRef]
13. Gao, P.; Zhang, J.; Guo, Z.; Gao, J.; Xu, D.; Ma, Y.; Zhang, L.; Wang, Y. Experimental and quantum chemical calculations investigations of morpholine-based ionic liquids as extractants for efficient extraction of nitrogen heterocyclic neutral compounds. *Fuel* **2023**, *333*, 126446. [CrossRef]
14. Ji, Y.; Hou, Y.; Ren, S.; Wu, W. Highly efficient separation of indole from model wash oil using tetraethyl ammonium amino acid ionic liquids. *Sep. Purif. Technol.* **2021**, *258*, 117997. [CrossRef]
15. Liu, Q.; Zhang, T.; Gao, P.; Gao, J.; Xu, D.; Zhao, P.; Zhang, L.; Wang, Y. Separation of indole by designed ionic liquids with dual functional chemical sites: Mechanism exploration and experimental validation. *J. Environ. Chem. Eng.* **2021**, *9*, 105971. [CrossRef]
16. Gao, P.; Yang, L.; Wang, J.; Gao, J.; Xu, D.; Ma, L.; Zhang, L.; Wang, Y. Integrated investigation for extractive denitrogenation of fuel oils with eco-friendly piperazine-based ionic liquids. *Fuel* **2023**, *337*, 127187. [CrossRef]
17. Uemasu, I. Effect of methanol-water mixture solvent on concentration of indole in coal tar using β-cyclodextrin as complexing agent. *J. Jpn. Pet. Inst.* **1991**, *34*, 371–374. [CrossRef]
18. Uemasu, I.; Nakayama, T. Concentration of indole in coal tar using α-cyclodextrin as the host for inclusion complexation. *J. Incl. Phenom. Mol. Recognit. Chem.* **1989**, *7*, 327–331. [CrossRef]
19. Ukegawa, K.; Matsumura, A.; Kodera, Y.; Kondo, T.; Nakayama, T.; Tanabe, H.; Yoshida, S.; Mito, Y. Solvent extraction of nitrogen compounds from a coal tar fraction. (Part 1). Effect of extraction conditions on the extraction rate and the selectivities of nitrogen compounds. *J. Jpn. Pet. Inst.* **1990**, *33*, 250–254. [CrossRef]
20. Feng, Y.; Yang, E.; Dang, L.; Wei, H. Liquid–liquid phase equilibrium for ternary mixtures of formamide (or ethylene glycol, or monoethanolamine) + indole + 2-methylnaphthalene at 308.15 K. *Fluid Phase Equilibria* **2015**, *398*, 10–14. [CrossRef]
21. Egashira, R.; Nagai, M. Separation of nitrogen heterocyclic compounds contained in coal tar absorption oil fraction by solvent extraction. *J. Jpn. Pet. Inst.* **2000**, *43*, 339–345. [CrossRef]
22. Kim, S.J.; Chun, Y.J. Separation of nitrogen heterocyclic compounds from model coal tar fraction by solvent extraction. *Sep. Sci. Technol.* **2005**, *40*, 2095–2109.
23. Kodera, Y.; Ukegawa, K.; Mito, Y.; Komoto, M.; Ishikawa, E.; Nakayama, T. Solvent extraction of nitrogen compounds from coal liquids. *Fuel* **1991**, *70*, 765–769. [CrossRef]
24. Kim, S.J. Separation and purification of indole in model coal tar fraction of 9 compounds system. *Polycycl. Aromat. Compd.* **2019**, *39*, 60–72. [CrossRef]
25. Kim, S.J. Experimental study on enrichment of indole in wash oil by a combined process of extraction and re-Extraction. *Processes* **2023**, *11*, 3097. [CrossRef]

processes

MDPI

Article

Adsorption–Desorption Process to Separate Dyes from Tanning Wastewaters

Paolo Trucillo *, Amedeo Lancia and Francesco Di Natale

Department of Chemical, Material and Industrial Production Engineering, University of Naples Federico II, Piazzale V. Tecchio, 80, 80125 Napoli, Italy; lancia@unina.it (A.L.); fdinatal@unina.it (F.D.N.)
* Correspondence: paolo.trucillo@unina.it; Tel.: +39-329-65-66-043

Abstract: Wastewater production is a major environmental issue for the leather and textile industries: in a modern plant, several synthetic dyes are used in separated coloring batches whose wastewaters are usually mixed, diluted with other process water streams, and sent to a unique wastewater treatment plant. This includes specific physical and biochemical tertiary treatments to remove dyes efficiently. One of the main difficulties of these processes is the presence of multiple dyes, which cannot be treated with the same efficiency as a "wide-spectrum" process. This work explores the possibility of using conventional granular activated carbon (GAC) and a new polyurethane foam (PUF) for the adsorption of an acid red dye in the wastewater of a specific coloring batch of the tanning industry. The aim of this work is twofold: on the one hand, we aim to explore the performance of the new PUF sorbent; on the other hand, we aim to explore the possibility of using adsorption as an optimized pre-treatment for single-dye batches, which may take advantage of the presence of a single type of target dye and its higher concentration. The effluent is then sent to the wastewater treatment plant for further depuration.

Keywords: granular activated carbon; polyurethane foam; adsorption; tanning; wastewaters; dyes

1. Introduction

The fashion and related industries such as garments, footwear, and accessories have been significantly affected by globalization [1–3]; therefore, hundreds of companies and brands all over the world have emerged thanks to the work of thousands of valuable designers and numerous prestigious design schools [4]. However, while design is predominant in Western countries [5,6], textile production is still considered an Asiatic domain [7,8] due to the cheapest manufacturing cost [9,10].

According to the Annual Fashion Talk released by Mediobanca, in 2019, the world fashion industry was worth USD 471 billion, summing up the revenues of the 80 biggest manufacturing industries worldwide. Among these, Italy was the most represented country with the 10 most famous brands [11–13]. Recently, the Global Fashion Industry (source: https://fashionunited.com, accessed on 15 December 2019), estimated the overall value of brands, and assets of the global fashion industry to be around USD 3 trillion. Despite this high value and economic yearly income, the fashion sector generated significant environmental issues due to the intense use of toxic chemicals [14,15], with a subsequent necessity to modify processes within sustainable and environmentally friendly limits [16,17]. It was estimated that in 2017, about 80 thousand million garments were sold worldwide; this substantial increase in consumption resulted in a 75% increase in used clothes disposal, which without a specific recycling process, was destined for landfill disposal or thermal incineration [18]. This caused manufacturing industries to adjust dramatically to the increased request of the market. Nowadays, the estimated yearly consumption of dyes is around 10,000 tons in textile industries [19], thus resulting in an even higher environmental impact [20].

The fashion industry distinguishes itself with the use of diverse production methods and technological advancements [21,22]; among those, dyeing and weaving produce the largest number of pollutants [23,24], which increase the level of toxicity and non-recyclability during disposal [25,26]. Nowadays, the production of 1 kg of fabric requires an average amount of 200 L water and an amount of chemicals between 100 g to 1 kg (i.e., up to 100% of fabric weight, on a mass basis) [27–30]. This inhomogeneity in wastewater composition is also due to different worldwide regulations [31–33] and the high diversity of textile wastes [34,35]. Since the dye binding process is not particularly efficient, this results in the loss of between 10% and 50% of dyes, but also other substances such as formaldehyde, chlorine, and heavy metals. The disposal of these compounds in rivers and lakes creates further negative effects on living organisms, which can be quantified only with specific eco-toxicological measurements [36,37]. Focusing on the dyeing process, 1 kg of produced fabric generates from 20 to 100 kg of spent dyes, thus resulting in several washing post-processing steps [38–42]. Therefore, the textile dyeing and finishing industry created a huge pollution problem, as it is one of the most-discussed secondary pollutants of textile wastewater in applications related to agricultural irrigations [43–45].

In the late 1990s, dye removal methods included only preliminary water purification processes such as equalization and sedimentation [46–48] due to the absence of clearly defined boundaries regarding the release of dye effluents into the environment. After the definition of the permissible dye effluent release standards, more effective dye removal methods were introduced, such as chemical–physical or biological plants with activated sludge [49–52]. Moreover, the necessity to remove high percentages of dyes and surfactants led companies to try to improve the purification yields of these traditional processes by adding specific products. Among the proposed techniques, separation using polymeric porous membranes or composites provided several advantages such as high selectivity, low energy consumption, and moderate cost [53–56]. Additionally, oxidation, electrocoagulation, and biofilm techniques were utilized to degrade or separate contaminants found in industrial wastewater [57–59]. The results obtained using this system are encouraging, but a complementary treatment process is needed to remove residual impurities; moreover, these methods are expensive and do not guarantee a high and selective removal of dyes [60–62].

Among the separation processes, several adsorption methods have been developed for the treatment of contaminants in diverse environmental applications, with activated carbon emerging as a widely favored choice. Nevertheless, it is worth delving into a comparative exploration of various adsorption techniques aimed at purifying wastewater and mitigating the impacts of these contaminants [63]. Activated carbon, renowned for its exceptional adsorption properties, plays a pivotal role in wastewater treatment plants. Its porous structure and high surface area make it an effective adsorbent for a wide spectrum of contaminants. However, activated carbon is not the sole contender in the arena of adsorption processes. Other materials such as polyurethanes, zeolites, clay minerals, and metal oxides also exhibit remarkable adsorption capacities. Furthermore, adsorption processes can be customized based on the specific wastewater composition and the target contaminants. Factors such as pH, temperature, and contact time can be adjusted to optimize adsorption efficiency. Additionally, advancements in adsorbent modification techniques, including surface functionalization or the use of nanostructured materials, have expanded the toolkit for wastewater treatment. This work represented a first attempt to create a method for the use of alternative materials in a single or combined use to depurate wastewater from contaminants.

Adsorption separates dyes from textile wastewaters with the selective deposition of the dye's molecules on the surface of an adsorbent material. This type of treatment is particularly suitable for organic substances, such as solvents, surfactants, and pesticides, as well as dyes [64,65]. The method for adsorption dye removal could be considered an outstanding process in the case that it selectively separates one dye or a mixture of dyes. In general, for the adsorption of organic compounds, adsorption can also be repeated several times, after the regeneration and reuse of the adsorbent material, until it becomes spent. This also permits a reduction in process costs in terms of fresh materials involved.

However, the number of regeneration cycles depends on various factors, including the nature and concentration of pollutants and the adsorption energy bonds. It is well-established that some dyes can be deposited on the adsorbent through physical adsorption pathways including the formation of a "condensed" phase on its surface, while in some other cases, chemisorption mechanisms involving site-specific interactions occur.

In this work, we report the first experimental data on the use of a new sorbent, namely, a polyurethane foam (PUF) for the treatment of a specific water-based solution produced during tanning processes. The use of foams in the treatment of wastewater is a promising option in the field of environmental protection and sustainable water management. Foams play a crucial role in facilitating the removal of contaminants and pollutants from wastewater streams [66]. These foam-based treatment methods are highly effective in separating suspended solids, oils, grease, and even certain dissolved contaminants from water, thus contributing to the purification of wastewater [67].

In particular, the use of polyurethanes in wastewater treatment represents an innovative and versatile approach to addressing environmental challenges. Polyurethanes, with their exceptional uptake capacities, have proven to be valuable materials in various stages of wastewater treatment processes. They are used for the fabrication of membranes and adsorbents with tailored properties, which are capable of selectively removing pollutants such as dyes, heavy metals, organic compounds, and microorganisms from wastewater streams [68,69].

This work (performed in collaboration with the company DMD S.p.A., Solofra, Avellino, Italy) concerns the use of new (the PUF) and conventional (the GAC) adsorbent materials to depurate the wastewater produced by a single-dye coloring batch to allow a more targeted pre-treatment of the dye. The aim is to provide a selective recovery of dyes and to reduce the amount of dye that is sent to the company's wastewater treatment plants. In fact, the presence of multiple dye streams, each with specific chemical composition and characteristics, and their overall dilution with the other process waters makes the tertiary treatment of these wastewaters particularly complex and expensive. The idea behind this approach is that it can be easier to treat the wastewater of each dyeing process separately, targeting the treatment to its specific chemistry. This work focused on the adsorption of dyes on two types of adsorbent materials: activated carbons [70–73], already studied and used in traditional purification processes, and polyurethane foams (PUF) [74], explored as an alternative adsorbent. The preparation of the model dyeing solution used in the tanning process was replicated in our laboratory. Starting from this, adsorption tests at 20 °C and 40 °C were performed, also investigating the effect of chemical additives generally used in the dyeing step (ammonia, fats, formic acid). In addition to the adsorption process, the desorption reverse process was also analyzed, with the final aim of understanding whether and how to dispose of the adsorbent material or to regenerate and reuse it in a subsequent adsorption cycle.

2. Materials and Methods

2.1. Materials

In this work, adsorption experiments were performed either in aqueous solutions or in model dyeing solutions containing fat-liquoring agents, as used in industrial tanning processes. "Acid red 97" (obtained by DMD Solofra S.p.A., Avellino, Italy) was used as a dyeing agent for this work. This kind of dye is particularly suitable for chrome-tanned leather. The authors only received its commercial nomenclature; therefore, it was not possible to report specific and detailed information about the formulation, but a UV-Vis spectrum obtained on the dye was provided, working in collaboration with DMD S.p.A, Solofra (AV), Italy. For the preparation of the aqueous solutions, the dye was simply dissolved in distilled water. In contrast, the preparation of the model tanning solution required several additional chemicals, such as Lipoderm N, ammonia, Coripol DX 1202, formic acid, and distilled water. Sorbents utilized for adsorption tests were Filtercarb GCC 1240 and polyurethane. The characteristics of each used compound are reported in the following paragraphs.

"Lipoderm N" (BASF, Ludwigshafen, Germany) is an anionic emulsifier with a fat-liquoring action; its effect is considered necessary since animal skin loses most of its natural fats and oils during the tanning stage. Therefore, this emulsifier is put in contact with the leather matrix, preventing the adhesion of fibers [75,76] and favoring the penetration of dye into the leather. According to the BASF datasheet, the liquid form of Lipoderm N is characterized by a yellowish-brown color and pH of 8; moreover, it has an active content of approximately 50% on a mass basis, and its suggested stocking conditions are between 0 °C and 35 °C. This compound can be easily diluted in water, and its solutions are generally resistant to acids, alkalis, and salts.

Ammonia (Sigma Aldrich, Milan, Italy) is one of the auxiliaries used during the dyeing process to adjust the pH from acid to basic. In fact, at the beginning of the process, the leather that is obtained from the previous tanning steps has a pH of 3–4; then, with the addition of ammonia, the pH becomes close to 8. When the solution is basic, the dye is conveyed into the fiber. Indeed, in this step, the fiber allows the dye to penetrate within the cross-section of the leather.

Coripol DX 1202 (TFL, Rheinfelden, Germany) was used as a synthetic fat-liquoring agent. This white/yellowish anionic compound appears as an emulsion and is based on sulfated high molecular hydrocarbons. One of the properties of Coripol is its high heat resistance and good stability in mineral tanning floats. It is possible to dilute it in water under stirring at 60 °C. By combining it properly with the individual components of the fat-liquoring mixture, it is possible to reach practically any kind of softness or surface effects. Its pH is approximately 8, which is the same as the compound whose commercial name is Lipoderm N.

Formic acid (Thermo Fisher Scientific, Waltham, MA, USA), 85% *w*/*w* in water, was used as a reactive to adjust the acidity at the end of the dyeing protocol and to further improve the color penetration into fibers. Formic acid is used in the dyeing process to fix the color of the leather; in particular, it has an inverse role with respect to ammonia. After addition, the pH of the solution becomes acid again, and the fibers close, entrapping the dye inside the pores and the section of leather.

Two adsorbent materials were used to perform and compare adsorption experiments: granular activated carbon and polyurethane foam [77,78]. The activated carbon used in this work is FILTERCARB GCC 1240, which is used in granules of 1–2 mm diameter. It is generally used for water filtration processes and was obtained by Carbonitalia S.r.l. (Vezzano Ligure, Italy). This material is produced from coconut charcoal, physically activated with water vapor to develop a large active surface, which makes it suitable for the purification of water and organic liquids of the chemical and food industry (oil, liqueurs, glycerin, acids). Filtercarb GCC 1240 is an adsorbent characterized by a large specific surface and finds applications in numerous fields, such as pharmaceutical, food, catalysis, gas storage, and electrode materials, and also in the removal of odor from liquid and gaseous phases and the elimination of organic pollutants from drinking water and wastewaters [79,80]. The granular activated carbon was pre-washed before adding it to colored solutions.

Polyurethane is a leading member of the wide-ranging and highly diverse family of polymers or plastics. In this work, polyurethane was used in slices of cubic shape (about 1×1 cm). Its cellular-like structure is expanded by adding to the formation reaction a blowing agent that volatilizes because of the heat generated during the polymerization reaction. Polyurethane (PUF) has been used as an adsorbent in the treatment of contaminated water and effluent because of its low cost and the possibility of using it without pre-treatments [81,82]. In addition, PUF belongs to classes of substances characterized by both polar and nonpolar groups. Chemical and physical properties of the material used in this work has been reported in Table 1.

Table 1. Chemical and physical properties of used materials.

Material	Molecular Weight [g/mol]	Color	CAS Number	Bulk Density [kg/m^3]	Water Solubility
Acid Red 97	699	red-yellowish	10169-02-5	1579	8.85 g/L
Lipoderm N	*	opaque white	*	*	*
Ammonia	17	colorless	7664-41-7	0.73	31% w/w
Formic acid	46	colorless	64-18-6	1.22	Highly miscible
Filtercarb GCC 1240	*	black	*	530	Not miscible
Polyurethane	312	red-yellowish	25036-33-3	870	Not miscible
Coripol DX 1202	*	opaque white	*	*	*

* Information not provided by the manufacturer.

2.2. Methods

The experimental work was preceded by the preparation of either water-dyeing or fat-liquoring model dyeing solutions. Then, the experiments were divided into two macro-steps: adsorption experiments of dye with granular activated carbon and polyurethane, using the previously prepared dyeing solutions; secondly, desorption of dye from spent sorbents was performed. A sketch of the methodology is provided in Figure 1. A further description of the methodology is reported in the following sub-sections.

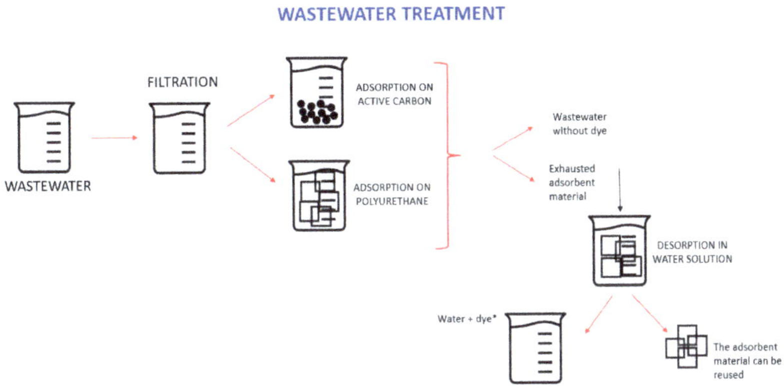

Figure 1. Description of the procedure used in this work for the treatment of wastewater, from preliminary filtration to adsorption and desorption process units. * On the basis of the selective capacity of the adsorbent material, here we may have other compounds reported in Table 1.

2.2.1. Dye Preparation Solutions

We followed a simplified protocol of a typical dyeing recipe provided to us by DMD Solofra S.p.A. and replicated it to simulate the composition of a typical tanning solution. In Table 2, a description of the four main steps involved in leather dyeing preparation is reported. However, in this study, we prepared dyeing solutions, as indicated in Table 2, but we did not use any leather scraps since the goal of this work was to adsorb dyes on active carbons and try to regenerate sorbents using desorption processes. In Table 2, all the percentages reported theoretically refer to the mass of leather, which, for simplicity, is set to a reference value of 5 g. We decided to work in the worst conditions, meaning that we considered the case in which it is possible to find all the chemical additives used in the dyeing phase in the simulated wastewater.

According to the recipe reported above, the first step consists of the addition of the fat-liquoring agent and ammonia to the water in order theoretically to prepare the leather (not used in this study) for the addition of dye. To reproduce the stirring occurring on a large scale in tanning drums, the solutions are stirred for 60 min. In the second step, the addition of dye occurs, with a continuous magnetic rotating plate for 30 min. In the third step, the fattening agent is added during another 30 min stirring. In the fourth and final step, formic acid is added to the solution; this has the function of narrowing the fibers and, consequently, fixing the dye deeply. According to this recipe, 3% of dye on a mass basis is added to the solution.

Table 2. Simplified model dyeing solution preparation (mass percentages per unit leather mass).

Mass Ratio	Steps of Preparation	Role of Additive
	1st step—60 min stirring at 200 rpm *	
600% *w/w*	Distilled water	Diluent
1% *w/w*	Lipoderm N	Emulsifier
3% *w/w*	Ammonia	pH corrector
	2nd step—addition of dye with 30 min stirring at 200 rpm	
3% *w/w*	Acid Red 97	Coloring agent
	3rd step—pre-fixing with 30 min stirring at 200 rpm	
3% *w/w*	Coripol DX 1202	Emulsifier
	4th step—fixing with 60 min stirring at 200 rpm	
5% *w/w*	Formic acid diluted in water 1:1 *v/v*	pH corrector

* Note that this first step is also characterized by the addition of 5 g leather; however, in this study, leather is not involved since the authors focused on the recovery and eventual reuse of the model solution.

2.2.2. Adsorption Experiments

The adsorption experiments are batch tests carried out in a PID-controlled oven at a fixed temperature. A fixed volume of the target solutions is placed in contact with a given mass of sorbent. For the kinetic tests, the experiments were performed setting the mass of GAC at 0.5 g and the mass of PUF at 0.1 g. In contrast, the initial dye concentration within the solution was varied according to the following indications: setting a volume of 30 mL of distilled water, different samples were prepared at 6 different dye concentrations, corresponding to dye concentration between 10 and 200 mg/kg. For the adsorption isotherms, the dosage and the concentration of the dye were varied to cover a representative concentration range.

Dye concentration measurements (in mg per kg of solutions) were performed using a spectrophotometer HACH (Loveland, CO, USA) mod. DR/2010 operating in the visible region, equipped with square-based glass cuvettes for blank and sample absolute absorbance measurement. As it is possible to see in Figure 2a, Acid Red 97's maximum absorbance peak was detected at 500 nm. Calibration lines were obtained on diluted Acid Red 97 solutions (Figure 2b), whose starting concentrations were known. In particular, the dye was dissolved first in water (round dots) and then in the model solution including tanning additives (square dots). These solutions were diluted 1:10 *v/v* in distilled water before absorbance measurements.

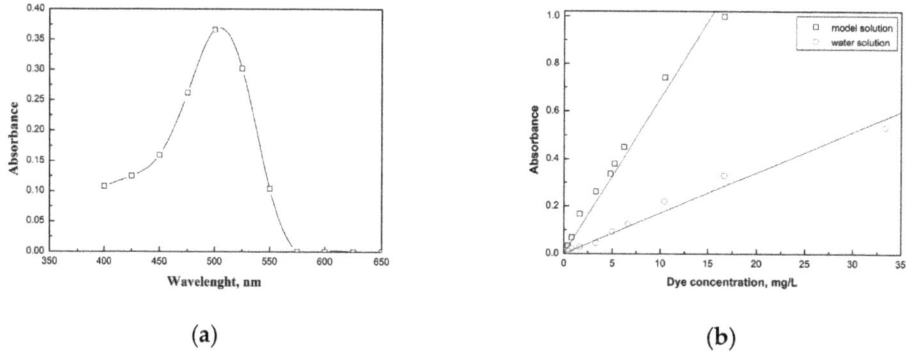

Figure 2. (**a**) UV-Vis spectrum of Acid Red 97. (**b**) Calibration curves of dye concentrations in water and model solutions.

The dye concentration and adsorption uptake expressed in these experiments were correlated by the following equation:

$$q(t) = \frac{V_a}{m}(C_0 - C(t)) \tag{1}$$

where $q(t)$ is the amount of dye adsorbed at time t, m is the mass of the sorbent, V_a is the volume of the solution, C_0 is the initial dye concentration, and $C(t)$ is the concentration of dye at time t. Adsorption isotherms were fitted using the Henry model as follows:

$$q_e = K\ C_e \tag{2}$$

where C_e is the dye concentration at equilibrium and q_e is the dye adsorption uptake at equilibrium.

2.2.3. Desorption Experiments

In this work, desorption tests were performed both in clean distilled water and in the clean solution obtained following the recipe described above, where "clean" refers to a total absence of the dye in the starting solutions. These tests were aimed at studying the possibility of reusing the solution in a new cycle of the tanning process, thus reducing fresh reagent consumption. In detail, a solution with a dye concentration of 70 mg/kg was put in contact with a given mass of sorbent until reaching uptake equilibrium conditions. Then, the adsorbent was separated from the solution and inserted into a newly prepared clean model solution. Then, the behavior of the adsorbent materials was investigated by changing the volume of this solution (6 mL, 9 mL, and 12 mL, respectively) at the temperature of 40 °C. While higher temperatures can be surely more effective for desorption, this temperature has been considered to contain the energy costs and the evaporative losses. The amount of dye desorbed from GAC to the receiving liquid medium was determined as a function of time, using the following equation:

$$q_d(t) = q_a - \frac{V_r}{m} C_a(t) \tag{3}$$

where $q_d(t)$ is the residual amount of dye on the sorbent at time t (mg/g), V_r is the volume of the receiving liquid medium, and $C_a(t)$ is the desorbed dye concentration in the liquid phase at time t (mg/kg). PUF was separated from the dyeing solutions after the adsorption experiments and was observed using a stereomicroscope, model SZX-T, Optika, Ponteranica, Italy.

During the experiments, we noted the presence of very fine PUF particles in the final solutions after centrifugation. Therefore, the solution was further filtered to be sure to remove these residues.

3. Results and Discussion

This first section concerns the adsorption of Acid Red 97 on activated carbon (GAC) and polyurethane foam (PUF), as reported in Figures 3 and 4.

Acid Red 97 dissolved in distilled water (pH = 8) was adsorbed on Filtercarb GCC 12 × 40. The kinetic tests are reported in Figure 3a,b. Figure 3a shows the time courses of Acid Red 97 concentration, $c(t)$, while Figure 3b represents its uptake on the activated carbon, $q(t)$, in distilled water during the batch adsorption tests performed at 20 °C. The experiments revealed that adsorption takes place over a long time, reaching equilibrium conditions after about 11 days. The dye uptake is around 9 mg/g for a residual concentration of about 55 mg/kg. As a qualitative representation of the experiments performed, Figure 4 reports the time evolution of color intensities in the test samples at the beginning (upper figure, at t = 0) and end of the adsorption treatment (lower figure, at t = 11 days). The efficacy of adsorption on activated carbon is evident: after about 11 days, the most concentrated tests with, respectively, an initial dye concentration of 202 mg/kg, 150 mg/kg, and 70 mg/kg, become almost transparent, while the three less concentrated samples (41 mg/kg, 30 mg/kg and 18 mg/kg) become transparent.

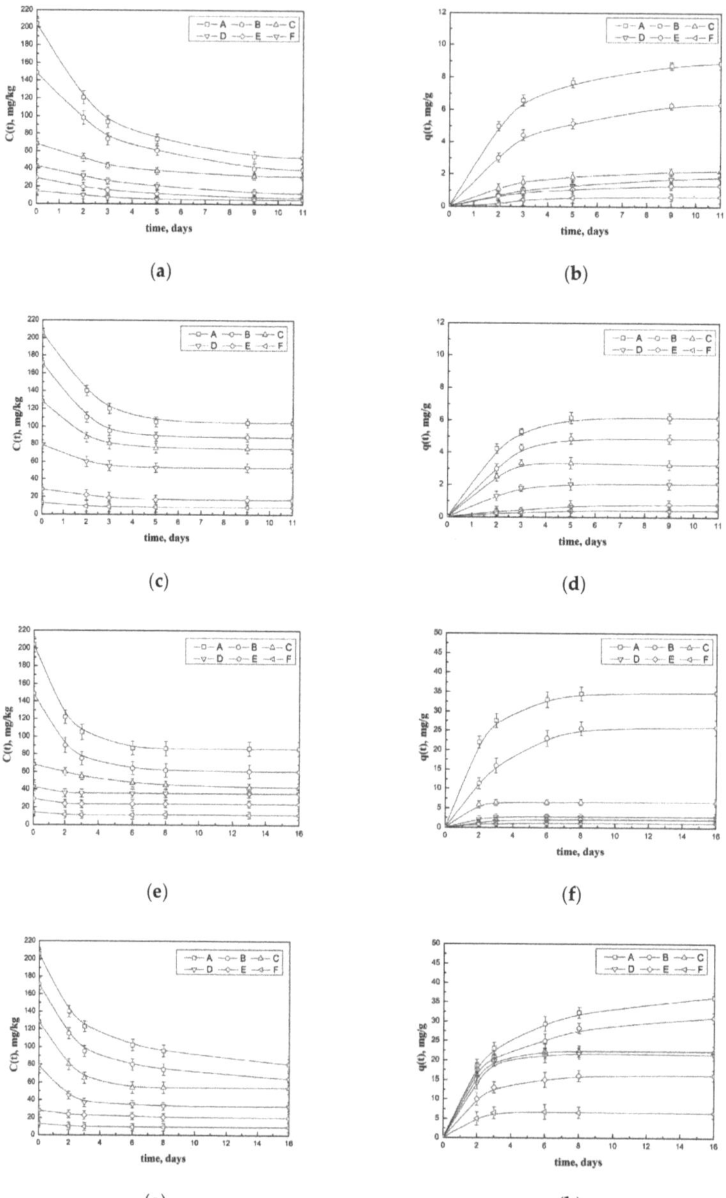

Figure 3. Test performed at 20 °C with Acid Red 97: (**a**) residual concentration in the distilled water solution in contact with GAC vs. test time and (**b**) adsorption uptake on GAC in the distilled water solution vs. test time. Test performed at 20 °C with Acid Red 97: (**c**) residual concentration in the model dyeing solution in contact with GAC vs. test time and (**d**) adsorption uptake of residual Acid Red 97 on GAC in the model dyeing water solution vs. test time. Test performed at 20 °C with Acid Red 97: (**e**) residual concentration in the distilled water solution in contact with PUF vs. test time and (**f**) adsorption uptake on PUF in the distilled water solution vs. test time. Test performed at 20 °C with Acid Red 97: (**g**) residual concentration in the model dyeing solution in contact with PUF vs. test time and (**h**) uptake of residual Acid Red 97 on PUF in the model dyeing solution vs. test time.

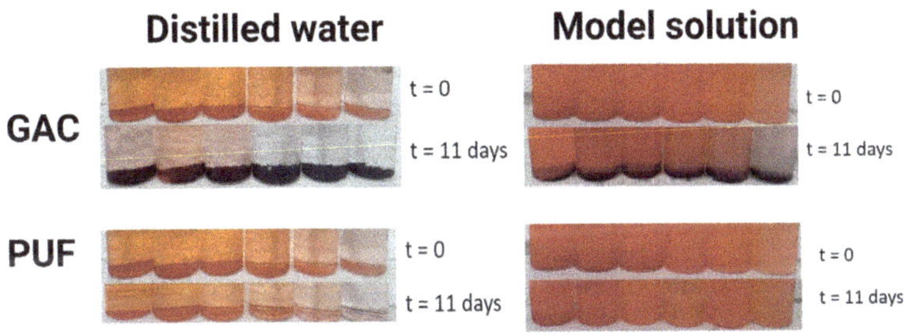

Figure 4. Test performed at 20 °C with Acid Red 97. Sample color intensity evolution intensities from the beginning (t = 0) to the end (t = 11 days) of the adsorption treatment using different adsorbent/solution couples.

Figure 3c,d shows the time courses of the Acid Red 97 concentration, $c(t)$, and its uptake on the activated carbon (GAC), $q(t)$, in the model dyeing solution during the batch adsorption tests performed at 20 °C. The mass of the sorbent was 0.5 g, the volume of the dyeing solution was 30 mL, and the pH was equal to 8, as in the previous set of experiments. The experimental results confirmed the general trend previously observed for the adsorption in the distilled water solution and indicated a lower adsorption efficiency, reaching, for the highest dye concentration, an uptake of around 6 mg/g for a residual concentration of about 100 mg/kg. In particular, the most concentrated starting solutions (205 mg/kg, 170 mg/kg, and 130 mg/kg, respectively) lost part of their color intensity without losing their opacity; the same behavior was encountered for the less concentrated samples. The experiments reported in Figure 3c,d revealed faster adsorption dynamics, with equilibrium conditions approached after around 5 days for all the samples, instead of 11 days, as observed in the case of distilled water. This result probably mirrors the competition between fats and dye on the surface of the activated carbon. The corresponding image in Figure 4 shows the time evolution of color intensities in the test samples at the beginning and end of the adsorption treatment. In this case, the solution color appears more opaque due to the presence of fattening agents: the color of the clean model solution is very close to the one shown for the lower dye concentration with GAC after 11 h.

In the following experiments, the granular activated carbon was substituted with PUF (Figure 3e–h) to compare the effect of another adsorbent material on distilled water plus dye solutions and on model dyeing solutions with fattening agents. The trend behavior of this new sorbent material was investigated. However, some differences arose from the use of a lower amount of PUF (0.1 g), which derived from the practical problem that it was not possible to set 0.5 g as the mass of PUF used in all the following experiments since the volume occupied by this material was much larger than 0.5 g GAC mass. A comparable mass of PUF would not have allowed a good bathing of the sorbent in the dyeing solution.

Figure 3e,f describes the time courses of the Acid Red 97 concentration and its uptake on the polyurethane foam (PUF) in distilled water during the batch adsorption tests performed at 20 °C in a total volume of 30 mL (pH was 7.8). As for the GAC, the experiments shown in Figure 4 revealed that adsorption took place over a long time, reaching equilibrium conditions after about 11 days. In these last experiments, the dye uptake is higher than that observed for the activated carbon, reaching up to 35 mg/g for a residual concentration of 85 mg/kg. Moreover, the corresponding image in Figure 4 shows the time evolution of color intensities in the test samples at the beginning (t = 0) and end (t = 11 days) of the adsorption treatment. Again, dye concentrations visibly decrease from left to right. In this case, due to the lower weight of PUF than GAC, the sorbent material is not immediately visible in the glass vial since it is floating on the upper part of the solution; however, it is still completely submerged.

Figure 3g,h shows the time courses of the Acid Red 97 concentration, $c(t)$, and of its uptake on the polyurethane foam (PUF), $q(t)$, in the model dyeing solution. The adsorption data indicated that, differently from the activated carbon, the adsorption of Acid Red 97 on PUF is not affected by the presence of other species in the dyeing solution.

In all the cases, the adsorption kinetics appear quite slow. In this work, we used the Lagergren model with the experimental equilibrium data and fitting the experiments with the sole kinetic constant. Despite a good fitting capacity, we are not able to describe the dataset in a consistent way. The long characteristic time suggests that, for the GAC, the adsorption is limited by diffusion in the pore structure while, for the PUF, the large pore structure probably links the low adsorption rate with surface reaction kinetics. Further studies are needed to interpret this aspect.

The adsorption isotherms for Acid Red 97 in distilled water and the model solution at 20 and 40 °C tested with GAC and PUF are shown in Figure 5. The isotherms show an almost linear trend, which is well-described by the Henry law presented in Section 2, whose parameters are reported in Table 3. Other models can be used, but the significance of the additional fitting parameters is questionable.

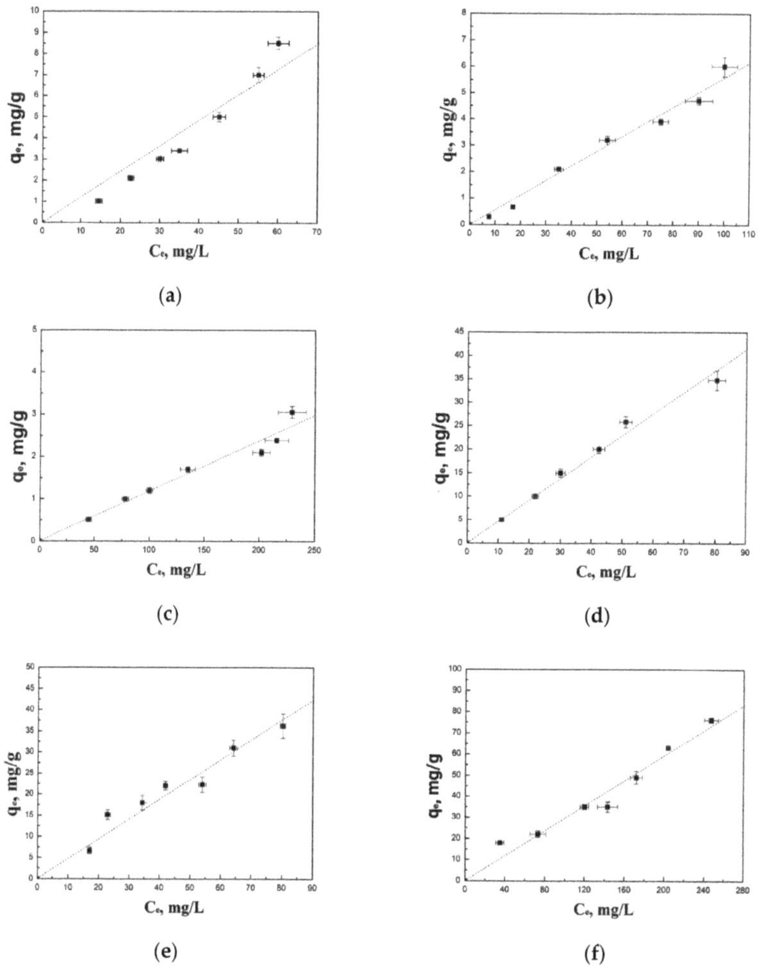

Figure 5. Adsorption isotherms of Acid Red 97 over (**a**) GAC in distilled water (DW) at 20 °C, (**b**) GAC in the model solution (MD) at 20 °C, (**c**) GAC in the model solution at 40 °C, (**d**) PUF in distilled water (DW) at 20 °C, (**e**) PUF in the model solution (MD) at 20 °C, and (**f**) PUF in the model solution at 40 °C.

Table 3. Henry model parameters obtained from fitting on isotherms.

Solution	Ads* Material	Temperature, °C	Henry Constant	R^2, %
Aqueous	GAC	20	0.121	93.4
Model	GAC	20	0.056	98.5
Model	GAC	40	0.012	96.7
Aqueous	PUF	20	0.459	98.6
Model	PUF	20	0.469	95.7
Model	PUF	40	0.296	96.9

*Ads: adsorbent material; R^2: mean squared error.

The experiments revealed that the adsorption isotherm at T = 20 °C with distilled water and the model solution have quite different behavior; however, the isotherm at 40 °C with the model solution is less favorable. As expected, due to the effect of temperature in an exothermic process, the adsorption capacity at 40 °C is far lower than that observed at 20 °C.

The same construction of isotherms is reported for the adsorption experiments performed with PUF at 20 °C in distilled water and using the model solution at 20 °C and 40 °C. At 20 °C, the use of PUF did not show a significant difference between the adsorption isotherm in distilled water and the same isotherm with the model solution. In this case, at a constant temperature, the adsorption is as favorable as using the model solution, without being affected by the presence of the additional species in the model dyeing solution. On the other hand, the adsorption isotherm for PUF at 40 °C in the model solution is less affected by a temperature change from 20 °C to 40 °C than the activated carbon.

The Henry law isotherm can be seen as the first portion of the Langmuir model:

$$\lim_{c\to 0} q = q_{max}\frac{Kc}{1+Kc} \cong q_{max}Kc = Hc \tag{4}$$

where q_{max} is the maximum adsorption capacity of the sorbent. In the case of the adsorption of a specific compound, such as a specific molecule or an ion, on a single specific active site, the Langmuir constant (K) corresponds to the equilibrium constant for the adsorption reaction and can be written as:

$$K = exp\left(-\frac{\Delta G^\circ}{RT}\right) \tag{5}$$

Therefore, the relation between Henry constant and temperature can be written as:

$$H = q_{max}\, exp\left(-\frac{\Delta G^\circ}{RT}\right) \tag{6}$$

Therefore, if at least two values of the Henry constant (H_1 and H_2) at two temperatures (T_1 and T_2) are known, one can derive an estimation of the ΔG° and q_{max} as:

$$\Delta G^\circ = \frac{Rln\left(\frac{H_1}{H_2}\right)}{\left(\frac{1}{T_2}-\frac{1}{T_1}\right)} \tag{7}$$

$$q_{max} = H_1 exp\left(\frac{\Delta G^\circ}{RT_1}\right) = H_2 exp\left(\frac{\Delta G^\circ}{RT_2}\right) \tag{8}$$

While this method is rigorously valid for the case of adsorption of one compound on one active site, it may be able to describe the behavior of more complex systems if they do not deviate too much from the ideal behavior. When applied to our data, the model indicates, for PUF, a value of ΔG° of −17.55 kJ/mol and a q_{max} = 347.9 mg/g. For GAC, the values are inconsistent. This is expected because PUF tests for the model aqueous solution and for the model dying solution show similar results, indicating that PUF is selective toward the dye and it is not affected by the other species in the liquid phase. Furthermore, due to the PUF chemical structure, the predominance of a single kind of active site is a reasonable assumption. On the other hand, the adsorption of the GAC reveals a high variability with the composition of the matrix and with the temperature, and several kinds of active surface sites can be expected. Therefore, the same inconsistencies of the ΔG° and q_{max} values further indicate that the dye adsorption process for GAC involves multiple active sites and that the interactions with the other components of the liquid solution cannot be neglected.

The limited variation in the adsorption capacity as a function of temperature suggests that the regeneration of the spent PUF is not feasible. To obtain an effective desorption, a significant reduction in the adsorption isotherm is needed.

Desorption tests on spent activated carbon were carried out, starting from a sample of GAC used for the adsorption of Acid Red 97 in the model dyeing solution.

We performed three desorption tests starting from the same adsorption test solution (same volume); however, the following desorption step occurred in three different volumes. To explain the experimental procedure, the following letters (reported in Figure 6) define the consequential steps of this process:

(A) A preliminary model solution of 30 mL containing an initial dye concentration of 80 mg/kg was prepared. In these conditions, without putting the solution in contact with GAC, the initial uptake capacity is referred to as 0 mg/kg. Then, 2 g of GAC (4 times larger than the previous adsorption experiments) was added to the solution in order to obtain a solid/liquid ratio of around 67 g/L.

(B) The equilibrium adsorption uptake was reached at 3.53 mg/g, at a concentration of 10.9 mg/kg at the temperature of 20 °C.

(C) The GAC adsorbent spent was then separated from the solution, dried, and put in contact with a fresh solution to perform the desorption step (in this case, the $c(t)$ becomes equal to zero).

(D) One-third of the spent GAC was added to the desorption liquid (volume of 6 mL), reaching a final concentration of 172 mg/kg, corresponding to about 1.47 mg/g residual uptake.

(E) One-third of the spent GAC was added to the desorption liquid (volume of 9 mL), reaching a final concentration of 174 mg/kg, corresponding to about 0.39 mg/g residual uptake.

(F) One-third of the spent GAC was added to the desorption liquid (volume of 12 mL), reaching a final concentration of 173 mg/kg, corresponding to almost no residual uptake.

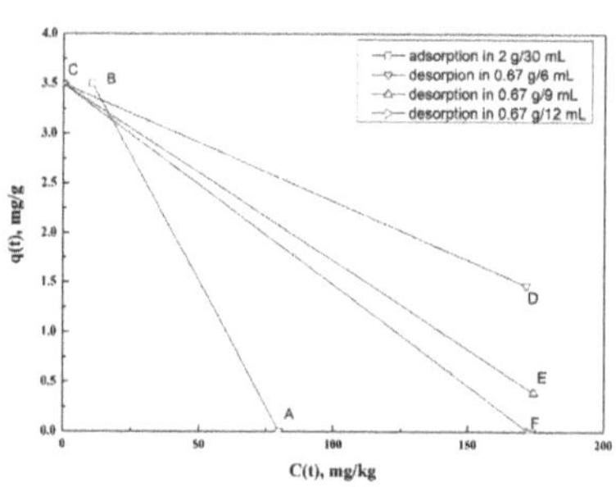

Figure 6. Adsorption and desorption test on Acid Red 97 adsorption on GAC using dye-free model dyeing solution at 40 °C as desorption media and using distiller water at 40 °C as desorption media (points D, E, and F overlap in terms of concentration).

Figure 6 shows the adsorption–desorption tests. In detail, the A to B segment is related to the adsorption process; the B to C segment is related to GAC addition to clean solution; the C to D segment is related to desorption in a new fresh volume of 6 mL; the C to E segment is related to desorption in a new fresh volume of 9 mL; and the C to F segment is related to desorption in a new fresh volume of 12 mL.

Figure 6 shows that the worst operating conditions are defined by the letter D, corresponding to about 1.5 mg/g residual uptake, while better performances are observed for E and F. When the tests were carried out with distilled water at 40 °C, all the points, D, E, and F, approached the Acid Red 97 isotherm. When the tests were carried out with the clean model solution, point D appeared very close to the corresponding 40 °C isotherm, but the E and F points were below the isotherm. Such behavior is unexpected and probably mirrors the existence of specific chemical interactions between the dye and the other components of the model solution, which enforce desorption efficiency thanks to complexation mechanisms. It is worth noting that the liquid produced by desorption in the clean model solution can be used to prepare a fresh batch for a new tanning process.

This experimental result indicates that, despite the lower adsorption capacity, the use of GAC can be a valuable option to reduce the content of Acid Red 97 in tannery wastewater plants while restoring other components that can be useful for the production process.

4. Conclusions

Considering the generally high cost of wastewater treatment [83–91], in this work, we investigated the possible on-site depuration of exhaust dye solutions used in the leather industry before discharging them to the traditional sewage system. This work aimed to study the adsorption treatment of the effluent of a specific coloring drum used in the leather industry in place of testing the mixture of diluted dyes transferred to a wastewater treatment plant. This approach gives the chance to reduce the concentration of the effluents before they reach the plant, which can simplify the treatment of the other process waters while taking benefits from the presence of a single dye at higher concentration levels. The coloring batch process unit only generates excess dye and fattening agents as wastes; therefore, it could be easier to recover those materials instead of sending them to general plant wastes. In the experiments, a real dyeing solution (dyes and fattening agents) was prepared following the coloring recipe provided by an Italian manufacturer.

The experiments use two sorbents, a polyurethane foam (PUF) and granular activated carbon (GAC). The experiments revealed slow adsorption kinetics: for GAC, the adsorption rate is probably limited by diffusion in the pores, and the foam kinetics is probably limited by the surface reaction rate. Further studies are needed to investigate this issue.

The experiments indicate that the PUF has a far larger adsorption capacity with respect to GAC, but GAC may be effectively desorbed, thus opening the possibility for a cyclic use of the sorbent and the reutilization of the solution for future tanning processes. Of course, this possibility requires new in-field investigations. It is finally worth comparing the performances of the PUF and GAC with those of other sorbents: despite the huge number of studies on dye adsorption, the large differences in dye typologies and wastewater solutions make the comparison cumbersome [92,93]. In the range of concentrations studied therein, the sorbent adsorption capacity ranks low with respect to other sorbents, but the linear trend of adsorption isotherms indicated that the attainment of saturation levels is still far, suggesting that there is room for further exploitation of the PUF and GAC in this specific treatment. Furthermore, this also suggests that other sorbents can be proficiently used to improve the single-dye batch treatment process.

Author Contributions: Conceptualization, A.L. and F.D.N.; methodology, P.T.; software, P.T.; validation, P.T., A.L. and F.D.N.; formal analysis, F.D.N.; investigation, P.T. and F.D.N.; resources, P.T.; data curation, A.L., P.T. and F.D.N.; writing—original draft preparation, P.T., A.L. and F.D.N.; writing—review and editing, A.L. and F.D.N.; supervision, A.L.; project administration, F.D.N.; funding acquisition, P.T. All authors have read and agreed to the published version of the manuscript.

Funding: This research received no external funding.

Data Availability Statement: Not applicable.

Acknowledgments: The authors kindly acknowledge the society DMD Solofra S.p.A. and, in particular, Maffei, for his kind assistance during the experimental campaign and for sharing with us the useful information on the simplified recipe for the preparation of the model dyeing solutions. The authors also acknowledge Caterina De Ponte for her help in performing the experiments, which were also part of her master's degree thesis project.

Conflicts of Interest: The authors declare no conflict of interest.

References

1. Laing, R.M.; Sleivert, G.G. Clothing, textiles, and human performance. *Text. Prog.* **2002**, *32*, 1–122. [CrossRef]
2. Bonetti, E. Strategic groups in the fashion industry. *Int. J. Bus. Glob.* **2014**, *13*, 153–172. [CrossRef]
3. Mabeleng, L.B. An Assessment of the Role of the Textile and Clothing Industry in the South Africa Economy. Doctoral Dissertation, North-West University, Potchefstroom, South Africa, 2021.
4. Burns, L.D.; Mullet, K.K.; Bryant, N.O. *The Business of Fashion: Designing, Manufacturing, and Marketing*; Bloomsbury Publishing USA: New York, NY, USA, 2016.
5. Ledezma, V. Globalization and fashion: Too fast, too furious. *Laurier Undergrad. J. Arts* **2017**, *4*, 9.
6. Narumi, H. Fashion orientalism and the limits of counter culture. *Postcolonial Stud. Cult. Politics Econ.* **2000**, *3*, 311–330. [CrossRef]
7. Kim, J.O.; Traore, M.K.; Warfield, C. The textile and apparel industry in developing countries. *Text. Prog.* **2006**, *38*, 1–64. [CrossRef]
8. Yu, H.L.; Kim, C.; Lee, J.; Hong, N. An analysis of modern fashion designs as influenced by Asian ethnic dress. *Int. J. Consum. Stud.* **2001**, *25*, 309–321. [CrossRef]
9. Elson, D.; Pearson, R. 'Nimble fingers make cheap workers': An analysis of women's employment in third world export manufacturing. *Fem. Rev.* **1981**, *7*, 87–107. [CrossRef]
10. Pollin, R.; Burns, J.; Heintz, J. Global apparel production and sweatshop labour: Can raising retail prices finance living wages? *Camb. J. Econ.* **2004**, *28*, 153–171. [CrossRef]
11. Barbaresco, G.; Salerno, E. *Mid-Sized Companies According to Mediobanca-Unioncamere*; Mid-Sized Manufacturing Companies: The New Driver of Italian Competitiveness; Springer: Milano, Italy, 2013; pp. 13–40. [CrossRef]
12. Martina, M. How do we talk about fashion in Italy? The big players and independent publishers from 2000 to today: Transformations and orientations. *Film Fash. Consum.* **2016**, *5*, 83–102. [CrossRef]
13. Radwan, M.; Kamal, M.; Khavarinezhad, S.; Calandra, D. Influencing Factors on Modest Fashion Market: A Case Study. International. *J. Appl. Res. Manag. Econ.* **2019**, *2*, 12–22. [CrossRef]
14. Patti, A.; Cicala, G.; Acierno, D. Eco-sustainability of the textile production: Waste recovery and current recycling in the composites world. *Polymers* **2020**, *13*, 134. [CrossRef] [PubMed]
15. Zhou, Q.; Le, Q.V.; Meng, L.; Yang, H.; Gu, H.; Yang, Y.; Chen, X.; Lam, S.S.; Sonne, C.; Peng, W. Environmental perspectives of textile waste, environmental pollution and recycling. *Environ. Technol. Rev.* **2022**, *11*, 62–71. [CrossRef]
16. Dissanayake, D.G.K.; Sinha, P. Sustainable waste management strategies in the fashion industry sector. *Int. J. Environ. Sustain.* **2012**, *8*, 77–90. [CrossRef]
17. Targosz-Wrona, E. Ecolabelling as a Confirmation of the Application of Sustainable Materials in Textiles. *Fibres Text. East. Eur.* **2009**, *17*, 75.
18. Chavero, S.T. The unsustainability of fast fashion. *Datatèxtil* **2017**, *36*, 56–62.
19. Al-Tohamy, R.; Ali, S.S.; Li, F.; Okasha, K.M.; Mahmoud, Y.A.G.; Elsamahy, T.; Iiao, H.; Fu, Y.; Sun, J. A critical review on the treatment of dye-containing wastewater: Ecotoxicological and health concerns of textile dyes and possible remediation approaches for environmental safety. *Ecotoxicol. Environ. Saf.* **2022**, *231*, 113160. [CrossRef]
20. Parmar, S.; Daki, S.; Bhattacharya, S.; Shrivastav, A. Microorganism: An ecofriendly tool for waste management and environmental safety. In *Development in Wastewater Treatment Research and Processes*; Elsevier: Amsterdam, The Netherlands, 2022; pp. 175–193. [CrossRef]
21. Bullon, J.; González Arrieta, A.; Hernández Encinas, A.; Queiruga Dios, A. Manufacturing processes in the textile industry. Expert Systems for fabrics production. *ADCAIJ Adv. Distrib. Comput. Articial Intell. J.* **2017**, *6*, 17–23.
22. Macchion, L.; Moretto, A.; Caniato, F.; Caridi, M.; Danese, P.; Vinelli, A. Production and supply network strategies within the fashion industry. *Int. J. Prod. Econ.* **2015**, *163*, 173–188. [CrossRef]
23. Hauser, P.J. Reducing Pollution and Energy Requirements in Cotton Dyeing. *Text. Chem. Color. Am. Dyest. Report.* **2000**, *32*, 44–48.
24. Mukherjee, S. Environmental and social impact of fashion: Towards an eco-friendly, ethical fashion. *Int. J. Interdiscip. Multidiscip. Stud.* **2015**, *2*, 22–35.
25. Correia, V.M.; Stephenson, T.; Judd, S.J. Characterisation of textile wastewaters—A review. *Environ. Technol.* **1994**, *15*, 917–929. [CrossRef]
26. Nidheesh, P.V.; Couras, C.; Karim, A.V.; Nadais, H. A review of integrated advanced oxidation processes and biological processes for organic pollutant removal. *Chem. Eng. Commun.* **2022**, *209*, 390–432. [CrossRef]
27. Madhav, S.; Ahamad, A.; Singh, P.; Mishra, P.K. A review of textile industry: Wet processing, environmental impacts, and effluent treatment methods. *Environ. Qual. Manag.* **2018**, *27*, 31–41. [CrossRef]

28. Phillips, B.J.; McQuarrie, E.F. Contesting the social impact of marketing: A re-characterization of women's fashion advertising. *Mark. Theory* **2011**, *11*, 99–126. [CrossRef]
29. Karthik, T.; Gopalakrishnan, D. Environmental analysis of textile value chain: An overview. In *Roadmap to Sustainable Textiles and Clothing*; Springer: Singapore, 2014; pp. 153–188. [CrossRef]
30. Roy Choudhury, A.K. Environmental impacts of the textile industry and its assessment through life cycle assessment. In *Roadmap to Sustainable Textiles and Clothing*; Springer: Singapore, 2014; pp. 1–39. [CrossRef]
31. Li, X.; Wang, L.; Ding, X. Textile supply chain waste management in China. *J. Clean. Prod.* **2021**, *289*, 125147. [CrossRef]
32. Kamau, E.C. Pollution Control in Developing Countries with a case study on Kenya. A need for consistent and stable regimes. *Rev. Int. Direito Cid.* **2010**, *9*, 29–42.
33. Bhuiya, M.H. Upcycling the Garment Solid Waste in Bangladesh. Ph.D. Dissertation, Tallinn University of Technology, Tallinn, Estonia, 2017.
34. Zhang, Y.Q.; Lykaki, M.; Markiewicz, M.; Alrajoula, M.T.; Kraas, C.; Stolte, S. Environmental contamination by microplastics originating from textiles: Emission, transport, fate and toxicity. *J. Hazard. Mater.* **2022**, *430*, 128453. [CrossRef]
35. Khattab, T.A.; Abdelrahman, M.S.; Rehan, M. Textile dyeing industry: Environmental impacts and remediation. *Environ. Sci. Pollut. Res.* **2020**, *27*, 3803–3818. [CrossRef]
36. Atangana, E.; Oberholster, P.J. Using heavy metal pollution indices to assess water quality of surface and groundwater on catchment levels in South Africa. *J. Afr. Earth Sci.* **2021**, *182*, 104254. [CrossRef]
37. Hellawell, J.M. Toxic substances in rivers and streams. *Environ. Pollut.* **1988**, *50*, 61–85. [CrossRef]
38. Chequer, F.D.; De Oliveira, G.R.; Ferraz, E.A.; Cardoso, J.C.; Zanoni, M.B.; De Oliveira, D.P. Textile dyes: Dyeing process and environmental impact. *Eco-Friendly Text. Dye. Finish.* **2013**, *6*, 151–176. [CrossRef]
39. Chen, H.L.; Burns, L.D. Environmental analysis of textile products. *Cloth. Text. Res. J.* **2006**, *24*, 248–261. [CrossRef]
40. Hussain, T.; Wahab, A. A critical review of the current water conservation practices in textile wet processing. *J. Clean. Prod.* **2018**, *198*, 806–819. [CrossRef]
41. Thadepalli, S.; Roy, S. Implications of Sustainability on Textile Fibres and Wet Processing, Barriers in Implementation. In *Sustainable Approaches in Textiles and Fashion*; Springer: Singapore, 2018; pp. 133–156.
42. Singha, K.; Pandit, P.; Maity, S.; Sharma, S.R. Harmful environmental effects for textile chemical dyeing practice. In *Green Chemistry for Sustainable Textiles*; Woodhead Publishing: Cambridge, UK, 2021; pp. 153–164.
43. Verma, R.K.; Sankhla, M.S.; Rathod, N.V.; Sonone, S.S.; Parihar, K.; Singh, G.K. Eradication of fatal textile industrial dyes by wastewater treatment. *Biointerface Res. Appl. Chem.* **2021**, *12*, 567–587. [CrossRef]
44. Jolly, Y.N.; Islam, A.; Mustafa, A.I. Characterization of dye industry effluent and assessment of its suitability for irrigation purpose. *J. Bangladesh Acad. Sci.* **2009**, *33*, 99–106. [CrossRef]
45. Sen, S.K.; Patra, P.; Das, C.R.; Raut, S.; Raut, S. Pilot-scale evaluation of bio-decolorization and biodegradation of reactive textile wastewater: An impact on its use in irrigation of wheat crop. *Water Resour. Ind.* **2019**, *21*, 100106. [CrossRef]
46. Lin, S.H.; Peng, C.F. Treatment of textile wastewater by electrochemical method. *Water Res.* **1994**, *28*, 277–282. [CrossRef]
47. Malliaros, C.; Guitonas, A. Pre-treatment and elimination systems of toxic industrial waste and sludges. The case study of the department of Attika. *Water Sci. Technol.* **1997**, *36*, 91–100. [CrossRef]
48. Babu, B.R.; Parande, A.; Raghu, S.; Kumar, T.P. Textile technology. *Technology* **1995**, *11*, 110–122.
49. Saleh, I.A.; Zouari, N.; Al-Ghouti, M.A. Removal of pesticides from water and wastewater: Chemical, physical and biological treatment approaches. *Environ. Technol. Innov.* **2020**, *19*, 101026. [CrossRef]
50. Haddad, M.; Abid, S.; Hamdi, M.; Bouallagui, H. Reduction of adsorbed dyes content in the discharged sludge coming from an industrial textile wastewater treatment plant using aerobic activated sludge process. *J. Environ. Manag.* **2018**, *223*, 936–946. [CrossRef]
51. Ciardelli, G.; Corsi, L.; Marcucci, M. Membrane separation for wastewater reuse in the textile industry. *Resour. Conserv. Recycl.* **2001**, *31*, 189–197. [CrossRef]
52. Ciardelli, G.; Capannelli, G.; Bottino, A. Ozone treatment of textile wastewaters for reuse. *Water Sci. Technol.* **2001**, *44*, 61–67. [CrossRef] [PubMed]
53. Liu, X.; Wang, L.; Zhou, X.; He, X.; Zhou, M.; Jia, K.; Liu, X. Design of polymer composite-based porous membrane for in-situ photocatalytic degradation of adsorbed organic dyes. *J. Phys. Chem. Solids* **2021**, *154*, 110094. [CrossRef]
54. Hu, F.; Fang, C.; Wang, Z.; Liu, C.; Zhu, B.; Zhu, L. Poly (N-vinyl imidazole) gel composite porous membranes for rapid separation of dyes through permeating adsorption. *Sep. Purif. Technol.* **2017**, *188*, 1–10. [CrossRef]
55. Zirehpour, A.; Rahimpour, A. Membranes for wastewater treatment. *Nanostructured Polym. Membr.* **2016**, *2*, 159–208. [CrossRef]
56. Vatanpour, V.; Nekouhi, G.N.; Esmaeili, M. Preparation, characterization and performance evaluation of ZnO deposited polyethylene ultrafiltration membranes for dye and protein separation. *J. Taiwan Inst. Chem. Eng.* **2020**, *114*, 153–167. [CrossRef]
57. Chen, G. Electrochemical technologies in wastewater treatment. *Sep. Purif. Technol.* **2004**, *38*, 11–41. [CrossRef]
58. Wang, Z.; Xue, M.; Huang, K.; Liu, Z. Textile dyeing wastewater treatment. *Adv. Treat. Text. Effl.* **2011**, *5*, 91–116. [CrossRef]
59. Singh, K.; Arora, S. Removal of synthetic textile dyes from wastewaters: A critical review on present treatment technologies. *Crit. Rev. Environ. Sci. Technol.* **2011**, *41*, 807–878. [CrossRef]
60. Qasem, N.A.; Mohammed, R.H.; Lawal, D.U. Removal of heavy metal ions from wastewater: A comprehensive and critical review. *Npj Clean Water* **2021**, *4*, 36. [CrossRef]

61. Särkkä, H.; Vepsäläinen, M.; Sillanpää, M. Natural organic matter (NOM) removal by electrochemical methods—A review. *J. Electroanal. Chem.* **2015**, *755*, 100–108. [CrossRef]
62. Kobya, M.; Bayramoglu, M.; Eyvaz, M. Techno-economical evaluation of electrocoagulation for the textile wastewater using different electrode connections. *J. Hazard. Mater.* **2007**, *148*, 311–318. [CrossRef]
63. Suwannahong, K.; Wongcharee, S.; Kreetachart, T.; Sirilamduan, C.; Rioyo, J.; Wongphat, A. Evaluation of the Microsoft Excel Solver Spreadsheet-Based Program for nonlinear expressions of adsorption Isotherm models onto magnetic nanosorbent. *Appl. Sci.* **2021**, *11*, 7432. [CrossRef]
64. Russo, M.E.; Di Natale, F.; Prigione, V.; Tigini, V.; Marzocchella, A.; Varese, G.C. Adsorption of acid dyes on fungal biomass: Equilibrium and kinetics characterization. *Chem. Eng. J.* **2010**, *162*, 537–545. [CrossRef]
65. Russo, M.E.; Di Natale, F.; Marzocchella, A.; Varese, G. Dyes biosorption of textile wastewaters in a lab-scale fluidised bed. In Proceedings of the MFIP12: 12th International Conference on Multiphase Flow in Industrial Plants, Ischia, Italy, 21–23 September 2011.
66. Buckley, T.; Xu, X.; Rudolph, V.; Firouzi, M.; Shukla, P. Review of foam fractionation as a water treatment technology. *Sep. Sci. Technol.* **2022**, *57*, 929–958. [CrossRef]
67. Hailan, S.M.; Ponnamma, D.; Krupa, I. The separation of oil/water mixtures by modified melamine and polyurethane foams: A review. *Polymers* **2021**, *13*, 4142. [CrossRef]
68. Amin, M.T.; Alazba, A.A.; Manzoor, U. A review of removal of pollutants from water/wastewater using different types of nanomaterials. *Adv. Mater. Sci. Eng.* **2014**, 825910. [CrossRef]
69. Dasa, P.; Duttab, S. Sustainable membranes with FNs: Current and emerging research trends. In *Membranes with Functionalized Nanomaterials: Current and Emerging Research Trends in Membrane Technology*; Elsevier: Amsterdam, The Netherlands, 2022; p. 159. [CrossRef]
70. Mezohegyi, G.; van der Zee, F.P.; Font, J.; Fortuny, A.; Fabregat, A. Towards advanced aqueous dye removal processes: A short review on the versatile role of activated carbon. *J. Environ. Manag.* **2012**, *102*, 148–164. [CrossRef]
71. Simpson, D.R. Biofilm processes in biologically active carbon water purification. *Water Res.* **2018**, *42*, 2839–2848. [CrossRef]
72. Wang, H.; Ho, L.; Lewis, D.M.; Brookes, J.D.; Newcombe, G. Discriminating and assessing adsorption and biodegradation removal mechanisms during granular activated carbon filtration of microcystin toxins. *Water Res.* **2007**, *41*, 4262–4270. [CrossRef]
73. Walker, G.M.; Weatherley, L.R. Biological activated carbon treatment of industrial wastewater in stirred tank reactors. *Chem. Eng. J.* **1999**, *75*, 201–206. [CrossRef]
74. Simón, D.; De Lucas, A.; Rodríguez, J.F.; Borreguero, A.M. Glycolysis of high resilience flexible polyurethane foams containing polyurethane dispersion polyol. *Polym. Degrad. Stab.* **2016**, *133*, 119–130. [CrossRef]
75. Cuq, M.H.; Benjelloun-Mlayah, B.; Delmas, M. Oil extracted from seal hides: Characterization and use as leather fat liquor. *J. Am. Oil Chem. Soc.* **1998**, *75*, 1015–1019. [CrossRef]
76. Sardari, A.; Sabbagh Alvani, A.A.; Ghaffarian, S.R. Preparation of castor oil-based fatliquoring agent via a Pickering emulsion method for use in leather coating. *J. Coat. Technol. Res.* **2019**, *16*, 1765–1772. [CrossRef]
77. Elhadiri, N.; Benchanaa, M.; Chikri, R. Activated carbon for dyes removal: Modeling and understanding the adsorption process. *J. Chem.* **2020**, *2020*, 2096834. [CrossRef]
78. Maddalena, R.L.; McKone, T.E.; Kado, N.Y. Simple and rapid extraction of polycyclic aromatic hydrocarbons collected on polyurethane foam adsorbent. *Atmos. Environ.* **1998**, *32*, 2497–2503. [CrossRef]
79. Ferreiro, C.; Villota, N.; de Luis, A.; Lombraña, J.I. Analysis of the effect of the operational conditions in a combined adsorption–ozonation process with granular activated carbon for the treatment of phenol wastewater. *React. Chem. Eng.* **2020**, *5*, 760–778. [CrossRef]
80. Ying, W.C.; Zhang, W.; Chang, Q.G.; Jiang, W.X.; Li, G.H. Improved methods for carbon adsorption studies for water and wastewater treatment. *Environ. Prog.* **2006**, *25*, 110–120. [CrossRef]
81. Ozsoy, H.D.; van Leeuwen, J.H. Removal of color from fruit candy waste by activated carbon adsorption. *J. Food Eng.* **2010**, *101*, 106–112. [CrossRef]
82. Vona, A.; Di Martino, F.; Garcia-Ivars, J.; Picó, Y.; Mendoza-Roca, J.A.; Iborra-Clar, M.I. Comparison of different removal techniques for selected pharmaceuticals. *J. Water Process Eng.* **2015**, *5*, 48–57. [CrossRef]
83. Ahmad, A.; Jamil, S.N.A.M.; Shean Yaw Choong, T.; Abdullah, A.H.; Mastuli, M.S.; Othman, N.; Jiman, N. Green flexible polyurethane foam as a potent support for Fe-Si adsorbent. *Polymers* **2019**, *11*, 2011. [CrossRef]
84. Lefebvre, L.; Kelber, J.; Jierry, L.; Ritleng, V.; Edouard, D. Polydopamine-coated open cell polyurethane foam as an efficient and easy-to-regenerate soft structured catalytic support (S2CS) for the reduction of dye. *J. Environ. Chem. Eng.* **2017**, *5*, 79–85. [CrossRef]
85. Selvasembian, R.; Gwenzi, W.; Chaukura, N.; Mthembu, S. Recent advances in the polyurethane-based adsorbents for the decontamination of hazardous wastewater pollutants. *J. Hazard. Mater.* **2021**, *417*, 125960. [CrossRef]
86. Anglada, A.; Urtiaga, A.; Ortiz, I. Contributions of electrochemical oxidation to waste-water treatment: Fundamentals and review of applications. *J. Chem. Technol. Biotechnol.* **2019**, *84*, 1747–1755. [CrossRef]
87. Crini, G.; Lichtfouse, E.; Wilson, L.D.; Morin-Crini, N. Conventional and non-conventional adsorbents for wastewater treatment. *Environ. Chem. Lett.* **2019**, *17*, 195–213. Available online: https://hal.science/hal-02082916 (accessed on 1 January 2020). [CrossRef]

88. Crini, G. Non-conventional low-cost adsorbents for dye removal: A review. *Bioresour. Technol.* **2006**, *97*, 1061–1085. [CrossRef]
89. Robinson, T.; McMullan, G.; Marchant, R.; Nigam, P. Remediation of dyes in textile effluent: A critical review on current treatment technologies with a proposed alternative. *Bioresour. Technol.* **2001**, *77*, 247–255. [CrossRef]
90. Suwannahong, K.; Sirilamduan, C.; Deepatana, A.; Kreetachat, T.; Wongcharee, S. Characterization and optimization of polymeric bispicolamine chelating resin: Performance evaluation via RSM using copper in acid liquors as a model substrate through ion exchange method. *Molecules* **2022**, *27*, 7210. [CrossRef]
91. Trucillo, P.; Lancia, A.; Di Natale, F. Recovery of platinum from diesel catalysts by combined use of H2O2/HCl leaching and adsorption. *J. Environ. Chem. Eng.* **2022**, *10*, 107730. [CrossRef]
92. Dutta, S.; Gupta, B.; Srivastava, S.K.; Gupta, A.K. Recent advances on the removal of dyes from wastewater using various adsorbents: A critical review. *Mater. Adv.* **2021**, *2*, 4497–4531. [CrossRef]
93. Agarwala, R.; Mulky, L. Adsorption of Dyes from Wastewater: A Comprehensive Review. *ChemBioEng Rev.* **2023**, *10*, 326–335. [CrossRef]

processes

MDPI

Review

Smart Card-Based Vehicle Ignition Systems: Security, Regulatory Compliance, Drug and Impairment Detection, Through Advanced Materials and Authentication Technologies

Vincenzo Vitiello [1], Alessandro Benazzi [2] and Paolo Trucillo [3,*]

[1] Inventori Cavensi, Via XXV Luglio 87, 84013 Cava De' Tirreni, Italy; enzo.vitiello15@gmail.com
[2] Slim!Architetti, Via Savio 1087, 47522 Cesena, Italy; alessandro@slimarchitetti.it
[3] Dipartimento di Ingegneria Chimica, dei Materiali e della Produzione Industriale, University of Naples Federico II, P.le V. Tecchio 80, 80125 Napoli, Italy
* Correspondence: paolo.trucillo@unina.it; Tel.: +39-329-65-66-043

Abstract: This study investigates the integration of smart card readers into vehicle ignition systems as a multifaceted solution to enhance security, regulatory compliance, and road safety. By implementing real-time driver verification, encryption protocols (AES-256, RSA), and multifactor authentication, the system significantly reduces unauthorized vehicle use and improves accident prevention. A critical advancement of this research is the incorporation of automated drug and impairment detection to prevent driving under the influence of substances, including illicit drugs and prescription medications. Risk models estimate that drug-related accidents could be reduced by 7.65% through the integration of these technologies into vehicle ignition systems, assuming high compliance rates. The study evaluates drug applications leveraging the same sensor-based monitoring technologies as used for impairment detection. These systems can facilitate the real-time tracking of medication intake and physiological responses, offering new possibilities for safety applications in medical transportation and assisted driving technologies. High-performance polymers such as polyetheretherketone (PEEK) enhance the durability and thermal stability of smart card readers, while blockchain-based verification strengthens data security and regulatory compliance. Despite challenges related to cost (USD 100–300 per unit) and adherence to ISO standards, these innovations position smart card-based ignition systems as a comprehensive, technology-driven approach to vehicle security, impairment prevention, and medical monitoring.

Keywords: smart card readers; vehicle ignition systems; automotive security; multifactor authentication; encryption protocols; blockchain technology; CAN bus compatibility; driver credential verification; automotive cybersecurity frameworks

1. Introduction

Ensuring regulatory compliance and enhancing vehicle security are critical challenges in modern transportation [1,2]. Unauthorized vehicle access, expired licenses, and non-compliance with safety regulations pose significant risks to road safety. Traditional enforcement methods rely on manual inspections and random checks, which are often inefficient and fail to provide real-time enforcement mechanisms.

These challenges include widespread non-compliance with mandatory vehicle inspections, delayed or avoided payment of vehicle ownership taxes, and expired or invalid driver's licenses. Additionally, there is a critical issue of license–class mismatches, where drivers operate vehicles beyond their authorized classification. For example, a driver holding only a standard passenger vehicle license may illegally operate a heavy-duty truck, creating severe regulatory violations and increasing road safety risks. Addressing these concerns requires an integrated and automated system capable of real-time verification and enforcement, which is the focus of this study [3–5].

Understanding the magnitude of non-compliance is essential to contextualize the urgency of this issue. Table 1 provides statistical insights into non-compliance rates across different regions, illustrating the prevalence of expired licenses, missing vehicle inspections, and unpaid ownership taxes. These figures highlight the limitations of current enforcement mechanisms and demonstrate the need for automated solutions that can systematically detect and address these violations. By presenting these data, the study establishes a quantitative foundation for evaluating the effectiveness of smart card-based authentication in improving compliance and road safety.

Table 1. Estimates of non compliance in vehicle regulations.

Region	Non-Compliance with Property Tax (%)	Non-Compliance with Insurance (%)	Non-Compliance with Inspection (%)	Expired Driver's License (%)	Age-Related Ineligibility (%)
Italy	15%	10%	20%	8%	5%
Europe	12%	8%	18%	7%	4%
Worldwide	20%	15%	25%	10%	6%

An important aspect of ensuring regulatory compliance and vehicle security is the ability to adapt enforcement mechanisms to emerging transportation trends. The rise of autonomous vehicles, shared mobility services, and digitally integrated transportation systems necessitates the implementation of authentication solutions that can dynamically verify driver and vehicle credentials. Traditional enforcement methods often fail to account for these evolving mobility models, leaving gaps in compliance monitoring. By integrating smart card-based authentication with digital infrastructure, the real-time validation of driver eligibility, tax and insurance status, and vehicle roadworthiness can be achieved. This shift towards intelligent compliance frameworks not only enhances security, but also streamlines administrative processes, reducing the burden on law enforcement and regulatory bodies. Moreover, leveraging technologies such as blockchain and AI-driven risk assessment models can improve fraud detection and predictive compliance monitoring, paving the way for a more adaptive and responsive automotive regulatory environment.

Currently, the verification of these aspects relies on random checks conducted by law enforcement. This approach allows many violations not to be detected; in some cases, this may result in dangerous consequences for drivers, passengers, and pedestrians [6]. Uninspected vehicles may have mechanical failures, expired licenses reflect the inadequate assessment of a driver's competence, and mismatched licenses increase the risk of accidents due to the improper handling of vehicles [7]. Addressing these issues requires more robust and systematic control mechanisms to ensure compliance and enhance overall road safety, and of course, this cannot be guaranteed by human control alone [8–10]. At present, the estimates of vehicles that are non-compliant to Italian, European and worldwide regulations [11–18] are indicated in Table 1.

To mitigate these issues, implementing a more centralized and automated monitoring system could significantly improve compliance. For instance, integrating databases for vehicle registration, inspection status, tax payments, and driver licensing into a unified platform would allow for real-time checks and automated alerts for overdue requirements [19–22].

Beyond the technical integration of vehicle data, the effectiveness of smart card readers in vehicle systems is contingent upon the infrastructure and digital preparedness of municipal facilities. The capacity of municipalities to implement real-time data-sharing networks, ensure up-to-date vehicle records, and provide responsive law enforcement mechanisms significantly influences the efficacy of such systems. In jurisdictions where municipal infrastructure is advanced, smart card-based verification can seamlessly interact with centralized transportation databases, leading to improved compliance enforcement and reduced administrative burdens. Conversely, in areas with outdated infrastructure or fragmented databases, the adoption of such technologies may face operational challenges, including inconsistent data synchronization and limited real-time enforcement capabilities. Addressing these issues requires strategic investments in digital infrastructure and inter-agency cooperation between transport authorities, law enforcement, and smart technology providers. This system could also enable the use of license plate recognition technology to flag non-compliant vehicles during routine traffic flow rather than relying solely on random inspections [23]. By streamlining verification processes and making them proactive rather than reactive, authorities could reduce the number of violators escaping detection and enhance the overall safety and reliability of the automotive system for all road users.

This study proposes a smart card-based vehicle authentication system designed to enhance security, compliance, and road safety through real-time driver verification, encryption protocols, and automated impairment detection. The proposed solution aims to reduce unauthorized vehicle use, ensure that only licensed and compliant drivers operate vehicles, and integrate with existing regulatory frameworks to improve enforcement efficiency.

2. Smart Card Readers in Vehicle Systems

2.1. *Enhancing Security and Compliance*

Recent research has explored the integration of smart card readers into vehicle systems, emphasizing both technological advancements and practical implementations. Key studies have demonstrated the critical role of robust encryption protocols, such as AES-256 [24] and RSA, in securing data exchanges during authentication processes [25]. Proximity-based authentication systems, which enhance convenience while maintaining security, are also gaining traction in practical applications in vehicles [26]. Furthermore, innovative approaches like Internet of Things (IoT)-based driver monitoring systems and blockchain-enabled decentralized verification frameworks are redefining security paradigms, ensuring transparency and resistance to tampering. Emerging trends in multifactor authentication, combining smart card usage with biometric verification, provide an additional layer of security and reliability, addressing vulnerabilities in current systems. Together, these advancements highlight the potential of integrated smart card technologies to transform vehicle access and operation, aligning security, compliance, and user convenience within next-generation automotive ecosystems [27].

An additional layer of security for vehicle access control could be implemented through Two-Factor Authentication (2FA), requiring drivers to validate their identity using a second independent verification method beyond the smart card. For instance, after inserting the smart card, drivers could be required to authenticate via a biometric scan (fingerprint or facial recognition) or enter a one-time passcode (OTP) sent to a registered mobile device. This approach significantly reduces the risks associated with stolen or cloned smart cards, preventing unauthorized individuals from bypassing security measures. A comparative study conducted in Japan and South Korea on fleet vehicle security systems showed that integrating 2FA with smart card authentication reduced vehicle theft by 43% and unauthorized vehicle use by 38% over a 12-month period. While this method enhances security, it also raises concerns regarding user convenience and potential delays in authentication, making it crucial to strike a balance between robust security and seamless usability in real-world automotive applications.

2.2. Implementation and Integration

The integration of smart card readers into vehicle ignition systems represents an innovative approach in the automotive industry, merging security, regulatory compliance, and user convenience into a unified system. Unlike traditional immobilizers and keyless entry mechanisms, this innovation introduces the real-time verification of driver credentials, ensuring that only authorized and eligible individuals can operate vehicles. The use of advanced encryption protocols (for example, AES-256 and RSA) combined with multifactor authentication provides a robust defense against unauthorized access, while the exploration of blockchain-based frameworks sets this system apart as a pioneer in data transparency and security. Furthermore, this paper uniquely addresses the compatibility challenges with modern vehicle electronic architectures like CAN bus systems, offering standardized solutions for seamless integration. By emphasizing the potential for contactless and biometric technologies, the research not only tackles current safety and regulatory gaps, but also anticipates future advancements, positioning the proposed system as a cornerstone in the evolution of intelligent and secure transportation ecosystems. This novel combination of novel technologies and practical automotive solutions highlights a significant leap forward in redefining the standards of vehicle access and operation.

While specific numerical data quantifying the effectiveness of smart card readers in enhancing vehicle security and compliance are limited, several authoritative sources underscore their critical role in safeguarding connected vehicles. The European Union Agency for Cybersecurity (ENISA) emphasizes the importance of robust authentication mechanisms, such as smart card readers, to protect against unauthorized access and cyber threats in smart cars [28]. Similarly, McKinsey & Company highlights the increasing significance of cybersecurity in the automotive industry's digital transformation, noting that connected cars can have up to 150 electronic control units, with projections of approximately 300 million lines of software code by 2030 [29]. This complexity necessitates advanced security measures, including the integration of smart card readers, to mitigate potential vulnerabilities.

2.3. Security Challenges and Compliance Strategies

However, beyond encryption-based protection, smart card authentication systems remain vulnerable to relay attacks, man-in-the-middle (MITM) attacks, and hardware tampering, all of which require additional mitigation strategies. Relay attacks exploit proximity-based authentication by relaying authentication signals between the smart card and the vehicle, effectively bypassing security controls. To counteract this, time-bound cryptographic challenges, distance bounding protocols, and radio-frequency fingerprinting can differentiate legitimate signals from replayed ones. MITM attacks, where an attacker intercepts and manipulates communication between the smart card reader and the ECU, necessitate end-to-end encryption with mutual authentication and secure key exchange protocols such as Diffie–Hellman or Elliptic Curve Cryptography (ECC), so as to ensure integrity and confidentiality in data transmission. Lastly, hardware tampering—where attackers physically modify the smart card reader or inject malicious components—can be mitigated through tamper-resistant hardware designs, including secure enclaves, epoxy-coated circuitry, and active intrusion detection sensors. Additionally, compliance with ISO 21434 cybersecurity standards [30] ensures that these security measures are aligned with the industry's best practices for automotive cybersecurity.

Furthermore, Giesecke + Devrient (G + D) reported that connected cars generate up to 25 GB of data every hour, underscoring the need for effective data protection solutions, such as smart card-based systems, to ensure cybersecurity in smart vehicles. While these sources highlight the importance of smart card readers, further empirical studies are needed to provide precise numerical assessments of their impact on vehicle security and compliance [31].

2.4. Smart Card-Based Compliance and Operational Control

An innovative solution could involve the use of advanced card readers paired with smart cards, which would be able to block the car in case of rules violations; this is currently already in use for other applications [32–34]. These are not merely traditional cards, but sophisticated smart cards capable of real-time verification of the driver's identity, license validity, payment status, and—most importantly—the driver's eligibility to operate the specific vehicle type [29–32]. This system would work by requiring the driver to insert their smart card into the vehicle's reader before starting the engine. If all checks are successfully verified, the vehicle will be enabled to start. If any requirement fails, the vehicle remains immobilized or may even shut down if already in use. This technology could serve as an effective preventive measure, ensuring compliance with regulations and significantly reducing the risks associated with non-compliance.

2.5. Smart Card Readers in Fleet Management and Regulatory Compliance

A notable implementation of smart card reader technology can be found in corporate fleet management systems, where companies use smart card authentication to regulate vehicle access based on driver credentials and compliance status. Fleet operators in Germany and the Netherlands have deployed contactless smart card-based ignition systems, ensuring that only authorized personnel with valid driving credentials can operate company-owned vehicles. These systems integrate biometric verification and real-time data synchronization with central compliance databases to check for driver fitness, drug/alcohol testing compliance, and adherence to licensing requirements. A comparative study between fleet operators using these authentication measures and those relying on traditional keys found a 32% reduction in unauthorized vehicle use and a 19% decrease in accidents due to driver impairment or fatigue [33–40] The purpose of this approach is to create a proactive, technology-driven system that ensures full compliance with automotive regulations, thereby enhancing road safety and reducing administrative burdens on law enforcement. By leveraging smart cards and real-time verification systems, this solution aims to minimize human error, prevent unauthorized vehicle use, and avoid non-compliance with legal requirements.

2.6. Adoption Challenges and Future Perspectives

Currently, the cost of integrating such devices into vehicles is relatively affordable, with estimates ranging from ISD 100 to 300 per unit, depending on the complexity of the features included. This cost includes several key components, such as manufacturing Costs (50–60%), installation costs (20–30%) and maintenance and software updates (10–20%). The largest portion of the cost is attributed to the production of the smart card reader and authentication system. This includes the fabrication of high-performance polymer housings (e.g., PEEK), the embedded microcontrollers, secure chipsets, and encryption-enabled firmware. The integration of advanced security features such as AES-256 encryption and biometric authentication can increase manufacturing costs, depending on the level of complexity. The process of integrating the smart card reader into the vehicle's electronic control unit (ECU) and CAN bus architecture contributes to the overall cost. This includes hardware connectors, secure software deployment, and labor costs for vehicle

adaptation. Ensuring compatibility with various vehicle models may also require additional engineering and compliance efforts. Finally, long-term expenses include periodic firmware updates to counter cybersecurity threats, the calibration of biometric authentication modules, and potential component replacements due to wear and tear. Over-the-air (OTA) software updates and blockchain-based verification systems can also introduce additional costs, depending on the security framework implemented. Despite these costs, the long-term benefits outweigh the initial investment. Comparative studies indicate that smart card-based ignition systems can reduce unauthorized vehicle use by 32% and driver impairment-related accidents by 19%.

While this represents an initial investment for manufacturers and drivers, the long-term benefits in terms of enhanced safety, reduced enforcement costs, and improved regulatory compliance make it a highly cost-effective solution. Ultimately, the goal is to provide a safer, more reliable, and efficient transportation ecosystem where both drivers and pedestrians can benefit from reduced risks and improved accountability.

2.7. Barriers to Adoption and Market Challenges

Currently, there are no countries producing vehicles equipped with card reader systems capable of blocking the car in case of failure in verifying the driver's license or age (see the sketch of Figure 1). The lack of a widespread adoption of smart card-based ignition systems can be attributed to several factors, including additional manufacturing and installation costs, challenges with integration with existing vehicle architectures, and the need for compliance with stringent regulatory frameworks such as UNECE Regulation No. 116 and FMVSS 114 [41,42]. Moreover, consumer adoption has been slow due to concerns regarding usability, potential failures in emergency situations, and the availability of alternative authentication technologies such as keyless entry and biometric verification. However, similar technologies, such as electronic immobilizers, are already in use to prevent vehicle ignition without the correct key. Additionally, some companies are developing advanced authentication systems, including biometric identification and facial recognition, to enhance vehicle security.

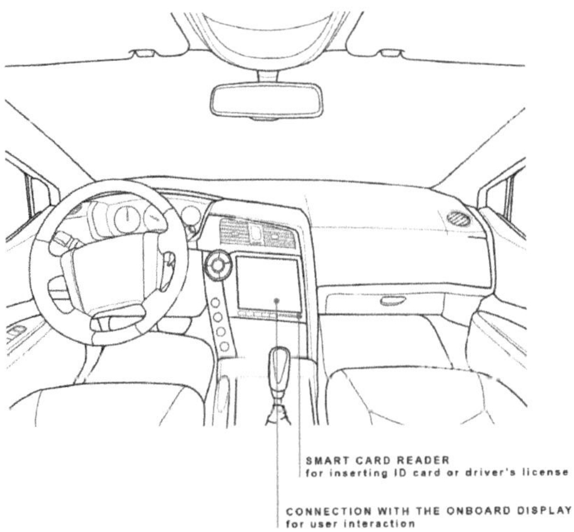

Figure 1. Smart card reader system integrated with onboard display.

While these advancements are promising, the widespread adoption of card readers for the real-time verification of driver credentials and age is not yet standard practice in the automotive industry. This highlights a significant opportunity for innovation and market differentiation, as such systems could address critical safety and regulatory challenges while offering additional value to consumers and manufacturers.

2.8. Potential Impact

In addition to improving regulatory compliance and road safety, these integrated systems could significantly reduce the global number of traffic accidents and vehicle thefts. By requiring real-time verification before a vehicle can start, unauthorized users, including potential thieves, would be unable to operate the vehicle without the corresponding smart card and matching credentials. This added layer of security would act as a powerful deterrent against theft and unauthorized use. Furthermore, by ensuring that only eligible and qualified drivers can operate vehicles, the likelihood of accidents caused by unfit drivers or improperly maintained vehicles would decrease, leading to safer roads and reduced economic and social costs associated with accidents and vehicle theft.

Figure 2 illustrates a conceptual user interface (UI) for a smart card-integrated vehicle ignition system, designed to enhance security and operational efficiency in automotive access control. The interface features a streamlined layout incorporating essential authentication elements, system status indicators, and user interaction components. The central component is the smart card authentication prompt, which ensures that only authorized users can initiate the vehicle ignition sequence. Additionally, status notification icons provide real-time feedback, including authentication success or failure, encryption status and multifactor authentication (MFA) indicators, which notify the user if additional verification steps, such as biometric authentication or smartphone-based validation, are required. The connectivity and system health status section displays icons representing the vehicle's integration with existing electronic architectures, such as the CAN bus system, ensuring compatibility and smooth operation. Moreover, user feedback and alerts are included to notify users of potential security concerns, such as unauthorized card detection, system errors, or regulatory compliance warnings. Future enhancements suggested by the UI concept include the integration of contactless smart card readers and smartphone/smartwatch-based authentication, reflecting the evolving nature of vehicle access technologies.

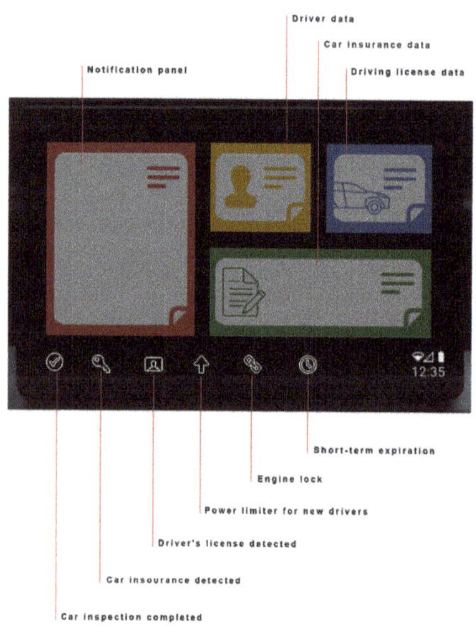

Figure 2. Conceptual user interface for a smart card-based vehicle ignition system.

While the integration of smart card readers in vehicle ignition systems is highly effective for ensuring security and compliance among vehicle owners, it is important to acknowledge that not all individuals own vehicles. An alternative approach could involve integrating smart authentication systems with mobile communication devices, such as personal smartphones, to allow broader accessibility. Mobile authentication, particularly through NFC-based digital identity verification, could enable non-car-owners to access shared or rental vehicles in a secure manner. However, compared to vehicle-integrated smart card readers, mobile-based authentication presents certain security risks, including susceptibility to relay attacks, malware threats, and unauthorized access through compromised applications. Additionally, vehicle-integrated systems benefit from direct connection to the onboard electronic control unit (ECU), ensuring more robust security measures through encrypted authentication and real-time compliance verification. While mobile-based systems offer flexibility and convenience, vehicle-integrated smart card readers provide a higher level of security and regulation enforcement, making them more suitable for critical applications such as ignition control and driver impairment prevention.

3. Hardware Integration

The integration of smart card readers into vehicle ignition systems presents a transformative step forward in enhancing both safety and security. These systems are designed not only to address the challenges of regulatory compliance, but also to deter theft and ensure only qualified drivers operate the vehicle. By integrating real-time verification capabilities, these systems could revolutionize how we approach vehicle access and operation.

The integration process requires advanced hardware configurations. Central to this design is the connection of the smart card reader to the vehicle's onboard electronic control unit (ECU). This setup enables the card reader to transmit signals to the ECU, determining whether to initiate or terminate engine functions based on the verification outcome. Such an approach ensures seamless communication between the authentication system and the vehicle's core operational mechanisms [43].

Current research demonstrates a growing adoption of these systems in secure fleet management and luxury vehicles. Keyless ignition, already prevalent in high-end models, serves as a foundation for implementing more advanced technologies, such as RFID-enabled cards and biometric smart cards. For instance, proximity-based ignition systems could easily be expanded to incorporate card authentication, offering a dual layer of security and convenience [44–46].

However, implementing a blockchain-based authentication system presents challenges related to real-time verification delays and network failure management. The latency in transaction validation can impact on user experience, especially in high-frequency access scenarios such as vehicle ignition systems. To mitigate these issues, strategies such as node redundancy, edge computing for pre-processing requests, and hybrid architectures combining blockchain with traditional databases can be adopted to ensure operational continuity in the case of network failures.

As defined above, the adoption of these systems would bring about several advantages, including improved road safety, reduced vehicle theft, and enhanced regulatory compliance. However, challenges remain, such as ensuring the affordability of these systems for mass-market adoption and addressing potential issues related to data security and user privacy. Overcoming these issues will require collaboration between automotive manufacturers, technology providers, and regulatory bodies. As discussed in previous sections, the integration of smart card readers aligns with a broader vision of a safer and more reliable transportation ecosystem. By implementing such systems, manufacturers can contribute to reducing the global number of accidents and thefts while fostering innovation in vehicle security technologies. A list of possible prototypal systems has been provided in Table 2.

Table 2. System features and applications [47–51].

Feature	Description	Current Applications	Potential Benefits
Smart Card Reader	Reads driver credentials and verifies compliance in real time	Secure fleet management, luxury cars	Enhanced compliance and security
Connection to ECU	Interfaces with the vehicle's electronic control unit for engine management	High-end vehicles, concept models	Seamless vehicle operation control
RFID/Proximity Cards	Enables wireless authentication for added convenience	Proximity-based ignition systems	Dual-layer security and user-friendliness
Biometric Smart Cards	Incorporates fingerprint or facial recognition for driver verification	Emerging prototypes	Advanced security and personalized access

4. Security

As discussed in previous chapters, the integration of smart card readers into automotive systems provides a significant method to improve safety and regulatory compliance. However, the implementation of these systems also raises significant security concerns. To ensure the reliability and safety of these technologies, a robust framework is necessary to address potential vulnerabilities such as unauthorized access, card cloning, and signal interception.

Modern encryption protocols have played a primary role in safeguarding communication between the smart card and the vehicle's control system. Commonly utilized encryption methods, such as AES-256 and RSA, provide high levels of security by encrypting data exchanges to prevent interception and unauthorized use [52–54]. These protocols ensure that only authorized credentials can enable the vehicle's ignition, adding a significant layer of protection against cyber threats.

One of the most promising advancements in this field is the integration of multifactor authentication (MFA) [55–57]. By combining smart card usage with secondary biometric verification—such as fingerprint scanning or facial recognition, the system creates a dual-layer defense against unauthorized access. This approach significantly reduces the likelihood of security breaches, as it requires not only the possession of the smart card, but also verification of the driver's unique biological features.

Emerging research highlights the potential use of blockchain technology in further enhancing the security of smart card-based ignition systems. By employing decentralized verification mechanisms, blockchain reduces the risk of unauthorized tampering and ensures that all data exchanges are securely recorded in an immutable ledger. This innovative approach could provide a transparent and tamper-proof solution to manage authentication processes.

A pioneering example of blockchain-based smart card integration in vehicle compliance can be found in a pilot project conducted in Estonia in 2023. The country, known for its advanced digital governance, implemented blockchain-secured vehicle registration and compliance verification systems, where each driver's license, insurance status, and drug test results are securely stored and authenticated via a decentralized ledger. When a driver inserts a smart card into a vehicle's ignition system, the system performs an instant verification of their compliance status via blockchain nodes. A preliminary assessment found that non-compliance rates dropped by 21%, while law enforcement agencies reported a 35% reduction in time spent on manual vehicle compliance checks. This study demonstrates the efficiency of real-time, tamper-proof verification systems in enhancing road safety while reducing administrative burdens.

While these technologies offer robust solutions to security concerns, they also introduce challenges related to implementation costs, system complexity, and user adoption (Table 3). Overcoming these barriers will require collaborative efforts between automotive manufacturers, cybersecurity experts, and regulatory bodies to create standardized frameworks and cost-effective solutions [58–64].

Table 3. Security features and technologies.

Feature	Description	Benefits	Challenges
AES-256/RSA Encryption	Encrypts data exchanges between smart card and ECU	Prevents interception and data breaches	Computational overhead in real-time systems
Multifactor Authentication	Combines smart card with biometric verification	Dual-layer security and enhanced reliability	Higher implementation costs and complexity
Blockchain Technology	Decentralized verification using immutable ledgers	Reduces tampering risks and ensures transparency	Limited adoption and scalability concerns
Cybersecurity Frameworks	Establishes standardized protocols for secure implementation	Streamlined deployment and user confidence	Requires global collaboration and regulation

By addressing these security concerns, the integration of smart card-based ignition systems can achieve its full potential, providing a secure, efficient, and reliable solution for the automotive industry. The next steps require a strategic alignment between technological advancements, practical considerations, and regulatory requirements to ensure that these systems achieve widespread adoption. This means that while innovative technologies such as encryption, multifactor authentication, and blockchain provide robust solutions, they must also be designed to be cost-effective, user-friendly, and easily integrated into existing automotive systems. Additionally, regulatory frameworks need to be developed or updated to standardize the use of these technologies, ensuring they meet safety and privacy standards while addressing the diverse needs of manufacturers, governments, and consumers. Achieving this balance will be critical to encouraging the automotive industry to adopt these solutions on a global scale, making vehicles safer and more secure for everyone.

5. Drug and Impairment Detection Systems

Driving under the influence of substances, such as smart and/or illicit drugs, prescription medications, and cognitive enhancers, significantly compromises road safety by impairing essential cognitive and motor functions. This paper explores the specific impacts of these substances on driving performance and examines the role of automated systems in mitigating associated risks. Through an analysis of current technologies and their effectiveness, it is possible to provide a mathematical estimation of potential risk reduction, distinguishing between reductions achieved through legal compliance measures and those specifically targeting substance-induced impairments.

A future advancement could involve integrating the existing system with physiological monitoring and behavioral analysis to enhance the detection of driver impairment related to drug use. This integrated system will be characterized by a complex merging of advanced materials and technologies based on infrared eye-tracking cameras, heart rate variability sensors, and facial expression analysis, hopefully powered by machine learning algorithms. By continuously assessing driver alertness, pupil dilation, gaze stability, and response time, the system will be available to identify deviations from normal driving conditions, which may be related to an altered condition in the driver.

Additionally, chemical breath analysis sensors, such as alcohol breathalyzers, are being developed to detect volatile organic compounds (VOCs) that correlate with drug use and abuse. However, a lot of work must still be performed, and several issues should be addressed first. Hypothetically, these technologies could be integrated with smart card-based ignition systems to ensure that the vehicle can only be used by drivers who possess the required physiological and cognitive standards. By utilizing real-time data processing, the system can issue warnings, limit vehicle functionality, or, in critical cases, prevent ignition entirely.

This is particularly important since substance-impaired driving remains a critical concern globally, contributing to a substantial number of traffic accidents and fatalities. Substances ranging from illicit drugs to prescription medications and cognitive enhancers can adversely affect a driver's ability to use a vehicle safely. While traditional preventive measures have primarily focused on legal enforcement and public education, their effectiveness is often limited by challenges in enforcement and compliance. However, advancements in technology present new opportunities for proactive prevention through automated systems capable of detecting impairment in real time and restricting vehicle operation accordingly.

Various substances can impair driving abilities in multiple ways. For example, cannabis consumption has been associated with impairments in tracking, attention, reaction time, short-term memory, hand-eye coordination, vigilance, time and distance perception, decision-making, and concentration, all of which are critical for safe driving. Stimulants such as cocaine, ecstasy, and amphetamines may not impair basic driving skills but can lead to overestimations of driving abilities and increased risk-taking behaviors, thereby elevating accident risk.

Opioids, including morphine, can cause drowsiness and cognitive impairments, potentially doubling the risk of vehicle crashes. Benzodiazepines and certain antidepressants may also impair motor skills and reaction times, adversely affecting driving performance.

Smart drugs (Nootropics), substances intended to enhance cognitive function, such as certain stimulants, may have side effects including increased risk-taking and impaired judgment, potentially compromising driving safety.

Technological interventions have been developed to detect driver impairment and prevent vehicle operation under unsafe conditions, such as Ignition Interlock Devices (IIDs). These are traditionally used to prevent alcohol-impaired driving. IIDs require a breath sample before allowing engine ignition. While effective for alcohol detection, their applicability to drug impairment is limited due to the lack of immediate and reliable breath tests for many drugs. Moreover, Driver Monitoring Systems (DMS) utilize in-vehicle cameras and sensors to monitor driver behavior and physiological signs. Machine learning algorithms analyze data to detect signs of impairment, such as delayed reaction times

or erratic movements. Studies have demonstrated that DMS can reliably detect alcohol impairment, with potential applicability to other substances. Lastly, Advanced Driver Assistance Systems' (ADAS) features like lane departure warnings, adaptive cruise control, and automatic emergency braking can compensate for some driver errors, potentially reducing accidents caused by impaired driving. However, these systems do not prevent impaired individuals from driving, but may mitigate the consequences.

A 2022 study conducted by the National Highway Traffic Safety Administration (NHTSA) in the U.S. evaluated the effectiveness of Driver Monitoring Systems (DMS) in identifying impairment due to drugs and alcohol. The study compared infrared-based eye-tracking systems and machine learning-driven facial recognition software across a sample of 500 drivers over a six-month period. The results show that infrared-based DMS achieved 87% accuracy rate in detecting alcohol impairment, but this dropped to 73% when identifying drug-related impairment. In contrast, machine-learning algorithms that combined facial expression analysis with steering behavior data achieved an overall 91% accuracy rate in detecting impairment, regardless of whether the driver was under the influence of alcohol, cannabis, or prescription medication. These findings highlight the potential of AI-enhanced DMS for use in preventing drug-impaired driving, while also identifying areas for improvement in current technology.

To quantify the potential impacts of automated systems on reducing drug-impaired driving risks, we consider the following factors: baseline risk (BR), this being the initial probability of accidents due to drug-impaired driving without intervention; system effectiveness (SE), consisting of the probability that the automated system correctly identifies impairment and prevents vehicle operation; compliance rate (CR), this being the proportion of drivers who adhere to system requirements and do not attempt to circumvent them.

The risk reduction (RR) can be calculated using Equation (1),

$$RR = BR \times SE \times CR \tag{1}$$

where BR represents the baseline risk, SE the system effectiveness and CR the compliance rate. Assuming that BR = 0.10 (10% baseline risk of accidents due to drug impairment), SE = 0.85 (85% effectiveness in detecting and preventing impaired driving) and CR = 0.90 (90% compliance among drivers). This calculation suggests a 7.65% reduction in accident risk due to the implementation of automated prevention systems.

Among the assumptions, BR = 0.10, studies have indicated that approximately 10% of drivers involved in fatal accidents test positive for drugs; SE = 0.85, since driver monitoring systems indicate that machine learning algorithms can detect alcohol impairment with an accuracy of up to 88%; CR = 0.90, since, while exact compliance rates vary, studies suggest that the majority of drivers adhere to in-vehicle monitoring systems, with compliance rates estimated around 90%.

To ensure the robustness of the 7.65% risk reduction estimate, a sensitivity analysis was conducted by varying key parameters (baseline risk, system effectiveness, and compliance rate) to evaluate their impact on the final result. If the baseline risk (BR) of drug-impaired accidents increases from 10% to 15%, reflecting a higher prevalence of drug use among drivers, the estimated reduction in accident risk would increase proportionally to 11.48%. Conversely, if system effectiveness (SE) declines from 85% to 75%, due to environmental factors affecting sensor accuracy or driver countermeasures, the risk reduction would decrease to 6.75%. Similarly, if the compliance rate (CR) drops to 80%, because of drivers bypassing monitoring systems, the accident reduction would fall to 6.12%. These findings indicate that maintaining high system reliability and compliance rates is essential for maximizing the benefits of automated impairment detection technologies. Future research should explore methods to enhance detection accuracy, such as multi-sensor fusion (infrared eye-tracking combined with physiological monitoring) and machine learning-driven behavioral profiling, to mitigate potential reductions in system performance under real-world conditions.

It is essential to differentiate between risk reductions achieved through legal compliance measures and those specifically targeting drug impairment. Smart card readers ensuring valid licenses, up-to-date taxes, and insurance primarily address administrative compliance. While they ensure that only authorized individuals operate vehicles, they do not directly impact impairment-related risks. Technologies like DMS and IIDs directly target and reduce risks associated with impaired driving by preventing the vehicle from operating when impairment is detected.

6. Compatibility

Integrating smart card readers into automotive systems enhances safety and regulatory compliance, but introduces security challenges such as unauthorized access, card cloning, and signal interception [65]. Robust security frameworks and technologies, including modern encryption protocols like AES-256 and RSA, protect data exchanges between smart cards and vehicle electronic control units (ECUs), preventing breaches and ensuring system reliability.

Multifactor authentication (MFA) adds a second layer of security by combining smart card use with biometric verification, such as fingerprint scanning or facial recognition, reducing risks associated with lost or stolen cards. Blockchain technology further strengthens security by providing a decentralized, tamper-proof method for verifying and recording authentication data, ensuring transparency and immutability. Together, these measures create a robust and trustworthy framework for smart card-based vehicle access.

An aspect of implementing smart card readers in vehicles is ensuring compatibility with the vehicle's existing electronic architecture. Most modern vehicles utilize CAN (Controller Area Network) bus systems to facilitate communication between various electronic components. The primary challenge is to integrate the smart card reader with the CAN bus in a way that avoids introducing latency or communication errors. The integration of smart card readers with CAN bus systems must account for latency, power consumption, and real-time response constraints. CAN bus communication introduces inherent delays due to arbitration and message prioritization, which may affect authentication speed. Experimental benchmarks indicate an average transmission latency of 1–5 ms, depending on bus load, which is generally acceptable for ignition systems, but may introduce slight delays under heavy network traffic. Additionally, smart card readers contribute to overall power consumption, typically in the range of 150–300 mW, necessitating optimization strategies such as low-power standby modes. Ensuring compliance with ISO 11898 [66] standards and implementing real-time scheduling techniques, such as time-triggered communication protocols, can enhance performance while maintaining reliability. Seamless integration is essential to maintain the vehicle's performance and reliability [67,68].

In other words, vehicles have electronic systems that "talk" to each other using a network called the CAN bus. Adding a smart card reader means ensuring it can "speak the same language" as the CAN bus without causing delays or mistakes. To address these challenges, emerging studies recommend adopting standardized communication protocols, such as ISO 7816 [69] for smart cards and ISO 21434 [30] for automotive cybersecurity [70,71]. These standards ensure secure and efficient data exchange between the smart card reader and the vehicle's systems. Compatibility testing frameworks are being developed to test the seamless operation of smart card readers across multiple vehicle models, reducing the risk of errors and ensuring optimal performance.

Implementing these solutions comes with associated costs. The integration of a smart card reader compatible with the CAN bus architecture typically requires an investment of USD 100–300 per vehicle, depending on the level of system sophistication. Additional costs for compatibility testing and adherence to standardized protocols may add USD 50–100 per unit. While these expenses represent a significant upfront investment, they are justified by the long-term benefits of enhanced security, reduced non-compliance, and improved user confidence. These concepts are summarized in Table 4.

Table 4. Compatibility features and costs.

Feature	Description	Benefits	Estimated Cost per Vehicle
CAN Bus Integration	Ensures smart card reader communicates effectively with vehicle systems	Reliable performance and no latency	USD 100–300
ISO 7816 Protocol	Standardized communication for smart cards	Secure and efficient data exchange	Included in implementation cost
ISO 21434 Protocol	Cybersecurity standards for vehicle systems	Protection against unauthorized access	USD 50–100
Compatibility Testing Framework	Verifies seamless operation across vehicle models	Reduced errors and increased reliability	USD 50–100

7. Challenges and Legal Implications

Ensuring the long-term reliability of smart card readers in automotive environments requires rigorous durability testing under extreme conditions. Standardized tests evaluate resistance to heat, humidity, and mechanical stress, aligning with ISO 16750-3 (mechanical loads), ISO 16750-4 (climatic loads), and IEC 60068-2-6 (vibration tests) [72–74]. Laboratory simulations expose smart card housings to temperatures up to 85 °C, relative humidity of 95%, and vibration profiles replicating road-induced stress (5–2000 Hz). Recent studies indicate that high-performance polymers such as PEEK and PPS maintain structural integrity beyond 1000 thermal cycles, while epoxy-based EMI shielding coatings show minimal degradation after 500 h of humidity exposure. These findings support the use of advanced materials for smart card readers in demanding automotive environments.

The integration of smart card readers with vehicle ignition systems involves navigating a complex legal and regulatory landscape [19,75]. Modifying a vehicle's ignition system may avoid warranties or conflict with regional automotive regulations, making compliance a critical aspect of implementation. Understanding and adhering to these regulations is essential for manufacturers to ensure market access and consumer trust.

In the European Union, UNECE Regulation No. 116 sets strict security standards for vehicle anti-theft systems [76,77]. This regulation mandates that any modifications to a vehicle's security features, including the integration of smart card readers, must meet rigorous performance and reliability requirements. For example, the regulation specifies tests for tamper resistance, durability, and operational functionality under various environmental conditions. Non-compliance with UNECE 116 can result in legal penalties and restrictions on vehicle sales within the European market, emphasizing the need for manufacturers to integrate smart card readers in alignment with these standards.

Several regions have explored smart card-based vehicle authentication through pilot programs and regulatory frameworks. While smart card-based vehicle authentication systems are not yet widely adopted in consumer vehicles, similar technologies have been implemented in fleet management and commercial transportation. For example, corporate fleet security systems in Germany and the Netherlands already use smart card authentication combined with biometric verification to restrict unauthorized access to company-owned vehicles. Additionally, some high-end automotive manufacturers are integrating facial recognition and fingerprint authentication into their vehicle entry and ignition systems. However, the proposed system differentiates itself by offering a holistic approach that integrates compliance verification, drug and impairment detection, and blockchain-enhanced security within a single framework. Unlike existing solutions, which often address security or compliance in isolation, the proposed system ensures that all regulatory, security, and driver wellness parameters are simultaneously validated before granting vehicle access.

A notable case is Germany's Federal Motor Transport Authority (KBA), which conducted a 2022 study on integrating smart card authentication with electronic vehicle registration (EVR). The study evaluated compliance with UNECE No. 116 and demonstrated that digital authentication could streamline registration checks and reduce unauthorized vehicle use by 31%.

Similarly, Japan's Ministry of Land, Infrastructure, Transport and Tourism (MLIT) launched a smart key verification pilot in 2023, testing the integration of JASO-approved contactless smart card readers with commercial fleet vehicles. The pilot showed a 22% reduction in unauthorized fleet access and provided insights into security challenges related to data privacy regulations. These case studies illustrate the growing regulatory interest in smart card-based vehicle authentication and highlight the need for standardized approval processes.

Different regions worldwide enforce varying standards for vehicle security and ignition systems (Table 5). For examples, in the United States of America, The Federal Motor Vehicle Safety Standards (FMVSS) include guidelines for vehicle systems but do not yet explicitly address smart card-based ignition systems. However, manufacturers are required to ensure that any new security features comply with general safety regulations, such as FMVSS 114, which pertains to theft prevention. In Japan, the Japanese Automotive Standards Organization (JASO) emphasizes both safety and technological innovation. JASO regulations encourage advanced anti-theft systems, and smart card readers could align with their focus on integrating next-generation vehicle technologies. In China, the National Standards of the People's Republic of China (GB standards) include stringent anti-theft requirements and data security provisions. Compliance with these standards is necessary for any vehicle system that involves digital communication, such as smart card-based ignition. In India, the Automotive Industry Standards (AIS) mandate anti-theft and safety protocols, with AIS-140 specifically addressing security in vehicles used for public transport [78]. While private vehicle regulations are less explicit, smart card systems would likely need to align with general safety norms.

In addition to regulatory compliance, liability issues can arise in the event of system failures or unauthorized access. For instance, if a smart card reader fails to authenticate a valid user, it could lead to customer dissatisfaction or even legal claims. Conversely, successful unauthorized access due to system vulnerabilities could result in breaches of privacy or theft, exposing manufacturers to significant liability.

Future research should focus on embedding fail-safe mechanisms to address these risks. Fail-safe systems ensure that in the event of a malfunction, the vehicle's essential functions remain operational, preventing users from being stranded or exposed to dangerous situations. Moreover, advanced cybersecurity protocols, such as encryption and blockchain, are being explored to enhance system resilience against unauthorized access.

Table 5. Regulatory comparisons and challenges [79–82].

Region	Key Regulation	Applicability to Smart Cards	Challenges
European Union	UNECE Regulation No. 116	Mandates anti-theft standards	Stringent compliance testing and certification
United States	FMVSS (e.g., FMVSS 114)	General theft prevention guidelines	Lack of explicit smart card-specific standards
Japan	JASO Standards	Supports next-gen vehicle technologies	Balancing innovation with traditional regulatory frameworks
China	GB Standards	Includes digital security requirements	Adapting to evolving data privacy laws
India	AIS Standards (e.g., AIS-140)	Emphasizes anti-theft in public transport	Limited specificity for private vehicles

8. Materials for Smart Card Readers in Automotive Systems

The integration of smart card readers into vehicle ignition systems relies heavily on the use of innovative materials to increase durability, and to guarantee high performance and compliance with automotive standards. Advanced materials have been designed to face and solve challenges related to thermal resistance, mechanical strength, electromagnetic interference shielding, and overall system reliability. The proper choice of materials significantly influences the properties of smart card readers in automotive applications. For example, advanced conductive polymers are nowadays employed in several emerging technologies; therefore, manufacturers are developing innovative systems in the automotive industry, while enhancing user experience and safety.

8.1. High-Performance Polymers

High-performance polymers such as polyetheretherketone (PEEK) and polyphenylene sulfide (PPS) are widely utilized in smart card reader housings and internal components. These materials offer exceptional thermal stability, resistance to chemicals, and mechanical strength, making them suitable for harsh automotive environments. Their lightweight nature also contributes to reducing the overall weight of the vehicle, aligning with industry trends toward fuel efficiency and reduced emissions [83].

8.2. Conductive Materials for EMI Shielding

To ensure the uninterrupted operation of smart card readers, shielding against electromagnetic interference is critical. Materials such as copper and aluminum alloys are commonly employed as EMI shields. Additionally, conductive coatings, including silver-filled epoxies and carbon-based nanomaterials, are applied to polymeric housings to enhance conductivity while maintaining lightweight properties [84].

8.3. Transparent Conductive Films

In cases where the smart card reader includes a touch-sensitive or visual interface, transparent conductive films made of indium tin oxide (ITO) or silver nanowires are utilized. These materials provide excellent optical transparency and electrical conductivity, enabling intuitive user interfaces while maintaining system performance [85].

8.4. Thermally Conductive Materials

To address the problem of heat dissipation in smart card readers, thermally conductive materials such as graphite-based composites and phase-change materials are integrated into the design. These materials enhance heat management, ensuring reliable performance in high-temperature automotive environments [86].

8.5. Advanced Adhesives and Encapsulation Materials

Adhesives and encapsulants based on silicone and epoxy chemistry are essential for protecting the delicate electronics within smart card readers. These materials provide mechanical stability, moisture resistance, and vibration damping, extending the lifespan of the device in demanding automotive conditions [87].

8.6. Future Trends in Materials for Smart Card Readers

Emerging materials such as graphene and other 2D materials are showing promise for next-generation smart card reader technologies. Their superior electrical, thermal, and mechanical properties could enable the development of thinner, lighter, and more efficient devices, paving the way for innovations in automotive security and convenience [88]. The new paragraph addresses the security risks of contactless smart cards and smartphone-based authentication, focusing on NFC relay attacks (where attackers intercept and relay authentication signals) and malware threats (which can steal credentials or manipulate biometric verification). To mitigate these risks, it recommends implementing Secure Element (SE) chips and Host Card Emulation (HCE) protections for NFC security, as well as time-based cryptographic challenges and distance-bounding protocols to detect unauthorized relays. For smartphone authentication, it suggests using Trusted Execution Environments (TEE) and AI-driven anomaly detection to identify suspicious activity. These measures enhance the security of next-generation authentication systems while maintaining user convenience in automotive applications.

9. Conclusions

The integration of smart card readers in vehicle ignition enhances security, compliance, and user convenience (see Figure 3). However, challenges remain, including regulatory hurdles, system compatibility, and adoption costs. Existing authentication methods lack robust credential verification, while smart card systems must address data security, reliability, and global regulations to ensure successful implementation [89–93].

Looking ahead, contactless and smartphone-based technologies offer exciting opportunities to further simplify and enhance vehicle access and ignition systems. Recent research highlights the role of smart transportation systems in encouraging energy-saving behaviors among users. The study by Gajdzik et al. (2024) demonstrates how integrating smart technologies with a user-centric model [94], such as the UTAUT framework, can significantly enhance adoption rates and promote sustainable urban mobility. This aligns with our findings, emphasizing the importance of designing authentication systems that not only improve security and compliance, but also support broader sustainability initiatives in the automotive sector.

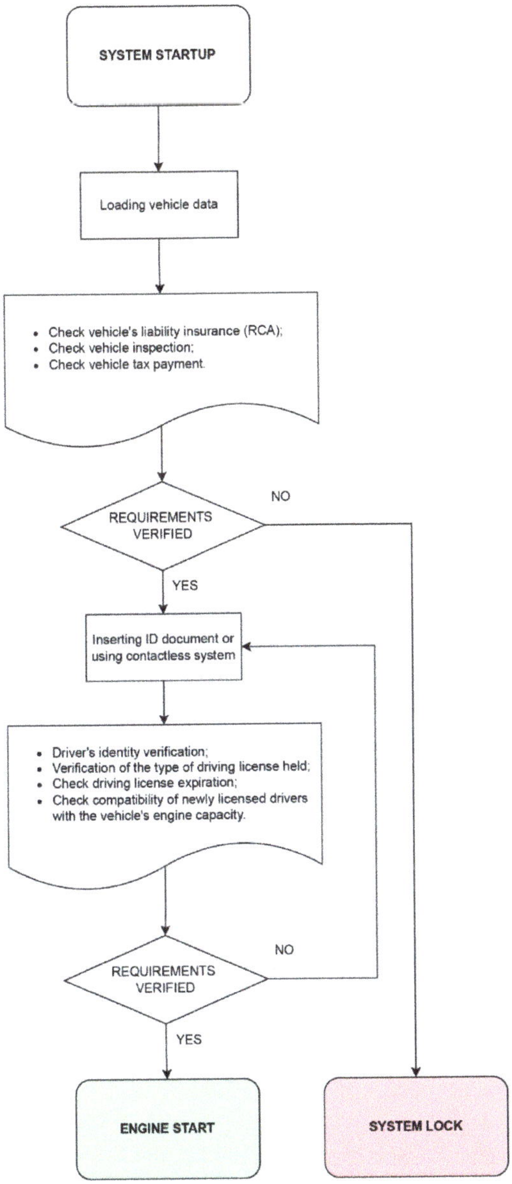

Figure 3. A decisional sketch for the vehicle permission verification.

10. Future Perspectives

These innovations may include contactless smart card readers and/or smartphone and smartwatch integration. These systems could enable seamless authentication without requiring physical card insertion. By allowing proximity-based interaction, they reduce wear and tear on hardware and improve user convenience. Moreover, using smartphones and smartwatch integration, vehicles could incorporate authentication mechanisms linked to personal devices, such as smartphones or smartwatches. These systems would use encrypted communication to validate credentials and offer an additional layer of biometric security, such as fingerprint or facial recognition, directly through the user's device. Additionally, using decentralized data management could enhance data security and streamline verification processes. This approach ensures transparency and reduces tampering risks, providing a robust framework for future systems.

While these advancements promise substantial benefits, they also necessitate addressing critical challenges related to cost and accessibility, data privacy and security, as well as global standardization. Ensuring affordability for mass-market adoption without compromising functionality is essential. Safeguards must be implemented to protect sensitive user data, ensuring they remain secure and are not misused by third parties. Additionally, effective collaboration between regulatory bodies is required to establish unified standards that accommodate the diverse automotive markets and technological landscapes worldwide.

Author Contributions: Conceptualization, V.V. and P.T.; methodology, V.V.; software, A.B.; validation, P.T. and A.B.; formal analysis, V.V.; investigation, V.V.; resources, P.T.; data curation, P.T.; writing—original draft preparation, V.V. and P.T.; writing—review and editing, P.T. and A.B.; visualization, A.B.; supervision, P.T.; project administration, V.V. and P.T.; funding acquisition, P.T. All authors have read and agreed to the published version of the manuscript.

Funding: This research received no external funding.

Data Availability Statement: Dataset available on request from the authors.

Acknowledgments: We would like to thank all the minds that, every day, never stop thinking about how to make the world a better place. Their contribution is essential for the progress of the scientific community and, even more profoundly, for humanity.

Conflicts of Interest: Author Vincenzo Vitiello was employed by Inventori Cavensi. Author Alessandro Benazzi was employed by Slim!Architetti. The remaining author declares that the research was conducted in the absence of any commercial or financial relationships that could be construed as a potential conflict of interest.

Abbreviations

The following abbreviations are used in this manuscript:

AES	Advanced Encryption Standard
CAN	Controller Area Network
ECU	Electronic Control Unit
FMVSS	Federal Motor Vehicle Safety Standards
GB	Guobiao Standards (National Standards of the People's Republic of China)
ISO	International Organization for Standardization
JASO	Japanese Automotive Standards Organization
MFA	Multifactor Authentication
NFC	Near Field Communication
RSA	Rivest–Shamir–Adleman (encryption algorithm)
UI	User Interface
UNECE	United Nations Economic Commission for Europe
V2X	Vehicle-to-Everything Communication

References

1. Lee, D.; Hess, D.J. Regulations for on-road testing of connected and automated vehicles: Assessing the potential for global safety harmonization. *Transp. Res. Part A Policy Pract.* **2020**, *136*, 85–98. [CrossRef]
2. Khan, M.N.; Das, S. Advancing traffic safety through the safe system approach: A systematic review. *Accid. Anal. Prev.* **2024**, *199*, 107518. [CrossRef] [PubMed]
3. Wegman, F. The future of road safety: A worldwide perspective. *IATSS Res.* **2017**, *40*, 66–71. [CrossRef]
4. Tapia, J.L.; Duñabeitia, J.A. Driving safety: Investigating the cognitive foundations of accident prevention. *Heliyon* **2023**, *9*, e21355. [CrossRef]

5. Chen, Y.S.; Cheng, C.H. A Delphi-based rough sets fusion model for extracting payment rules of vehicle license tax in the government sector. *Expert Syst. Appl.* **2010**, *37*, 2161–2174. [CrossRef]
6. Beck, K.H. Lessons learned from evaluating Maryland's anti-drunk driving campaign: Assessing the evidence for cognitive, behavioral, and public health impact. *Health Promot. Pract.* **2009**, *10*, 370–377. [CrossRef]
7. Montero-Salgado, J.P.; Muñoz-Sanz, J.; Arenas-Ramírez, B.; Alén-Cordero, C. Identification of the mechanical failure factors with potential influencing road accidents in Ecuador. *Int. J. Environ. Res. Public Health* **2022**, *19*, 7787. [CrossRef]
8. Marusin, A.; Marusin, A.; Danilov, I. A method for assessing the influence of automated traffic enforcement system parameters on traffic safety. *Transp. Res. Procedia* **2018**, *36*, 500–506. [CrossRef]
9. Saha, S. Automated traffic law enforcement system: A feasibility study for the congested cities of developing countries. *Int. J. Innov. Technol. Interdiscip. Sci.* **2020**, *3*, 346–363.
10. Kerimov, M.; Safiullin, R.; Marusin, A.; Marusin, A. Evaluation of functional efficiency of automated traffic enforcement systems. *Transp. Res. Procedia* **2017**, *20*, 288–294. [CrossRef]
11. Iarrocci, G.; Cattani, G. *Analisi dei Dati Italiani del Trasporto su Strada 2000–2005–2007*; Istituto Superiore per la Protezione e la Ricerca Ambientale (ISPRA): Livorno, Italy, 2009.
12. Liu, Z.; Li, R.; Wang, X.C.; Shang, P. Noncompliance behavior against vehicle restriction policy: A case study of Langfang, China. *Transp. Res. Part A Policy Pract.* **2020**, *132*, 1020–1033. [CrossRef]
13. Wu, R.; Zhang, S.; Yang, L.; Wu, X.; Yang, Z.; Zhang, X.; Zhang, D.; Huang, J.; Wu, Y. Corporate average fuel consumption evaluation and non-compliance disaggregation based on real-world data. *Appl. Energy* **2023**, *347*, 121353. [CrossRef]
14. Fedeli, S.; Giuriato, L. Value added tax non-compliance in the car market. *Fisc. Stud.* **2023**, *44*, 85–104. [CrossRef]
15. Watson-Brown, N.; Truelove, V.; Senserrick, T. Self-Regulating compliance to enhance safe driving behaviours. *Transp. Res. Part F Traffic Psychol. Behav.* **2024**, *105*, 437–453. [CrossRef]
16. Poulter, D.R.; Chapman, P.; Bibby, P.A.; Clarke, D.D.; Crundall, D. An application of the theory of planned behaviour to truck driving behaviour and compliance with regulations. *Accid. Anal. Prev.* **2008**, *40*, 2058–2064. [CrossRef]
17. Zador, P.L.; Ahlin, E.M.; Rauch, W.J.; Howard, J.M.; Duncan, G.D. The effects of closer monitoring on driver compliance with interlock restrictions. *Accid. Anal. Prev.* **2011**, *43*, 1960–1967. [CrossRef] [PubMed]
18. Freund, D.M. *Foundations of Commercial Vehicle Safety: Laws, Regulations, and Standards*; SAE International: Warrendale, PA, USA, 2007.
19. McLachlan, S. How might Driver Licensing and Vehicle Registration evolve if we adopt Autonomous Cars and Digital Identification? *arXiv* **2022**, arXiv:2202.09861.
20. Sankhe, S.; Malhotra, P.; Siddiqui, A.A.; Shaikh, A.R.; Mulla, R.; Khan, J. A Blockchain based solution to manage vehicle documents using QR-Code. In Proceedings of the 2023 6th International Conference on Advances in Science and Technology (ICAST), Mumbai, India, 8–9 December 2023; pp. 7–12.
21. Ugwuanyi, D.; Martin, O.; Chukwuemeka, E. The revance of electronic governance and E-driving licence: The nexus. *Arab. Group J.* **2017**, *6*, 81–105. [CrossRef]
22. Chowdhury, M.; Dey, K.; Apon, A. (Eds.) *Data Analytics for Intelligent Transportation Systems*; Elsevier: Amsterdam, The Netherlands, 2024.
23. Huang, Y.; Organ, B.; Zhou, J.L.; Surawski, N.C.; Hong, G.; Chan, E.F.C. Remote sensing of on-road vehicle emissions: Mechanism, applications and a case study from Hong Kong. *Atmos. Environ.* **2018**, *182*, 58–74. [CrossRef]
24. Advanced Encryption Standard (AES). AES-256. Available online: https://www.nist.gov/publications/advanced-encryption-standard-aes-0 (accessed on 1 March 2025).
25. Ryandika, D.G.; Prabowo, W.A. Two-Stage Encryption for Strengthening Data Security in Web-Based Databases: AES-256 and RSA Integration. In Proceedings of the 2023 IEEE International Conference on Communication, Networks and Satellite (COMNETSAT), Malang, Indonesia, 23–25 November 2023; pp. 486–492.
26. Pérez, J.; Gutiérrez, M. Proximity-based smart card authentication for vehicle access control. *IEEE Trans. Veh. Technol.* **2021**, *70*, 7563–7574.
27. Mohammed, K.; Abdelhafid, M.; Kamal, K.; Ismail, N.; Ilias, A. Intelligent driver monitoring system: An Internet of Things-based system for tracking and identifying the driving behavior. *Comput. Stand. Interfaces* **2023**, *84*, 103704. [CrossRef]
28. Školc, G.; Markelj, B. Smart cars and information security. *J. Crim. Justice Secur.* **2018**, *2*, 218–236.
29. Deichmann, J.; Klein, B.; Scherf, G.; Stützle, R. *The Race for Cybersecurity: Protecting the Connected Car in the Era of New Regulation*; McKinsey Company: New York, NY, USA, 2019.
30. *ISO/SAE 21434:2021*; Road Vehicles—Cybersecurity Engineering. International Organization for Standardization: Geneva, Switzerland, 2021.
31. Scalas, M.; Giacinto, G. Automotive cybersecurity: Foundations for next-generation vehicles. In Proceedings of the 2019 2nd International Conference on new Trends in Computing Sciences (ICTCS), Amman, Jordan, 9–11 October 2019; pp. 1–6.

32. Busold, C.; Taha, A.; Wachsmann, C.; Dmitrienko, A.; Seudié, H.; Sobhani, M.; Sadeghi, A.R. Smart keys for cyber-cars: Secure smartphone-based NFC-enabled car immobilizer. In Proceedings of the third ACM conference on Data and application security and privacy, New York, NY, USA, 18–20 February 2013; pp. 233–242.
33. European Road Transport Research Advisory Council (ERTRAC). *Report on Authentication Measures and Fleet Safety*; ERTRAC: Brussels, Belgium, 2023.
34. Li, W.; Zhang, Y.; Wang, X. Automotive cybersecurity and smart card integration: A systematic review. *J. Automot. Technol.* **2022**, *45*, 245–260.
35. Gurulian, I.; Shepherd, C.; Markantonakis, K.; Akram, R.N.; Mayes, K. When Theory and Reality Collide: Demystifying the Effectiveness of Ambient Sensing for NFC-based Proximity Detection by Applying Relay Attack Data. *arXiv* **2016**, arXiv:1605.00425.
36. Sánchez-García, J.; García-Campos, J.M.; Reina, D.G.; Toral, S.L.; Barrero, F. On-siteDriverID: A secure authentication scheme based on Spanish eID cards for vehicular ad hoc networks. *Future Gener. Comput. Syst.* **2016**, *64*, 50–60. [CrossRef]
37. Amaxilatis, D.; Tselios, C.; Akrivopoulos, O.; Chatzigiannakis, I. On the design of a Fog computing-based, driving behaviour monitoring framework. *arXiv* **2020**, arXiv:2010.09421.
38. Wolf, M.; Weimerskirch, A.; Wollinger, T. State of the art: Embedding security in vehicles. *EURASIP J. Embed. Syst.* **2007**, *2007*, 74706. [CrossRef]
39. Dodge, M.; Kitchin, R. The automatic management of drivers and driving spaces. *Geoforum* **2007**, *38*, 264–275. [CrossRef]
40. Dimple, B.; Chary, M.V.; Reddy, J.N.; Dileep, A. Authenticated access control for vehicle ignition system by smart card and fingerprint technology. *IOSR J. Electron. Commun. Eng.* **2015**, *10*, 45–48.
41. Economic and Social Council. Protection of Motor Vehicles Against Unauthorized Use: Proposal for Amendments to Regulation No. 116. ECE/TRANS/WP.29/GRSG/2010/8. 2010. Available online: https://digitallibrary.un.org/record/684996?v=pdf (accessed on 1 March 2025).
42. FMVSS 114. Theft Protection and Rollaway Prevention. Available online: https://www.ntea.com/NTEA/Member_benefits/Technical_resources/FMVSSguide/FMVSS114.aspx (accessed on 1 March 2025).
43. Haider, A.; Khan, A.H.; Denai, M. A Smart Wireless Car Ignition System for Vehicle Security. Advances in Automobile Engineering. *Adv. Automob. Eng.* **2017**, *6*, 1000169. [CrossRef]
44. Ravi, K.S.; Varun, G.H.; Vamsi, T.; Pratyusha, P. RFID based security system. *Int. J. Innov. Technol. Explor. Eng.* **2013**, *2*, 132–134.
45. Farooq, U.; ul Hasan, M.; Amar, M.; Hanif, A.; Asad, M.U. RFID based security and access control system. *Int. J. Eng. Technol.* **2014**, *6*, 309. [CrossRef]
46. Ramkumar, M. Fingerprint based driving licensing authentication system using FPGA implementation. *Int. J. Eng. Sci. Res. Technol.* **2014**, *3*, 2006–2009.
47. Ashwin, S.; Loganathan, S.; Kumar, S.S.; Sivakumar, P. Prototype of a fingerprint based licensing system for driving. In Proceedings of the 2013 International Conference on Information Communication and Embedded Systems (ICICES), Chennai, India, 21–22 February 2013; pp. 974–987.
48. Dhomne, S.; Bulkunde, P.; Lohakare, S.; Ukey, A.; Gajbiye, S.; Deolekar, S.; Shambarkar, N. Smart Ignition System in Automobile Industries. *IJIRT J.* **2019**, *5*, 410–416.
49. Ali, A.M.; Awad, H.M.; Abdalgader, I.K. Authenticated Access Control for Vehicle Ignition System by Driver's License and Fingerprint Technology. In Proceedings of the 2020 International Conference on Computer, Control, Electrical, and Electronics Engineering (ICCCEEE), Khartoum, Sudan, 26 February–1 March 2021; pp. 1–6.
50. Sushmitha, N.; Supriya, B.; Prajeeshan, R.A. Bio-metric automobile security. *Int. J. Sci. Eng. Technol. Res.* **2015**, *4*, 3550–3554.
51. Zhou, Y.; Tang, X.; Zhang, Y. A Hybrid Encryption Algorithm Based on RSA and AES for Wireless Sensor Networks. In Proceedings of the 2018 IEEE International Conference on Smart Internet of Things (SmartIoT), Xi'an, China, 17–19 August 2018; pp. 136–141.
52. Wu, Y.; Xiong, L.; Wang, C.; Xu, Y. Efficient Secure Mechanisms for In-Vehicle Ethernet in Autonomous Vehicles. *Electronics* **2024**, *13*, 3625. [CrossRef]
53. Yahaya, A.S.; Javaid, N.; Zeadally, S.; Farooq, H. Blockchain based optimized data storage with secure communication for Internet of Vehicles considering active, passive, and double spending attacks. *Veh. Commun.* **2022**, *37*, 100502. [CrossRef]
54. Ometov, A.; Bezzateev, S.; Mäkitalo, N.; Andreev, S.; Mikkonen, T.; Koucheryavy, Y. Multi-factor authentication: A survey. *Cryptography* **2018**, *2*, 1. [CrossRef]
55. Ometov, A.; Bezzateev, S. Multi-factor authentication: A survey and challenges in V2X applications. In Proceedings of the 2017 9th International Congress on Ultra Modern Telecommunications and Control Systems and Workshops (ICUMT), Munich, Germany, 6–8 November 2017; pp. 129–136.
56. Burton, S.L. Advancing Cybersecurity: Strategic Insights Into Multifactor Authentication. *Organ. Readiness Res. Secur. Manag. Decis. Mak.* **2025**, *8*, 247–282.
57. Zhang, K.; Ni, J.; Yang, K.; Liang, X.; Ren, J.; Shen, X. Security and Privacy in Smart City Applications: Challenges and Solutions. *IEEE Commun. Mag.* **2017**, *55*, 122–129. [CrossRef]

58. Kebande, V.R.; Awaysheh, F.M.; Ikuesan, R.A.; Alawadi, S.A.; Alshehri, M.D. A blockchain-based multi-factor authentication model for a cloud-enabled internet of vehicles. *Sensors* **2021**, *21*, 6018. [CrossRef] [PubMed]
59. Almadani, M.S.; Alotaibi, S.; Alsobhi, H.; Hussain, O.K.; Hussain, F.K. Blockchain-based multi-factor authentication: A systematic literature review. *Internet Things* **2023**, *23*, 100844. [CrossRef]
60. Khan, S.K.; Shiwakoti, N.; Stasinopoulos, P.; Chen, Y.; Warren, M. Cybersecurity Framework for Connected and Automated Vehicles: A Modeling Perspective. *Transp. Policy* **2025**, *162*, 47–64. [CrossRef]
61. Kifor, C.V.; Popescu, A. Automotive cybersecurity: A Survey on frameworks, standards, and testing and monitoring technologies. *Sensors* **2024**, *24*, 6139. [CrossRef] [PubMed]
62. Zhang, H.; Pan, Y.; Lu, Z.; Wang, J.; Liu, Z. A cyber security evaluation framework for in-vehicle electrical control units. *IEEE Access* **2021**, *9*, 149690–149706. [CrossRef]
63. Bushager, A.F. Smart Card Systems: Managing Risks and Modelling Security Protocols Using Systemc and Transaction Level Modelling. Ph.D. Thesis, University of Southampton, Southampton, UK, 2011.
64. Bozdal, M.; Samie, M.; Aslam, S.; Jennions, I. Evaluation of can bus security challenges. *Sensors* **2020**, *20*, 2364. [CrossRef]
65. Schmittner, C.; Griessnig, G.; Ma, Z. Status of the Development of ISO/SAE 21434. In Proceedings of the Systems, Software and Services Process Improvement: 25th European Conference, EuroSPI 2018, Bilbao, Spain, 5–7 September 2018; Proceedings 25. Springer International Publishing: Berlin/Heidelberg, Germany, 2018; pp. 504–513.
66. *ISO 11898-1:2024*; Road Vehicles—Controller Area Network (CAN)—Part 1: Data Link Layer and Physical Signalling. International Organization for Standardization: Geneva, Switzerland, 2024.
67. Benadjila, R.; Renard, M.; Elbaze, D.; Trébuchet, P. LEIA: The Lab Embedded ISO7816 Analyzer A Custom Smartcard Reader for the ChipWhisperer. In Proceedings of the Symposium on Information and Communications Technology Security, Rennes, France, 5–7 June 2019.
68. Tiberti, W.; Civino, R.; Gavioli, N.; Pugliese, M.; Santucci, F. A Hybrid-Cryptography Engine for Securing Intra-Vehicle Communications. *Appl. Sci.* **2023**, *13*, 13024. [CrossRef]
69. *ISO/IEC 7816-4:2020*; Identification cards—Integrated Circuit Cards—Part 4: Organization, Security and Commands for Interchange. International Organization for Standardization: Geneva, Switzerland, 2020.
70. Tuohy, S.; Glavin, M.; Hughes, C.; Jones, E.; Trivedi, M.; Kilmartin, L. Intra-Vehicle Networks: A Review. *IEEE Trans. Intell. Transp. Syst.* **2015**, *16*, 534–545. [CrossRef]
71. Abdelhalim, A.; Bailey, L.; Dalphy, E.; Raboy, K. Data Enforced: An Exploratory Impact Analysis of Automated Speed Enforcement in the District of Columbia. *arXiv* **2021**, arXiv:2106.09933.
72. *ISO 16750-3:2023*; Road vehicles—Environmental Conditions and Testing for Electrical and Electronic Equipment—Part 3: Mechanical Loads. International Organization for Standardization: Geneva, Switzerland, 2023.
73. *ISO 16750-4:2023*; Road vehicles—Environmental Conditions and Testing for Electrical and Electronic Equipment—Part 4: Climatic Loads. International Organization for Standardization: Geneva, Switzerland, 2023.
74. *IEC 60068-2-6:2007*; Environmental Testing—Part 2–6: Tests—Test Fc: Vibration (Sinusoidal). International Electrotechnical Commission: London, UK, 2007.
75. Dukarski, J. *Unsettled Legal Issues Facing Data in Autonomous, Connected, Electric, and Shared Vehicles*; SAE Technical Paper No. EPR2021019; SAE International: Warrendale, PA, USA, 2021.
76. Ahmad, U.; Han, M.; Jolfaei, A.; Jabbar, S.; Ibrar, M.; Erbad, A.; Song, H.H.; Alkhrijah, Y. A comprehensive survey and tutorial on smart vehicles: Emerging technologies, security issues, and solutions using machine learning. *IEEE Trans. Intell. Transp. Syst.* **2024**, *25*, 15314–15341. [CrossRef]
77. Weber, J.; Weber, J. Primary or Customer Relevant Complete Vehicle Characteristics. *Automot. Dev. Process. Process. Success. Cust. Oriented Veh. Dev.* **2009**, *7*, 107–286.
78. *AIS-140*; Intelligent Transportation Systems (ITS)—Requirements for Public Transport Vehicle Operation. Automotive Research Association of India (ARAI): Pune, India, 2018.
79. Dabaghchian, M.; Alipour-Fanid, A.; Zeng, K. Intelligent Policing Strategy for Traffic Violation Prevention. *arXiv* **2019**, arXiv:1909.09291.
80. Popović, V.M.; Damjanović, M.Z.; Blagojević, I.A.; Simović, S.S. Technical regulations and conditions for importing passenger vehicles on the territory of Southeast Europe. *FME Trans.* **2011**, *39*, 105–116.
81. Balasundaram, E.; Nedunchezhian, C.; Arumugam, M.; Asaikannu, V. Recent Advances in Intelligent Transportation Systems in India: Analysis, Applications, Challenges, and Future Work. In *Machine Intelligence, Big Data Analytics, and IoT in Image Processing: Practical Applications*; Wiley: Hoboken, NJ, USA, 2023; pp. 323–339.
82. Das, H.S.; Rahman, M.M.; Li, S.; Tan, C.W. Electric vehicles standards, charging infrastructure, and impact on grid integration: A technological review. *Renew. Sustain. Energy Rev.* **2020**, *120*, 109618. [CrossRef]
83. Zheng, J.; Wang, Y. Advanced Polymer Applications in Automotive Electronics. *J. Appl. Polym. Sci.* **2023**, *140*, 3456–3462.

84. Kim, H.J.; Park, S. EMI Shielding in Automotive Electronics Using Nanocomposite Materials. *Sens. Actuators A Phys.* **2024**, *212*, 117338.
85. Lee, S.; Cho, K. Advances in Transparent Conductive Films for Automotive Applications. *Adv. Mater. Interfaces* **2022**, *9*, 2200123.
86. Patel, R.; Gupta, V. Thermal Management Solutions for Automotive Electronics. *J. Therm. Anal. Calorim.* **2023**, *145*, 987–995.
87. Chen, Z.; Li, M. Encapsulation Techniques for Durable Automotive Electronics. *IEEE Trans. Compon. Packag. Manuf. Technol.* **2024**, *14*, 101–108.
88. Smith, T.J.; Zhang, Y. Exploring the Potential of Graphene in Automotive Electronics. *Carbon* **2023**, *201*, 122–130.
89. Kim, A.; Bogard, D.; Perlman, D.; Harrington, R. *Review of Federal Motor Vehicle Safety Standards (FMVSS) for Automated Vehicles: Identifying Potential Barriers and Challenges for the Certification of Automated Vehicles Using Existing FMVSS*; No. DOT-VNTSC-OSTR-16-03; John A. Volpe National Transportation Systems Center (US): Cambridge, MA, USA, 2016.
90. Rathore, R.S.; Hewage, C.; Kaiwartya, O.; Lloret, J. In-vehicle communication cyber security: Challenges and solutions. *Sensors* **2022**, *22*, 6679. [CrossRef] [PubMed]
91. Lee, T.Y.; Lin, I.A.; Liao, R.H. Design of a FlexRay/Ethernet Gateway and Security Mechanism for In-Vehicle Networks. *Sensors* **2020**, *20*, 641. [CrossRef] [PubMed]
92. Khan, J.; Lim, D.W.; Kim, Y.S. Intrusion Detection System CAN-Bus In-Vehicle Networks Based on the Statistical Characteristics of Attacks. *Sensors* **2023**, *23*, 3554. [CrossRef] [PubMed]
93. Bari, B.S.; Yelamarthi, K.; Ghafoor, S. Intrusion Detection in Vehicle Controller Area Network (CAN) Bus Using Machine Learning: A Comparative Performance Study. *Sensors* **2023**, *23*, 3610. [CrossRef]
94. Gajdzik, B.; Awdziej, M.; Jaciow, M.; Lipowska, I.; Lipowski, M.; Szojda, G.; Tkaczyk, J.; Wolniak, R.; Wolny, R.; Grebski, W.W. Encouraging Residents to Save Energy by Using Smart Transportation: Incorporating the Propensity to Save Energy into the UTAUT Model. *Energies* **2024**, *17*, 5341. [CrossRef]

processes

MDPI

Review

A Critical Review of Systems for Bioremediation of Tannery Effluent with a Focus on Nitrogenous and Sulfurous Species Removal and Resource Recovery

Philadelphia V. Ngobeni [1,2], Ashton B. Mpofu [1], Amrita Ranjan [1] and Pamela J. Welz [1,*]

1 Applied Microbial and Health Biotechnology Institute, Cape Peninsula University of Technology, Bellville Campus, Symphony Way, Cape Town 7350, South Africa
2 Water Research Group, Department of Civil Engineering, University of Cape Town, Rondebosch, Cape Town 7700, South Africa
* Correspondence: welzp@cput.ac.za

Abstract: Tanneries generate copious amounts of potentially toxic sludge and effluent from the processing of skins and hides to leather. The effluent requires remediation before discharge to protect the receiving environment. A range of physicochemical methods are used for pre- and post-treatment, but biological secondary remediation remains the most popular choice for the reduction of the organic and macronutrient fraction of tannery effluent. This review provides an update and critical discussion of biological systems used to remediate tannery effluent. While the conventional activated sludge process and similar technologies are widely used by tanneries, they have inherent problems related to poor sludge settling, low removal efficiencies, and high energy requirements. Treatment wetlands are recommended for the passive polishing step of beamhouse effluent. Hybrid systems that incorporate anoxic and/or anaerobic zones with sludge and/or effluent recycling have been shown to be effective for the removal of organics and nitrogenous species at laboratory scale, and some have been piloted. Novel systems have also been proposed for the removal and recovery of elemental sulfur and/or energy and/or process water in support of a circular economy. Full-scale studies showing successful long-term operation of such systems are now required to convince tanneries to modernize and invest in new infrastructure.

Keywords: activated sludge; aeration; anaerobic digestion; beamhouse; hybrid; macronutrient; membrane bioreactor; tanning; treatment wetland; wastewater

Abbreviations

AD = anaerobic digestion; AS = activated sludge; BAF = biological aerated filter; BOD_5 = 5-day biological oxygen demand; BNR = biological nutrient removal; BSO = biological sulfide oxidation; BSR = biological sulfate reduction; CAS = convectional activated sludge; COD = chemical oxygen demand; CW = constructed wetland; DO = dissolved oxygen; EO = electrochemical oxidation; HA = hydrolysis and acidification; HLFCR = hybrid linear flow channel reactor; HRT = hydraulic retention time; HSSF = horizontal subsurface flow; MBBR = moving bed bioreactor; MBR = membrane bioreactors; ML = mixed liquor; MLVSS = mixed liquor volatile suspended solids; OLR = organic loading rate; OUR = oxygen utilization rate; RAS = return activated sludge; RO = reverse osmosis; SBR = sequencing batch reactor; SOB = sulfur oxidizing bacteria; SRT = solids retention time; STR = stirred tank reactor; SWWS = secondary wastewater sludge, TAN = total ammonia nitrogen; TDS = total dissolved solids; TKN = total Kjeldahl nitrogen; TN = total nitrogen; TOC = total organic carbon; TW = treatment wetland; TSS = total suspended solids; TWW = tannery wastewater; TWWTP = tannery wastewater treatment plant; UASB = upflow anaerobic sludge blanket; VOA = volatile organic acids; WAS = waste activated sludge; WWTP = wastewater treatment plant.

1. Introduction

Despite the emergence of alternative materials, the durability, flexibility, and aesthetic appeal of leather have led to a sustained increase in the demand for this product [1]. However, there are significant environmental concerns due to inadequate waste management by many tanning and leather-finishing facilities [2,3]. Among other concerns, high volumes of toxic tannery wastewater (TWW) are disseminated to the environment through larger tanneries and thousands of artisanal (micro-) tanneries [4–6]. Traditional and unsustainable tanning methods are still widely practiced, especially in micro-tanneries [4]. It has been shown that the improper discharge of tannery wastewater (TWW) has negatively impacted the quality of soil and ground and surface water in India and Pakistan [5]. For example, high concentrations of toxic metals, including chromium (Cr), were measured in an area in India that had historically been irrigated with TWW [6]. Consequently, tanneries worldwide face mounting pressure to embrace more sustainable practices.

Tannery wastewater is usually highly saline and contains varying concentrations of total suspended solids (TSS), organics, metals, and inorganics from beamhouse and tanyard operations, which is discussed in more detail in Section 2 [7]. Tanneries are water-intensive. In a study conducted in Bangladesh, it was calculated that the wet processes in tanneries accounted for 97% of the total water footprint of leather, which also includes drinking water and irrigation water for the feed crops of the animals [8]. Studies suggest that TWW from some processes can be successfully re-used in other tannery processes, thereby reducing the amount of TWW being discharged [7,9]. Irrespective of the volume, it is imperative that TWW is treated to comply with local discharge regulations [5,6] and that the industry at large adopts more modern, effective, and sustainable processes and TWW treatment methods [4,10].

In most larger tanneries, the quality of TWW is improved via a combination of primary and tertiary physicochemical and biological processes before discharge. Physicochemical treatment processes are important for the holistic remediation of TWW. These include coagulation/flocculation, flotation, electrocoagulation, advanced oxidation processes, membrane separation, absorption, photocatalytic treatment, ozonation, wet air oxidation, and thermal catalysis [11–16]. An example of how primary and secondary (biological) processes are typically combined in a conventional TWW treatment facility is shown in Figure 1.

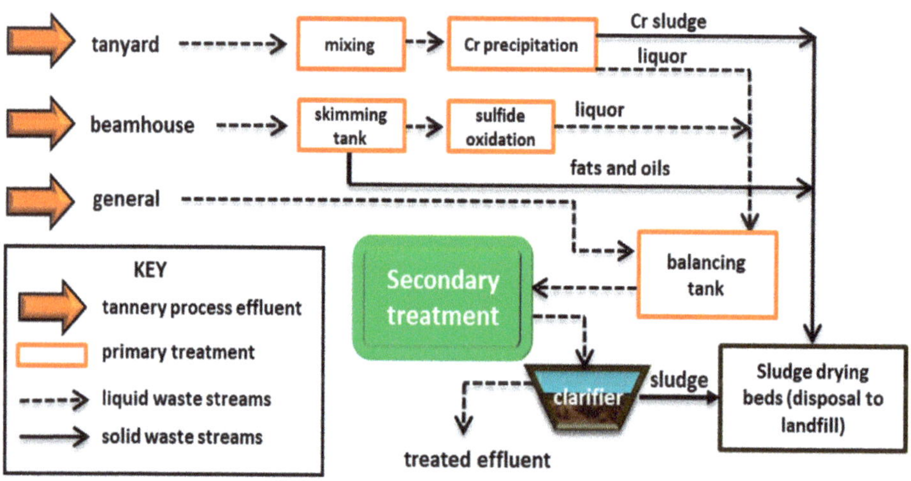

Figure 1. Set-up of a typical wastewater treatment plant at a tannery that employs wet-blue tanning (adapted from [2]).

Recent reviews on the topic of TWW treatment include descriptions of primary, secondary, and tertiary treatment technologies [11–13]. Due to the all-encompassing nature of these reviews, they contain limited information on the biological remediation of TWW. A more comprehensive and up-to-date appraisal of biological TWW treatment systems is, therefore, warranted as the subject was last reviewed in 2011 [14]. This manuscript includes (i) a short explanation of TWW from beamhouse and tanning operations, including both wet-blue and vegetable tanning; (ii) a comprehensive evaluation of the operation and performance of secondary TWW remediation systems, with a focus on the removal of organics, nitrogenous, and sulfurous compounds; and (iii) discussions on opportunities for using biological systems for recovering resources from TWW in support of a bio-circular economy.

2. Characteristics of Tannery Effluent

Tannery operations generate significant volumes of TWW, characterized by high concentrations of various pollutants. While the volume and character of TWW varies from tannery to tannery, it has been estimated that a metric ton of raw hide/skin yields 450–730 kg of solid waste, approximately 500 kg of wet sludge, and 20–40 m^3 of complex effluent containing residual processing chemicals [2,7]. Beamhouse operations consist of processes that pre-treat the skins or hides before tanning, namely, soaking, liming, unhairing, fleshing, deliming and bating, and pickling (Figure 2). Salt is used to preserve skins and hides, but if green (unsalted) hides are processed, the effluent is less saline. The solids consist of organic as well as inorganic matter, with most of the organics consisting of fats and proteins removed from the hides and skins during unhairing and fleshing [2,7]. The exact nature of the TSS in the beamhouse effluent depends on the types of skins or hides that are processed and seasonal factors [2,7].

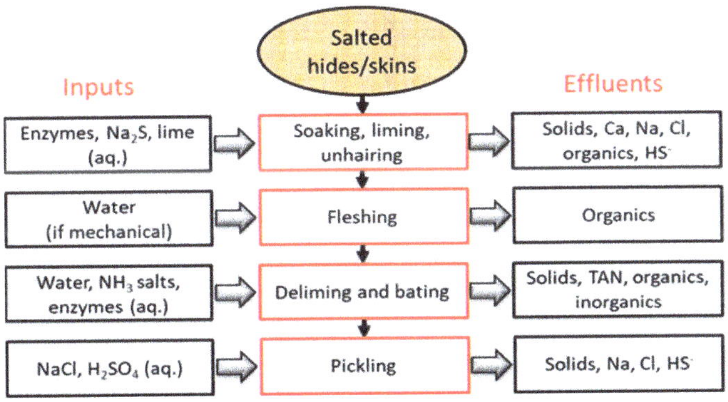

Figure 2. Schematic showing conventional inputs and main effluent constituents from beamhouse unit operations. TAN = total ammonia nitrogen.

Conventional wet-blue tanning employs Cr, which can be converted into the highly carcinogenic hexavalent form Cr(VI) in the environment. Although tannery wastewater treatment plants (TWWTPs) usually precipitate and recycle Cr, it may persist in the final effluent, sometimes in high concentrations (Table 1). The effluents from non-Cr tanning processes (e.g., wet-white tanning with glutaraldehyde and vegetable tanning) areis, therefore, perceived as less toxic [15]. However, wet-blue tanning is still widely applied because it produces consistently high-quality leather products. Fortunately, alternative processes that can equal wet-blue in terms of leather quality are slowly gaining industry traction [15,16].

Overall, beamhouse operations account for over 80% of the organic load, up to 70% of the total ammonia nitrogen (TAN), and most of the salinity of mixed TWW [3,7,17,18]. Tanyard effluent contains dyes, higher amounts of SO_4^{2-} than beamhouse effluent [3], and high concentrations of Cr or tannins emanate from wet-blue and vegetable tanning, respectively. Tannin concentrations as high as 19.7 g/L have been measured in effluent from vegetable tanning [19].

The effluent from each beamhouse and tanning unit operation has been characterized [20]. While this is important to confirm the etiology of each pollutant, in the 'real world', the streams from the beamhouse are typically combined, as are those from tanning. The beamhouse and tanning effluent may later be blended into a general effluent stream after some form of physicochemical treatment (Figure 1). Most tanneries limit the number of parameters that are routinely measured in the general TWW to those required for legislative purposes [2,7]. These include temperature, pH, TSS, biological oxygen demand (BOD) and/or COD, sulfate (SO_4^{2-}) sulfide (S^2), Cr((VI) and/or (III)), Cl, and ammonia nitrogen (NH_3-N) [11]. Academic studies typically report remediation efficiencies obtained from combined TWW effluent streams [7], but a few studies have focused on the treatment of beamhouse or tanning effluent as separate streams (Table 1). Considerable inter-tannery TWW variations occur in both, which is clear from the tabulated results. It is also well accepted that there are daily and seasonal intra-tannery variations in the quality and quantity of TWW [7].

Table 1. Selected parameters (measured averages) in beamhouse and tanning effluents.

pH Units	TSS g/L	COD g/L	BOD_5 g/L	TKN mg/L	NH_3 mg/L	SO_4^{2-} g/L	Na mg/L	Cl^- mg/L	Cr g/L	Country	Reference
					Beamhouse effluent						
6.4	0.03	-	-	268	96	-	-	-	-	Spain	[18]
12.0	4.32	40.3	-	3570	-	5.53	5683	-	-	Morocco	[21]
-	1.06	1.15	-	109	-	0.87	-	1700	-	Spain	[22]
					Chrome tanning effluent						
4.1	0.46	0.39	0.12	-	-	0.05	-	-	2.00	Brazil	[23]
3.6	0.04	4.19	0.02	-	-	0.25	-	-	2.13	Egypt	[24]
3.5	2.00	1.70	0.65	-	-	-	-	-	-	Sudan	[25]
					Vegetable tanning effluent						
3.5	3.30	25.5	4.05	-	-	7.40	-	-	-	India	[19]
7.1	5.30	7.63	3.04	-	860	0.02	-	741	-	Cameroon	[26]
4.5	1.85	27.0	-	-	-	3.93	-	-	-	India	[27]
6.0	3.21	24.3	2.80	37.2	16.8	0.03	259	751	-	Ghana	[28]

Total dissolved solids (TDS); total suspended solids (TSS); total organic carbon (TOC); chemical oxygen demand (COD); 5-day biological oxygen demand (BOD_5); total Kjeldahl nitrogen (TKN); ammonia (NH_3), sulfate (SO_4^{2-}), sodium (Na), chloride (Cl^-), chromium (Cr).

3. Bioremediation of Tannery Wastewater

3.1. Introduction

In comparison to most physicochemical TWW treatment methods, biological treatment methods require little or no chemical inputs, are more economical, and generate less potentially toxic sludge [29]. All biological remediation strategies are designed to reduce the organic load in TWW and ammonia (NH_3) in the case of aerated systems. More recently, biological removal of S species has also been advocated [30,31]. Nutrient cycling is complex, and there are an exhaustive number of chemical reactions that can occur involving carbon (C), sulfur (S), nitrogen (N), and phosphorus (P) in wastewater treatment plants (WWTPs) [32–35]. Tannery effluents only contain negligible amounts of phosphorus (P), so in contrast to domestic and many other forms of industrial effluents, there is little focus on the secondary removal of this macronutrient [26,33]. On the contrary, P is sometimes added to balance microbial nutrient requirements [33]. The removal of P is, therefore, not considered in this review, which focusses on the most common reactions involving N and S cycling shown in Figure 3.

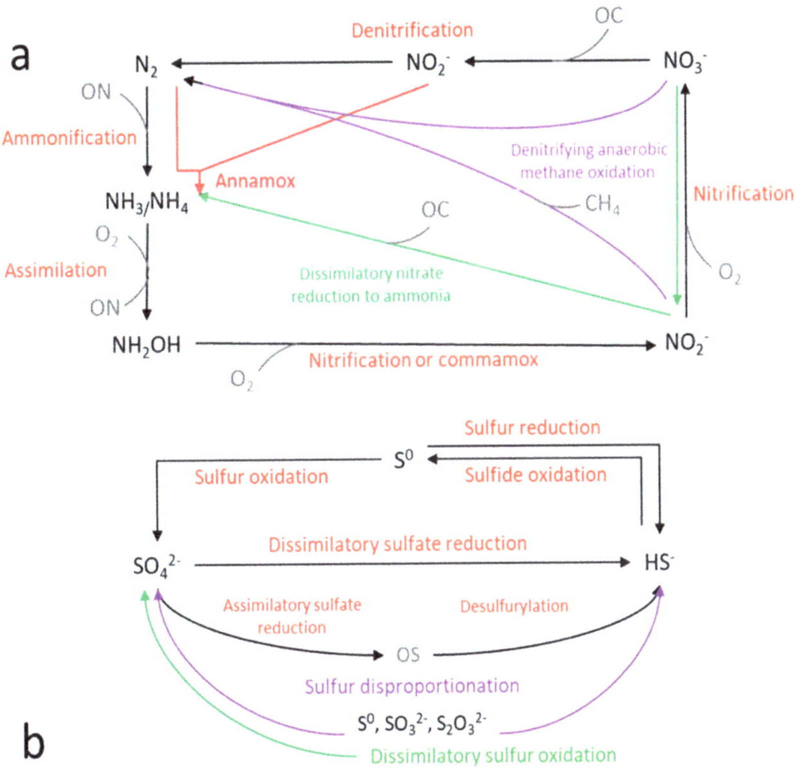

Figure 3. Major biological nitrogen (**a**) and sulfur (**b**) cycling pathways taking place in wastewater treatment plants. Adapted from Meng et al. [32] and Lin et al. [34]. OC = organic carbon, ON = organic nitrogen, OS = organic sulfur.

Under anaerobic/anoxic conditions, TWW particulates are typically broken down more effectively than under aerobic conditions, and denitrification can take place in the absence of oxygen (O_2). Apart from nitrification and denitrification, other pathways for N conversions exist in WWTPS, including anaerobic ammonium oxidation (ANNAMOX) and denitrifying anaerobic methane oxidation (DAMO), shown in Figure 3. The denitrification of TWW is theoretically not limited by the lack of organic electron donors, which is roughly determined by the COD to TN ratio, with a reported threshold of >3.5 [36]. The ratios measured in fourteen studies reviewed by Mpofu et al. [7] ranged from as low as 5 to as high as 1980, all above the threshold. However, there are drawbacks associated with a lack of O_2. Biological sulfate reduction (BSR) is promoted, and SO_4^{2-} is converted to toxic hydrogen sulfides (HS^-/H_2S) that can pollute the atmosphere [30,37]. Secondly, some organic molecules, such as aromatics from TWW, may be recalcitrant in anaerobic/anoxic environments [30,37], although others, including tannins from vegetable tanning, may be more biodegradable under anaerobic conditions [38]. Given that aerobic and anaerobic/anoxic systems have advantages and disadvantages for the remediation of TWW, there is a move towards adopting hybrid biological technologies to maximize TWW bioremediation. Apart from improving removal efficiencies, new TWW bioremediation strategies seek to recycle water and nutrients and/or produce energy or value-added products [31]. This step toward a circular bioeconomy offers economic and environmental benefits for the modern era [39,40].

Biological systems such as conventional activated sludge (CAS) and its variants [41], anaerobic digestion (AD), membrane bioreactors (MBR), and treatment wetlands (TWs) have been applied in the bioremediation of TWW and are critically discussed in Section 3.

3.2. *Conventional and Hybrid Activated Sludge*

3.2.1. Conventional Activated Sludge Systems

In CAS systems, influent wastewater continuously enters an aerated reactor and is remediated as it flows in a linear manner (plug flow) through the reactor. The mixed liquor (ML) from CAS reactors flows to clarifiers, where the solids settle out gravitationally from the clarified effluent. The settled sludge contains functional microbial species in flocs, and a portion of the sludge, known as the return activated sludge (RAS), is fed back to the reactor while the rest is wasted (waste-activated sludge, WAS). Recycling ratios of ML and RAS are important operational parameters that require periodic adjustments to maximize system performance.

The CAS process is widely applied in TWWTPs across the globe, but the systems generate significant quantities of secondary wastewater sludge (SWWS), are energy intensive, and contribute to global warming. It is estimated that 1000 W/hour of electricity is required for aeration to remove ~106 mg of BOD with a generation of 106 mg of CO_2 [42]. In addition, issues with filamentous overgrowth, poor removal efficiencies, and poor floc settling in clarifiers treating TWW have been reported [2,43]. Ultimately, these drawbacks, coupled with limited potential for resource recovery, make reliance on CAS increasingly unsustainable for tanneries in the context of modern environmental concerns [44,45].

Nonetheless, attempts have been made to improve the efficiency of the CAS process. In one study, a full-scale 2-stage CAS system treating TWW combined with domestic wastewater was bioaugmented with 'beneficial' microorganisms [40]. Good COD, S^{2-}, and TN removal efficiencies, with 99% removal of NH_3, were reported (Table 2), but the system lacked comparison with a non-augmented system. Although nitrates/nitrites (NO_3^-/NO_2^-) were not measured, it was assumed that denitrification was limited by the high concentrations (1–5 mg/L) of dissolved oxygen (DO) of and the residual N (14.6 mg/L) was due to the presence of NO_3^-/NO_2^-. Under the high-DO conditions, 99% removal of 2.8 ± 0.3 mg HS^-/L was achieved, but the influent and effluent SO_4^{2-} concentrations were not measured, so it was not clear whether removal was due to oxidation and/or atmospheric losses and/or precipitation as metal S^{2-} as previously described [46].

De Gisi et al. [47] conducted a pilot study using CAS as a pre-treatment step to specifically reduce the organic fraction of highly saline and sulfurous re-tanning TWW before reverse osmosis (RO). Flocculation and sand filtration were incorporated after CAS to enhance process efficiency. The authors did not report on N and S removal from the CAS reactor, but 54 to 74% COD removal was achieved (Table 2). Despite the energy-intensive nature of the overall process, the membranes functioned well, removing almost all the SO_4^2, NH_4^+, and NO_3^-. The RO permeate was suitable for reuse, which is particularly advantageous in regions facing water scarcity.

3.2.2. Hybrid Activated Sludge Systems

While CAS systems can achieve high nitrification rates unless anoxic zones are created within the systems for denitrification and/or DAMO, TN removal rates are poor, and high concentrations of NO_3^- and some NO_2^- are found in effluents [32]. Biological nutrient removal (BNR) WWTP configurations achieve higher TN removal by nitrification–denitrification (aerobic–anoxic) or denitrification–nitrification (anoxic–aerobic). The latter always necessitates recycling of ML from the aerobic to the anoxic zone. Simple configurations consist of two zones (e.g., modified Ludzack–Ettinger) or three zones (e.g., University of Cape Town, 3-stage Bardenpho process configurations) [32,48]. Additional anaerobic zones are incorporated in others, such as the 5-stage Bardenpho configuration, especially when an anaerobic zone is required for the removal of P. However, enhanced biological P removal is not relevant for TWW for reasons alluded to in Section 3.1.

To reduce energy consumption for aeration, enhance the biodegradability of TWW and/or improve removal of total nitrogen (TN), pilot and laboratory-scale studies have been conducted on hybrid systems that incorporate anoxic and/or anaerobic reactors up-front of CAS reactors (Table 2). Some of the complex organics found in TWW can be quite recalcitrant, which led a group of researchers to investigate whether the addition of an upstream anaerobic hydrolysis and acidification (HA) reactor would improve the biodegradability of the CAS influent [43]. They did not report on CAS removal efficiencies per se but found that low temperatures significantly reduced the COD removal efficiency of the HA reactor (from 30 to 40% at temperatures between 15 °C and 25 °C to <15% at temperatures < 10 °C). Others also employed AD before CAS to treat high-strength raw TWW without physicochemical intervention [49]. The clarified CAS effluent was then polished in a series of TWs, but the individual performances of the different units were not evaluated. There was also no apparent recycling of RAS or ML needed to retain functional and acclimated microbial communities. Nonetheless, the integrated system (including the TWs) achieved high overall COD removal rates (97%, influent: 12.5 ± 3.9 g/L), nitrification, and SO_4^{2-} removal (Table 2), but the average TN (62 mg/L) in the TW effluent was still marginally above the stipulated discharge limit of 60 mg/L.

A hybrid anoxic–aerobic system focused on COD and TN removal by incorporating an upstream anoxic reactor for pre-denitrification was piloted [50]. To allow for nitrification, the ML from the CAS reactor and clarifier sludge were recycled to the head of the anoxic reactor at rates of 100–200% and 100–150%, respectively. It was found that high organic loading rates (OLR) and low DO levels (2 mg/L) hindered nitrification but that when operational parameters were adjusted (OLR 0.72 kgCOD/$m^3 \cdot day^{-1}$), the system functioned effectively in removing 95–98% COD (influent: 5.5 ± 1.2 g/L) and 95% NH_3. Of interest, the authors found that the presence of Cr (23.3–42.5 mg/L) did not adversely affect nitrification rates.

Other studies by Sodhi et al. [51–53] on hybrid CAS systems have been conducted at laboratory-scale (Table 2). Although outcomes require validation at pilot scale, some promising results were obtained. The first "MANODOX" system consisted of four sequentially operated biological reactors, namely an aerobic moving bed bioreactor (MBBR), followed by AD, anoxic, and CAS reactors with RAS sent to the anoxic, CAS, and MBBR reactors [51,53]. The performance of the system was compared to a stand-alone CAS system run in parallel, and significantly higher N removal rates were achieved due to denitrification in the MANODOX system. The main focus of the 320-day study was to reduce the volume of SWWS and a notable 72% reduction was achieved when compared to the stand-alone CAS. The authors later determined that removal efficiency in the MANODOX system was not significantly affected by variable OLR within the range tested (1.47–2.01 kgCOD/$m^3 \cdot day^{-1}$) and that the accumulation of exopolysaccaharides (EPS) was three times lower in the SWWS from the MANODOX system than single stage CAS [53]. Although the MANADOX system showed promising results, the overall process consisted of many unit operations that may not be feasible at scale. The same authors studied and compared two simpler hybrid system configurations with stand-alone CAS, which also mainly focused on SWWS volume reduction [52]. The first consisted of an anoxic zone followed by CAS (An-CAS), while the second consisted of upstream CAS followed by AD and oxic reactors (CAS-OSA). The effect of OLR (up to 1.89 kgCOD/$m^3 \cdot day^{-1}$) was studied [52]. When compared to CAS, the systems were more resistant to shock loading, and the SWWS volume was reduced by 21% and 52%, respectively, by the An-CAS and CAS-OSA configurations. While this was less than the 72% achieved by the MANADOX system, running such systems in tanneries would incur far lower operational and maintenance costs, which merits piloting the technologies with a view to full-scale implementation [52].

Table 2. Summary of studies on treatment of tannery wastewater using conventional and hybrid activated sludge systems.

TWW	Pre-Treatment	Anaerobic/Anoxic	Selected Operational Parameters (CAS)	Selected Influent Parameters	Removal Efficiency	Country [Ref]
Full-scale system						
70% TWW 30% DWW	"Semi-finished"	None	2-stage CAS HRT: 2.5 and 0.4 days DO: 1–5 mg/L	COD: 2.08 ± 0.52 g/L TN: 61.9 ± 25.1 mg/L NH_3-N: 54.2 ± 22.3 mg/L HS^-: 2.8 ± 0.3 mg/L	95% COD removal 76% TN removal 98% NH_3-N removal 99% HS^- removal	China [40]
Pilot scale systems						
Re-tanning TWW	Screening → equalization → pH adjustment	None	HRT: 30 hrs DO: 4.0–4.9 F/M: 0.37–0.75 kgCOD/kgMLVSS·day^{-1}	COD: 5.5 ± 1.2 g/L NH_3-N: 80–160 mg/L NO_3^-: 200–510 mg/L SO_4^{2-}: 0.9–2.3 g/L Cl^-: 1.2–2.1 g/L	54–74% COD removal	Italy [47]
Raw TWW	Biological	Stirred anoxic reactor	HRT: 40 hrs DO: 2.2–5.8 mg/L OLR: 0.72–1.13 1.9 $kgCODm^{-3}$·day^{-1}	COD: 5.5 ± 1.2 g/L NH_3-N: 80–160 mg/L SO_4^2: 0.36–0.68 g/L	95–98% COD removal 46–95% NH_3-N removal	Ethiopia [50]
Raw TWW	Screening → Biological	AD	HRT: 24 hrs	COD: 12.5 ± 3.9 g/L TN: 125–258 mg/L NH_3-N: 287 ± 178 mg/L SO_4^2: 0.80–0.51 g/L	97% COD removal 70% TN removal 85% NH_3-N removal 96% SO_4^{2-} removal	Ethiopia [49]
Laboratory studies						
Raw TWW	Equalization → C&F→ Biological	MBBR, AD, anoxic	HRT: 30 hrs DO: 1.8–2.5 mg/L SRT: 11–19 days	COD: 1.6 ± 2.2 g/L (range: 1.6–2.3 g/L)	Effluent COD: <0.2 g/L	India [51]
Raw TWW	Equalization → C&F → Biological	(1) Anoxic (2) AD, oxic	HRT: 30 hrs DO: 1.5–2.5 mg/L SRT: (1) 26–34 days, (2) 21–26 days	COD: 1.9 ± 0.1 g/L (range: 1.7–2.1 g/L)	Effluent COD: 1) 0.25 ± 0.44 g/L 2) 0.16 ± 0.29 g/L	India [52]

CAS = conventional activated sludge; COD = chemical oxygen demand; C&F = coagulation and flocculation; DO = dissolved oxygen; DWW = domestic wastewater; HRT = hydraulic retention time; MBBR = moving bed bioreactor; OLR = organic loading rate; SRT = solids retention time; TN = total nitrogen.

3.3. Laboratory Sequencing Batch Reactors and Other Hybrid Systems

Aerobic sequencing batch reactors (SBRs) combine the aeration tank and clarifier in one unit, operating in feed, react, settle, and decant cycles (Figure 4). The react step is aerated and mixed, and the duration of each step, as well as the amount of ML that is retained between cycles, can be manipulated to achieve optimal performance [54]. Similar to CAS systems, settling problems due to poor floc formation may be experienced in SBR systems treating TWW, and interventions such as the addition of polyelectrolytes or TWW dilution may be needed to reduce settling times to practical levels [55]. To the best of our knowledge, only laboratory-based SBR systems treating TWW have been described in the literature, suggesting that they may not perform well when scaled up. One study employed synthetic TWW only. Although a wide range of operational parameters were tested and good sludge granulation and removal efficiencies were reported, the synthetic TWW consisted mostly of milk powder and ammonium sulfate ($(NH_4)_2SO_4$) [56], so it is difficult to extrapolate the results to real TWW given the complexity of this waste stream. Another study used a temperature controlled (30 °C) and bioaugmented system, which would not be practical or economical to operate in the 'real world' [14].

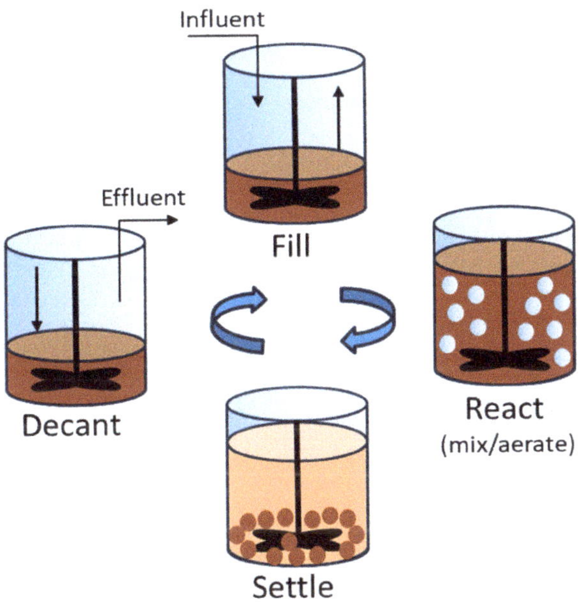

Figure 4. Schematic of the four cycles of simple aerobic sequencing batch reactors.

Studies reporting on the performance of stand-alone SBRs or hybrid SBR systems for bioremediation of real TWW under different operational conditions are presented in Table 3. Good organic removal rates were achieved in all. The most comprehensive study was conducted by Liu et al. [57] using an integrated system comprised of an upflow anaerobic sludge blanket (UASB) reactor followed by an SBR, electrochemical oxidation (EO), and a biological aerated filter (BAF), with equalization tanks between [57]. The system achieved 99% COD removal (influent 4.20–4.80 g/L), with the UASB contributing 50% and the SBR 38% to the overall removal. As with hybrid CAS systems, the results clearly demonstrated the effectiveness of combining different biological processes, and the final effluent complied with the discharge standards of the Chinese leather industry [57]. Most notably, the authors found that (i) a considerable portion of the readily biodegradable organics was removed in the UASB operated at optimal OLR of 4.56 ± 0.20 g/L and hydraulic retention time

(HRT) of 48 hr, (ii) the biodegradability of the TWW improved within the UASB, similar to the findings of Wang et al. [43] with a CAS system with upstream anaerobic HA reactor, (iii) the SBR was useful for additional removal of organics and nitrification, and (iv) UASB treatment led to more stable nitrification in the SBR. In addition, 78.3 ± 1.6% 81.5 ± 2.2% of the SO_4^{2-} (influent 334–428 mg/L) and S^- (influent 42–65 mg/L) were removed in the UASB, which would likely have a positive impact on downstream microbial activities in the SBR. It was found that the S^{2-} was immobilized as highly insoluble precipitates of metal salts in the anaerobic sludge.

A study using combined effluent from 128 tanneries in India demonstrated the practical implications of measuring the oxygen utilization rate (OUR) via a respirometer. This parameter was robust for assessing the activity of functional microbial consortia involved in metabolizing organics in TWW [54]. The system achieved 83–99% NH_3-N and 80–82% COD removal. The OUR showed a strong correlation with total COD removal rates and provided better insights into COD removal compared to measurements of different COD fractions (soluble, particulate, total) [54]. In a subsequent study, the same authors investigated nitrification–denitrification in SBRs using synthetic and real TWW [58]. They observed that nitrification occurred within the first 5 h of the mixed and aerated 'react' cycle but was unstable, possibly due to inhibitors in the TWW. In contrast, denitrification was stable during the static anoxic 4 h feed and 1 h settle/decant periods. The system achieved optimum nitrification and denitrification of 6.9 mg NH_4- N/g mixed liquor volatile suspended solids (MLVSS)·h^{-1} and 6.24 mg NO_3-N/gMLVSS·h^{-1}, respectively.

Denitrification has also been reported in other systems, including hybrid linear channel reactors (HLFCRs) that function on the principle that anoxic conditions exist in the bottom layers of the reactors, while more oxygenic conditions exist in the upper layer of the bulk liquid [31]. The authors reported an average 71% reduction in NO_3^- (influent: 11.5 ± 0.9 mg/L) and 89% reduction in NO_2^- (influent: 4.5 ± 1.2 mg/L) from partially treated mixed TWW. Other researchers studying the denitrification of TWW used fixed film reactors containing polymer balls operated in series [59]. The first two reactors were mixed and were operated to achieve HA of particulates, while the third was anoxic and unmixed for denitrification of TWW pre-treated by coagulation, precipitation, and biological desulfurization. At HRT of 3–6 hrs, 56–69% of the total organic N was converted to NH_3. The abundance of electron donors from HA of endogenous organic matter ensured complete denitrification, reaching a rate of 76.3 mg/L·hr^{-1}. Although the free NH_3 may have contributed to buffering in the denitrification reactor, the concentrations in the final effluent were high (up to 900 mg/L), so additional remediation would be required for nitrification–denitrification to improve the removal of TN.

3.4. Systems for Biological Sulfate Reduction and/or Sulfide Oxidation and Sulfur Recovery

It is important to understand the status of S species in TWW during remediation. Under anaerobic conditions, SO_4^{2-} is converted into the poisonous, corrosive, and flammable H_2S, which may be in solution, volatilized as a toxic air pollutant, or dissolved as highly corrosive HS^-/S^{2-} [46]. Even after aerobic TWW treatment, toxic H_2S gas can be re-formed in the environment or municipal sewage systems after discharge. Dissolved and total S has been measured in four spatial areas from sewers receiving effluent from tanneries [46]. Values ranged from 97.6 ± 170 mg/L to 135 ± 210 mg/L (total S) and 1.2 ± 2.6 mg/L to 40.4 ± 82.8 with an upper limit of 360 mg/L for dissolved S [46]. Concentrations of H_2S in the sewer headspace up to 3 g/L were measured, all values far exceeding the literature values for municipal sewers [46]. The authors proposed S^{2-} ppt. with iron (Fe) salts as a mitigation measure to prevent the build-up of H_2S gas and to protect the sewage system from corrosion [46].

Table 3. Performance of laboratory sequencing batch reactors treating tannery wastewater.

TWW Origination	PRE-Treatment	Selected Operational Parameters	Relevant Influent Parameters	Optimal Performance	Country [Ref]
* TWW	Polyelectrolytes, TWW dilution	6 L SBR HRT: 48 hr MLVSS/MLSS: 0.85	$COD_{soluble}$: 1.5–4.0 g/L BOD: 0.48–1.23 g/L	75–80% COD removal	Italy [55]
* TWW	No details provided	10 L SBR at 30 °C pH 7 Bioaugmented HRT: 5-days	COD: 6.24 g/L OLR: 2 $kgCOD/m^3 \cdot day^{-1}$	75% COD removal	India [14]
TWW combined from 128 tanneries	Coagulation, Cr ppt.	8 L SBR 12 hr cycle	COD: 1.91 ± 0.17 g/L NH_3-N: 120 ± 15 mg/L OLR: 1.9 $kgCODm^{-3} \cdot day^{-1}$	80–82% COD removal 83–99% NH_3-N removal	India [54]
TWW combined from 90 tanneries (wet-blue to finished leather)	Coagulation	6 L SBR 12 hr cycle 4:7:1 (feed:react:decant) 50% ML retained	COD: 1.64 ± 0.21 g/L NH_3-N: 132 ± 16 mg/L OLR: 1.9 $kgCODm^{-3} \cdot day^{-1}$	Nitrification: 6.9 mg NH_4-N/gMLVSS·h^{-1} Denitrification: 6.24 mg NO_3-N/g VSS h^{-1}	India [58]
* TWW	Screening (coarse and fine) UASB	React 8–20 hr, Settle 0.5 hr SRT: 30-day MLSS: 4 g/L	COD: 4.20–4.70 g/L NH_3-N: 274–317 mg/L	38% COD removal (SBR) 99% COD removal (system) 84% NH_3-N removal	China [59]

* TWW = tannery wastewater (no details provided); BOD = biological oxygen demand; COD = chemical oxygen demand; DOC = dissolved organic carbon; HRT = hydraulic retention time; MLVSS = mixed liquor volatile suspended solids; MLSS = mixed liquor suspended solids; NH_3-N = ammonia as nitrogen; OLR = organic loading rate; SBR = sequencing batch reactor; UASB = upflow anaerobic sludge blanket.

The first study to understand BSR during remediation TWW was conducted in 1996 [60]. The authors used pilot systems consisting of stirred tank reactors (STRs) followed by suspended fixed film bed reactors operated in upflow mode to compare the BSR of TWW from three different tanneries. Using multiple regression analysis, they found no significant differences in the origin of the TWW on BSR rates, indicating that the results could be extrapolated to other tanneries. However, this was not the case with COD removal, which differed in the TWW from different origins. The pH had a notable effect on BSR in the STR (Table 4). A similar study was performed to ascertain whether TWW would be a relevant carbon source for BSR in acid mine drainage [61]. The authors compared the performance of a UASB and a STR operated with sludge recycling from a small clarifier. The systems were operated at OLRs of 0.4–1.0 gCOD/L·day^{-1} and 0.2–10 gCOD/L·day^{-1}, respectively, and the highest BSR rates were obtained in the UASB (Table 4). The S^{2-} concentration in the influent was high (average 1.3 g/L), with 7–8% in the form of H_2S. Neither of these studies determined whether S^{2-} was removed via volatilization or precipitation into the solids fraction.

Another group of researchers found that sulfate-reducing bacteria (SRB) out-competed methanogens in a UASB-treating TWW with a low COD:SO_4^{2-} ratio of 1.4 (range 1.1–4.6) [62]. Half-inhibition constants of NH_3 and SO_4^{2-} of 180 mg/L and 480 mg/L, respectively, were calculated for BSR [62]. In contrast to other studies, the authors found that anaerobic treatment did not increase the biodegradability of the TWW. Competition between sulfidogens and methanogens during the remediation of TWW has also been studied in terms of electron flows diverted to each group in an advanced facultative pond [63]. It was found that the relative electron flow towards BSR (59–83%) was higher than the flow towards methanogenesis (17–41%), and the flow of electrons towards SRB increased when the SO_4^{2-} increased and/or the COD:SO_4^{2-} ratio decreased. Other studies have shown that although sulfidogens and methanogens require organic substrates, both processes can take place simultaneously with high CH_4 yields provided there are sufficient electron donors and the SO_4^{2-} concentration in the substrate is not too high [44,64]. For example, it was found that methanogenesis was only inhibited with TWW SO_4^{2-} concentrations $\geq$1.96 g/L during AD of secondary TWW sludge from a CAS reactor [64]. In this instance, the concentration of total organic carbon (TOC) was the most significant driver of the BSR bacterial and methanogenic archaeal community structures in anaerobic sequencing batch reactors (ASBRs) [65].

Recovery of S species from TWW has been advocated in support of a circular economy. For example, SO_4^{2-} (22.5 g/L) from TWW has been crystallized into gypsum using Ca compounds as initiators [66]. Physicochemical conversions such as these are energy- and resource-intensive as they typically require numerous unit operations, and ancillary waste streams are inevitable. It has been proposed that biological sulfide oxidation (BSO) can be utilized as a cheaper and more environmentally friendly alternative [18,19,63,67,68]. It was found that much of the S^{2-} from BSR was converted to elemental S (S^0) in an advanced facultative pond by an abundance of pink photosynthetic sulfur bacteria in the upper layer of the pond, and the authors suggested that this could be harvested [63]. Biological sulfide oxidation was also studied in a laboratory-aerated STR inoculated with sludge from a tannery WWTP and fed with sodium sulfide (Na_2S) supplemented with macronutrients. The authors focused on the molecular identification of relevant bacterial species by cloning and sequencing 16S rRNA gene amplicons and verifying these using fluorescent in situ hybridization. They also used culture-dependent techniques to isolate sulfur-oxidizing bacteria (SOB) and found that different species of the saline-tolerant genus Halothiobacillus dominated the SOB population.

More recently, HLFCRs have been proposed as passive systems for simultaneous partial organic remediation and removal and recapture of S species [30,31]. The reactors are operated in plug-flow mode that promotes BSR in anoxic conditions in the bulk liquid and partial S^{2-}/HS^- oxidation to S^0 in the interface between the bulk liquid and the atmosphere once a floating S biofilm (FSB) has been established [30,31]. It was shown that functional SRB and SOB endogenous to the TWW used in the study were selected over those from saline-adapted inocula from sulfidogenic estuaries, obviating the need for bioaugmentation [68]. The FSB can be periodically harvested as a bio-S product that contains organic C and has superior qualities to highly leachable inorganic fertilizer equivalents [30]. Near-complete S^{2-}/HS^{-} removal can be achieved in HLFCRs, and the treated effluent is amenable to AD because it is less toxic but still contains sufficient organic substrate [30]. In a later study, a pilot hybrid HLFCR–anaerobic SBR system recovered 21% of the inlet S in the FSB and 238 mL $CH_4/gCOD_{added}$. It was calculated that a medium-sized tannery treating 2258 m^3 beamhouse effluent could generate 3420 m^3CH_4, 50 m^3 irrigation water, and 31 tons of biofertilizer, promoting a circular bioeconomy and net positive tannery operations [31]. Methanogenic archaea were not active in the HLFCRs, but both SRB and methanogens were active in the anaerobic SBRs [44].

3.5. Anaerobic Digestion

While AD allows for the recovery of energy in support of a bio-circular economy, it is not widely applied as a stand-alone technology for TWW remediation because sensitive functional microbes are inhibited by inorganic S and N species, volatile organic acids (VOAs), and/or heavy metals in concentrations typically found in TWW [7,31,65,68]. This can be overcome by pre-treatment to reduce the concentration of inhibitors and/or by co-digesting TWW with other substrates [30,69]. In a recent manuscript, researchers [7] advocated for the application of AD integrated with other forms of remediation in TWWTPs in developing countries, offering opportunities to establish biorefineries for resource recovery and the promotion of sustainable economic development. Readers are referred to this review for details of previous studies on AD of TWW, which mostly reported biogas and/or CH_4 yields and COD removal efficiencies. Details of non-methanogenic hybrid bioremediation systems incorporating anaerobic reactors for HA and/or sulfidogenesis are included in Section 3.2–3.4. In terms of N and S removal during AD, 49–85% reduction in $SO_4{}^{2-}$ while co-digesting ostrich TWW and slaughterhouse wastewater blended at different ratios (%v/v) and inoculum to substrate ratios (2–5) has been reported [64]. When beamhouse and tanning effluent was blended in different ratios (%v/v), 7–81% and 34–85% decreases in $NO_3{}^{2-}$ and $SO_4{}^{2-}$ were measured [69].

3.6. Membrane Bioreactors

Membrane bioreactors decouple solids retention time (SRT) and HRT and are not reliant on clarifiers like traditional suspended growth systems. They also have lower spatial footprints, generally operate more stably, and are more conducive to recovery and the reuse of process water when coupled with RO [70–72]. Despite their advantages, MBRs have not been introduced in tanneries ostensibly due to high capex and operational costs, unresolved problems with fouling caused by the high amounts of organic and inorganic suspended solids in TWW, and the need to periodically regenerate the membranes [73,74]. Moktadir et al. [72] recently reviewed laboratory studies on a variety of MBR-based technologies for the remediation of TWW, and readers are referred to this publication for further details. In essence, hybrid MBR technologies provide promising results for COD and N reduction from TWW, and of the different options, the authors advocate that MBBRs have the greatest potential for successful remediation of TWW [72], but the technology still needs to be tested in the field.

Table 4. Systems for biological sulfate reduction and/or sulfide oxidation.

TWW Origination	Reactor/s	Operational Parameters	Relevant Influent Parameters	Optimal Performance	Country [Ref]
Mixed raw TWW 3 tanneries (ABC)	Pilot STR-UFFR Intermittent UFFR 7.9 L	35-day operation Temp: UFFR 34 °C pH: 5.6–7.0 HRT: 3.5 day	COD: 8.20 ± 6.19, 5.97 ± 3.08, 2.99 ± 2.87 g/L (A,B,C) SO_4^{2-}: 1.00 ± 0.55, 1.25 ± 0.85, 0.75 ± 00.29 g/L (A,B,C)	STR SO_4^{2-} removal: 5%, 38%, 45% (pH 5, 6, 7) UFFR SO_4^{2-} removal: 43%, 24%, 20% (pH 5, 6, 7)	South Africa [60]
Mixed raw TWW	Pilot UASB, STR Continuous UASB/STR: 1.5 m^3	58-day operation Temp: ambient pH: 7.9–8.2 HRT: 4 days	pH: 7.5 COD: 5.32 g/L SO_4^{2-}: 3.19 g/L	Removal: UASB SRR: 0.6 g SO_4^{2-}/L·day^{-1} UASB ORR: 0.5 $gCOD^-$/L·day^{-1}	South Africa [61]
Settled mixed TWW (vegetable tanning)	Pilot UAF Continuous 52 L	160-day operation Temp: 35 °C ± 0.5 pH: 7.3 ± 0.2 HRT: 2.2 ± 0.2 days	COD: 2.53 ± 0.70 g/L SO_4^{2-}: 1.81 ± 0.60 g/L HS^-: 10 ± 5.5 mg/L	COD removal 42% SO_4^{2-} removal 53%	Italy [62]
Synthetic N & P supplemented	Aerated laboratory CSTR Continuous 450 L	53-day operation Temp: 10.7 ± 2.7 °C pH: 2–4 HRT: NG	SO_4^{2-}: 1.61 ± 0.37 g/L	SOR: 22 mg HS^-/L·day^{-1}	Italy [67]
Mixed raw TWW (wet-blue tanning)	Pilot AFP Continuous 23 m^3	Temp: ambient pH: 8 HRT: 3–8 days	Loading rates SO_4^{2-}: 6–182 g/m^3·day^{-1} COD: 0.132–2.27 g/m^3·day^{-1}	Removal: SO_4^{2-}: 0.385–2.65 g/L COD: 0.723–8.22 g/L	Ethiopia [63]
Mixed TWW (wet-blue tanning)	Laboratory HLFCR in series Continuous 4 L working volume	104-day operation Temp: Ambient pH: 7.5 HRT: 4-days	COD: 7.0–27 g/L SO_4^{2-}: 2.50 g/L HS^-: 0.35 g/L	Removal: SO_4^{2-}: 80% HS^-: >97%	South Africa [30]
Mixed raw TWW (wet-blue tanning)	Laboratory HLFCR in series Continuous 16.2 L working volume	76-day operation Temp: ambient pH: 7.0–7.7 HRT: 4-days	COD: 22.8 ± 3.7 g/L SO_4^{2-}: 1.95 ± 0.31 g/L HS^-: 1.12 ± 0.00 g/L	Removal: SO_4^{2-}: 54% HS^-: 96%	South Africa [31,44]

(C) STR = (continuously) stirred tank reactor; UFFR = upflow fixed film reactor; HRT = hydraulic retention time; COD = chemical oxygen demand; UASB = upflow anaerobic sludge blanket; SRR = sulfate reduction rate; ORR = organic removal rate; UAF = upflow anaerobic filter; SOR = sulfide oxidation rate; NG = not given; AFP = advanced facultative pond; HLFCR = hybrid linear flow channel reactor.

3.7. Treatment Wetlands

Treatment wetlands, formerly known as constructed wetlands (CWs), are passive treatment systems that can 'polish' TWW to meet legislated requirements for discharge to the environment for reuse via irrigation, as evidenced by studies conducted in Ethiopia [75,76], Spain [77], and Peru [78]. A major advantage of well-acclimated TWs is that they can produce effluent of a consistent quality when remediating wastewater, such as TWW, that varies in composition and volume [77]. A few pilot studies have investigated the performance of TWs for tertiary treatment of TWW (Table 5), comparing different factors, including hydraulic retention times (HRT) [75,79,80], OLR [79,81], plant species [78,81,82], and media substrate types [76,78,83–85].

Macronutrient and TSS removal are typically the primary foci of studies for the remediation of TWW in TWs. Organics and N and S compounds can theoretically be mineralized, the latter two via nitrification–denitrification and BSR-BSO, respectively [75,86]. The plants and media used in TWs need to be 'fit for purpose'. In line with conventional TWs, different forms of gravel have been employed as the substrate in most pilot TW systems treating TWW (Table 5). In some cases, sand has been added as a top layer to improve plant germination [77,81]. A more expansive approach is to employ hybrid TW systems to maximize functionality. Saaed et al. [84] employed different flow regimes and media in a three-stage pilot TW system (Table 5). The use of coco-peat in the primary vertical flow system created oxygenic conditions for nitrification and aerobic organic biodegradation.

It is preferable to select non-invasive plant species that are resilient to TWW and suited to the prevailing climatic conditions [78]. Phragmites and Typha species are popular choices (Table 5). Arundo donax, Canna indica, Sarcocornia fruticosa, and Stenotaphrum secundatum have also been studied, and Isolepis cernua has been acclimated to pre-treated TWW, while Nasturtium aquaticum was unable to acclimate [78–82]. In another study, four plant species showed varying degrees of stress to raw TWW (Echinochloa pyramidalis > Cyprus latifolius > Typha domingensis > Pennisetum purpureum) but adapted well when TWW was diluted by 50% [76].

Based on the studies conducted to date, the COD concentrations in the diluted or treated TWW used as influent to the TWs ranged from 1.14 $\pm$ 0.3 to 1.14 to 11.6 $\pm$ 6 g/L [75,84]. The highest COD removal rate (771 kg COD/ha/day) but the lowest COD removal efficiency (53%) was measured in a two-stage horizontal subsurface flow (HSSF) system [85]. In this study, it is possible that the removal efficiency could be improved by increasing the HRT, but it also highlights the fact that readily biodegradable organics are typically removed in upstream secondary treatment systems (in this case, two-stage AD). Anomalous removal rates can, therefore, be found because of the high proportion of more recalcitrant organics in the pre-treated TWW. Four of the studies included data on the removal of TN and/or other forms of N (TKN, NH_4^+, NO_3^-), and in each case, the final effluent met the discharge standards of the country where the study was conducted. Although studies rarely include results on S removal, some results are highly promising [75]. Removal rates of 78% and 93% in influent SO_4^{2-} and S^{2-}, respectively, were obtained in a TW planted with Phragmites karka [75]. Lower SO_4^{2-} removal rates were achieved in systems planted with the grasses Leptochloa fusca (42%) and Brachiara mutica (25%) [87].

Table 5. Tertiary treatment of tannery wastewater in treatment wetlands (leather finishing effluent excluded).

TW Type	TWW	Media	Plants	Influent Parameters	Average Removal Performance	Country [Ref]
Pilot HSSF	50%	Basalt gravel	*Pennisetum purpureum*, *Typha domingensis*, *Cyprus latifolius*, *Echinochloa pyramidalis*	COD: 1.19 ± 0.6 g/L NO_3^--N: 30 ± 8 mg/L TSS: 427 ± 306 mg/L	79–84% COD (334–355 kg COD/ha/day) 63–71% % NO_3^--N 69–71% TSS	Ethiopia [76]
Pilot HSSF in series	Treated: 2-stage AD	Basalt gravel	*Phragmites karka*	COD: 1.14 ± 0.3 g/L TN: 220 ± 18 mg/L SO_4^{2-}: 433 ± 162 mg/L S^{2-}: 6.6 ± 0.4 mg/L TSS: 427 ± 306 mg/L Cr: 11.7 ± 7.0	93% COD (537 kg COD/ha/day) 78% TN 78% SO_4^{2-} 93% S^{2-} TSS NG 97% Cr	Ethiopia [75]
Pilot HSSF	Treated: PC, DAF	Granitic gravel 5–8 mm	*Typha latifolia*	COD: 2.1 g/L TSS: 208 mg/L Cr: 1.1 mg/L	53% COD (771 kg COD/ha/day) 69% TSS 50% Cr	Argentina [85]
Pilot HSSF batch mode	Treated: PC, secondary	Limestone gravel 23–40 cm, sand (top)	*Phragmites australis*	TKN: 816 ± 12 mg/L Cr: 0.23 ± 0.0 mg/L	10% TKN 48% Cr	Spain [77]
Lab-scale VF → HSSF → VF	"Raw"	Peat → slag 20 mm → pea gravel 1.2–2.3 mm	*Phragmites australis*	COD: 11.6 ± 6 g/L NH_4^+: 111 ± 39 mg/L NO_3^-: 66 ± 35 mg/L TSS: 27.6 ± 10.2 g/L	98% COD (377 kg COD/ha/day) 86% NH_4^+ 50% NO_3^- 55% TSS	Bangladesh [84]
Pilot HSSF → FWSF	Treated: PC	Gravel and sand	*Isolepsis cernua* → *Nasturtium aquaticum*	COD: 2.4 ± 1.3 mg/L TSS: 272 ± 118 mg/L Cr: 8.11 ± 4.86 mg/L	89% COD 90% TSS 100% Cr	Peru [78]

HSSF = horizontal subsurface flow; VF = vertical flow; FWSF = free water surface flow; TWW = tannery wastewater; AD = anaerobic digestion; PC = physicochemical; DAF = dissolved air flotation; COD = chemical oxygen demand; = NO_3^--N nitrate as nitrogen; TSS = total suspended solids; TN = total nitrogen; SO_4^{2-} = sulfate; S^{2-} = sulfide; TKN = total Kjeldahl nitrogen; NG = not given.

Although Cr can be adsorbed onto the medium or absorbed by plants, and good removal rates can be obtained (Table 5), a major drawback is that the Cr removal functionality can be reversed if adsorption sites are expended and/or if there is a change in redox status that causes desorption, and/or if the plants senesce [86]. Large amounts of ancillary toxic waste may be generated, requiring specialized landfills for disposal. It can, therefore, be contended that while TWs are viable options for polishing beamhouse and general waste streams from tanneries, they should be used with caution for treating streams from wet-blue tanning unless complete physicochemical Cr removal is conducted upstream. Another concern is that none of the published studies have focused on the removal of Na from TWW. Beamhouse effluent can contain high levels of salts from the soaking process (Section 2). Sodium does not partition into the substrate of CWs [86,88] and can cause sodicity in the receiving environment. The use of halophytic plants to remove Na may be an option [86] but would require monitoring and regular plant removal.

The advantages of TWs are that harvested macrophyte biomass can be used as a soil conditioner or green fertilizer, reducing secondary pollution risks [89]. The biomass can also be converted into solid fuel or biogas using low-maintenance technologies [90]. Treated effluent can be used for agricultural irrigation or low-grade process water, addressing increasing water demands.

4. Conclusions and Recommendations

Tanneries are one of the most polluting industries. Biological treatment of TWW forms an important link in ameliorating the negative effect of TWW on the environment. Biological systems can also be used to assist in recovering resources such as energy and S^0 from TWW in support of a circular economy. Promising hybrid systems and other novel systems have been described in the literature, but tanneries still tend to rely on older technologies such as CAS that have inherent problems. There is a need for long-term and credible testing of systems that have proven successful at laboratory and then pilot scale in the 'real world' in order to provide evidence that such systems offer environmental and economic benefits. To reduce the financial burden on tanneries for research, government funding agencies should consider co-funding to support this important economic sector.

Author Contributions: Conceptualization, P.V.N., A.B.M., A.R. and P.J.W.; methodology, P.V.N., A.B.M., A.R. and P.J.W.; writing—original draft preparation, P.V.N., A.B.M., A.R. and P.J.W.; writing—review and editing, P.V.N., A.B.M., A.R. and P.J.W. All authors have read and agreed to the published version of the manuscript.

Funding: This research received no external funding.

Data Availability Statement: Not Applicable.

Conflicts of Interest: The authors declare no conflicts of interest.

References

1. Hira, A.; Pacini, H.; Attafuah-Wadee, K.; Sikander, M.; Oruko, R.; Dinan, A. Mitigating Tannery Pollution in Sub-Saharan Africa and South Asia. *J. Dev. Soc.* **2022**, *38*, 360–383. [CrossRef]
2. Swartz, C.D.; Jackson-Moss, C.; Roswell, R.; Mpofu, A.B.; Welz, P.J. *NATSURV 10: Water and Wastewater Management in the Tanning and Leather Finishing Industry*, 2nd ed.; WRC TT 713/17; Water Research Commission: Pretoria, South Africa, 2017; ISBN 978-1-4312-0881-4.
3. Buljan, J.; Kral, I. *The Framework for Sustainable Leather Manufacturing*, 2nd ed.; Beachcroft-Shaw, H., Ed.; The United Nations Industrial Development Organization: Vienna, Austria, 2019.
4. Gatto, A.; Parziale, A. Towards a green and just industry? Insights from traditional leather districts in Southern Italy. *Sci. Tot. Environ.* **2024**, *942*, 171552. [CrossRef] [PubMed]
5. Ali, H.Q.; Yasir, M.U.; Farooq, A.; Khan, M.; Salman, M.; Waqar, M. Tanneries impact on groundwater quality: A case study of Kasur city in Pakistan. *Environ. Monit. Assess* **2022**, *194*, 823. [CrossRef] [PubMed]
6. Dotaniya, M.; Meena, V.; Rajendiran, S.; Coumar, M.V.; Saha, J.; Kundu, S.; Patra, A. Geo-accumulation indices of heavy metals in soil and groundwater of Kanpur, India under long term irrigation of tannery effluent. *Bull. Environ. Contam. Toxicol.* **2017**, *98*, 706–711. [CrossRef] [PubMed]

7. Mpofu, A.B.; Oyekola, O.O.; Welz, P.J. Anaerobic Treatment of Tannery Wastewater in the Context of a Circular Bioeconomy for Developing Countries. *J. Clean. Prod.* **2021**, *296*, 126490. [CrossRef]
8. Humayra, S.; Hossain, L.; Hasan, S.R.; Khan, M.S. Water footprint calculation, effluent characteristics and pollution impact assessment of leather industry in Bangladesh. *Water* **2023**, *15*, 378. [CrossRef]
9. De Aquim, P.M.; Hansen, E.; Gutterres, M. Water re-use: An alternative to minimize the environmental impact on the leather industry. *J. Environ. Manag.* **2019**, *230*, 456–463. [CrossRef] [PubMed]
10. Moniro, U.; Mostafa, M.G. Leather industrial effluent and environmental concerns: A review. *Sustain. Water Res. Manag.* **2023**, *9*, 181. [CrossRef]
11. Bhardwaj, A.; Kumar, S.; Singh, D. Tannery Effluent Treatment and Its Environmental Impact: A Review of Current Practices and Emerging Technologies. *Water Qual. Res. J.* **2023**, *58*, 128–152. [CrossRef]
12. Nigam, M.; Mishra, P.; Kumar, P.; Rajoriya, S.; Pathak, P.; Singh, S.R.; Kumar, S.; Singh, L. Comprehensive Technological Assessment for Different Treatment Methods of Leather Tannery Wastewater. *Environ. Sci. Pollut. Res.* **2022**, *30*, 124686–124703. [CrossRef]
13. Zhao, J.; Wu, Q.; Tang, Y.; Zhou, J.; Guo, H. Tannery Wastewater Treatment: Conventional and Promising Processes, an Updated 20-Year Review. *J. Sci. Eng.* **2022**, *4*, 10. [CrossRef]
14. Durai, G.; Rajasimman, M.; Rajamohan, N. Aerobic Digestion of Tannery Wastewater in a Sequential Batch Reactor by Salt-Tolerant Bacterial Strains. *Appl. Water Sci.* **2011**, *1*, 35–40. [CrossRef]
15. Shi, J.; Sheng, L.; Salmi, O.; Masi, M.; Puig, R. Life Cycle Assessment Insights into Nanosilicates-Based Chrome-Free Tanning Processing towards Eco-Friendly Leather Manufacture. *J. Clean. Prod.* **2024**, *434*, 139892. [CrossRef]
16. Baquero, G.; Sorolla, S.; Cuadros, R.; Ollé, L.; Bacardit, A. Analysis of the Environmental Impacts of Waterproofing versus Conventional Vegetable Tanning Process—A Life Cycle Analysis Study. *J. Clean. Prod.* **2021**, *325*, 129344. [CrossRef]
17. Yang, F.; Huang, Z.; Huang, J.; Wu, C.; Zhou, R.; Jin, Y. Tanning Wastewater Treatment by Ultrafiltration: Process Efficiency and Fouling Behavior. *Membranes* **2021**, *11*, 461. [CrossRef] [PubMed]
18. Marsal, A.; Hernández, E.; Cuadros, S.; Puig, R.; Bautista, E.; Font, J. Recovery of Proteins from Wastewater of Tannery Beamhouse Operations: Influence on the Main Pollution Parameters. *Water Sci. Technol.* **2010**, *62*, 658–666. [CrossRef] [PubMed]
19. Balakrishnan, A.; Kanchinadham, S.B.K.; Kalyanaraman, C. Studies on the Effect of Pre-Treatment of Vegetable Tanning Process Wastewater Prior to Biological Treatment. *J. Environ. Chem. Eng.* **2020**, *8*, 104020. [CrossRef]
20. *UNIDO 2000*; The Scope for Decreasing Pollution Load in Leather Processing (US/RAS/92/120/11-51). United Nations Industrial Development Organization—Regional Programme for Pollution Control in the Tanning Industry in South-East Asia: Vienna, Austria, 2000.
21. Majouli, A.; Tahiri, S.; Younssi, S.A.; Loukili, H.; Albizane, A. Treatment of Effluents Coming from Beamhouse Section of Tannery by Microfiltration through Cordierite/Zirconia and Alumina Tubular Ceramic Membranes. *J. Mater. Environ. Sci.* **2012**, *3*, 808–815.
22. Goltara, A.; Martinez, J.; Mendez, R. Carbon and Nitrogen Removal from Tannery Wastewater with a Membrane Bioreactor. *Water Sci. Technol.* **2003**, *48*, 207–214. [CrossRef]
23. Mella, B.; Glanert, A.C.; Gutterres, M. Removal of Chromium from Tanning Wastewater and Its Reuse. *Proc. Saf. Environ. Prot.* **2015**, *95*, 195–201. [CrossRef]
24. Abdulla, H.M.; Kamal, E.M.; Mohamed, A.H.; El-Bassuony, A.D. Chromium Removal from Tannery Wastewater Using Chemical and Biological Techniques Aiming Zero Discharge of Pollution. In Proceedings of the Fifth Scientific Environmental Conference, Houston, TX, USA, 12–16 July 2010; pp. 171–183.
25. Islam, B.I.; Musa, A.E.; Ibrahim, E.H.; Sharafa, S.A.A.; Elfaki, B.M. Evaluation and Characterization of Tannery Wastewater. *J. Forest Prod. Ind.* **2014**, *3*, 141–150.
26. Paltahe, A.; Cornelius, T.; Sambo, B.; Christian, D.; Téri, T.; Rallet, D.; Wahabou, A. Physico-Chemical Characterization of Local Tannery Waste Water Before and After Flocculation Treatment. *Int. J. Chem.* **2019**, *11*, 77. [CrossRef]
27. Borchate, S.S.; SKulkarni, D.G.; Kore, S.V.; Kore, V.S. Application of coagulation-flocculation for vegetable tannery wastewater. *Int. J. Eng. Sci. Technol.* **2012**, *4*, 1944–1948.
28. Appiah-Brempong, M.; Essandoh, H.M.K.; Asiedu, N.Y.; Dadzie, S.K.; Momade, F.W.Y. Artisanal Tannery Wastewater: Quantity and Characteristics. *Heliyon* **2022**, *8*, e08680. [CrossRef] [PubMed]
29. Goswami, S.; Mazumder, D.; IPA-Under Creative Commons License 3.0. Scope of Biological Treatment for Composite Tannery Wastewater. *Int. J. Environ. Sci.* **2014**, *5*, 607–622. [CrossRef]
30. Horn, E.J.; Oyekola, O.O.; Welz, P.J.; van Hille, R.P. Biological Desulfurization of Tannery Effluent Using Hybrid Linear Flow Channel Reactors. *Water* **2021**, *14*, 32. [CrossRef]
31. Mpofu, A.B.; Kaira, W.M.; Holtman, G.A.; Oyekola, O.O.; van Hille, R.P.; Welz, P.J. Resource Recovery from Tannery Wastewater Using an Integrated Biological System: Towards a Circular Bioeconomy and Net Positive Tannery Operations. *J. Clean. Prod.* **2023**, *387*, 135872. [CrossRef]
32. Meng, X.; Huang, Z.; Ge, G. Upgrade and Reconstruction of Biological Processes in Municipal Wastewater Treatment Plants. *Desalination Water Treat* **2024**, *317*, 100299. [CrossRef]
33. Zhao, C.; Chen, W. A Review for Tannery Wastewater Treatment: Some Thoughts under Stricter Discharge Requirements. *Environ. Sci. Pollut. Res.* **2019**, *26*, 26102–26111. [CrossRef]

34. Lin, S.; Mackey, H.R.; Hao, T.; Guo, G.; van Loosdrecht, M.C.M.; Chen, G. Biological Sulfur Oxidation in Wastewater Treatment: A Review of Emerging Opportunities. *Water Res.* **2018**, *143*, 399–415. [CrossRef]
35. Hao, T.; Xiang, P.; Mackey, H.R.; Chi, K.; Lu, H.; Chui, H.; van Loosdrecht, M.C.M.; Chen, G.-H. A Review of Biological Sulfate Conversions in Wastewater Treatment. *Water Res.* **2014**, *65*, 1–21. [CrossRef] [PubMed]
36. Daigger, G.T. Oxygen and Carbon Requirements for Biological Nitrogen Removal Processes Accomplishing Nitrification, Nitritation, and Anammox. *Water Environ. Res.* **2014**, *86*, 204–209. [CrossRef] [PubMed]
37. Reemtsma, T.; Jekel, M. Dissolved Organics in Tannery Wastewaters and Their Alteration by a Combined Anaerobic and Aerobic Treatment. *Water Res.* **1997**, *31*, 1035–1046. [CrossRef]
38. Ramirez Canon, A.; Angelis-Dimakis, A.; Ospina-Mora, D.C. Evaluation of the Aerobic and Anaerobic Degradation of an Industrial Effluent from Vegetable Tannery Processing of Leather on Batch Reactors. *Glob. NEST J.* **2020**, *23*, 22–28. [CrossRef]
39. Dhir, B. Bioremediation Technologies for the Removal of Pollutants. In *Advances in Environmental Biotechnology*; Kumar, R., Sharma, A.K., Ahluwalia, S.S., Eds.; Springer: Singapore, 2017; pp. 69–91.
40. Cheng, Y.; Chon, K.; Ren, X.; Kou, Y.; Hwang, M.-H.; Chae, K.-J. Bioaugmentation Treatment of a Novel Microbial Consortium for Degradation of Organic Pollutants in Tannery Wastewater under a Full-Scale Oxic Process. *Biochem. Eng. J.* **2021**, *175*, 108131. [CrossRef]
41. Xiang, S.; Liu, Y.; Zhang, G.; Ruan, R.; Wang, Y.; Wu, X.; Zheng, H.; Zhang, Q.; Cao, L. New Progress of Ammonia Recovery during Ammonia Nitrogen Removal from Various Wastewaters. *World J. Microbiol. Biotechnol.* **2020**, *36*, 144. [CrossRef] [PubMed]
42. Devi, A.; Verma, M.; Saratale, G.D.; Saratale, R.G.; Ferreira LF, R.; Mulla, S.I.; Bharagava, R.N. Microalgae: A Green Eco-Friendly Agents for Bioremediation of Tannery Wastewater with Simultaneous Production of Value-Added Products. *Chemosphere* **2023**, *336*, 139192. [CrossRef] [PubMed]
43. Wang, K.; Li, W.; Gong, X.; Li, X.; Liu, W.; He, C.; Wang, Z.; Minh, Q.N.; Chen, C.-L.; Wang, J.-Y. Biological Pretreatment of Tannery Wastewater Using a Full-Scale Hydrolysis Acidification System. *Int. Biodeterior. Biodegrad.* **2014**, *95*, 41–45. [CrossRef]
44. Welz, P.J.; De Jonge, N.; Lilly, M.; Kaira, W.; Mpofu, A.B. Integrated Biological System for Remediation and Valorization of Tannery Wastewater: Focus on Microbial Communities Responsible for Methanogenesis and Sulfidogenesis. *Bioresour. Technol.* **2024**, *395*, 130411. [CrossRef]
45. Kehrein, P.; van Loosdrecht, M.; Osseweijer, P.; Garfí, M.; Dewulf, J.; Posada, J. A Critical Review of Resource Recovery from Municipal Wastewater Treatment Plants—Market Supply Potentials, Technologies and Bottlenecks. *Environ. Sci.* **2020**, *6*, 877–910. [CrossRef]
46. Matos, R.V.; Peixeiro, M.; Ferreira, F.; Matos, J.S. Model-Driven Strategies for Sulfide Control in a Regional Wastewater System Receiving Tannery Effluents in Portugal. *Water* **2021**, *13*, 2838. [CrossRef]
47. De Gisi, S.; Galasso, M.; De Feo, G. Treatment of Tannery Wastewater through the Combination of a Conventional Activated Sludge Process and Reverse Osmosis with a Plane Membrane. *Desalination* **2009**, *249*, 337–342. [CrossRef]
48. Welz, P.J.; Thobejane, M.P.; van Blerk, G.N. Ammonium Oxidizing Bacterial Populations in South African Activated Sludge Wastewater Treatment Plants. *Water Environ. Res.* **2023**, *95*, e10945. [CrossRef] [PubMed]
49. Desta, A.F.; Assefa, F.; Leta, S.; Stomeo, F.; Wamalwa, M.; Njahira, M.; Appolinaire, D. Microbial Community Structure and Diversity in an Integrated System of Anaerobic-Aerobic Reactors and a Constructed Wetland for the Treatment of Tannery Wastewater in Modjo, Ethiopia. *PLoS ONE* **2014**, *9*, e115576. [CrossRef] [PubMed]
50. Leta, S.; Assefa, F.; Gumaelius, L.; Dalhammar, G. Biological Nitrogen and Organic Matter Removal from Tannery Wastewater in Pilot Plant Operations in Ethiopia. *Appl. Microbiol. Biotechnol.* **2004**, *66*, 333–339. [CrossRef]
51. Sodhi, V.; Bansal, A.; Jha, M.K. Excess Sludge Disruption and Pollutant Removal from Tannery Effluent by Upgraded Activated Sludge System. *Bioresour. Technol.* **2018**, *263*, 613–624. [CrossRef] [PubMed]
52. Sodhi, V.; Bansal, A.; Jha, M.K. Minimization of Excess Bio-Sludge and Pollution Load in Oxic-Settling-Anaerobic Modified Activated Sludge Treatment for Tannery Wastewater. *J. Clean. Prod.* **2020**, *243*, 118492. [CrossRef]
53. Sodhi, V.; Bansal, A.; Jha, M.K. Investigation of Activated Sludge Characteristics and Their Influence on Simultaneous Sludge Minimization and Nitrogen Removal from an Advanced Biological Treatment for Tannery Wastewater. *Environ. Technol. Innov.* **2021**, *24*, 102013. [CrossRef]
54. Ganesh, R.; Balaji, G.; Ramanujam, R.A. Biodegradation of Tannery Wastewater Using Sequencing Batch Reactor—Respirometric Assessment. *Bioresour. Technol.* **2006**, *97*, 1815–1821. [CrossRef]
55. Balaguer-Arnandis, E.; Cuartas-Uribe, B.; Bes-Piá, M.A.; Mendoza-Roca, J.A.; Galiana-Aleixandre, M.V. Performance Improvement of a Sequencing Batch Reactor for Treating Tannery Wastewaters. *Chem. Eng. Technol.* **2017**, *40*, 1666–1673. [CrossRef]
56. Melesse, A.G.; Velmurugan, N.; Shanmugham Venkatachalam, S.; Pothanamkandathil Chacko, S.; Demissie, B.A. Startup of Granulation of Sludge in Sequencing Batch Airlift Reactor for Simultaneous Removal of Nitrogen and Organic Carbon from Tannery Wastewater. *J. Water Proc. Eng.* **2020**, *38*, 101605. [CrossRef]
57. Liu, W.-H.; Zhang, C.-G.; Gao, P.-F.; Liu, H.; Song, Y.-Q.; Yang, J.-F. Advanced Treatment of Tannery Wastewater Using the Combination of UASB, SBR, Electrochemical Oxidation and BAF. *J. Chem. Technol. Biotechnol.* **2017**, *92*, 588–597. [CrossRef]
58. Ganesh, R.; Sousbie, P.; Torrijos, M.; Bernet, N.; Ramanujam, R.A. Nitrification and Denitrification Characteristics in a Sequencing Batch Reactor Treating Tannery Wastewater. *Clean. Technol. Environ. Policy* **2015**, *17*, 735–745. [CrossRef]
59. Zhao, G.; Dai, M.; Du, Q.; Yang, H. Application of Immobilized Biological Fillers for the Hydrolytic Acidification and Denitrification of Sulfide-Containing Tannery Wastewater. *Biochem. Eng. J.* **2024**, *208*, 109342. [CrossRef]

60. Genschow, E.; Hegemann, W.; Maschke, C. Biological Sulfate Removal from Tannery Wastewater in a Two-Stage Anaerobic Treatment. *Water Res.* **1996**, *30*, 2072–2078. [CrossRef]
61. Boshoff, G.; Duncan, J.; Rose, P.D. Tannery Effluent as a Carbon Source for Biological Sulphate Reduction. *Water Res.* **2004**, *38*, 2651–2658. [CrossRef] [PubMed]
62. Mannucci, A.; Munz, G.; Mori, G.; Lubello, C. Factors affecting biological sulphate reduction in tannery wastewater treatment. *Environ. Eng. Manag.* **2014**, *13*, 1005–1012. [CrossRef]
63. Tadesse, I.; Green, F.B.; Puhakka, J.A. The Role of Sulphidogenesis in Anaerobic Treatment Phase of Tannery Wastewater Treatment in Advanced Integrated Wastewater Pond System. *Biodegradation* **2003**, *14*, 219–227. [CrossRef] [PubMed]
64. Mpofu, A.B.; Kibangou, V.A.; Kaira, W.M.; Oyekola, O.O.; Welz, P.J. Anaerobic Co-Digestion of Tannery and Slaughterhouse Wastewater for Solids Reduction and Resource Recovery: Effect of Sulfate Concentration and Inoculum to Substrate Ratio. *Energies* **2021**, *14*, 2491. [CrossRef]
65. Alex Kibangou, V.; Lilly, M.; Busani Mpofu, A.; de Jonge, N.; Oyekola, O.O.; Jean Welz, P. Sulfate-Reducing and Methanogenic Microbial Community Responses during Anaerobic Digestion of Tannery Effluent. *Bioresour. Technol.* **2022**, *347*, 126308. [CrossRef]
66. Jennita Jacqueline, P.; Saravanakumar, M.P. Removal and Recovery of Sulphate from RO Rejects Tannery Wastewater by Double-Jacketed Agitated Crystallizer via Gypsum Crystallization. *Chem. Eng. J.* **2024**, *486*, 150341. [CrossRef]
67. Giordano, C.; Spennati, F.; Melone, A.; Petroni, G.; Verni, F.; Munz, G.; Mori, G.; Vannini, C. Biological Sulfur-Oxidizing Potential of Primary and Biological Sludge in a Tannery Wastewater Treatment Plant. *Water Air Soil Pollut.* **2015**, *226*, 391. [CrossRef]
68. Horn, E.J.; van Hille, R.P.; Oyekola, O.O.; Welz, P.J. Functional Microbial Communities in Hybrid Linear Flow Channel Reactors for Desulfurization of Tannery Effluent. *Microorganisms* **2022**, *10*, 2305. [CrossRef] [PubMed]
69. Mpofu, A.B.; Kaira, W.M.; Oyekola, O.O.; Welz, P.J. Anaerobic Co-Digestion of Tannery Effluents: Process Optimisation for Resource Recovery, Recycling and Reuse in a Circular Bioeconomy. *Proc. Saf. Environ. Prot.* **2022**, *158*, 547–559. [CrossRef]
70. Fernández-Medrano, V.; Cuartas-Uribe, B.; Bes-Piá, M.A.; Mendoza-Roca, J.A. Application of Nanofiltration and Reverse Osmosis Membranes for Tannery Wastewater Reuse. *Water* **2022**, *14*, 2035. [CrossRef]
71. Mendoza-Roca, J.A.; Galiana-Aleixandre, M.V.; Lora-García, J.; Bes-Piá, A. Purification of Tannery Effluents by Ultrafiltration in View of Permeate Reuse. *Sep. Purif. Technol.* **2010**, *70*, 296–301. [CrossRef]
72. Moktadir, M.A.; Maliha, M.; Tujjohra, F.; Munmun, S.A.; Alam, M.S.; Islam, M.A.; Rahman, M.M. Treatment of Tannery Wastewater by Different Membrane Bioreactors: A Critical Review. *Environ. Adv.* **2024**, *15*, 100478. [CrossRef]
73. Banerjee, S.; Santra, B.; Kar, S.; Banerjee, D.; Ghosh, S.; Majumdar, S. Performance Assessment of the Indigenous Ceramic UF Membrane in Bioreactor Process for Highly Polluted Tannery Wastewater Treatment. *Environ. Sci. Pollut. Res.* **2022**, *29*, 48620–48637. [CrossRef] [PubMed]
74. Tran, C.S.; Vo TK, Q.; Dang, T.B.; Nguyen, P.T.; Nguyen, K.Q.; Hoang, Q.H.; Le, L.T.; Nguyen, T.T.; Bui, X.T. Anaerobic Baffled Reactor Coupled with Membrane Bioreactor Treating Tannery Wastewater. *Case Stud. Chem. Environ. Eng.* **2022**, *5*, 100185. [CrossRef]
75. Alemu, T.; Lemma, E.; Mekonnen, A.; Leta, S. Performance of Pilot Scale Anaerobic-SBR System Integrated with Constructed Wetlands for the Treatment of Tannery Wastewater. *Environ. Process.* **2016**, *3*, 815–827. [CrossRef]
76. Alemu, A.; Gabbiye, N.; Lemma, B. Evaluation of Tannery Wastewater Treatment by Integrating Vesicular Basalt With Local Plant Species in a Constructed Wetland System. *Front. Environ. Sci.* **2021**, *9*, 1–10. [CrossRef]
77. García-Valero, A.; Martínez-Martínez, S.; Faz, Á.; Terrero, M.A.; Muñoz, M.Á.; Gómez-López, M.D.; Acosta, J.A. Treatment of WASTEWATER from the Tannery Industry in a Constructed Wetland Planted with Phragmites Australis. *Agronomy* **2020**, *10*, 176. [CrossRef]
78. Zapana JS, P.; Arán, D.S.; Bocardo, E.F.; Harguinteguy, C.A. Treatment of Tannery Wastewater in a Pilot Scale Hybrid Constructed Wetland System in Arequipa, Peru. *Int. J. Environ. Sci. Technol.* **2020**, *17*, 4419–4430. [CrossRef]
79. Calheiros, C.S.C.; Rangel, A.O.S.S.; Castro, P.M.L. Constructed Wetland Systems Vegetated with Different Plants Applied to the Treatment of Tannery Wastewater. *Water Res.* **2007**, *41*, 1790–1798. [CrossRef]
80. Calheiros, C.S.C.; Rangel, A.O.S.S.; Castro, P.M.L. Evaluation of Different Substrates to Support the Growth of Typha Latifolia in Constructed Wetlands Treating Tannery Wastewater over Long-Term Operation. *Bioresour. Technol.* **2008**, *99*, 6866–6877. [CrossRef] [PubMed]
81. Calheiros, C.S.C.; Rangel, A.O.S.S.; Castro, P.M.L. The Effects of Tannery Wastewater on the Development of Different Plant Species and Chromium Accumulation in Phragmites Australis. *Arch. Environ. Contam. Toxicol.* **2008**, *55*, 404–414. [CrossRef]
82. Calheiros, C.S.C.; Quitério, P.V.B.; Silva, G.; Crispim, L.F.C.; Brix, H.; Moura, S.C.; Castro, P.M.L. Use of Constructed Wetland Systems with Arundo and Sarcocornia for Polishing High Salinity Tannery Wastewater. *J. Environ. Manage* **2012**, *95*, 66–71. [CrossRef] [PubMed]
83. Dotro, G.; Palazolo, P.; Larsen, D. Chromium Fate in Constructed Wetlands Treating Tannery Wastewaters. *Water Environ. Res.* **2009**, *81*, 617–625. [CrossRef]
84. Saeed, T.; Afrin, R.; Muyeed, A.A.; Sun, G. Treatment of Tannery Wastewater in a Pilot-Scale Hybrid Constructed Wetland System in Bangladesh. *Chemosphere* **2012**, *88*, 1065–1073. [CrossRef] [PubMed]
85. Dotro, G.; Castro, S.; Tujchneider, O.; Piovano, N.; Paris, M.; Faggi, A.; Palazolo, P.; Larsen, D.; Fitch, M. Performance of Pilot-Scale Constructed Wetlands for Secondary Treatment of Chromium-Bearing Tannery Wastewaters. *J. Hazard Mater.* **2012**, *239–240*, 142–151. [CrossRef]

86. Mader, A.E.; Holtman, G.A.; Welz, P.J. Treatment Wetlands and Phyto-Technologies for Remediation of Winery Effluent: Challenges and Opportunities. *Sci. Total Environ.* **2022**, *807*, 150544. [CrossRef] [PubMed]
87. Ashraf, S.; Naveed, M.; Afzal, M.; Seleiman, M.F.; Al-Suhaibani, N.A.; Zahir, Z.A.; Mustafa, A.; Refay, Y.; Alhammad, B.A.; Ashraf, S.; et al. Unveiling the Potential of Novel Macrophytes for the Treatment of Tannery Effluent in Vertical Flow Pilot Constructed Wetlands. *Water* **2020**, *12*, 549. [CrossRef]
88. Holtman, G.A.; Haldenwang, R.; Welz, P.J. Biological Sand Filter System Treating Winery Effluent for Effective Reduction in Organic Load and PH Neutralisation. *J. Water Process. Eng.* **2018**, *25*, 118–127. [CrossRef]
89. Song, U.; Park, H. Importance of Biomass Management Acts and Policies after Phytoremediation. *J. Ecol. Environ.* **2017**, *41*, 13. [CrossRef]
90. Avellán, T.; Gremillion, P. Constructed Wetlands for Resource Recovery in Developing Countries. *Renew. Sustain. Energ. Rev.* **2019**, *99*, 42–57. [CrossRef]

processes

MDPI

Review

Advancing Wastewater Treatment: A Comparative Study of Photocatalysis, Sonophotolysis, and Sonophotocatalysis for Organics Removal

Szabolcs Bognár [1], Dušica Jovanović [1], Vesna Despotović [1], Nina Finčur [1], Predrag Putnik [2,*] and Daniela Šojić Merkulov [1,*]

[1] Department of Chemistry, Biochemistry and Environmental Protection, University of Novi Sad Faculty of Sciences, Trg Dositeja Obradovića 3, 21000 Novi Sad, Serbia; sabolc.bognar@dh.uns.ac.rs (S.B.); dusica.jovanovic@dh.uns.ac.rs (D.J.); vesna.despotovic@dh.uns.ac.rs (V.D.); nina.fincur@dh.uns.ac.rs (N.F.)

[2] Department of Food Technology, University North, Trg Dr. Žarka Dolinara 1, 48000 Koprivnica, Croatia

* Correspondence: pputnik@alumni.uconn.edu (P.P.); daniela.sojic@dh.uns.ac.rs (D.Š.M.)

Abstract: Clear and sanitarily adequate water scarcity is one of the greatest problems of modern society. Continuous population growth, rising organics concentrations, and common non-efficient wastewater treatment technologies add to the seriousness of this issue. The employment of various advanced oxidation processes (AOPs) in water treatment is becoming more widespread. In this review, the state-of-the-art application of three AOPs is discussed in detail: photocatalysis, sonophotolysis, and sonophotocatalysis. Photocatalysis utilizes semiconductor photocatalysts to degrade organic pollutants under light irradiation. Sonophotolysis combines ultrasound and photolysis to generate reactive radicals, enhancing the degradation of organic pollutants. Sonophotocatalysis synergistically combines ultrasound with photocatalysis, resulting in improved degradation efficiency compared to individual processes. By studying this paper, readers will get an insight into the latest published data regarding the above-mentioned processes from the last 10 years. Different factors are compared and discussed, such as degradation efficiency, reaction kinetics, catalyst type, ultrasound frequency, or water matrix effects on process performance. In addition, the economic aspects of sonophotolysis, photocatalysis, and sonophotocatalysis will be also analyzed and compared to other processes. Also, the future research directions and potential applications of these AOPs in wastewater treatment will be highlighted. This review offers invaluable insights into the selection and optimization of AOPs.

Keywords: organic pollutants; water purification; advanced oxidation processes; photocatalysis; sonophotolysis; sonophotocatalysis; economy aspects

1. Introduction

Environmental pollution refers to the introduction of various compounds (gas, liquid, or solid) or forms of energy into the environment at a rate that exceeds the environment's capacity to eliminate them. Due to environmental pollution, a wide spectrum of harmful effects can be observed, such as health issues or biodiversity loss [1]. All natural resources (soil, water, and air) are exposed to the dreadful effects of environmental pollution; however, water pollution and pure water scarcity are globally the most threatening ones. Water pollution is a severe problem both in urban and rural areas. Interaction with contaminated water can result in various infections and parasitic illnesses, and it can multiply the number of industrial effluents, heavy metals, or algal toxins [2]. Based on a UN report from 2023, 26% of the global population is facing pure water scarcity, while 46% of the population has a lack of access to adequately managed sanitation. It is expected that by 2050, 2.4 billion people will be facing water scarcity. In addition, extreme and prolonged droughts are also stressing ecosystems, with severe consequences for the living world [3].

Water pollution is mainly the result of various human activities and facilities (e.g., farming, industry, healthcare). The level of organic pollution, for instance in rivers, results from two opposing processes: pollutant input and natural purification. Urban and agricultural wastewater discharges are the primary sources of organic pollutants, expected to rise with urbanization and intensified farming. While pollution originates at discharge points, its effects propagate downstream, affecting both communities and ecosystems as pollutants travel through river networks. The severity of downstream impacts hinges on the river's ability to self-purify through dilution from runoff and degradation by microorganisms [4–6]. The present persistent organics are also known as emerging organic pollutants (EOPs). Several sources of EOP emissions have been identified; however, effluent discharges from wastewater treatment plants are the primary contributors. These substances are consistently detected in wastewater samples, both pre- and post-treatment, typically in a concentration range from ng/L to μg/L. The composition and concentration of EOPs in raw wastewater is largely influenced by the socioeconomic demographics of the contributing population. Conversely, the concentration of EOPs in treated effluents depends on the initial pollution level of incoming waters and the efficiency of the purification process [7,8]. Furthermore, the possible bioaccumulation and biomagnification of the mentioned EOPs makes them extremely hazardous to the environment [9]. Namely, as one ascends the food chain, concentrations of EOPs typically increase. Consequently, species occupying the upper levels of the food chain, such as fish, predatory birds, mammals, and humans, exhibit the highest levels of these chemicals, placing them at a heightened risk of experiencing acute and chronic adverse effects [10]. Thus, the appearance of EOPs results in significant health issues for human beings, fauna, flora, and the marine ecosystem [9]. EOPs encompass a wide array of compounds from various chemical classes, while the most common ones include pharmaceuticals (e.g., antibiotics, hormones), personal care products (ingredients found in cosmetics, soaps, fragrances, etc.), pesticides and their metabolites, plasticizers, and organic colors [9,11,12].

Taking all the negative impacts into account, it is obvious that EOPs must be removed from the environment, and their discharge to the environment has to be discontinued. There are various conventional water treatments available to ensure safe drinking water and a pure aquatic environment for the global community [13]. In response to the adverse impacts of polluted water, numerous nations globally have implemented increasingly stringent regulations and restrictions on effluent emissions. The approach to water treatment varies among countries, with each employing unique combinations of processes based on regulatory constraints, the utilization of the best available technology, and the characteristics of the treated water [14]. In general, there are three types of usual water treatment lines: (i) simple physical treatment and disinfection; (ii) normal treatment, chemical and disinfection; and (iii) physical treatment, advanced chemistry, refining and disinfection [15]. The simple disinfection techniques include ultraviolet (UV) irradiation, chemical methods that include the usage of chlorine, chloramines, and unscented bleach, then distillation and ozonation, along with boiling, in times of emergency. Shock chlorination stands out as the prevalent sanitizing treatment for wells [15]. The simple physical treatment targets high-quality surface waters with minimal turbidity fluctuations and applies to all groundwater, particularly karstic waters with low turbidity. While these waters share similarities with the previous category, their suspended matter concentrations necessitate prior physical treatment. Coagulation occurs before filtration (coagulation in the filter). Typically, closed-type filters are utilized, due to their compact dimensions and ability to facilitate high filtration rates. Presently, an effective substitute approach is the utilization of ultrafiltration membranes, accompanied by disinfection [15]. If the normal treatment, chemical and disinfection, is being observed, this treatment targets surface waters abundant in suspended particles and organic substances, surpassing the standards for drinking water due to the presence of micropollutants. Additionally, it is suitable for waters with elevated levels of iron and manganese. The pre-oxidation stage serves to oxidize ammoniacal nitrogen (when chlorine is the oxidant), dissolved iron, and manganese, leading to the formation of precipitates. It also aids in algae removal and safeguards settling tanks. Pre-oxidation plays a vital role in enhancing the coagulation–flocculation process [15]. In addition, the physical treatment, advanced chemistry, and refining and disinfection techniques are thoroughly developed and applicable to surface waters, rich in organic matter, dyes, and micropollutants. However, the above-mentioned EOPs cannot be effectively removed by these techniques [15].

Thus, in the quest for sustainable solutions to environmental challenges, advanced oxidation processes (AOPs) have emerged as powerful tools in the purification of water, air, and soil. AOPs represent a cutting-edge approach to (waste)water treatment and pollution remediation, harnessing the potent reactivity of reactive oxygen species, such as hydroxyl radicals ($HO^{\bullet}$), to degrade and transform a wide array of organic and inorganic contaminants [16]. Over the years, various AOPs have been introduced and studied for degrading numerous EOPs found in (waste)water. These processes involve cavitation induced by ultrasonic irradiation [17–20], photocatalytic oxidation [21–26], and Fenton chemistry that relies on the reaction of iron(II) sulfate with hydrogen peroxide (H_2O_2), i.e., Fenton's reagent [27,28]. Additionally, the synergy of AOPs leads to the development of hybrid methods, including ultrasound-assisted Fenton [29], sonophotocatalysis [30,31], photo-Fenton [32,33], and ozone/H_2O_2 [34–36], to achieve enhanced oxidation efficiency. These hybrid approaches are designed to overcome the limitations and challenges associated with individual AOPs, particularly in targeting specific pollutants [37]. Previous research by Elkacmi and Bennajah presented a literature review on AOPs applications for detoxifying olive mill wastewater, covering chemical, photochemical, sonochemical, and electrochemical technologies, along with their combination with biological and other techniques. It also addressed the influence of operating parameters on these processes [38]. Additionally, the study by Babu Ponnusami et al. focused on integrating AOPs and biological processes in wastewater treatment, evaluating their advancements, feasibility, and practicality, and recommending their combined use to achieve treatment goals, while considering economic and operational factors [39]. Furthermore, Yu et al. demonstrated recent advancements in using encapsulated transition-metal nanoparticle catalysts for AOPs targeting organic pollutant degradation. The authors discussed the structure, composition, synthesis methods, applications in various AOPs, and highlighted major challenges and opportunities associated with these catalysts, providing insights for future research and development [40].

This review aims to give readers an overview about the state-of-the-art application and efficiency of photocatalysis, sonophotolysis, and their combination, i.e., sonophotocatalysis, in (waste)water treatment for organic pollutants removal. By exploring these innovative methods, it provides valuable insights for researchers and professionals dedicated to purifying water contaminated with various organic pollutants.

2. Advanced Oxidation Processes

In the Introduction, it was mentioned that AOPs are advanced and efficient techniques, which are being used, for instance, in organic pollutants removal. AOPs are new green chemical technologies that are promising and sustainable alternatives to conventional techniques. AOPs are based on the formation of highly reactive oxygen species like $HO^{\bullet}$, hydroperoxyl radicals ($HO_2^{\bullet}$), sulfate radicals ($SO_4^{\bullet-}$), and superoxide radical anions ($O_2^{\bullet-}$) that degrade hazardous pollutants by ISO 9001:2015 standards by utilizing renewable and clean solar energy [41]. These techniques minimize the formation of sludge and other hazardous byproducts, reducing disposal costs and environmental impact. The economic feasibility of AOPs presents challenges due to high capital and operational costs, while their effectiveness and potential for integration into sustainable treatment systems make them a valuable tool for advanced wastewater management. By optimizing costs, improving energy efficiency, and leveraging policy support, AOPs can play a crucial role in achieving sustainable water treatment and protecting environmental and public health.

AOPs are typically categorized according to the radical formation method, including chemical, photochemical, radiation-induced, cavitation, and electrochemical processes [42]. The classification of conventional and advanced AOPs techniques is presented in Figure 1.

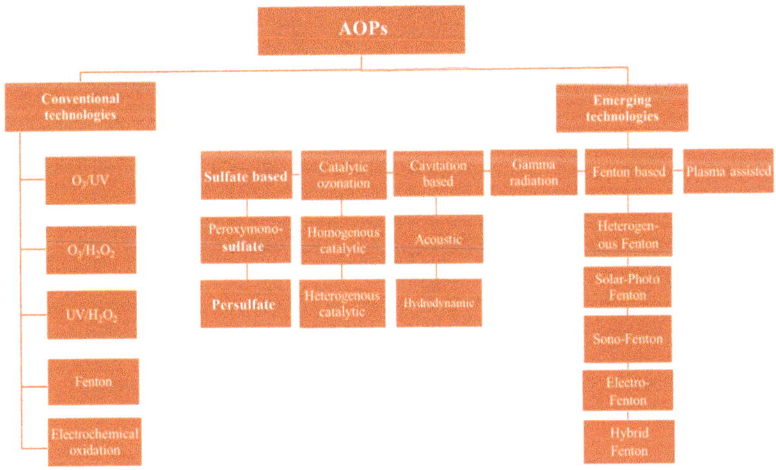

Figure 1. The classification of conventional and advanced AOPs techniques. Reprinted with permission from Ref. [42], copyright Elsevier.

This review is focusing on AOPs techniques where the reactive species are generated by cavitation and photochemical routes, as well as on their synergistic combination. The input data (article title, abstract, keywords) were extracted from academic papers indexed in Scopus with the search terms "photocatalysis/sonophotolysis/sonophotocatalysis" + "advanced oxidation processes" + "water" + "organics OR organic pollutant *". The search was set to include only articles/reviews papers (excluding book chapters and proceedings). The number of publications about photocatalysis, sonophotolysis, and sonophotocatalysis is continuously increasing. In the last 10 years (the time period was set from 2014 to 2024), 688 research studies were published in the case of photocatalysis, 3 studies regarding the application of sonophotolysis, and 8 articles about the employment of sonophotocatalysis in the degradation of organic pollutants in (waste)water. The annual distribution of these articles is shown in Figure 2.

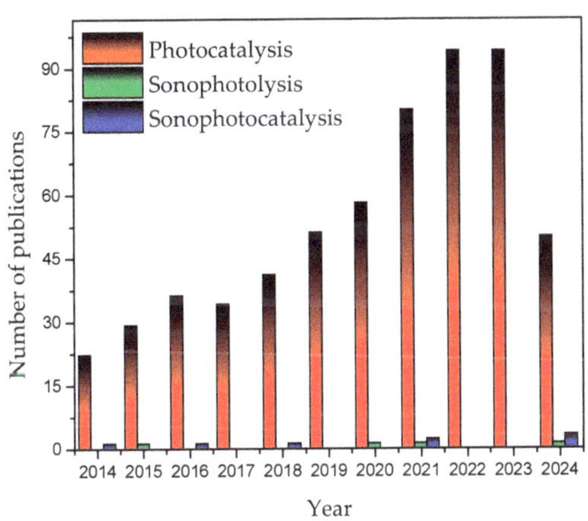

Figure 2. The number of publications on photocatalysis, sonophotolysis, and sonophotocatalysis from 2014 to 2024 based on SCOPUS.

2.1. Heterogeneous Photocatalysis

Photocatalysis, another type of AOPs, is the combination of photochemistry and catalysis. Photocatalysis hinges on the necessity of both light and a catalyst to drive or expedite a chemical conversion. Essentially, it can be characterized as the "enhancement of a photoreaction in the presence of a catalyst". This definition encompasses photosensitization, wherein a chemical species undergoes photochemical modification due to the initial absorption of radiation by another chemical species referred to as the photosensitizer [43]. Photocatalysis can be divided into two types: homogeneous and heterogeneous. However, due to easier separation of catalyst particles from the reaction mixture, heterogeneous photocatalysis is more popular and practical. Thus, the further discussion in this review will cover this photocatalysis type [44].

The very first application of heterogeneous photocatalysis is dated to 1972, when Fujishima and Honda conducted photoelectrochemical water splitting using natural radiation [45]. Following this, in the late 1970s, intensive research in the field of heterogeneous photocatalysis commenced based on Fujishima and Honda's study, but in the absence of an electrochemical cell [46]. One of the numerous advantages of heterogeneous photocatalysis is the possibility of the complete mineralization of present pollutants in a gaseous or liquid phase into safe compounds such as water, carbon dioxide, and inorganic ions [47].

Heterogeneous photocatalysis revolves around photoreactions taking place specifically at the catalyst's surface. If the adsorbate undergoes photoexcitation initially and then interacts with the catalyst in its ground state, this process is termed a "sensitized photoreaction". Conversely, if the catalyst is photoexcited first, and then interacts with the adsorbate molecule in its ground state, it is labeled as a "catalyzed photoreaction". In most instances, when discussing heterogeneous photocatalysis, we are referring to semiconductor photocatalysis or semiconductor-sensitized photoreactions [43].

In an ideal photocatalytic process, organic pollutants undergo mineralization, transforming into carbon(IV) oxide (CO_2), water (H_2O), and mineral acids in the presence of catalysts and reactive oxidizing species. The initiation of photocatalytic reactions occurs as the catalyst particles absorb photons with energies higher than their bandgap energy, under illumination. Consequently, photo-induced electrons are transformed from the valence band (VB) to the conduction band (CB), generating positively charged holes (h^+_{VB}) and free electrons (e^-_{CB}) on the surface of the applied catalyst (Figure 3). It is crucial to mention that the photo-generated holes in the VB tend to recombine with the photo-excited electrons in the CB, dissipating energy as heat. Hence, the presence of oxygen as electron scavengers extends the recombination of e^-_{CB}–h^+_{VB} pairs, while producing $O_2^{\bullet-}$. The interaction of $O_2^{\bullet-}$ with OH^- may result in the generation of HO•. Notably, the HO• radicals serve as an immensely potent, non-selective oxidant, facilitating the partial or complete mineralization of organic compounds. Additionally, the substantial oxidative potential of the h^+_{VB} in the photocatalyst enables the direct oxidation of organic substances to reactive intermediaries [43]. The mentioned processes can be described as follows (Equations (1)–(6)):

$$\text{Catalyst} + hv \rightarrow h^+_{VB} + e^-_{CB} \tag{1}$$

$$h^+_{VB} + e^-_{CB} \rightarrow \text{heat} \tag{2}$$

$$e^-_{CB} + O_2 \rightarrow O_2^{\bullet-} \tag{3}$$

$$h^+_{VB} + \text{OH-} \rightarrow \text{HO}\bullet \tag{4}$$

$$\text{HO}\bullet + \text{R} - \text{H} \rightarrow \text{R}\bullet + H_2O \tag{5}$$

$$h^+_{VB} + \text{R} \rightarrow \text{R+} \rightarrow \text{Intermediates} \tag{6}$$

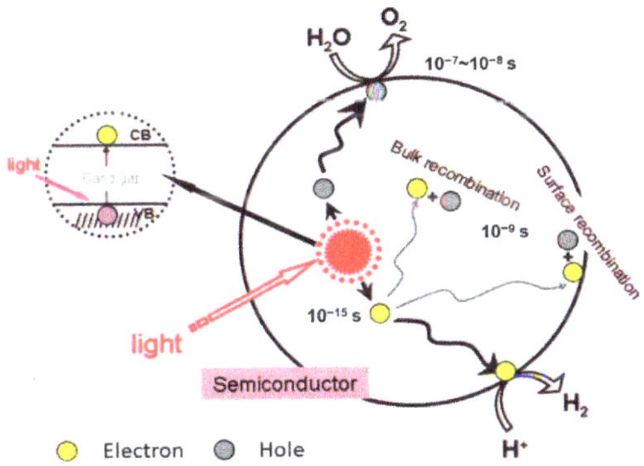

Figure 3. Mechanism of heterogeneous photocatalysis. Reprinted from Ref. [48] with permission, copyright Elsevier.

Heterogeneous photocatalysis with different photoactive materials can be efficiently employed in the removal of selected emerging organics, such as pharmaceutically active ingredients [22–25,49,50], pesticides [51–55], dyes [56–58], etc., from aquatic environments using simulated solar irradiation (SSI) or UV irradiation. Heterogeneous photocatalysis, while offering several advantages in environmental remediation and pollutant degradation, also comes with certain disadvantages: limited light absorption [59], catalyst recycling and separation challenges [60], surface recombination of charge carriers [61], potential toxicity of byproducts [62], and catalyst stability and durability [63]. Thus, it is necessary to improve the above-mentioned drawbacks.

2.2. Sonophotolysis

Since the early 20th century, ultrasound (US) has garnered significant attention for its ability to enhance chemical and physical effects in various processes. In the 1930s, it was observed that sonication lead to the breakdown of polymers [64]. Basically, ultrasound can be divided into three groups by intensity: low (20–100 kHz); medium (200–1000 kHz); and high (5000–10,000 kHz). In general, high-intensity US waves that come into contact with gases dissolved in liquid medium encourage acoustic cavitation, i.e., the formation, expansion, and implosive collapse of bubbles. US waves have cycles of compression and expansion. During expansion, bubbles can be generated if the waves have an intensity that can exceed the molecular forces of the liquid. These bubbles continually absorb energy from the alternating ultrasonic cycles of compression and expansion. Thus, bubbles grow (by diffusion of vapor or gas from the liquid medium) until they attain a critical size, at which point they collapse. This implosion creates a localized "hot spot" with extreme conditions of temperature (~5000 K), pressure (~1000 atm), and short life. Hence, water molecules and gases are being broken [64]. Additionally, the process can be further improved by introducing O_3, which thermally degrades within the microbubbles [42]. The mentioned processes can be described using the following Equations (7)–(14):

$$H_2O + \text{ultrasound} \rightarrow H^{\bullet} + HO\bullet \tag{7}$$

$$O_2 + \text{ultrasound} \rightarrow 2\,O\bullet \tag{8}$$

$$H_2O + O\bullet \rightarrow 2\,HO\bullet \tag{9}$$

$$O_2 + H\bullet \rightarrow O\bullet + HO\bullet \tag{10}$$

$$\text{Organic compounds} + HO\bullet \rightarrow \text{products} \tag{11}$$

$$O_3 + H_2O \rightarrow O_2 + 2\,HO\bullet \tag{12}$$

$$O_3 + HO\bullet + e- \rightarrow HO_2^- + O_2 \tag{13}$$

$$O_3 + HO_2^- \rightarrow HO\bullet + O_2^{\bullet-} + O_2 \quad (14)$$

There are various factors affecting the efficiency of sonochemical reactions: (a) ultrasound frequency—influences the cavitation process by altering the size of the bubbles and collapse time of the cavity [65]; (b) dissolved gas—the characteristics of dissolved gases, such as thermal conductivity or water solubility, have an impact on sonochemical activity (e.g., implosion temperature, heat transfer, etc.) [66]; (c) power input—an increase in ultrasonic power leads to higher levels of sonochemical activity in the liquid medium; regardless of the type of substance (volatile, hydrophobic, or hydrophilic), the response to ultrasonic power remains consistent [64]; (d) effect of bulk temperature—the highest temperature reached during bubble collapse is contingent upon the bulk temperature of the liquid [64]; and (e) pollutant concentration—since the pollutant concentration is dependent on the water source, it is an important factor. This influence is dependent on the type of organic pollutants (volatile or nonvolatile, hydrophilic or hydrophobic) [64].

The combination of ultrasound and light irradiation—sonophotolysis—is recognized as a highly effective reagent-free method for inactivating pathogenic microorganisms present in aqueous media, as well as for removing EOPs. While UV treatment has become a prevalent technology for water and wastewater disinfection, its efficacy can be significantly impacted by the quality of water and various constraints (light scattering and absorbance, cell shading and reactivation effects). In contrast, ultrasound disinfection is less affected by such factors. Therefore, ultrasonication can be regarded as a substitute standalone method, or be used in conjunction with UV radiation to enhance the overall treatment performance [67]. Moreover, the combination of these two techniques presents a more economically attractive option for wastewater treatment compared to using either technique individually. To reduce operational costs associated with ultrasound and UV treatment, researchers have explored combining these techniques with other AOPs, such as sono-hybrid and photo-hybrid processes [68]. The processes during sonophotolysis are represented in Figure 4. However, the number of studies is limited, i.e., there were three research articles published about organic pollutant removal using sonophotolysis in the last 10 years.

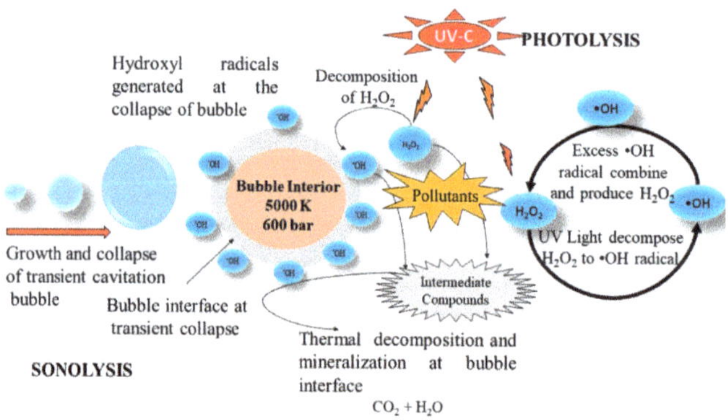

Figure 4. Processes during sonophotolysis. Reprinted with permission from Ref. [68], copyright Elsevier.

2.3. Sonophotocatalysis

The combination of sonolysis with photocatalysis facilitates a notably improved degradation of emerging pollutants. The heightened efficacy of sonophotocatalytic processes in eliminating toxic contaminants primarily stems from the synergistic interaction between photocatalysis and sonolysis. The fusion of these methodologies offers several advantages, including the enhanced formation of cavitation bubbles through ultrasound waves in the presence of solid catalysts, along with an increased production of ultrasonic cavitation bubbles and free radicals via the separation of e_{CB}^-–h_{VB}^+ pairs in the semiconductor photocatalyst. Additionally, ultrasound waves consistently cleanse the surface of the photocatalyst,

thereby boosting and sustaining its performance over an extended period (Figure 5). Moreover, the integration of both techniques facilitates the degradation of both hydrophobic and hydrophilic organic pollutants [69].

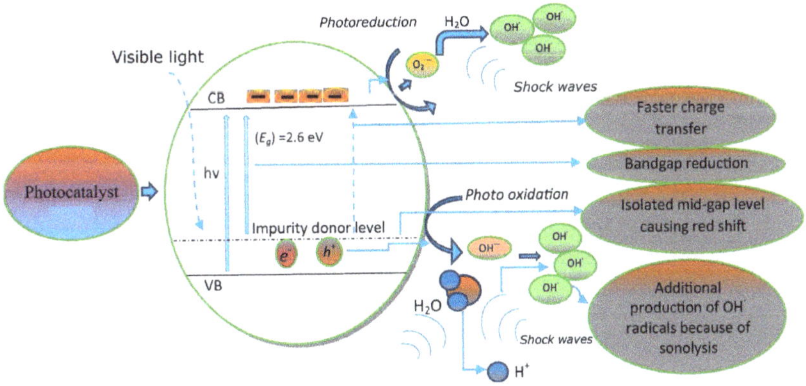

Figure 5. Mechanism of sonophotocatalysis. Reprinted with permission from Ref. [70], copyright Elsevier.

Apart from the irradiation sources, namely, ultrasound and light, the overall effectiveness of sonophotocatalysis is heavily reliant on the characteristics of the materials involved, known as sonophotocatalysts, and their proficiency in generating an adequate amount of reactive oxygen species. Hence, suitable sonophotocatalysts must possess the capability to responsively interact with both ultrasound irradiation and light, while preserving favorable chemical- and photo-stability, commendable electronic properties, and efficiency, along with minimal toxicity and cost-effectiveness. Semiconductor materials are frequently favored due to their pivotal role in reducing the energy barrier for the generation of cavitation bubbles in the process of sonocatalysis, alongside their ability to harvest light, facilitating the photogeneration of e^-_{CB}–h^+_{VB} pairs during the photocatalytic process [71].

Even though there is a limited number of articles about the employment of sonophotocatalysis in the removal of organic pollutants, the published studies showed promising results. Namely, various organics were effectively removed from the environment, for instance, methylene blue [72], phenol [17], phthalocyanine pigment [73], and 17β-estradiol [74].

The aim of this review is to give readers a comprehensive revision guide about the up-to-date achievements of photocatalysis, sonophotolysis, and sonophotocatalysis, with the most recent published studies.

3. State-of-the-Art Application of AOPs

The following provides the latest research data on photocatalysis, sonophotolysis, and the synergistic effects observed in the combined process known as sonophotocatalysis. A summary of the reviewed studies is represented in Table 1, while the main strengths and weaknesses of each individual process are given in Figure 6.

Table 1. Summary of efficiency of sonophotolysis, photocatalysis, and sonophotocatalysis.

Organic Pollutant	Type of *AOPs*	Removal Efficiency (%)	Reference
	Photocatalysis		
Alprazolam	Heterogeneous photocatalysis with ZnO and TiO_2 P25, under UV irradiation	100	[75]
Phenol	Heterogeneous photocatalysis with ZnO under UV irradiation	55	[17]
Mesotrione	Heterogeneous photocatalysis with ZnO and TiO_2 P25 under UV	100	[76]

Table 1. *Cont.*

Organic Pollutant	Type of *AOPs*	Removal Efficiency (%)	Reference
	Photocatalysis		
Alprazolam	Heterogeneous photocatalysis zinc–tin oxide nanocrystalline powders (both ternary and coupled binary) under UV irradiation	90–100 depending on catalyst type	[77]
Amitriptyline	Heterogeneous photocatalysis with ZnO/SnO_2, ZnO, and TiO_2 P25 under UV irradiation	80	[78]
Direct blue 71	Heterogeneous photocatalysis with Cu-doped ZnO under visible light	96	[79]
Alprazolam	Heterogeneous photocatalysis with ZnO and TiO_2 Degussa P25 under UVA, visible, and solar irradiation	100 (UV/ZnO)	[80]
Cefotaxime	Heterogeneous photocatalysis with ZnO under SSI	90.6	[81]
Atrazine	Heterogeneous photocatalysis with mixed oxide catalysts (ZnO/TiO_2) using various ZnO concentrations, under UV irradiation	97.5 (5% ZnO/TiO_2) 94 (10% ZnO/TiO_2)	[82]
Mesotrione	Heterogeneous photocatalysis with ZnO and TiO_2 under UV irradiation	40 (ground water and ZnO) 50 (river water and ZnO)	[83]
Acid red 18	Heterogeneous photocatalysis with ZnO-Ag-Nd under UV irradiation	100	[84]
Ibuprofen	Heterogeneous photocatalysis with TiO_2 and ZnO under UV irradiation	99	[85]
Two fungicides (vinclozoline and fenarimol) and four insecticides (malathion, fenotrothion, quinalphos, and dimethoate)	Heterogeneous photocatalysis with ZnO in pilot plant under artificial light	92 (DOC)	[86]
Methylene blue	Heterogeneous photocatalysis with reduced graphene oxide-N-ZnO, under visible irradiation	98.5	[87]
Selected organic compounds (tetrachlorethylene; chlorodifluoroacetamide; amphetamine; dibutyl phthalate; (2,3-dihydroxypropyl Z)-9-octadecenoate; fluoxetine; furazan; phenylpropanolamine; phthalic acid; 1,2-benzisothiazol-3-amine; 2,3-dihydroxypropyl elaidate)	Heterogeneous photocatalysis with ZnO/TiO_2 and TiO_2 catalysts, under SSI	85.5	[88]
Wastewater with various organics	Heterogeneous photocatalysis with ZnO immobilized on polystyrene pellets under UV irradiation	61.7 (TOC)	[89]
Two antibiotics (ciprofloxacin and ceftriaxone) and two herbicides (tembotrione and fluroxypyr).	Heterogeneous photocatalysis with TiO_2, ZnO, and MgO under UV and SSI	90–100 (depending on pollutant, under UV) 70–100 (depending on pollutant, under SSI)	[90]
Amitriptyline hydrochloride	Heterogeneous photocatalysis under UV and SSI using ZnO, TiO_2 P25, and TiO_2 Hombikat	30 (TOC)	[50]

Table 1. *Cont.*

Organic Pollutant	Type of *AOPs*	Removal Efficiency (%)	Reference
	Photocatalysis		
4-bromophenol and diethyl phthalate	Heterogeneous photocatalysis with nanocomposites composed of reduced graphene oxide and ZnO under UV irradiation	99 (4-bromophenol) 98.6 (diethyl phthalate)	[91]
Phenol	Heterogeneous photocatalysis with $CdO/ZnO/Yb_2O_3$ under SSI	71.5 97.8 (with H_2O_2)	[92]
p-nitrophenol	Heterogeneous photocatalysis under UV irradiation using ZnO	80	[93]
Penicillin G	Heterogeneous photocatalysis with graphitic carbon nitride–calcium or magnesium co-doped cobalt ferrite–zinc oxide nanocomposite under natural sunlight	74	[94]
Various organics	Heterogeneous photocatalysis with ZnO nanoparticles under natural sunlight	17.1 (COD) 71.7 (BOD)	[95]
Clomazone, amitriptyline, and sulcotrione	Heterogeneous photocatalysis with ZnO under SSI	20–70% (depending on the pollutant)	[96]
Phenol, o-cresol, toluene, and xylene	Heterogeneous photocatalysis with green ZnO under SSI	51 52 88 93	[97]
Methylene blue dye	Heterogeneous photocatalysis with Ag/ZnO-ZnS/PANI under UV irradiation	95	[31]
Methylene orange and nitrophenol	Heterogeneous photocatalysis with chromium-doped ZnO under UV irradiation	99 98.2	[98]
Phenol	Heterogeneous photocatalysis with ZnO under UV and solar irradiation	>25	[99]
Rhodamine B	Heterogeneous photocatalysis with ZnO under natural sunlight and UV irradiation	91 (sunlight) 99 (UV)	[100]
Docosane	Heterogeneous photocatalysis with ZnO nanorods under natural sunlight	68.5	[101]
Clomazone, ciprofloxacin, and 17α-ethynilestradiol	Heterogeneous photocatalysis with ZnO/MeOx nanopowders (ZnO/MgO, ZnO/CeO_2, and ZnO/ZrO_2) under SSI	77 86 71	[25]
Acid blue 25	Heterogeneous photocatalysis with TiO2-ZnO/coal fly ash under UV irradiation	98	[102]
	Sonophotolysis/sonocatalysis		
Ibuprofen Sulfamethoxazole	Sonolysis	97 92	[103]
Ciprofloxacin	Sonocatalysis	61	[104]
	Sonophotocatalysis		
Acid red 17	Sonophotocatalysis with Pt/CeO_2	90	[105]
Amoxicilin	Sonophotocatalysis with N-doped TiO_2	37	[19]
Flonicamid	Sonophotocatalysis with CuO, ZnO, and TiO_2	98.36 (COD, for TiO_2)	[106]
Tetracycline	Sonophotocatalysis with TiO_2 decorated on magnetic activated carbon	93	[107]

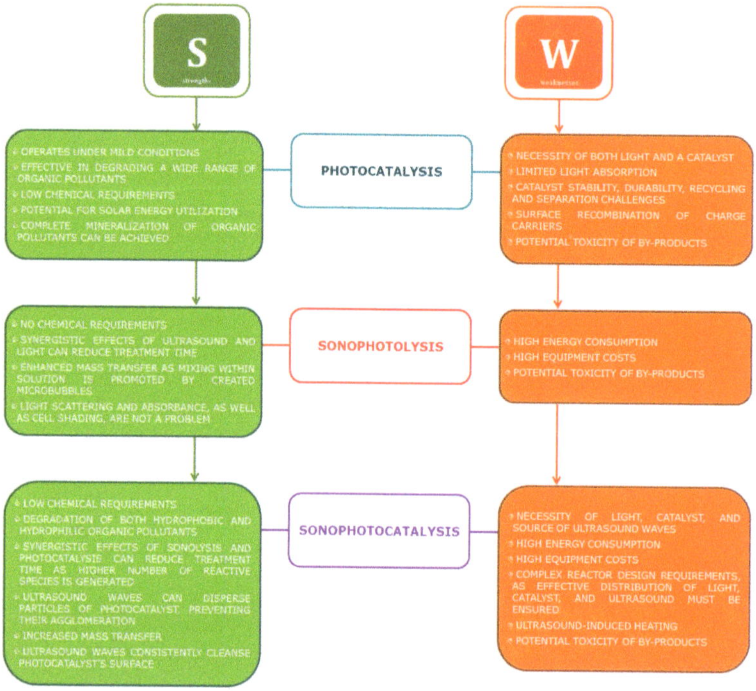

Figure 6. Strengths and weaknesses of selected AOPs.

3.1. *Photocatalysis*

Heterogeneous photocatalysis is a highly researched topic among scientists. By the application of an adequate semiconductor as a photocatalyst, promising results can be achieved in the removal of various organics from the environment, such as drugs, pesticides, or dyes. In this section, the latest results will be highlighted.

For instance, Ivetić et al. [75] synthesized Mg-doped ZnO nanocrystallites via a conventional solid-state reaction and used them in the degradation of the anxiolytic drug alprazolam, under UV irradiation. The impact of annealing temperature on the structural and optical properties of the resulting nanomaterial was examined with X-ray powder diffraction (XRD), scanning electron microscope (SEM), mercury intrusion porosimetry (MIP), Raman spectroscopy (Raman), and ultraviolet–visible diffuse reflectance spectroscopy (UV–Vis DRS). Moreover, the effectiveness of Mg-doped ZnO in the photocatalytic degradation of alprazolam was compared with the efficiency of pure ZnO and TiO_2 Degussa P25 photocatalysts. The obtained results showed a complete removal efficiency of alprazolam, both in the presence of the newly synthesized Mg-doped ZnO, annealed at 700 °C, and in the presence of commercially available ZnO and TiO_2 Degussa P25, after 60 min of UV irradiation.

Jyothi et al. [17] examined the effectiveness of various AOPs, including ZnO-mediated sono-/photocatalysis, for removing phenol from water at ambient conditions. Their findings indicated that phenol degradation followed the sequence sonophotocatalysis > photocatalysis > sonocatalysis > sonolysis > photolysis. Specifically, the employment of photocatalysis resulted in a 55% removal of phenol, under UV irradiation.

In the research carried out by Šojić et al. [76], the photocatalytic degradation of the herbicide mesotrione was investigated in aqueous suspensions of TiO_2 Degussa P25 and ZnO, considering various operational parameters, such as the type of catalyst and light source, catalyst loading, and initial pH. The findings clearly demonstrated that photocatalytic treatment utilizing TiO_2 Degussa P25 and ZnO with UV irradiation effectively removed mesotrione from water. Namely, complete removal was accomplished after 15 min of UV irradiation, while the mineralization of mesotrione was completed after about 4 h. Applying the liquid chromatography–electrospray ionization–tandem mass spectrometry (LC–ESI–MS/MS) method, several intermediates were identified, suggesting that the degradation pathways with TiO_2 Degussa P25 and ZnO may not be identical.

Additionally, Ivetić et al. [77] introduced the preparation and characterization of zinc–tin oxide nanocrystalline powders, both ternary and coupled binary types, via a straightforward solid-state mechanochemical method. The structural and optical properties of the resulting powder samples were investigated using XRD, SEM, Raman, and reflectance spectroscopy. The efficacy of the synthesized nanomaterials in the photocatalytic degradation of alprazolam under UV irradiation was assessed and compared with pure ZnO and SnO_2. The photocatalytic investigation revealed that mixed binary zinc–tin oxide catalysts displayed superior photocatalytic activity compared to their ternary counterparts.

Furthermore, Ivetić et al. [78] conducted a study involving the preparation of a ZnO/SnO_2 heterojunction through a straightforward three-step mechanochemical solid-state method. The phase composition, crystalline structure, morphology, and bandgap of the resulting coupled catalyst were extensively examined. The efficiency of these prepared materials was evaluated in the photocatalytic removal of amitriptyline under SSI and UV irradiation. The findings of this investigation demonstrate that ZnO/SnO_2 nanoparticles possess superior photocatalytic activity in comparison with both ZnO and the widely used TiO_2 Degussa P25 catalyst. Namely, 100% of amitriptyline was removed after 60 min of UV irradiation, while a slightly lower degradation efficiency (80%) was reached in the case of SSI.

In the study conducted by Thennarasu and Sivasamy [79], the detailed synthesis and characterization of Cu-doped ZnO were described. The synthesis involved the co-precipitation method, followed by a thorough characterization using various techniques, including XRD, field-emission scanning electron microscope (FE-SEM), transmission electron microscope (TEM), Fourier transform infrared spectroscopy (FT-IR), and UV–Vis DRS. The photocatalytic performance of the Cu-doped ZnO catalyst was evaluated in the degradation of direct blue 71 dye in an aqueous environment under visible light. Several factors, such as the pH of the aqueous suspension, duration of irradiation, quantity of photocatalyst used, and initial dye concentration, influenced the extent of degradation. The optimal pH for achieving maximum photocatalytic degradation was determined to be 6.8. Furthermore, it was found that 3 mg/mL of Cu-doped ZnO was the ideal amount for complete degradation of the investigated dye at a concentration of 0.01 g/L. The photocatalyst reusability was assessed, revealing that up to 96% of direct blue 71 dye was degraded even after three cycles of usage, employing visible light. Additionally, chemical oxygen demand (COD) and electrospray ionization–mass spectrometry analyses confirmed the complete mineralization of direct blue 71 dye molecules.

Finčur et al. [80] conducted a comprehensive investigation into the photocatalytic degradation of alprazolam, using heterogeneous photocatalysis, with ZnO and TiO_2 Degussa P25 as photocatalysts. The study explored various factors, including the type of irradiation (UVA, visible light, solar), photocatalyst type, photocatalyst loading, pH value, and the presence of $HO^{\bullet}$ radical and h^+_{VB} scavengers. The findings clearly demonstrate that the UV/ZnO system was more efficient in alprazolam removal, since a complete removal efficiency was found after 10 min of UV irradiation. A detailed analysis of degradation intermediates using LC–ESI–MS/MS suggested that the degradation pathways with ZnO and TiO_2 Degussa P25 might differ. Additionally, reutilization experiments with ZnO showed that the photocatalyst stayed effective after three runs.

León et al. [81] presented a study of the photocatalytic removal of the antibiotic cefotaxime from aqueous solutions utilizing SSI in the presence of ZnO. Photocatalytic experiments on cefotaxime (20.0 mg/L) were conducted in a sunlight simulator equipped with a xenon lamp. A central composite circumscribed experimental design was employed to evaluate the impact of the catalyst loading and initial pH value on cefotaxime removal efficiency. The acquired results established that the optimized conditions that led to the highest pollutant removal (90.6%) after 8 min of phototreatment were pH = 7.5, ZnO loading = 1.45 g/L, under SSI. In the scavenger experiments, it was concluded that both $HO^{\bullet}$ radicals and h^{+} participate in cefotaxime removal using ZnO. Lastly, a dissolved organic carbon (DOC) analysis confirmed that it was possible to reduce the organic matter present in the systems by photocatalytic treatment.

Silva et al. [82] carried out a study to assess the efficacy of mixed oxide catalysts (ZnO/TiO_2) with varying ZnO concentrations (5, 8, 10, and 15 wt. %) in the photocatalysis of atrazine in aqueous solutions under UV irradiation. The catalysts underwent preparation via wet impregnation and were subjected to characterization via parameters such as specific surface area (Brunauer–Emmett–Teller (BET) method), pore diameter, pore volume, XRD, thermogravimetric analysis (TGA), and SEM. Photocatalytic experiments were carried out in a batch-type reactor, and the resulting products were scrutinized using high-performance liquid chromatography (HPLC) and UV–Vis spectrophotometry at λ_{max} = 221 nm to track the atrazine's behavior throughout the process. The findings unveiled that the catalyst labeled as 5% ZnO/TiO_2 and 10% ZnO/TiO_2 exhibited the highest photocatalytic performance, achieving a complete degradation of atrazine and partial mineralization of the byproducts. Specifically, after 10 min of the process, the percentages of removal were recorded as 97.5 and 94% for the 5% ZnO/TiO_2 and 10% ZnO/TiO_2 catalysts, respectively.

The study of Šojić Merkulov et al. [83] sought to investigate how ground and river water matrices influence the photocatalytic removal of mesotrione, the active ingredient of Callisto®. The results showed that under UV irradiation, ZnO exhibited a higher efficiency in degrading mesotrione compared to TiO_2, in both ground and river water, whilst a comparable degradation efficiency was observed for both photocatalysts in distilled deionized water. The ZnO/SSI system reduced the concentration of mesotrione by approximately 40% and 50% in the ground and river water, respectively. Furthermore, ground and river water as the matrix significantly diminished the removal rate (approximately by 1.5 and 4 times for ZnO and TiO_2, respectively) during mesotrione photocatalytic oxidation under UV irradiation.

The well-known role of heterogeneous photocatalysis in solving water pollution issues was put to use by Azadi et al. [84] to remove the organic dye acid red 18. The process was carried out for 180 min in a semi-batch photoreactor using UV light, applying a zinc oxide–silver–neodymium (ZnO-Ag-Nd) nanocomposite, synthesized via the combustion method, and later characterized using XRD, FT-IR spectroscopy, and SEM. The degradation kinetics were evaluated by altering several experimental parameters (photocatalyst loading, initial pH value, and substrate concentration). The treatment process efficiency was determined by spectrophotometric analysis, following the decolorization of the solution at λ_{max} = 507 nm. After the optimization of the treatment conditions (catalyst loading = 0.08 mg/mL, pH value = 6.2, and low concentration of dye solution), total organic carbon (TOC) measurements were performed to assess the mineralization degree, i.e., the degradation of the dye after heterogeneous photocatalysis. The obtained results showed that the degradation degree was always below the degree of decolorization. Namely, after 180 min of treatment in the presence of ZnO-Ag-Nd under UV irradiation, around 65% of organic matter was transformed into inorganic, while the decolorization of the acid red 18 dye was almost 100%.

Tanveer et al. [85] studied the degradation of ibuprofen under UV and solar irradiation using two photocatalysts, TiO_2 and ZnO. Various catalyst loadings, ranging from 0.1 to 2.0 mg/mL, were tested for both types of catalysts, and the effect of pH value on degradation rate was examined across acidic, neutral, and basic pH. In addition to a degradation rate analysis, TOC and COD analyses were conducted under optimized conditions including catalyst loading, pH, and radiation source. An optimal ZnO loading of 1.0 mg/mL was identified for ibuprofen degradation in an aqueous environment. In addition, ZnO-based experiments demonstrated higher degradation rates under neutral conditions (pH 7.0). Furthermore, the degradation performance and TOC, COD removal

rates were higher under UV irradiation compared to solar setups, whether utilizing quartz or borosilicate assemblies. Overall, UV-based catalysis proved to be a more effective option for addressing pharmaceutical pollutants compared to solar photocatalysis. Namely, 99% of ibuprofen was removed after 15 min of UV irradiation with TiO_2, while the overall mineralization, based on TOC, after the same time was 32%.

In the work of Vela et al. [86], the photocatalytic removal of two fungicides (fenarimol and vinclozoline) and four insecticides (dimethoate fenotrothion, malathion, and quinalphos) under natural sunlight at a pilot plant scale was presented. The approach integrated $HO^{\bullet}$ radical- and sulfate radical-based AOPs, utilizing ZnO as a photocatalyst and $Na_2S_2O_8$ as an oxidant, respectively. Preliminary experiments involved optimizing catalyst loading, electron acceptor effects, and pH in a laboratory photoreactor under artificial light. Subsequently, the study included 200 mg/L of ZnO and 250 mg/L of $Na_2S_2O_8$ at a pH of about 7 for further experiments at pilot plant scale. The findings indicated a significant enhancement in the reaction rate of the targeted pesticides when utilizing the tandem $ZnO/Na_2S_2O_8$ system compared to photolytic testing. At the end of the treatment, the remaining DOC percentage was substantially below its initial amount, with an up to 92% reduction.

The study conducted by Suresh and Sivasamy [87] focuses on a novel nanocomposite photocatalyst, reduced graphene oxide–N-ZnO, which exhibits visible light activity. This photocatalyst was prepared using the hydrothermal technique, and characterization of the synthesized nanocomposite was carried out using various techniques including XRD, FT-IR, UV–Vis DRS, FE-SEM, atomic force microscopic (AFM), X-ray photoelectron spectroscopy (XPS), and BET analyses. The degradation of methylene blue under visible light supported the estimation of the reduced graphene oxide–N-ZnO nanocomposite's photocatalytic performance. The nanocomposite exhibited significantly enhanced degradation, achieving the upper limit of methylene blue degradation (98.5%) after 120 min of irradiation with visible light.

Ángel-Hernández et al. [88] employed a heterogeneous photocatalytic process in order to reduce the initial concentrations of various organics present in wastewater treatment plant (WWTP) effluent using ZnO/TiO_2 and TiO_2 catalysts, synthesized via the sol–gel method. Newly synthesized materials were characterized by XRD and SEM techniques. A total of eleven organic compounds (tetrachlorethylene; chlorodifluoroacetamide; amphetamine; dibutyl phthalate; (2,3-dihydroxypropyl Z)-9-octadecenoate; fluoxetine; furazan; phenylpropanolamine; phthalic acid; 1,2-benzisothiazol-3-amine; 2,3-dihydroxypropyl elaidate), detected via gas chromatography–mass spectrometry (GC–MS) analysis of the water sample, were subjected to photocatalytic removal using both artificial UV and natural solar light. Namely, a batch reactor was equipped with a UV lamp, whereas the solar reactor was utilizing natural sunlight. A solar collector with ZnO/TiO_2 proved to be the best option for several reasons. Firstly, the amount of total suspended solids removed after heterogeneous photocatalytic process was 85.5%. Secondly, the production price of the ZnO/TiO_2 catalyst was rather low. And finally, this treatment combination is simple, low-cost, and environmentally friendly, given that it demands electrical energy only for the stirring of the reaction mixture.

Caracciolo et al. [89] studied the photocatalytic treatment of four different water samples coming from the WWTP of leather industries, using a commercially available ZnO immobilized on polystyrene pellets (ZnO/PS). Photocatalytic degradation experiments were carried out in a cylindrical Pyrex photoreactor surrounded with four UV lamps placed at the same distance from the external photoreactor surface. The reaction progress was examined with regard to the residual COD and TOC. After 7 h of UV irradiation in the presence of ZnO/PS with 0.5 mg/mL photocatalyst loading, the average removal of pollutants present in four different wastewater samples amounted to 63.4% COD and 61.7% TOC.

Finčur et al. [90] reported the synthesis of TiO_2, ZnO, and MgO nanoparticles using the sol–gel method, followed by an investigation into their structural and morphological properties through XRD, FTIR, UV–Vis DRS, BET, and SEM/EDX techniques. A comparative analysis was conducted on the photocatalytic performance of these nanopowders in degrading two antibiotics (ceftriaxone and ciprofloxacin) and two herbicides (fluroxypyr and tembotrione). TiO_2 emerged as the most effective nanopowder under UV and SSI. Specifically, the introduction of $(NH_4)_2S_2O_8$ in low concentrations was found to accelerate the removal of both antibiotics and the herbicide fluroxypyr in the presence of TiO_2. LC–ESI–MS analysis identified several degradation intermediates of ciprofloxacin, tembotrione, and fluroxypyr, suggesting that $HO^{\bullet}$ radicals primarily drive the transformations of selected pollutants.

Work carried out by Finčur et al. [50] was focused on the investigation of the kinetics, mineralization, and toxicological effects of the antidepressant drug amitriptyline hydrochloride in UV- or solar-illuminated aqueous suspensions of ZnO, TiO_2 Degussa P25 and TiO_2 Hombikat. The findings suggest that ZnO effectively catalyzed the photodegradation of amitriptyline in the presence of oxygen and under solar light. The degradation rate was influenced by various parameters, including catalyst loading, the initial substrate concentration, and the presence or absence of electron acceptors such as molecular oxygen, $HO^{\bullet}$ radicals, and h^+ scavengers. The optimal loading of the photocatalyst was experimentally determined to be 1.0 mg/mL. Additionally, the degradation rate increased with higher initial concentrations of amitriptyline. The presence of H_2O_2 and $(NH_4)_2S_2O_8$ as electron acceptors initially decreased the reaction rate, while $KBrO_3$ slightly increased the degradation rate of amitriptyline. Moreover, ethanol inhibited the photodegradation of amitriptyline more than NaI, indicating that the reaction mechanism primarily relies on free $HO^{\bullet}$ radicals, with partial involvement of h^+_{VB}. Generally, a ~30% level of TOC decrease was found after 240 min of SSI.

The positive qualities of photocatalysis were also harnessed by Kumar et al. [91]. In their study of 4-bromophenol and diethyl phthalate removal from an aqueous environment, nanocomposites composed of reduced graphene oxide and ZnO (rGZ), synthesized with a high-temperature refluxing method, were used as photocatalysts. Techniques including XRD, FE-SEM, UV–Vis DRS, Raman, and FT-IR were used to study the properties of the nanocomposites. Degradation studies of the aqueous solutions of selected pollutants (10 ppm) were performed for 180 min under UV light, while an HPLC analysis was employed to follow 4-bromophenol and diethyl phthalate photocatalytic degradation. Several rGZ nanocomposites were prepared with an altered wt. % ratio of graphene oxide and ZnO, and among them, the superior photocatalytic efficiency in the degradation of both pollutants was displayed by rGZ nanocomposite with 5% of ZnO (rGZ-5). Subsequent photocatalytic degradation experiments were performed using different loadings of rGZ-5, and in the light of the obtained results, it was established that 0.8 mg/mL was the optimal loading. This setting brought forth the elimination of 99 and 98.6% of 4-bromophenol and diethyl phthalate, respectively.

The research of Li et al. [92] was focused on the sustainable heterogeneous photocatalytic treatment of phenol, which is a common organic persistent pollutant in industrial wastewaters. For this purpose the authors developed a cadmium oxide/zinc oxide/ytterbium(III) oxide ($CdO/ZnO/Yb_2O_3$) composite through a simple one-pot hydrophile synthesis pathway. The synthesized materials were then described in detail by UV–Vis DRS, FTIR, XRD, FE-SEM, TEM, energy-dispersive X-ray spectroscopy (EDS), and XPS techniques. The degradation of phenol (5.0 mg/L) was carried out at the natural pH value in a custom-made photoreactor under SSI. The degradation samples were analyzed at λ_{max} = 271 nm using UV–Vis absorption spectroscopy. After 15 min of photocatalytic treatment, the degradation of the phenol by the $CdO/ZnO/Yb_2O_3$ photocatalyst (0.67 mg/mL) reached 71.5%. Afterwards, the authors managed to improve the removal efficiency of phenol up to 97.8% by conducting photocatalytic experiments with the addition of H_2O_2 and isopropyl alcohol.

In the research conducted by Mahy et al. [93] the effectiveness of the UV-assisted heterogeneous photocatalysis of *p*-nitrophenol was explored in the presence of ZnO nanopar-

ticles, synthesized by a sol–gel method and characterized by XRD, BET, TEM, UV–Vis DRS, and XPS techniques. The photocatalytic degradation process of the selected pollutant (0.1 mmol/L) was conducted in a quartz sealed round-bottom flask that was exposed to two/four UV lamps after the addition of 10 mg of each ZnO nanomaterial. The reduction in the p-nitrophenol concentration was measured by UV–Vis spectroscopy at λ_{max} = 317 nm. The influence of the ZnO nanoparticles' distinctive morphology (nanotubes, nanorods, and nanospheres) on the photocatalytic activity was put to test. The following conclusion was drawn: with the increase in the photocatalyst particle size, its catalytic activity decreased. Namely, in the presence of Z19, which is the ZnO nanomaterial with the smallest particle size (8.3 nm), a 52% removal of *p*-nitrophenol was achieved under the illumination of two UV lamps. To enhance the photocatalytic degradation of p-nitrophenol in the presence of the same nanopowder, authors irradiated p-nitrophenol solution with four UV lamps and reached a removal efficacy equal to 80% after 7 h of the process. Z19 photocatalyst's reusability was inspected in three consecutive runs, and it was observed that the material kept its integrity for 21 h.

In the research by Baladi et al. [94], penicillin G was subjected to heterogeneous photocatalytic removal. The experiments were performed in an aqueous environment utilizing natural sunlight at room temperature, and in the presence of a graphitic carbon nitride–calcium or magnesium co-doped cobalt ferrite–zinc oxide nanocomposite (gCN-Ca, Mg doped CFO-ZnO), prepared via the hydrothermal method and characterized by powder XRD, FT-IR, Raman, FE-SEM, TEM, EDS, DRS, vibrating sample magnetometer (VSM), and photoluminescence (PL) techniques. By applying a magnetic field, the magnetic composites were effortlessly separated from the reaction mixture. Photocatalytic experiments aimed to investigate several experimental parameters such as irradiation time, initial pH value, and initial substrate concentration, as well as the ZnO ratio in the nanocomposites. The removal of the antibiotic was monitored using UV–Vis spectrometry. As expected, prolonged irradiation time led to an increase in the penicillin G degradation degree in the presence of all studied nanocomposites. Among the three examined novel materials with different ZnO content, the one with 33.3% of ZnO displayed the highest degradation efficiency of penicillin G, regardless of the photocatalytic treatment length. Next, the degradation of penicillin G in the presence of gCN-Ca, Mg-doped CFO-ZnO (33.3%) nanocomposite was favored in the acidic environment and at a lower initial antibiotic concentration. Therefore, the highest penicillin G degradation efficiency of 74% was accomplished under the following optimal conditions: time of irradiation = 120 min, pH value = 5, penicillin G concentration = 10 ppm, and gCN–CFO–ZnO (33.3%) loading = 1.0 mg/mL.

Tamashiro et al. [95], in their research study, represented the synthesis of ZnO nanoparticles, using the precipitation of zinc sulfate heptahydrate and sodium hydroxide. The synthesized photocatalyst was applied in heterogeneous photocatalysis for diminishing COD and biochemical oxygen demand (BOD), as well as for antimicrobial purposes. Microscopic analysis indicated the presence of *Saccharomyces cerevisiae* microorganisms in vinasse, with the minimum inhibitory concentration for ZnO nanoparticles determined as 1.56 mg/mL. Under sunlight exposure for 4 h, photocatalysis with 40 mg/L of ZnO nanoparticles led to a 17.1% and 71.7% reduction in COD and BOD, respectively. This research underscores the feasibility of ZnO nanoparticles utilization in vinasse treatment, promoting sustainable practices, and mitigating the environmental repercussions of fertigation.

Despotović et al. [96] showed the synthesis of ZnO nanoparticles via the precipitation method, using water and ethanol solutions of zinc acetate dihydrate and zinc nitrate hexahydrate as the corresponding metal precursors. As-synthesized catalysts were afterwards calcined at various temperatures, and their structure and morphology were characterized using diverse techniques such as XRD, BET, and SEM. Also, the photocatalytic performance of the newly synthesized nanoparticles under SSI was evaluated for the removal of the antidepressant drug amitriptyline and the pesticide clomazone. The results showed that ZnO nanoparticles prepared from the water solution of zinc acetate dihydrate and calcined at 500 °C exhibited the highest efficiency under SSI. Additionally, the impact of initial pH was investigated. It was observed that the initial pH had no effect on the removal of clomazone, while for amitriptyline, the reaction rate constant slightly increased within a pH range from approximately 7 to 10.

Solar-assisted heterogeneous photocatalysis was put to use in the study by El Golli [97], with the intention of removing four aromatic (toluene, phenol, o-cresol, and xylene) hydrocarbons, frequently found in refinery effluent. ZnO nanoparticles synthesized via a conventional chemical route (chem-ZnO) and green ZnO nanoparticles (green-ZnO), prepared via a green synthesis route using *Moringa oleifera* leaves extract, were applied as photocatalysts. Materials were characterized by UV–Vis, XRD, FE-SEM, TEM, BET, and Barrett–Joyner–Halenda (BJH) analyses. The sets of experiments were conducted in a borosilicate photoreactor equipped with a xenon lamp placed in a solar box to simulate sunlight. Following the removal of target pollutants, an HPLC analysis was employed. Through the catalyst adsorption and catalyst loading experiments, both conducted at three identical levels, the optimal catalyst loading was determined to be 0.25 mg/mL. The impact of the initial pH value on the removal efficiency of the target pollutants was studied at four levels in the presence of the catalyst at the optimal loading. It was concluded that a neutral pH value increased the degradation degree of all the studied aromatic hydrocarbons. And finally, in comparison with the chem-ZnO nanoparticles, the green-ZnO nanoparticles exhibited greater degradation effectiveness in the heterogeneous photocatalysis of o-cresol, phenol, toluene, and xylene, with a respective 51, 52, 88, and 93% removal efficiency after 180 min of the process.

As a promising AOP, photocatalysis was employed by Khan et al. [31] for the degradation of methylene blue dye, which has the status of a usual persistent organic pollutant in the textile industry. Used photocatalysts, silver-doped zinc oxide–zinc sulfide–polyaniline composites (Ag/ZnO-ZnS/PANI), were made through a simple and straightforward co-precipitation method, followed by ultrasonic-assisted Ag deposition and subsequent in situ oxidative polymerization. Different techniques like FTIR, XRD, SEM, EDS, and XPS were engaged to describe the properties of the new materials. The photocatalytic activity of several Ag/ZnO-ZnS/PANI photocatalysts was investigated using a digital UV light chamber with six UV lamps, whilst methylene blue removal was monitored at λ_{max} = 664 nm by a double-beam UV spectrophotometer. To optimize the photocatalytic process, the influence of several parameters, such as pH value, catalyst loading, dye concentration, and irradiation time, was studied. In light of the findings, the optimal process parameters were as follows: pH value = 6, methylene blue dye concentration = 10 mg/L, photocatalyst loading = 0.05 mg/mL, and reaction time = 90 min. To avoid the electron/hole recombination process, the effect of H_2O_2 addition in different concentrations was examined, and the optimal oxidant dose proved to be 3.0 mmol/L. The authors also compared the efficiency of both immobilized and suspended photocatalysts, and the first one demonstrated superior efficiency, removing 95% of methylene blue after the process of photocatalysis. Additionally, a reusability study of the various Ag/ZnO-ZnS/PANI composites was conducted under optimal conditions, and the results showed that the photocatalytic activity was preserved even after five consecutive runs. And lastly, radical-scavenging tests in the presence of isopropyl alcohol, ascorbic acid, disodium ethylene diamine tetraacetate, and potassium dichromate revealed that $HO^\bullet$ radicals play the main role in the photocatalytic degradation of methylene blue.

The research conducted by Pavithra and Raj [98] explores the development of nanoporous chromium-doped ZnO as a sustainable, energy-efficient, and stable photocatalyst. The porous chromium-doped ZnO nanostructures were produced using an ultrasonic-assisted co-precipitation method, whereas techniques such as XRD, FT-IR, SEM, TEM, high resolution TEM, and BET were used for the characterization of the prepared nanostructures. Also, methylene orange and nitrophenol were removed up to 99% and 98.2%, respectively, with half-life degradation rate constants of 22 min and 26 min, under UV irradiation. An analysis of TOC in the treated water confirmed the successful degradation of xenobiotic molecules, indicating the potential for reusing the treated water.

Sarvothaman et al. [99], in their work, investigated the efficiency of different AOPs, a cavitation-mediated pre-treatment of ZnO, and cavitation photocatalysis peroxide-based hybrid processes. The pre-treatment method resulted in a >25% enhancement in phenol oxidation compared to conventional ZnO photocatalysis alone. Additionally, hydrodynamic cavitation photocatalysis with a peroxide-based system exhibited a cavitational yield five times greater than its acoustic cavitation counterpart. In the case of photocatalysis, the effect of radiation type (UV and sunlight) was investigated, and the results showed that the rate constant obtained for phenol conversion demonstrates an approximately five-fold increase when exposed to UV light compared to natural solar light.

Furthermore, a Thongam and Chaturvedi [100] study addressed the primary hurdles encountered in deploying photocatalytic water treatment. This was achieved by modifying the slurry system, removing the need for external triggering sources, and repurposing face mask fabric coated with ZnO to serve as a floating photocatalyst. The face mask fabric was dip-coated with ZnO photocatalysts (with the variations in synthesis medium, diethylene glycol, *N*,*N*-dimethylformamide, or water, and methods, precipitation or solvothermal), to serve as a floating agent for rhodamine B degradation under natural sunlight. The results revealed that distinct morphological structures resembling cauliflower, hydrangea, and petals can be obtained through variations in the synthesis medium and methods. These variations were found to be contingent upon the solvent properties. In addition, the obtained results showed that the degradation efficiency of rhodamine B was approximately 91% after 100 min of treatment, comparable to the 99% efficiency observed in the UV light-illuminated slurry system.

In the study by Alsharyani and Muruganandam [101], photocatalytic degradation of organic docosane solution was carried out in the presence of hexagonal-shaped ZnO nanorods, obtained via a microwave-assisted hydrothermal synthesis method and later grown on substrates made of glass. SEM, XRD, UV–Vis, and PL techniques were utilized to characterize novel material. The photocatalytic degradation of docosane (10 ppm) was performed in a solar simulator equipped with a xenon lamp, whilst the effectiveness was monitored by GC-MS/MS analysis. It was found that after 5 h of irradiation, 68.5% of the docosane was removed from the aqueous solution, and that the initial pH value gradually decreased towards the end of the process. The beneficial presence of ZnO nanorods was later confirmed with a TOC analysis, when 60.5% more docosane was removed by photocatalysis compared to photolysis.

The research of Bognár et al. [25] aimed to explore the effectiveness of newly synthesized binary coupled ZnO/MeO_x nanomaterials (ZnO/MgO, ZnO/CeO_2, and ZnO/ZrO_2) in the photocatalytic degradation of the pesticide clomazone and two pharmaceutically active compounds, 17α-ethynilestradiol and ciprofloxacin, under varying experimental conditions, such as catalyst loading and initial pH. Nanopowders were prepared by a three-step mechanochemical-assisted calcination method and characterized using XRD, SEM-EDS, TEM, DLS, Raman, UV–Vis DRS, and zeta potential analysis. Chemometrics helped in defining optimal photocatalytic experimental conditions. Under optimal experimental conditions, the presence of ZnO/ZrO_2 resulted in the highest degradation efficiency, with 71% of EE2, 77% of CLO, and 86% of CIP removed after 120 min of SSI.

Yusuff et al. [102] showed the synthesis of different TiO_2-ZnO/coal fly ash (CFA) photocatalysts (ZnO/CFA, TiO_2/CFA, and TiO_2-ZnO/CFA) using sol-gel and impregnation techniques, and their application for degrading acid blue 25 dye from an aquatic environment, in a photoreactor that provides UV light. In addition, the chemical structure, functional groups, texture, and optical properties of the binary and ternary composites were assessed using various spectroscopic techniques (XRF, XRD, BET, FTIR, UV–Vis DRS, TEM, and EDS). The results indicated that TiO_2-ZnO/CFA exhibited a faster degradation of acid blue 25 (98%) compared to ZnO/CFA and TiO_2/CFA, due to its dualistic photocatalytic sites. In addition to the evaluation of TiO_2-ZnO/CFA reusability, the optimal experimental conditions (initial acid blue 25 concentration, flow rate, UV light intensity, and time of irradiation) required for achieving maximum removal efficiency were investigated.

3.2. Sonophotolysis

The first process which will be discussed in this review is sonophotolysis. However, in order to obtain a more detailed picture about the efficacy of ultrasound, some data will be given on sonolysis, as well.

First of all, in the study by Gao et al. [108], the inactivation of Enterobacter aerogenes in skim milk using both low-frequency (20 kHz) and high-frequency (850 kHz) ultrasonication was examined. Low-frequency acoustic cavitation inflicted lethal damage to the target, which proved more vulnerable to ultrasound in water than in skim milk due to the varying protein concentrations. However, even at powers as high as 50 W for 60 min, high-frequency US failed to inactivate E. aerogenes in milk. Interestingly, while the high-frequency US treatment of milk induced no physical alterations, low-frequency ultrasonication reduced particle size and milk viscosity.

Another antibacterial activity of US was observed in the study by Gemici et al. [109], who delved into the synergistic effects of US and UV processes in inactivating Escherichia coli in a simulated aqueous environment. Their findings showcased the potential of a hybrid antibacterial approach integrating silver columns with US and UV, offering an effective means of water disinfection, while mitigating environmental risks and overcoming individual limitations associated with traditional disinfection methods.

The first-time successful coupling of photo-Fenton processes and US was witnessed in the study by Giannakis et al. [110], for *Escherichia coli* inactivation in secondary treated effluent. They employed sequential high-frequency/low-power sonication, followed by mild photo-Fenton treatment under SSI. The study aimed to assess the individual contributions of Fenton reaction, US, and irradiation towards removal rates and long-term bacterial survival. The results highlighted a significant enhancement in treatment efficiency, with the coupled process achieving total inactivation within a 4 h treatment period. Furthermore, the study revealed the short-term disinfecting benefits of US and its adverse effects on long-term bacterial survival, along with the influence of irradiation.

On the other hand, Yasir et al. [103] investigated the degradation of ibuprofen and sulfamethoxazole using ultrasonic irradiation (1000 kHz) with and without single-walled carbon nanotubes (SWCNTs). In the absence of SWCNTs, the efficiency of degradation was minimal. However, when ultrasound was combined with SWCNTs, the degradation efficiency significantly improved. Under SWNTs (adsorption) reactions, removal rates for ibuprofen and sulfamethoxazole were 57% and 48%, respectively. Under US reactions alone, these rates increased to 77% and 70%. Remarkably, under US/SWNTs reactions, removal rates surged to 97% and 92%, respectively. The ultrasonic irradiation-assisted dispersion of SWCNTs bolstered oxidation and adsorption activities, contributing to enhanced pollutant removal. The synthesized TiO_2 and TiO_2/montmorillonite samples served as catalysts for the sonocatalytic degradation of ciprofloxacin.

One more successful drug removal was recognized in the research conducted by Hassani et al. [104]. The degradation efficiency of ciprofloxacin via sonocatalysis was influenced by solution pH, catalyst loading, initial pollutant concentrations, and ultrasonic power. Notably, the TiO_2/montmorillonite nanocomposite exhibited a higher degradation efficiency (61%) compared to the pristine TiO_2 sample. This enhancement can be attributed to the decrease in TiO_2 nanoparticle size facilitated by the immobilization process and the electron acceptor role of montmorillonite within the TiO_2/montmorillonite structure. Consequently, the TiO_2/montmorillonite nanocomposite emerges as a promising catalyst for the sonocatalytic degradation of ciprofloxacin.

3.3. Sonophotocatalysis

Bearing in mind the efficiency of sonophotolysis and photocatalysis, in this part of this review, readers will be informed about the triumphant application of sonophotocatalysis.

For instance, Khan et al. [105] examined the degradation of acid red 17 dye using a Pt/CeO_2 sonophotocatalyst through a photocatalytic and sonophotocatalytic process, under visible light. The remarkable sonophotodegradation of acid red 17 in the presence of the Pt/CeO_2 photocatalyst was attributed to the synergy of superoxides and additional free $HO^{\bullet}$ radicals produced by ultrasonic waves. Additionally, the Pt/CeO_2 sonophotocatalyst exhibited outstanding recyclability.

Next, Karim and Shriwastav [19] investigated the effectiveness of photocatalytic, sonocatalytic, and sonophotocatalytic oxidation methods for degrading amoxicillin under visible light, employing N-doped TiO_2 nanoparticles as the catalyst and low-frequency ultrasound. In a novel multifrequency reactor and under optimal conditions, photocatalysis and sonocatalysis achieved degradation efficiencies of 27% and 31%, respectively. However, the combination of visible light and ultrasound in the presence of N-doped TiO_2 resulted in better amoxicillin degradation, attributed to the catalyst's reduced bandgap, enhanced cavitation effect, sonoluminescence phenomenon, and improved pollutant mass transfer. Consequently, sonophotocatalysis exhibited a greater degree of degradation (37%). The degradation of amoxicillin across these three studied oxidation processes followed a pseudo-first-order kinetics model.

After that, combination approaches incorporating sonolysis and photolysis, in the presence of CuO, TiO_2, and ZnO catalysts, have been utilized to treat commercial flonicamid solutions in the research of Ayare and Gogate [106]. At optimal loading, an extent of COD reduction was reached with a combination of ultrasound and the mentioned catalysts, and the following values were determined: 62.07%, 73.73%, and 77.59% for the CuO, ZnO, and TiO_2 catalysts, respectively. The sonocatalytic treatment process efficiency surpassed the efficiency of sonolysis, with a COD removal rate of 77.59% observed for TiO_2 catalysts compared to 39.23% for sonolysis operated individually. A similar trend was observed when comparing photocatalysis with photolysis. Sonophotocatalytic oxidation, with a maximum COD reduction of 98.36% in the case of TiO_2, was identified as the most effective process in comparison with sonocatalysis and photocatalysis.

Moreover, a combined system comprising photocatalysis and sonocatalysis was utilized in the degradation of tetracycline antibiotic, employing TiO_2 decorated on magnetic activated carbon (MAC@T) in conjunction with UV and US irradiations. This hybrid system, MAC@T/UV/US, integrating adsorption, photocatalytic, and sonocatalytic processes, proved effective in efficiently degrading tetracycline. MAC@T demonstrated strong catalytic activity when combined with both US and UV irradiation. Under optimal conditions, during a 180 min treatment, 93% of tetracycline was removed, whilst a 50.4% of TOC removal efficiency was reached. In summary, the synergy of MAC@T composite and US/UV for improved catalytic removal efficiency represents a prosperous and promising technique, which enjoys excellent catalytic activity, easy recovery, high adsorption capacity, and notable durability and photocatalyst recyclability [107].

4. Cost Estimation and Constraints of Different AOPs

The comprehensive cost analysis of a treatment technology encompasses its capital, operational, and maintenance expenses. In the realm of industrial-scale systems, operational costs stem from diverse factors, including initial investments, equipment and installation costs, amortization, raw materials procurement, energy consumption, parts replacements, labor, and more [111,112]. For example, in environmental remediation practices, expenditure is typically benchmarked against a fixed reference level of pollutant removal, often measured by metrics such as chemical oxygen demand or total organic carbon [111]. Notably, AOPs have emerged as highly effective techniques for degrading a broad spectrum of organic compounds, often ensuring their thorough mineralization. In this section, the cost-effectiveness of heterogeneous photocatalysis, sonocatalysis, and sonophotocatalysis will be compared mutually and also to other AOPs, including UV photolysis, UV/H_2O_2 treatment, Fenton reaction, ozonation, and sonolysis.

Certainly, it is imperative to weigh both the effectiveness and limitations of AOPs, particularly regarding the operational pH range. Notably, heterogeneous systems exhibit efficacy across a wider pH spectrum, encompassing the typical pH range found in natural waters and wastewaters (pH 2–9). This stands in contrast to treatments like Fenton and ozonation, which require specific acidic or alkaline conditions. From an industrial and practical standpoint, this broad operational pH range is a crucial prerequisite [111].

Although photocatalysis, especially with TiO_2, is recognized as a relatively expensive AOP, it remains highly effective in removing pollutants [113]. In recent decades, photocatalysis has garnered significant attention for several compelling reasons. These include its cost-effectiveness regarding its remarkable capacity for photocatalyst reuse and recyclability, the generation of highly active radicals, minimal sludge production, and rapid mineralization rates [114]. However, limitations such as equipment costs, maintenance requirements, and scalability challenges need to be addressed for widespread implementation. In general, various factors contribute to the overall costs of sono-/photocatalytic processes. For instance, the reusability of catalysts across multiple cycles can significantly reduce material consumption. Moreover, harnessing natural sunlight irradiation instead of energy-intensive lamps (UV photolysis, UV/H_2O_2 treatment) holds promise for cost reduction in terms of electricity expense. However, when UV radiation is integrated into other AOPs, removal efficiencies usually increase, though this comes with higher operational costs.

Furthermore, while sonochemistry effectively degrades numerous organic compounds, it often achieves low levels of mineralization (<10%) due to the hydrophilic and nonvolatile nature of the generated products, hindering their complete elimination. Additionally, the operation of ultrasound entails high electrical energy consumption, leading to elevated economic costs. Consequently, there is a pressing need for short treatment times. However, these challenges can largely be addressed by integrating ultrasound with other AOPs or biological systems [64].

Additionally, the efficacy of sono-/photocatalytic processes may vary depending on factors like pollutant type, concentration, and environmental conditions, necessitating the careful consideration of application-specific factors. Ahmad et al. [115] investigated the ZnO-decorated multiwall carbon nanotubes-assisted degradation of rhodamine B using photocatalysis, sonocatalysis, and sonophotocatalysis. Sonophotocatalytic processes exhibited relatively shorter reaction times and higher reaction rate constants compared to individual processes.

Moreover, several studies have conducted analyses on the electrical energy consumption of photocatalytic and sonocatalytic degradation systems. Moradi et al. [116] determined the electrical energy consumption for selected previous investigations and provided a summary of fundamental parameters and data, taking account of the consumption of energy translated into cost values. It is noteworthy that, across all cases, the electrical energy output of sonophotocatalytic systems is lower than the combined costs of photocatalytic and sonocatalytic systems. This observation confirms the efficacy and cost-effectiveness of the integrated system. The decrease in electrical energy output is due to the synergistic interaction between the two radical-producing processes, which enhances degradation events and shortens the time needed for the reaction.

5. Conclusions and Future Perspectives

As the global population constantly grows and the necessity for pure and sanitarily adequate water increases, various innovative techniques are being applied to remove organic pollutants from the aqueous environment.

This review aimed to give readers an insight into up-to-date data about the application of AOPs, with special emphasize on sonophotolysis, photocatalysis, and their synergistic approach, sonophotocatalysis. These techniques are very popular and highly investigated, which is proved by the number of publications in the last 10 years. The application of sonophotolysis is a relatively new approach for organic pollutant removal. Even though this AOP can be efficiently applied for organic pollutant removal, there are some drawbacks which should be addressed in the future, such as energy consumption, complexity of operation, cavitation-induced damage, and environmental (noise pollution) and safety (thermal runaway due to the freed-up heat) concerns. Putting photocatalysis under the magnifying glass, it can be concluded that promising results can be achieved. According to the reviewed data, it can be assumed that a wide spectrum of organic pollutants can be efficiently removed under various experimental conditions. Consider, for instance, that 100% of mesotrione and 95% of atrazine pesticides can be degraded under UV and employing ZnO and TiO_2 as photocatalysts. Promising results are achieved in the field of pharmaceutical removal, as well. Namely, 80–100% of antibiotics and/or different endocrine disruptors can be successfully degraded depending on the operational conditions. According to the published data, a milestone has been achieved in the degradation of organic dyes too. To be exact, 90–100% of several dyes (e.g., methylene blue, methylene orange, acid blue 25, acid red 17, etc.) can be successfully removed by choosing the optimal photocatalytic conditions (catalyst type, irradiation source). Meanwhile, although the employment of freely available sunlight energy makes this process eco-friendly, the utilization of various semiconductors can also be harmful to the environment. Namely, the traditional synthesis of different nanomaterials that are being used as photocatalysts is increasing our footprint in the environment and making this process less favorable. Furthermore, the activity of the newly synthesized materials is often low under sunlight irradiation. Hence, in the future, advanced and green, possibly plant-based, catalysts should be developed with high photocatalytic activity under natural conditions. In addition, heterogeneous photocatalytic process optimization and revolutionized reactor designs with scale-up and commercialization can spread the application of this technique. Considering sonophotocatalysis, it can be stated that this synergistic approach can result in great removal efficiency for various organic pollutants. Specifically, employing sono-based AOPs, promising findings are achieved in the field of pharmaceutical removal. Widespread drugs, such as ibuprofen, ciprofloxacin, or amoxicillin, can be degraded in the range of 30–97% applying optimal experimental conditions. Furthermore, pesticides (e.g., flonicamid) can also be eliminated using sonophotocatalysis with different semiconductors. However, some drawbacks should be addressed to realize its full benefits and make it a more practical and sustainable technology, such as energy consumption, equipment cost, limited penetration depth, limited scalability, and environmental concerns.

Lastly, based on the economy aspects of these processes, it can be noted that the mentioned AOPs are economically more feasible if they are coupled. For instance, lower energy consumption can be observed for sonophotocatalysis than for sonophotolysis and photocatalysis, separately. Also, the investigated AOPs in this review possess lighter operational parameters, compared to other AOPs, such as photo-Fenton or UV/H_2O_2. However, different key factors should be discussed and solved in the future, such as scale-up, integration with other technologies, application in emerging fields, or resource recovery, in order to obtain a completely sustainable technique. Additionally, the future integration of electricity from renewable resources, such as solar cells, is expected to diminish the operational costs of sonophotocatalytic systems.

Author Contributions: Conceptualization, D.Š.M.; methodology, D.Š.M.; writing—original draft preparation, S.B., D.J., N.F., V.D. and D.Š.M.; writing—review and editing, P.P. and D.Š.M.; visualization, S.B.; supervision, D.Š.M.; funding acquisition, P.P. All authors have read and agreed to the published version of the manuscript.

Funding: This research was supported by the Science Fund of the Republic of Serbia (Grant No. 7747845, In situ pollutants removal from waters by sustainable green nanotechnologies—CleanNanoCatalyze).

Conflicts of Interest: The authors declare no conflicts of interest.

References

1. Britannica. Available online: https://www.britannica.com/explore/savingearth/pollution-overview (accessed on 20 April 2024).
2. Singh, S. Water pollution in rural areas: Primary sources and associated health issues. In *Water Resources Management for Rural Development*; Madhav, S., Srivastav, A.L., Chibueze Izah, S., Hullebusch, E.V., Eds.; Elsevier: Amsterdam, The Netherlands, 2024; pp. 29–44.

3. UNESCO Report. Available online: https://www.unesco.org/en/articles/imminent-risk-global-water-crisis-warns-un-world-water-development-report-2023 (accessed on 9 April 2024).
4. Nelson, K.L.; Murray, A. Sanitation for Unserved Populations: Technologies, Implementation Challenges, and Opportunities. *Annu. Rev. Environ. Resour.* **2008**, *33*, 119–151. [CrossRef]
5. Malaj, E.; von der Ohe, P.C.; Grote, M.; Kuhne, R.; Mondy, C.P.; Usseglio-Polatera, P.; Brack, W.; Schafer, R.B. Organic chemicals jeopardize the health of freshwater ecosystems on the continental scale. *Proc. Natl. Acad. Sci. USA* **2014**, *111*, 9549–9554. [CrossRef] [PubMed]
6. Wen, Y.; Schoups, G.; van de Giesen, N. Organic pollution of rivers: Combined threats of urbanization, livestock farming and global climate change. *Sci. Rep.* **2017**, *7*, 43289. [CrossRef] [PubMed]
7. Garcia-Corcoles, M.T.; Rodriguez-Gomez, R.; de Alarcon-Gomez, B.; Cipa, M.; Martin-Pozo, L.; Kauffmann, J.M.; Zafra-Gomez, A. Chromatographic methods for the determination of emerging contaminants in natural water and wastewater samples: A Review. *Crit. Rev. Anal. Chem.* **2019**, *49*, 160–186. [CrossRef] [PubMed]
8. Karpińska, J.; Kotowska, U. Removal of organic pollution in the water environment. *Water* **2019**, *11*, 2017. [CrossRef]
9. Aravind Kumar, J.; Krithiga, T.; Sathish, S.; Renita, A.A.; Prabu, D.; Lokesh, S.; Geetha, R.; Namasivayam, S.K.R.; Sillanpaa, M. Persistent organic pollutants in water resources: Fate, occurrence, characterization and risk analysis. *Sci. Total Environ.* **2022**, *831*, 154808. [CrossRef] [PubMed]
10. Shumbula, P.; Maswanganyi, C.; Shumbula, N. Type, sources, methods and treatment of organic pollutants in wastewater. In *Persistent Organic Pollutants (POPs)—Monitoring, Impact and Treatment*; Rashed, M., Ed.; IntechOpen: London, UK, 2022; pp. 1–20.
11. Otálora, A.; Lerma, T.A.; Arrieta-Urango, Y.; Palencia, M. Emerging organic pollutants in aqueous environments: Detection, monitoring, and removal techniques. *J. Sci. Technol. Appl.* **2021**, *10*, 92–153. [CrossRef]
12. Vasilachi, I.; Asiminicesei, D.; Fertu, D.; Gavrilescu, M. Occurrence and fate of emerging pollutants in water environment and options for their removal. *Water* **2021**, *13*, 181. [CrossRef]
13. CDC. Available online: https://www.cdc.gov/healthywater/drinking/public/water_treatment.html (accessed on 11 April 2024).
14. Yeoh, J.X.; Md. Jamil, S.N.A.; Syukri, F.; Koyama, M.; Nourouzi Mobarekeh, M. Comparison between Conventional treatment processes and advanced oxidation processes in treating slaughterhouse wastewater: A Review. *Water* **2022**, *14*, 3778. [CrossRef]
15. Cococeanu, A.L.; Man, T.E. Methods and characteristics of conventional water treatment technologies. In *Water Safety, Security and Sustainability: Threat Detection and Mitigation*; Vaseashta, A., Maftei, C., Eds.; Springer International Publishing: Cham, Germany, 2021; pp. 305–330.
16. Mahy, J.G.; Wolfs, C.; Vreuls, C.; Drot, S.; Dircks, S.; Boergers, A.; Tuerk, J.; Hermans, S.; Lambert, S.D. Advanced oxidation processes for waste water treatment: From laboratory-scale model water to on-site real waste water. *Environ. Technol.* **2021**, *42*, 3974–3986. [CrossRef]
17. Jyothi, K.P.; Yesodharan, S.; Yesodharan, E.P. Ultrasound (US), Ultraviolet light (UV) and combination (US+UV) assisted semiconductor catalysed degradation of organic pollutants in water: Oscillation in the concentration of hydrogen peroxide formed in situ. *Ultrason. Sonochem.* **2014**, *21*, 1787–1796. [CrossRef] [PubMed]
18. Villaroel, E.; Silva-Agredo, J.; Petrier, C.; Taborda, G.; Torres-Palma, R.A. Ultrasonic degradation of acetaminophen in water: Effect of sonochemical parameters and water matrix. *Ultrason. Sonochem.* **2014**, *21*, 1763–1769. [CrossRef]
19. Karim, A.V.; Shriwastav, A. Degradation of amoxicillin with sono, photo, and sonophotocatalytic oxidation under low-frequency ultrasound and visible light. *Environ. Res.* **2021**, *200*, 111515. [CrossRef] [PubMed]
20. Terki, M.; Triaa, S.; Ali, F.K.; Youcef, R.; Brahim, I.O.; Trari, M. Sono-assisted degradation of rhodamine B using the Fe modified MgO nanostructures: Characterization and catalytic activity. *React. Kinet. Mech. Catal.* **2023**, *136*, 1143–1155. [CrossRef]
21. Sahani, S.; Malika Tripathi, K.; Il Lee, T.; Dubal, D.P.; Wong, C.-P.; Chandra Sharma, Y.; Young Kim, T. Recent advances in photocatalytic carbon-based materials for enhanced water splitting under visible-light irradiation. *Energy Convers. Manag.* **2022**, *252*, 115133. [CrossRef]
22. Bognár, S.; Putnik, P.; Maksimović, I.; Velebit, B.; Putnik-Delić, M.; Šojić Merkulov, D. Sustainable removal of tolperisone from waters by application of photocatalysis, nanotechnology, and chemometrics: Quantification, environmental toxicity, and degradation optimization. *Nanomaterials* **2022**, *12*, 4199. [CrossRef] [PubMed]
23. Finčur, N.; Šojić Merkulov, D.; Putnik, P.; Despotović, V.; Banić, N.; Bognár, S.; Jovanović, D.; Panić, S.; Ivetić, T.; Abramović, B. Sunlight-driven degradation of alprazolam and amitriptyline by application of binary zinc oxide and tin oxide powders. *Separations* **2023**, *10*, 316. [CrossRef]
24. Šojić Merkulov, D.; Vlazan, P.; Poienar, M.; Bognár, S.; Ianasi, C.; Sfirloaga, P. Sustainable removal of 17α-ethynylestradiol from aqueous environment using rare earth doped lanthanum manganite nanomaterials. *Catal. Today* **2023**, *424*, 113746. [CrossRef]
25. Bognár, S.; Jovanović, D.; Putnik, P.; Despotović, V.; Ivetić, T.; Bajac, B.; Tóth, E.; Finčur, N.; Maksimović, I.; Putnik-Delić, M.; et al. Solar-driven removal of selected organics with binary ZnO based nanomaterials from aquatic environment: Chemometric and toxicological assessments on wheat. *J. Environ. Chem. Eng.* **2024**, *12*, 112016. [CrossRef]
26. Cao, J.; Wang, J.; Wang, Z.; Zubairu, S.M.; Ding, Y.; Zhu, G. In-situ construction of Z-scheme 2D/2D g-C_3N_4/BiOBr heterojunction with enhanced photocatalytic CO_2 reduction. *Surf. Interfaces* **2024**, *45*, 103875. [CrossRef]
27. Thomas, N.; Dionysiou, D.D.; Pillai, S.C. Heterogeneous Fenton catalysts: A review of recent advances. *J. Hazard. Mater.* **2021**, *404*, 124082. [CrossRef] [PubMed]

78. Ivetić, T.B.; Finčur, N.L.; Abramović, B.F.; Dimitrievska, M.; Štrbac, G.R.; Čajko, K.O.; Miljević, B.B.; Đačanin, L.R.; Lukić-Petrović, S.R. Environmentally friendly photoactive heterojunction zinc tin oxide nanoparticles. *Ceram. Int.* **2016**, *42*, 3575–3583. [CrossRef]
79. Thennarasu, G.; Sivasamy, A. Enhanced visible photocatalytic activity of cotton ball like nano structured Cu doped ZnO for the degradation of organic pollutant. *Ecotoxicol. Environ. Saf.* **2016**, *134*, 412–420. [CrossRef]
80. Finčur, N.L.; Krstić, J.B.; Šibul, F.S.; Šojić, D.V.; Despotović, V.N.; Banić, N.D.; Agbaba, J.R.; Abramović, B.F. Removal of alprazolam from aqueous solutions by heterogeneous photocatalysis: Influencing factors, intermediates, and products. *Chem. Eng. J.* **2017**, *307*, 1105–1115. [CrossRef]
81. León, D.E.; Zúñiga-Benítez, H.; Peñuela, G.A.; Mansilla, H.D. Photocatalytic removal of the antibiotic cefotaxime on TiO_2 and ZnO suspensions under simulated sunlight radiation. *Water Air Soil Pollut.* **2017**, *228*, 361. [CrossRef]
82. Silva, G.; De Souza, G.M.; Neto, A.A.; De Matos Jorge, L.M.; Santos, O.A. Influence of ZnO content in mixed oxides catalysts applied in the photocatalytic degradation of atrazine. *Chem. Eng. Trans.* **2017**, *57*, 637–642. [CrossRef]
83. Šojić Merkulov, D.; Lazarević, M.; Despotović, V.; Banić, N.; Finčur, N.; Maletić, S.; Abramović, B. The effect of inorganic anions and organic matter on mesotrione (Callisto®) removal from environmental waters. *J. Serbian Chem. Soc.* **2017**, *82*, 343–355. [CrossRef]
84. Azadi, M.; Hasani, A.H.; Olya, M.E.; Borghei, S.M. Application of ZnO-Ag-Nd nanocomposite as a new synthesized nanophotocatalyst for the degradation of organic compounds: Kinetic, thermodynamic and economic study. *Toxicol. Ind. Health* **2019**, *35*, 1–10. [CrossRef] [PubMed]
85. Tanveer, M.; Guyer, G.T.; Abbas, G. Photocatalytic degradation of ibuprofen in water using TiO_2 and ZnO under artificial UV and solar irradiation. *Water Environ. Res.* **2019**, *91*, 822–829. [CrossRef] [PubMed]
86. Vela, N.; Calín, M.; Yáñez-Gascón, M.J.; el Aatik, A.; Garrido, I.; Pérez-Lucas, G.; Fenoll, J.; Navarro, S. Removal of Pesticides with Endocrine Disruptor Activity in Wastewater Effluent by Solar Heterogeneous Photocatalysis Using $ZnO/Na_2S_2O_8$. *Water Air Soil Pollut.* **2019**, *230*, 134. [CrossRef]
87. Suresh, M.; Sivasamy, A. Fabrication of graphene nanosheets decorated by nitrogen-doped ZnO nanoparticles with enhanced visible photocatalytic activity for the degradation of Methylene Blue dye. *J. Mol. Liq.* **2020**, *317*, 114112. [CrossRef]
88. Ángel-Hernández, B.; Hernández-Aldana, F.; Pérez-Osorio, G.; Gutiérrez-Arias, G.E.M. Municipal wastewater treatment by photocatalysis: Comparison between UV lamp and solar radiation using TiO_2 and ZnO/TiO_2 synthesized catalysts. *Rev. Mex. Ing. Quim.* **2021**, *20*, Cat2438. [CrossRef]
89. Caracciolo, D.; Vaiano, V.; Gambicorti, T.; Sacco, O. Photocatalytic treatment of industrial wastewaters using structured photocatalysts. *Chem. Eng. Trans.* **2021**, *84*, 151–156.
90. Finčur, N.; Sfirloaga, P.; Putnik, P.; Despotović, V.; Lazarević, M.; Uzelac, M.; Abramović, B.; Vlazan, P.; Ianasi, C.; Alapi, T.; et al. Removal of emerging pollutants from water using environmentally friendly processes: Photocatalysts preparation, characterization, intermediates identification and toxicity assessment. *Nanomaterials* **2021**, *11*, 215. [CrossRef] [PubMed]
91. Kumar, S.; Kaushik, R.D.; Upadhyay, G.K.; Purohit, L.P. rGO-ZnO nanocomposites as efficient photocatalyst for degradation of 4-BP and DEP using high temperature refluxing method in in-situ condition. *J. Hazard. Mater.* **2021**, *406*, 124300. [CrossRef] [PubMed]
92. Li, Z.; Zhang, H.; Jiang, W. Research on the sustainable heterogeneous catalyst development for photocatalytic treatment of phenol. *Sustainability* **2021**, *13*, 4670. [CrossRef]
93. Mahy, J.G.; Lejeune, L.; Haynes, T.; Body, N.; De Kreijger, S.; Elias, B.; Marcilli, R.H.M.; Fustin, C.-A.; Hermans, S. Crystalline ZnO photocatalysts prepared at ambient temperature: Influence of morphology on p-nitrophenol degradation in water. *Catalysts* **2021**, *11*, 1182. [CrossRef]
94. Baladi, E.; Davar, F.; Hojjati-Najafabadi, A. Synthesis and characterization of g-C_3N_4-$CoFe_2O_4$-ZnO magnetic nanocomposites for enhancing photocatalytic activity with visible light for degradation of penicillin G antibiotic. *Environ. Res.* **2022**, *215*, 114270. [CrossRef]
95. Tamashiro, J.R.; Lima, I.S.; Paiva, F.F.G.d.; Silva, L.H.P.; Oliveira, D.V.M.d.; Baffa, O.; Kinoshita, A. Treatment of Sugarcane Vinasse Using Heterogeneous Photocatalysis with Zinc Oxide Nanoparticles. *Sustainability* **2022**, *14*, 16052. [CrossRef]
96. Despotović, V.; Finčur, N.; Bognar, S.; Šojić Merkulov, D.; Putnik, P.; Abramović, B.; Panić, S. Characterization and Photocatalytic performance of newly synthesized ZnO nanoparticles for environmental organic pollutants removal from water system. *Separations* **2023**, *10*, 258. [CrossRef]
97. El Golli, A.; Contreras, S.; Dridi, C. Bio-synthesized ZnO nanoparticles and sunlight-driven photocatalysis for environmentally-friendly and sustainable route of synthetic petroleum refinery wastewater treatment. *Sci. Rep.* **2023**, *13*, 20809. [CrossRef]
98. Pavithra, M.; M B, J.R. Reusable porous chromium- zinc oxide nano-sheets for efficient detoxification of xenobiotics through integrated advanced oxidation water clean-up process. *J. Hazard. Mater. Adv.* **2024**, *13*, 100403. [CrossRef]
99. Sarvothaman, V.P.; Velisoju, V.K.; Subburaj, J.; Panithasan, M.S.; Kulkarni, S.R.; Castano, P.; Turner, J.; Guida, P.; Roberts, W.L.; Nagarajan, S. Is cavitation a truly sensible choice for intensifying photocatalytic oxidation processes?—Implications on phenol degradation using ZnO photocatalysts. *Ultrason. Sonochem.* **2023**, *99*, 106548. [CrossRef]
100. Thongam, D.D.; Chaturvedi, H. Induced defect and ZnO nano-flower formation by N, N, dimethylformamide solvent for natural sunlight responsive floating photocatalytic advanced oxidation process. *Chemosphere* **2023**, *313*, 137600. [CrossRef] [PubMed]
101. Alsharyani, A.K.; Muruganandam, L. Fabrication of zinc oxide nanorods for photocatalytic degradation of docosane, a petroleum pollutant, under solar light simulator. *RSC Adv.* **2024**, *14*, 9038–9049. [CrossRef] [PubMed]

102. Yusuff, A.S.; Popoola, L.T.; Gbadamosi, A.O.; Igbafe, A.I. Coal fly ash-supported ZnO-promoted TiO_2 towards UV photocatalytic degradation of anthraquinone dye: Parametric optimization, kinetics and mechanism studies. *Mater. Today Commun.* **2024**, *38*, 107999. [CrossRef]
103. Al-Hamadani, Y.A.J.; Jung, C.; Im, J.-K.; Boateng, L.K.; Flora, J.R.V.; Jang, M.; Heo, J.; Park, C.M.; Yoon, Y. Sonocatalytic degradation coupled with single-walled carbon nanotubes for removal of ibuprofen and sulfamethoxazole. *Chem. Eng. Sci.* **2017**, *162*, 300–308. [CrossRef]
104. Hassani, A.; Khataee, A.; Karaca, S.; Karaca, C.; Gholami, P. Sonocatalytic degradation of ciprofloxacin using synthesized TiO_2 nanoparticles on montmorillonite. *Ultrason. Sonochem.* **2017**, *35*, 251–262. [CrossRef] [PubMed]
105. Khan, M.F.; Cazzato, G.; Saleemi, H.A.; Macadangdang, R.R., Jr.; Aftab, M.N.; Ismail, M.; Khalid, H.; Ali, S.; Bakhtiar, S.U.H.; Ismail, A.; et al. Sonophotocatalytic degradation of organic pollutant under visible light over Pt decorated CeO_2: Role of ultrasonic waves for unprecedented degradation. *J. Mol. Struct.* **2022**, *1247*, 131397. [CrossRef]
106. Ayare, S.D.; Gogate, P.R. Sonochemical, photocatalytic and sonophotocatalytic oxidation of flonicamid pesticide solution using different catalysts. *Chem. Eng. Process.* **2020**, *154*, 108040. [CrossRef]
107. Kakavandi, B.; Bahari, N.; Rezaei Kalantary, R.; Dehghani Fard, E. Enhanced sono-photocatalysis of tetracycline antibiotic using TiO_2 decorated on magnetic activated carbon (MAC@T) coupled with US and UV: A new hybrid system. *Ultrason. Sonochem.* **2019**, *55*, 75–85. [CrossRef]
108. Gao, S.; Hemar, Y.; Lewis, G.D.; Ashokkumar, M. Inactivation of Enterobacter aerogenes in reconstituted skim milk by high- and low-frequency ultrasound. *Ultrason. Sonochem.* **2014**, *21*, 2099–2106. [CrossRef]
109. Gemici, B.T.; Karel, F.B.; Karaer, F.; Koparal, A.S. Water disinfection with advanced methods: Successive and hybrid application of antibacterial column with silver, ultrasound and UV radiation. *Appl. Ecol. Environ. Res.* **2018**, *16*, 4667–4680. [CrossRef]
110. Giannakis, S.; Papoutsakis, S.; Darakas, E.; Escalas-Canellas, A.; Petrier, C.; Pulgarin, C. Ultrasound enhancement of near-neutral photo-Fenton for effective *E. coli* inactivation in wastewater. *Ultrason. Sonochem.* **2015**, *22*, 515–526. [CrossRef] [PubMed]
111. Huddersman, K.; Ekpruke, A.; Asuelimen, L. Application of AOPs in the treatment of OSPAR chemicals and a comparative cost analysis. *Crit. Rev. Environ. Sci. Technol.* **2019**, *49*, 277–317. [CrossRef]
112. Mahbub, P.; Duke, M. Scalability of advanced oxidation processes (AOPs) in industrial applications: A review. *J. Environ. Manag.* **2023**, *345*, 118861. [CrossRef] [PubMed]
113. Cuerda-Correa, E.M.; Alexandre-Franco, M.F.; Fernández-González, C. Advanced oxidation processes for the removal of antibiotics from water. An Overview. *Water* **2019**, *12*, 102. [CrossRef]
114. Moradi, S.; Isari, A.A.; Hayati, F.; Rezaei Kalantary, R.; Kakavandi, B. Co-implanting of TiO_2 and liquid-phase-delaminated g-C_3N_4 on multi-functional graphene nanobridges for enhancing photocatalytic degradation of acetaminophen. *Chem. Eng. J.* **2021**, *414*, 128618. [CrossRef]
115. Ahmad, M.; Ahmed, E.; Hong, Z.L.; Ahmed, W.; Elhissi, A.; Khalid, N.R. Photocatalytic, sonocatalytic and sonophotocatalytic degradation of Rhodamine B using ZnO/CNTs composites photocatalysts. *Ultrason. Sonochem.* **2014**, *21*, 761–773. [CrossRef]
116. Moradi, S.; Rodriguez-Seco, C.; Hayati, F.; Ma, D. Sonophotocatalysis with photoactive nanomaterials for wastewater treatment and bacteria disinfection. *ACS Nanosci. Au* **2023**, *3*, 103–129. [CrossRef]

MDPI AG
Grosspeteranlage 5
4052 Basel
Switzerland
Tel.: +41 61 683 77 34

Processes Editorial Office
E-mail: processes@mdpi.com
www.mdpi.com/journal/processes

www.ingramcontent.com/pod-product-compliance
Lightning Source LLC
Chambersburg PA
CBHW061618220926
51850CB00005B/535

* 9 7 8 3 7 2 5 8 6 1 1 1 8 *